se

Healthcare Common Procedure Coding System

Medicare's National Level II Codes

HCPCS
2006

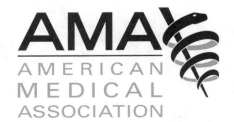

AMA
AMERICAN MEDICAL ASSOCIATION

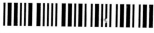

Eighteenth edition © 2005 Ingenix Publishing Group

First printing November 2005

OP095106
ISBN 1-57947-688-0

Special Reports
Special reports, code changes and regulatory information can be found by visiting www.ama-assn.org/go/cpt.
Click on 2006 HCPCS Special Announcements and Reports.

To stay current on important HCPCS regulatory developments go to http://www.cms.hhs.gov/medicare/hcpcs.

Additional copies of this publication may be ordered by telephoning (800) 621-8335 or by writing to the following address:

American Medical Association
Order Department
PO Box 930876
Atlanta, GA 31193-0876

DISCLAIMER

This publication is based on the Healthcare Common Procedure Coding System (HCPCS) developed by the Centers for Medicare and Medicaid Services (CMS). It is designed to be a current, authoritative source regarding HCPCS codes and every reasonable effort has been made to ensure the accuracy and completeness of the codes, symbols, and illustrations. However, the American Medical Association (AMA) makes no guarantee, warranty, or representation that this compilation is accurate, complete, or without errors.

It is understood that the American Medical Association is not rendering any legal or other professional services or advice in providing these codes and that the AMA bears no liability for any results or consequences which may arise from the use of this book.

Introduction

Organization of HCPCS

The American Medical Association (AMA) 2006 *HCPCS Level II* book contains mandated changes and new codes for use as of January 1, 2006. Deleted codes have also been indicated and cross-referenced to active codes when possible. New codes have been added to the appropriate sections, eliminating the time-consuming step of looking in two places for a code. However, keep in mind that the information in this book is a reproduction of the 2006 HCPCS; additional information on coverage issues may have been provided to Medicare contractors after publication. All contractors periodically update their systems and records throughout the year. If this book does not agree with your contractor, it is either because of a mid-year update or correction, or a specific local or regional coverage policy.

To make this year's HCPCS book even more useful, we have included codes noted in addendum B of the November 2005 OPPS update as published in the *Federal Register* and from transmittals through 2005 that include codes not discussed in other CMS documents. The sources for these codes are often noted in blue beneath the description.

Index

Since HCPCS is organized by code number rather than by service or supply name, the index enables the coder to locate any code without looking through individual ranges of codes. Just look up the medical or surgical supply, service, orthotic, prosthetic, or generic or brand name drug in question to find the appropriate codes. This index also refers to many of the brand names by which these items are known.

Table of Drugs

The brand names listed are examples only and may not include all products available for that type of drug. Our table of drugs lists HCPCS codes from any available sections including A codes, C codes, J codes, S codes, and Q codes under brand and generic drug names with amount, route of administration, and code numbers. While we try to make the table comprehensive, it is not all-inclusive.

Color-coded Coverage Instructions

The AMA HCPCS Level II codebook provides colored symbols for each coverage and reimbursement instruction. A legend to these symbols is provided on the bottom of each two-page spread.

How to Use the AMA HCPCS Level II Book

Blue Color Bar—Special Coverage Instructions
A blue bar for "special coverage instructions" over a code means that special coverage instructions apply to that code. These special instructions are also typically given in the form of Medicare Pub.100 reference numbers. The appendixes provide the full text of the cited Medicare Pub.100 references.

A4211 Supplies for self-administered injections

Yellow Color Bar—Carrier Discretion
Issues that are left to "contractor discretion" are covered with a yellow bar. Contact the contractor for specific coverage information on those codes.

A4248 Chlorhexidine containing antiseptic, 1 ml

Red Color Bar—Not Covered by or Invalid for Medicare
Codes that are not covered by or are invalid for Medicare are covered by a red bar. The pertinent Medicare Internet-only manuals (pub. 100) reference numbers are also given explaining why a particular code is not covered. These numbers refer to the appendixes, where we have listed the Medicare references.

A4223 Infusion supplies not used with external infusion pump, per cassette or bag (list drugs separately)

The HCPCS Level II codes follow the AMA CPT code book conventions to indicate new, revised, and deleted codes.

- A black circle (●) precedes a new code.
- A black triangle (▲) precedes a code with revised terminology or rules.
- A circle (○) precedes a reinstated code.
- Codes deleted from the 2005 active codes appear with a strike-out.

●	A4411	Ostomy skin barrier, solid 4x4 or equivalent, extended wear, with built-in convexity, each
▲	A4641	Radiopharmaceutical, diagnostic, not otherwise classified
○	J7620	Albuterol, up to 2.5 mg and ipratropium bromide, up to 0.5 mg, non-compounded
	~~A4260~~	~~Levonorgestrel (contraceptive) implants system, including implants and supplies~~ See code(s) J7306.

Quantity Alert
Many codes in HCPCS report quantities that may not coincide with quantities available in the marketplace. For instance, a HCPCS code for an ostomy pouch with skin barrier reports each pouch, but the product is generally sold in a package of 10; "10" must be indicated in the quantity box on the CMS claim form to ensure proper reimbursement. This symbol indicates that care should be taken to verify quantities in this code.

☑ A4207 Syringe with needle, sterile 2 cc, each

♀ Female Only
This icon identifies procedures that should only be reported for female patients.

♂ Male Only
This icon identifies procedures that should only be reported for male patients.

A Age Edit
This icon denotes codes intended for use with a specific age group, such as neonate, newborn, pediatric, and adult. Carefully review the code description to assure the code you report most appropriately reflects the patient's age.

M Maternity
This icon identifies procedures that by definition should only be used for maternity patients generally between 12 and 55 years of age.

1-9 ASC Groupings
Codes designated as being paid by ASC groupings that were effective at the time of printing are denoted by the group number.

DMEPOS
Use this icon to identify when to consult the CMS DMEPOS for payment of this durable medical item.

Skilled Nursing Facility (SNF)
Use this icon to identify certain items and services not covered under the Skilled Nursing Facility Prospective Payment System (SNFPPS).

AMA provides explanatory information in blue beneath many codes. These annotations help you better understand the code and its billing.

Drugs commonly reported with a code are listed underneath by brand or generic name.

"See" references help you determine related or alternate codes for the supply or service.

CMS does not use consistent terminology when a code for a specific procedure is not listed. The code description may include any of the following terms: unlisted, not otherwise classified (NOC), unspecified, unclassified, other, and miscellaneous. If you are sure there is no code for the service or supply provided or used, be sure to provide adequate documentation to the payer. Check with the payer for more information.

A4280 Adhesive skin support attachment for use with external breast prosthesis, each ♀

A4326 Male external catheter specialty type with integral collection chamber, each ♂

D8010 Limited orthodontic treatment of the primary dentition A

H1001 Prenatal care, at-risk enhanced service; antepartum management M

G0105 Colorectal cancer screening; colonoscopy on individual at high risk 2

A4322 Irrigation syringe, bulb or piston, each

A0999 Unlisted ambulance service ⊘

J7191 Factor VIII (anti-hemophilic factor (porcine), per IU
Use this code for Hyate:C. Medicare jurisdiction: local contractor.

J7193 Factor IX (antihemophilic factor, purified, non-recombinant) per IU
Use this code for AlphaNine SD, Mononine.

J7502 Cyclosporine, oral, 100 mg
Use this code for Neoral, Sandimmune, Gengraf, Sangcya.
See also code: C9438

A0999 Unlisted ambulance service

APC Status Indicators

Ⓐ-Ⓨ *APC Status Indicators*

Status indicators identify how individual HCPCS Level II codes are paid or not paid under the OPPS. The same status indicator is assigned to all the codes within an APC. Consult the payer or resource to learn which CPT codes fall within various APCs. Status indicators for HCPCS and their definitions are below:

Ⓐ   Indicates services that are paid under some other method such as the DMEPOS fee schedule or the physician fee schedule

Ⓑ   Indicates codes not allowed or paid under OPPS

Ⓒ   Indicates inpatient services that are not paid under the OPPS

Ⓔ   Indicates services for which payment is not allowed under the OPPS. In some instances, the service is not covered by Medicare. In other instances, Medicare does not use the code in question but does use another code to describe the service

Ⓕ   Indicates corneal tissue acquisition costs, certain CRNA services and hepatitis B vaccines that are paid at reasonable cost

Ⓖ   Indicates a current drug or biological for which payment is made under the transitional pass-through provisions

Ⓗ   Indicates either a device paid under pass-through provisions; or brachytherapy sources and radiopharmaceuticals that are paid at reasonable cost

Ⓚ   Indicates non-pass-through drugs and biologicals. Effective July 1, 2001, co-payments for these items and the service of the administration of the items are aggregated and may not exceed the inpatient hospital deductible.

Ⓛ   Indicates influenza or pneumococcal pneumonia vaccine paid as of reasonable cost with no deductable or coinsurance

Ⓜ   Indicates that this code should not be reported by hospitals to their fiscal intermediary

Ⓝ   Indicates services that are incidental, with payment packaged into another service or APC group

Ⓟ   Indicates services paid only in partial hospitalization programs

Ⓢ   Indicates significant procedures for which payment is allowed under the hospital OPPS but to which the multiple procedure reduction does not apply

Ⓣ   Indicates surgical services for which payment is allowed under the hospital OPPS. Services with this payment indicator are the only ones to which the multiple procedure payment reduction applies.

Ⓥ   Indicates visits for which payment is allowed under the hospital OPPS

Ⓧ   Indicates ancillary services for which payment is allowed under the hospital OPPS

Ⓨ   Indicates nonimplantable durable medical equipment (DME) that is billed by providers other than home health agencies to the DMERC

The "Q" icon is not included because there are no codes that have a "Q" status indicator in the 2006 HCPCS Level II code set.

Ⓐ   A4321   Therapeutic agent for urinary catheter irrigation

Ⓑ   A4550   Surgical trays

Ⓒ   G0341   Percutaneous islet cell transplant, includes portal vein catheterization and infusion

Ⓔ   A0021   Ambulance service, outside state per mile, transport (Medicaid only)

Ⓕ   V2785   Processing, preserving and transporting corneal tissue

Ⓖ   C9113   Injection, pantoprazole sodium, per vial

Ⓗ   A9505   Thallium Tl-201 thallous chloride, diagnostic, per millicurie

Ⓚ   A9535   Injection, methylene blue, 1 ml

Ⓛ   G0008   Administration of influenza virus vaccine when no physician fee schedule service on the same day

Ⓜ   G0333   Dispense fee initial 30 day

Ⓝ   A4220   Refill kit for implantable infusion pump

Ⓟ   G0177   Training and educational services related to the care and treatment of patient's disabling mental health problems per session (45 minutes or more)

Ⓢ   C1300   Hyperbaric oxygen under pressure, full body chamber, per 30 minute interval

Ⓣ   C9724   Endoscopic full-thickness plication in the gastric cardia using endoscopic plication system (EPS); includes endoscopy

Ⓥ   G0101   Cervical or vaginal cancer screening; pelvic and clinical breast examination

Ⓧ   C8952   Therapeutic, prophylactic or diagnostic injection; intravenous push

Ⓨ   A4222   Infusion supplies for external drug infusion pump, per cassette or bag (list drugs separately)

MED: This notation precedes an instruction pertaining to this code in the Centers for Medicare and Medicaid Services' (CMS) Publication 100 (Pub 100) electronic manual or in a National Coverage Determinatuion (NCD). These CMS sources, formerly called the *Medicare Carriers Manual* (MCM) and *Coverage Issues Manual* (CIM), present the rules for submitting these services to the federal government or its contractors and are included in the appendix of this book

A4300   Implantable access catheter, (e.g. venous, arterial, epidural subarachnoid, or peritoneal, etc.) external access
MED: 100-2, 15, 120

AHA: *American Hospital Association Coding Clinic for HCPCS* citations help you find expanded information about specific codes and their usage.

A4290   Sacral nerve stimulation test lead, each
AHA: 1Q, '02, 9

Current as of 11/23/2005

About HCPCS Codes

The AMA does not develop or maintain HCPCS Level II codes. The federal government does.

Any supplier or manufacturer can submit a request for coding modification to the HCPCS Level II national codes. A document explaining the HCPCS modification process, as well as a detailed format for submitting a recommendation for a modification to HCPCS Level II codes, is available on the HCPCS website at http://www.cms.hhs.gov/medicare/hcpcs/. Besides the information requested in this format, a requestor should also submit any additional descriptive material, including the manufacturer's product literature and information that is believed would be helpful in furthering CMS's understanding of the medical features of the item for which a coding modification is being recommended. The HCPCS coding review process is an ongoing, continuous process.

Requests for coding modifications should be sent to the following address:

Alpha-Numeric HCPCS Coordinator
Center for Medicare Management
Centers for Medicare and Medicaid Services
C5-08-27
7500 Security Boulevard
Baltimore, MD 21244-1850

How to Use HCPCS Level II

Coders should keep in mind, however, that the insurance companies and government do not base payment solely on what was done for the patient. They need to know why the services were performed. In addition to using the HCPCS coding system for procedures and supplies, coders must also use the ICD-9-CM coding system to denote the diagnosis. This book will not discuss ICD-9-CM codes, which can be found in a current ICD-9-CM code book for diagnosis codes. To locate a HCPCS Level II code, follow these steps:

To locate a HCPCS Level II code, follow these steps:

1. Identify the services or procedures the patient received.
    Example:

    Patient administered PSA exam.

2. Look up the appropriate term in the index.
    Example:

    >   **Screening**
    >   prostate

    Coding Tip: Coders who are unable to find the procedure or service in the index can look in the table of contents for the type of procedure or device to narrow the code choices. Also, coders should remember to check the unlisted procedure guidelines for additional choices.

3. Assign a tentative code.
    Example:

    Codes G0103

    Coding Tip: To the right of the terminology, there may be a single code or multiple codes, a cross-reference or an indication that the code has been deleted. Tentatively assign all codes listed.

4. Locate the code or codes in the appropriate section. When multiple codes are listed in the index, be sure to read the narrative of all codes listed to find the appropriate code based on the service performed.
    Example:

    >   G0103   Prostate cancer screening; prostate specific antigen test (PSA), total

5. Check for color bars, symbols, notes, and references.
    Example:

    > Ⓐ   G0103   Prostate cancer screening; prostate specific antigen test (PSA), total   ♂
    >   **MED: 100-3, 210.1; 100-4, 18, 50**

6. Review the appendixes for the reference definitions and other guidelines for coverage issues that apply.

7. Determine whether any modifiers should be used.

8. Assign the code.
    Example:

    The code assigned is G0103.

Coding Standards

Levels of Use

Coders may find that the same procedure is coded at two or even three levels. Which code is correct? There are certain rules to follow if this should occur.

When both a CPT and a HCPCS Level II code have virtually identical narratives for a procedure or service, the CPT code should be used. If, however, the narratives are not identical (for example, the CPT code narrative is generic, whereas the HCPCS Level II code is specific), the Level II code should be used.

Be sure to check for a national or local code when a CPT code description contains an instruction to include additional information, such as describing specific medication. For example, when billing Medicare or Medicaid for supplies, avoid using CPT code 99070, supplies and materials (except spectacles), provided by the physician over and above those usually included with the office visit or other services rendered (list drugs, trays, supplies, or materials provided). There are many HCPCS Level II codes that specify supplies in more detail.

Special Reports

Submit a special report with the claim when a new, unusual, or variable procedure is provided or a modifier is used. Include the following information:

*   A copy of the appropriate report (e.g., operative, x-ray), explaining the nature, extent, and need for the procedure
*   Documentation of the medical necessity of the procedure
*   Documentation of the time and effort necessary to perform the procedure

10% LMD, J7100

2 Load, hook prosthesis, L6795

3-in-1 composite commode, E0164

5% dextrose/normal saline, J7042

5% dextrose/water, J7060

A

Abarelix, J0128

Abbokinase, J3364, J3365

Abciximab, J0130

Abdomen/abdominal
dressing holder/binder, A4462
pad, low profle, L1270

Abdominal binder
elastic, A4462

Abduction
control, each, L2624
pillow, E1399
rotation bar, foot, L3140-L3170

Abortion, S2260-S2267

Abscess, incision and drainage, D7510-D7520

Absorption dressing, A6251-A6256

Abutments
for implants, D6056-D6057
retainers for resin bonded "Maryland bridge," D6545

Accession of tissue, dental, D0472-D0474

Accessories
ambulation devices, E0153-E0159
artifcial kidney and machine (see also ESRD), E1510-E1699
beds, E0271-E0280, E0305-E0326
wheelchairs, E0950-E1010, E1050-E1298, E2201-E2226, E2300-E2367, K0001-K0108

Access system, A4301

AccuChek
blood glucose meter, E0607
test strips, box of 50, A4253

Accu Hook, prosthesis, L6790

Accurate
prosthetic sock, L8420-L8435
stump sock, L8470-L8485

Acetate concentrate for hemodialysis, A4708

Acetazolamide sodium, J1120

Acetylcysteine
inhalation solution, J7608
injection, J0132

Achromycin, J0120

Acid concentrate for hemodialysis, A4709

ACTH, J0800

Acthar, J0800

Actimmune, J9216

Action neoprene supports, L1825

Action Patriot manual wheelchair, K0004

Action Xtra, Action MVP, Action Pro-T, manual wheelchair, K0005

Active Life
convex one-piece urostomy pouch, A4421
flush away, A5051
one-piece
drainable custom pouch, A5061
pre-cut closed-end pouch, A5051
stoma cap, A5055

Acyclovir, J0133

Adalimumab, J0135

Adaptor
neurostimulator, C1883
pacing lead, C1883

Addition
cushion AK, L5648
cushion BK, L5646
harness upper extremity, L6675-L6676
to lower extremity prosthesis, K0670
wrist, flexion, extension, L6620

Adenocard, J0150

Adenosine, J0150-J0152

Adhesive
barrier, C1765
catheter, A4364
disc or foam pad, A5126
medical, A4364
Nu-Hope
1 oz bottle with applicator, A4364
3 oz bottle with applicator, A4364
ostomy, A4364
pads, A6203-A6205, A6212-A6214, A6219-A6221, A6237-A6239, A6245-A6247, A6254-A6256
remover, A4365, A4455
support, breast prosthesis, A4280
tape, A4450, A4452
tissue, G0168

Adjunctive services, dental, D9220-D9310

Adjustabrace 3, L2999

Adjustment, bariatric band, S2083

Administration, medication, T1502
direct observation, H0033

Adoptive immunotherapy, S2107

Adrenalin, J0170

Adrenal transplant, S2103

Adriamycin, J9000

Adrucil, J9190

AdvantaJet, A4210

AFO, E1815, E1830, L1900-L1990, L4392, L4396

Agalsidase beta, J0180

A-hydroCort, J1720

Aimsco Ultra Thin syringe, 1 cc or 1/2 cc, each, A4206

Air ambulance — *see also* **Ambulance**

Air bubble detector, dialysis, E1530

Aircast, L4350-L4380

Aircast air stirrup ankle brace, L1906

Air fluidized bed, E0194

Airlife Brand Misty-Neb nebulizer, E0580

Air pressure pad/mattress, E0186, E0197

AirSep, E0601

Air travel and nonemergency transportation, A0140

Airway device, E0485-E0486

Akineton, J0190

Alarm
enuresis, S8270
pressure, dialysis, E1540

Alatrofloxacin mesylate, J0200

Albumarc, P9041

Albumin, human, P9041, P9045-P9047

Albuterol
administered through DME, J7611, J7613

Alcohol
abuse service, H0047
pint, A4244
testing, H0048
wipes, A4245

Aldesleukin, J9015

Aldomet, J0210

Aldurazyme, J1931

Alefacept, J0215

Alemtuzumab, J9010
injection, S0088

Alferon N, J9215

Algiderm, alginate dressing, A6196-A6199

Alginate dressing, A6196-A6199

Alglucerase, J0205

Algosteril, alginate dressing, A6196-A6199

Alimta, J9305

Alkaban-AQ, J9360

Alkaline battery for blood glucose monitor, A4233-A4236

Alkeran, J8600

Allogenic cord blood harvest, S2140

Allograft
small intestine and liver, S2053
soft dental tissue, D4275

Alpha 1-proteinase inhibitor, human, J0256

Alteplase recombinant, J2997

Alternating pressure mattress/pad, E0180, E0181, E0277
pump, E0182

Alternative communication device, i.e., communication board, E1902

Alveoloplasty, D7310, D7320, D7321
with extraction(s), D7311

Alveolus, fracture, D7770

Amalgam, restoration, dental, D2140-D2161

Amantadine hydrochloride, G9017, G9033

Ambulance, A0021-A0999
air, A0436
disposable supplies, A0382-A0398
oxygen, A0422
response, treatment, no transport, A0998

Ambulation device, E0100-E0159

Ambulation stimulator
spinal cord injured, E0762

Amcort, J3302

A-methaPred, J2920, J2930

Amevive, J0215

Amifostine, J0207

Amikacin sulfate, J0278

Aminaid, enteral nutrition, B4154

Aminolevulinic acid, topical, J7308

Aminophylline/Aminophyllin, J0280

Amiodarone hydrochloride, J0282

Amirosyn-RF, parenteral nutrition, B5000

Amitriptyline HCl, J1320

Ammonia N-13
diagnostic imaging agent, A9526

Ammonia test paper, A4774

Amobarbital, J0300

Amphocin, J0285

Amphotericin B, J0285
cholesterol sulfate, J0288
lipid complex, J0287
liposome, J0289

Ampicillin sodium, J0290
  sodium/sulbactam sodium, J0295

Amputee
  adapter, wheelchair, E0959
  prosthesis, L5000-L7510, L7520, L7900,
    L8400-L8465
  stump sock, L8470
  wheelchair, E1170-E1190, E1200

Amygdalin, J3570

Amytal, J0300

Anabolin LA 100, J2320-J2322

Analgesia, dental, D9230, D9241, D9242
  non-intravenous conscious sedation,
    D9248

Anastrozole, S0170

Ancef, J0690

Anchor, screw, C1713

Andrest 90-4, J0900

Andro-Cyp, J1070-J1080

Andro-Estro 90-4, J0900

Androgyn L.A., J0900

Andro L.A. 200, J3130

Androlone
  -D 100, J2321

Andronaq
  -LA, J1070

Andronate
  -100, J1070
  -200, J1080

Andropository 100, J3120

Andryl 200, J3130

Anectine, J0330

Anergan (25, 50), J2550

Anesthesia
  dental, D9210-D9221
  dialysis, A4736-A4737

Angiography
  coronary arteries, S8093
  digital subtraction, S9022
  iliac artery, G0278
  magnetic resonance, C8901-C8914,
    C8918-C8920
  reconstruction, G0288
  renal artery, G0275

Anistreplase, J0350

Ankle-foot orthosis AFO; — *see also*
  Orthopedic shoe, and tibia, L1900-
    L1990, L2106-L2116
  Dorsiwedge Night Splint, L4398 or
    A4570 or, L2999
  Specialist
    Ankle Foot Orthosis, L1930
    Tibial Pre-formed Fracture Brace,
      L2116
  Surround Ankle Stirrup Braces with
    Floam, L1906

Antagon, S0132

Anterior-posterior orthosis
  lateral orthosis, L0520, L0560-L0565,
    L0700, L0710

Antibiotic home infusion therapy,
  S9494-S9504

Antibody testing, HIV-1, S3645

Anticeptic
  chlorhexidine, A4248

Anticoagulation clinic, S9401

Antiemetic drug, prescription
  oral, Q0163-Q0181

Antifungal home infusion therapy,
  S9494-S9504

Anti-hemophilic factor (Factor VIII),
  J7190-J7192

Anti-inhibitors, J7198

Anti-neoplastic drug, NOC, J9999

Antispas, J0500

Antithrombin III, J7197

Antiviral home infusion therapy, S9494-
  S9504

Anzemet, J1260

Apexifcation, dental, D3351-D3353

Apicoectomy, dental, D3410-D3426

A.P.L., J0725

Apnea monitor, E0618-E0619
  with recording feature, E0619
  electrodes, A4556
  lead wires, A4557

Apomorphine hydrochloride, S0167

Appliance
  cleaner, A5131
  orthodontic
    fixed, D8220
    removable, D8210
    removal, D7997
  pneumatic, E0655-E0673

Aprepitant, J8501

Apresoline, J0360

Aprotinin, J0365

AquaMEPHYTON, J3430

AquaPedic sectional gel flotation, E0196

Aqueous
  shunt, L8612

Ara-C, J9100

Aralen, J0390

Aramine, J0380

Aranesp
  ESRD, J0882
  non-ESRD, J0881

Arbutamine HCl, J0395

Arch support, L3040-L3100

Aredia, J2430

Argatroban, C9121

Argyle Sentinel Seal chest drainage unit,
  E0460

Aristocort
  forte, J3302
  intralesional, J3302

Aristospan
  Intra-articular, J3303
  Intralesional, J3303

Arm
  sling
    deluxe, A4565
    mesh cradle, A4565
    universal
      arm, A4565
      elevator, A4565
  wheelchair, E0973

Arrestin, J3250

Arrow, power wheelchair, K0014

Arsenic trioxide, J9017

Arthrocentesis, dental, D7870

Arthroereisis
  subtalar, S2117

Arthroplasty, dental, D7865

Arthroscopy
  dental, D7872-D7877
  knee
    harvest of cartilage, S2112
    removal loose body, FB, G0289

Arthroscopy — *continued*
  shoulder
    with capsulorrhaphy, S2300
    tenodesis, biceps, S2114

Arthrotomy, dental, D7860

Artifcial
  kidney machines and accessories (*see
    also* Dialysis), E1510-E1699
  larynx, L8500

Asparaginase, J9020

Aspart insulin, S5551

Aspiration, bone marrow, G0364

Assertive community treatment, H0039-
  H0040

Assessment
  audiologic, V5008-V5020
  family, H1011
  geriatric, S0250
  mental health, H0031
  speech, V5362-V5364

Assisted living, T2030-T2031

Assistive listening device, V5268-V5274
  alerting device, V5269
  cochlear implant assistive device, V5273
  TDD, V5272
  telephone amplifier, V5268
  television caption decoder, V5271

Asthma
  education, S9441

Astramorph, J2275

Atgam, J7504

Ativan, J2060

Atropine
  inhalation solution
    concentrated, J7635
    unit dose, J7636
  sulfate, J0460

Attends, adult diapers, A4335

Audiologic assessment, V5008-V5020

Audiometry, S0618

Auricular prosthesis, D5914, D5927

Aurothioglucose, J2910

Autoclix lancet device, A4258

Auto-Glide folding walker, E0143

Autolance lancet device, A4258

Autolet lancet device, A4258

Autolet Lite lancet device, A4258

Autolet Mark II lancet device, A4258

Autoplex T, J7198

Avastin, J9035, S0116

Avonex, J1825

Azacitidine, J9025

Azathioprine, J7500
  parenteral, J7501

Azithromycin
  injection, J0456
  oral, Q0144

Aztreonam, S0073

B

**Babysitter, child of parents in
treatment**, T1009

Back supports, L0100-L0710

Baclofen, J0475, J0476
  intrathecal, J0475-J0476

Bacterial sensitivity study, P7001

Bactocill, J2700

Demonstration project
chemotherapy assessment, G9021-G9032
low vision therapist, G9043
occupational therapist, G9041
orientation and mobility specialist, G9042
rehabilitation teacher, G9044

Dennis Browne, foot orthosis, L3140, L3150

Dentures (removable)
adjustments, D5410-D5422
complete, D5110-D5140
overdenture, D5860-D5861
partial, D5211-D5281
mandibular, D5226
maxillary, D5225
precision attachment, D5862
rebase, D5710-D5721
reline, D5730-D5761
repairs, D5510, D5520, D5610-D5650
temporary, D5810-D5821

DepAndro
100, J1070
200, J1080

Dep-Androgyn, J1060

DepMedalone
40, J1030
80, J1040

Depo
-Medrol, J1020, J1030, J1040
-Provera, J1051, J1055
-Testadiol, J1060
-Testosterone, J1070, J1080

Depo-estradiol cypionate, J1000

Depogen, J1000

Depoject, J1030, J1040

Depopred
-40, J1030
-80, J1040

Depotest, J1070, J1080

Depotestogen, J1060

Derata injection device, A4210

Dermagraft, J7342

Dermal tissue
human origin, J7342, J7350

Desensitizing medicament, dental, D9910

Desensitizing resin, dental, D9911

Desferal mesylate, J0895

Desmopressin acetate, J2597

Detector, blood leak, dialysis, E1560

Device
joint, C1776
ocular, C1784
reaching/grabbing, A9281
retrieval, C1773
tissue localization and excision, C1819
urinary incontinence repair, C1771, C2631

DeVilbiss
9000D, E0601
9001D, E0601

Dexacen-4, J1100

Dexamethasone
acetate, J1094
inhalation solution
concentrated, J7637
unit dose, J7638
oral, J8540
sodium phosphate, J1100

Dexasone, J1100

Dexferrum (iron dextran), J1751-J1752

Dexone, J1100

Dexrazoxane HCl, J1190

Dextran, J7100, J7110

Dextroamphetamine sulfate, S0160

Dextrose, S5010-S5014
saline (normal), J7042
water, J7060, J7070

Dextrostick, A4772

D.H.E. 45, J1110

Diabetes
alcohol swabs, per box, A4245
battery for blood glucose monitor, A4233-A4236
bent needle set for insulin pump infusion, A4231
blood glucose monitor, E0607
with integrated lancer, E2101
with voice synthesizer, E2100
blood glucose test strips, box of 50, A4253
drugs
Humalin, J1815, J1817
Humalog, J1817, S5551
insulin, J1815, J1817, S5551
Novolin, J1815, J1817
injection device, needle-free, A4210
insulin pump, external, E0784
infusion set, A4231
syringe with needle, A4232
lancet device, A4258
lancets, box of 100, A4259
non needle cannula for insulin infusion, A4232
retinal exam, S3000
shoe
fitting, A5500
inlay, A5508
insert, A5512-A5513
modification, A5503-A5507
syringe, disposable
box of 100, S8490
each, A4206
urine glucose/ketone test strips, box of 100, A4250

Diabetic management program
E/M of sensory neuropathy, G0246-G0247
follow-up visit to MD provider, S9141
follow-up visit to non-MD provider, S9140
foot care, G0247
group session, S9455
insulin pump initiation, S9145
nurse visit, S9460

Diagnostic
dental services, D0120-D0999
radiology services, D0210-D0340

Dialet lancet device, A4258

Dialysate
concentrate additives, A4765
peritoneal dialysis solution, A4720-A4726, A4766
solution, A4728
testing solution, A4760

Dialysis
access system, C1881
air bubble detector, E1530
anesthetic, A4736-A4737
bath conductivity, meter, E1550
blood leak detector, E1560
centrifuge, E1500
cleaning solution, A4674
concentrate
acetate, A4708
acid, A4709
bicarbonate, A4706-A4707
drain bag/bottle, A4911
emergency treatment, G0257
equipment, E1510-E1702
extension line, A4672-A4673
filter, A4680
fluid barrier, E1575

Dialysis — *continued*
heating pad, E0210
hemostats, E1637
home equipment repair, A4890
infusion pump, E1520
mask, surgical, A4928
peritoneal
clamps, E1634
pressure alarm, E1540
scale, E1639
shunt, A4740
supplies, A4671-A4918
surgical mask, A4928
syringe, A4657
tourniquet, A4929
unipuncture control system, E1580

Dialyzer, artificial kidney, A4690

Diamox, J1120

Diaper service, T4538

Diaphragm, contraceptive, A4266

Diazepam, J3360

Diazoxide, J1730

Dibent, J0500

Didanosine, S0137

Didronel, J1436

Dietary education, S9449, S9452

Dietary planning, dental nutrition, D1310

Diethylstilbestrol
diphosphate, J9165

Diflucan injection, J1450

Digital subtraction angiography, S9022

Digoxin, J1160

Digoxin immune fab, J1265

Dihydrex, J1200

Dihydroergotamine mesylate, J1110

Dilantin, J1165

Dilaudid, J1170

Dilomine, J0500

Dilor, J1180

Dimenhydrinate, J1240

Dimercaprol, J0470

Dimethyl sulfoxide (DMSO), J1212

Dinate, J1240

Dioval (XX, 40), J0970, J1380, J1390

Diphenacen-50, J1200

Diphenhydramine HCl, J1200
oral, Q0163

Dipyridamole, J1245

Disarticulation
lower extremities, prosthesis, L5000-L5999
upper extremities, prosthesis, L6000-L6692

Discoloration, dental, removal, D9970

Disease management program, S0317

Disetronic
glass cartridge syringe for insulin pump, each, A4232
H-Tron insulin pump, E0784
insulin infusion set with bent needle, with or without wings, each, A4231

Diskard head halter, E0940

Disk decompression, lumbar, S2348

Diskectomy, lumbar, S2350, S2351
single interspace, S2350

Disotate, J3520

Di-Spaz, J0500

Enema — *continued*
cancer screening, G0120

Enovil, J1320

Enoxaparin sodium, J1650

Enrich, enteral nutrition, B4150

Ensure, enteral nutrition, B4150
HN, B4150
Plus, B4152
Plus HN, B4152
powder, B4150

Enteral
administration services, feeding, S9340-S9343
feeding supply kit (syringe) (pump) (gravity), B4034-B4036
fiber or additive, B4104
formulae, B4150-B4162
electrolytes, B4102, B4103
for metabolic disease, B4157
intact nutrients, B4149, B4150, B4152
pediatric, B4158-B4162
gastronomy tube, B4086
nutrition infusion pump (with alarm) (without), B9000, B9002
supplies, not otherwise classified, B9998

Epinephrine, J0170

Epiribicin HCl, J9178

Epoetin alfa
ESRD, J0886
non-ESRD, J0885

Epoprostenol, J1325
dilutant, sterile, S0155
infusion pump, K0455

Equestrian/hippotherapy, S8940

Equilibration, dental, D9951-D9952

Erbitux, J9055

Ergonovine maleate, J1330

Ertapenem sodium, J1335

Erythromycin lactobionate, J1364

ESRD End Stage Renal Disease; — *see also* **Dialysis**
bundle demo/basic, G9013
expanded, G9014
counseling or assessment, G0308-G0319
home dialysis, G0320-G0327
machines and accessories, E1510-E1699
plumbing, A4870
services, E1510-E1699, G0308-G0327
supplies, A4651-A4913

Estra-D, J1000

Estradiol, J1000, J1060
cypionate and testosterone cypionate, J1060
L.A., J0970, J1380, J1390
L.A. 20, J0970, J1380, J1390
L.A. 40, J0970, J1380, J1390
valerate and testosterone enanthate, J0900

Estra-L (20, 40), J0970, J1380, J1390

Estra-Testrin, J0900

Estro-Cyp, J1000

Estrogen conjugated, J1410

Estroject L.A., J1000

Estrone (5, Aqueous), J1435

Estronol, J1435
-L.A., J1000

Ethanolamine oleate, J1430

Ethyol, J0207

Etidronate disodium, J1436

Etopophos, J9181, J9182
oral, J8560

Etoposide, J9181, J9182
oral, J8560

Evaluation
comprehensive, multi-discipline, H2000
dental, D0120-D0180
for power mobility device, G0372
self assessment, depression, S3005
team for handicapped, T1024

Everone, J3120, J3130

Exactech lancet device, A4258

Examination
breast, S0613
breast and pelvic, G0101
for college, S0622
initial Medicare, G0344
oral, D0120-D0160
related to surgical procedure, S0260

Excision, tissue localization, C1819

Exercise
class, S9451
equipment, A9300

Exo-Static overdoor traction unit, E0860

Exostosis (tuberosity) removal
lateral, D7471
osseous tuberosity, D7485
reduction of fibrous tuberosity, D7972

External
ambulatory infusion pump, E0781, E0784
counterpulsation, G0166
power, battery components, L7360-L7499
power, elbow, L7191
urinary supplies, A4356-A4359

External defibrillator
battery replacement, K0607
electrode replacement, K0609
garment replacement, K0608

Extractions, D7111-D7140
surgical, D7210-D7250

Extraoral films, D0250, D0260

Extremity belt/harness, E0945

Eye
lens (contact) (spectacle), S0500-S0514, V2100-V2615
pad, A6410-A6411
patch, A6410-A6411
prosthetic, V2623-V2629
service (miscellaneous), V2700-V2799

E-ZJect disposable insulin syringes, up to 1 cc, per syringe, A4206

E-ZJect Lite Angle lancets, box of 100, A4259

E-Z-lets lancet device, A4258

E-Z Lite wheelchair, E1250

F

Fabrazyme, J0180

Face tent, oxygen, A4619

Factor IX, anti-hemophilic factor, J7193-J7195

Factor VIII, anti-hemophilic factor, J7190-J7192

Factrel, J1620

Family stabilization, S9482

Famotidine, S0028

Fastodex, J9395

FDG, A9552

Fecal
occult blood test, G0107

Fee, coordinated care, G9009-G9012

Fentanyl citrate, J3010
and droperidol, J1810

Fern test, Q0114

Fertility services
donor service (sperm or embryo), S4025
in vitro fertilization, S4013-S4022
ovulation induction, S4042
sperm procurement, S4026, S4030-S4031

Fetal surgery, repair teratoma, S2405

Fiberotomy, dental, transeptal, D7291

Filgrastim (G-CSF), J1440, J1441

Filler, wound
alginate, A6199
foam, A6215
hydrocolloid, A6240-A6241
hydrogel, A6248
not elsewhere classified, A6261, A6262

Film
dressing, A6257-A6259
radiographic, dental, D0210-D0340

Filter
carbon, A4680
CPAP device, A7038-A7039
dialysis carbon, A4680
ostomy, A4368
tracheostoma, A4481
vena cava, C1880
ventricular assist device, Q0500

Finasteride, S0138

Finger
baseball splint, A4570
fold-over splint, A4570
four-pronged splint, A4570
splint, static, Q4049

Fisher & Paykel HC220, E0601

Fistula
cannulation set, A4730
oroantral, D7260
salivary, D7983

Fitness club membership, S9970

Fixed partial dentures (bridges), retainers
crowns, D6720-D6792
implant/abutment support, D6068-D6077
inlay/onlay, D6545-D6615
pontics, D6205-D6252
recementation, D6930
repair, D6980
resin bonded, D6545

Flap, gingival, D4240, D4241

Flashcast Elite casting material, A4590

Flexoject, J2360

Flexon, J2360

Flipper, dental prosthesis, D5820-D5821

Flolan, J1325

Flowmeter, E0440, E0555, E0580

Flow rate meter, peak, A4614

Floxuridine, J9200

Fluconazole, injection, J1450

Fludara, J9185

Fludarabine phosphate, J9185

Fluid barrier, dialysis, E1575

Flunisolide, J7641

Fluocinolone acetonide, C9225

Fluoride
custom tray/gel carrier, D5986
dispensing for home use, D9630
topical, D1201-D1205

Fluorine-18 fluorodeoxyglucose
contrast material, A9552
imaging using dual-head coincidence detection system, S8085

Graft, dental — *continued*
    maxillofacial soft/hard tissue, D7955
    ridge augmentation, D7950
    soft tissue, D4270-D4273
    soft tissue and pedicle, D4276

Graftjacket
    Reg Matrix, C9221
    SoftTis, C9222

Granisetron HCl, J1626, Q0166, S0091

Gravity traction device, E0941

Gravlee jet washer, A4470

Greissing, foot prosthesis, L5978

Guided tissue regeneration, dental,
    D4266-D4267

Guide wire, C1769

**Guilford multiple-post collar, cervical
orthosis**, L0190

Gynogen, J1380, J1390
    L.A. (10, 20, 40), J0970, J1380, J1390

H

Haberman Feeder, S8265

Habilitation, T2012-T2021

Hair analysis (excluding arsenic), P2031

Haldol, J1630
    decanoate (-50, -100), J1631

Hallus-valgus dynamic splint, L3100

Hallux prosthetic implant, L8642

Haloperidol, J1630
    decanoate, J1631

Halo procedures, L0810-L0859

Halter, cervical head, E0942

Handgrip (cane, crutch, walker), A4636

Hand restoration, L6900-L6915
    orthosis (WHFO), E1805, E1825, L3800-
        L3805, L3900-L3954
    partial prosthesis, L6000-L6020
    rims, wheelchair, E0967

Harness, E0942, E0944, E0945

Harvest
    bone marrow, G0267
    multivisceral organs, cadaver donor,
        S2055
    peripheral stem cell, G0267, S2150

Harvey arm abduction orthosis, L3960

Health club membership, S9970

Hearing devices, L8614, V5008-V5299
    accessories/supplies, V5267
    analog, V5242-V5251
    battery, V5266
    BICROS, V5210-V5230
    CROS, V5170-V5190
    digital, V5250-V5261
    dispensing fee, V5241
        BICROS, V5240
        monaural, V5241
        bilateral, V5110
        binaural
        CROS, V5200
        unspecified, V5090
    ear impression, V5275
    ear mold/insert, V5264-V5265
    programmable analog
        binaural, V5252-V5253
        monaural, V5244-V5247
            CIC, V5244

Heat
    application, E0200-E0239
    lamp, E0200, E0205
    pad, E0210, E0215, E0217, E0218,
        E0238, E0249
    units, E0239
        Hydrocollator, mobile, E0239
        Thermalator T-12-M, E0239

Heater (nebulizer), E1372

Heating pad, Dunlap, E0210
    for peritoneal dialysis, E0210

Heel
    elevator, air, E0370
    loop/holder, E0951
    pad, L3480, L3485
    protector, E0191
    shoe, L3430-L3485
    stabilizer, L3170

Helicopter, ambulance — *see also*
    Ambulance, A0431

Helmet
    with face guard, E0701
    cervical, L0100, L0110

Hemalet lancet device, A4258

Hematopoietic hormone administration,
    S9537

Hemin, J1640

Hemipelvectomy prosthesis, L5280

Hemisection, dental, D3920

Hemi-wheelchair, E1083-E1086

Hemodialysis
    acetate concentrate, A4708
    acid solution, A4709
    bicarbonate concentrate, A4706-A4707
    catheter, C1750, C1752
    drain bag/bottle, A4911
    machine, E1590
    mask, surgical, A4928
    protamine sulfate, A4802
    surgical mask, A4928
    tourniquet, A4929

Hemodialyzer, portable, E1635

Hemofl M, J7190

Hemophilia clotting factor, J7190-J7199

Hemostats, for dialysis, E1637

Hemostix, A4773

Heparin
    infusion pump (for dialysis), E1520
    lock flush, J1642
    sodium, J1644

HepatAmine, parenteral nutrition, B5100

Hepatic-aid, enteral nutrition, B4154

Hep-Lock (U/P), J1642

Herceptin, J9355

Hexadrol phosphate, J1100

Hexalite, A4590

Hexior power wheelchair, K0014

**High Frequency chest wall oscillation
equipment**, A7025-A7026, E0483

High osmolar contrast
    150-199 mgs iodine, Q9959
    200-249 mgs iodine, Q9960
    250-299 mgs iodine, Q9961
    300-349 mgs iodine, Q9962
    350-399 mgs iodine, Q9963
    400 or greater mgs iodine, Q9964
    up to 149 mgs iodine, Q9958

High risk area requiring escort, S9381

Hip
    Custom Masterhinge Hip Hinge 3, L2999
    disarticulation prosthesis, L5250, L5270
    Masterhinge Hip Hinge 3, L2999
    orthosis (HO), L1600-L1686

Hip-knee-ankle-foot orthosis (HKAFO),
    L2040-L2090

Histaject, J0945

Histerone (-50, -100), J3140

History and physical
    related to surgical procedure, S0260

Histrelin
    acetate injection, J1675
    implant, J9225

HIV-1 antibody testing, S3645

HKAFO, L2040-L2090

HN2, J9230

Holder
    heel, E0951
    toe, E0952

Hole cutter tool, A4421

Hollister
    belt adapter, A4421
    closed pouch, A5051, A5052
    colostomy/ileostomy kit, A5061
    drainable pouches, A5061
        with flange, A5063
    medical adhesive, A4364
    pediatric ostomy belt, A4367
    remover, adhesive, A4455
    skin barrier, A4362, A5122
    skin cleanser, A4335
    skin conditioning creme, A4335
    skin gel protective dressing wipes, A5120
    stoma cap, A5055
    stoma cap, A5055
    two-piece pediatric ostomy system,
        A5054, A5063, A5073
    urostomy pouch, A5071, A5072

Home health
    aide, S9122, T1030-T1031
        home health setting, G0156
    care
        certified nurse assistant, S9122,
            T1021
        home health aide, S9122, T1021
        nursing care, S9122-S9124, T1030-
            T1031
        re-certification, G0179-G0180
    gestational
        assessment, T1028
        delivery suppies, S8415
        diabetes, S9214
        hypertension, S9211
        pre-eclampsia, S9213
        preterm labor, S9208-S9209
    hydration therapy, S9373-S9379
    infusion therapy, S9325-S9379, S9494-
        S9497, S9537-S9810
    nursing services, S9212-S9213
    postpartum hypertension, S9212
    services of
        clinical social worker, G0155
        occupational therapist, G0152
        physical therapist, G0151
        skilled nurse, G0154
        speech/language pathologist, G0153
    transfusion, blood products, S9538
    wound care, S9097

Home uterine monitor, S9001

Hosmer
    baby mitt, L6870
    child hand, mechanical, L6872
    forearm lift, assist unit only, L6635
    gloves, above hands, L6890, L6895
    hand prosthesis, L6868
    hip orthotic joint, post-op, L1685
    hook
        with
            neoprene fingers, #88X, L6745
            neoprene fingers, #8X, L6740
            plastisol, #10P, L6750
        #5, L6705
        #5X, L6710
        #5XA, L6715
        child, L6755, L6765
        small adult, L6770
        stainless steel #8, L6735
            with neopren, L6780
        work, #3, L6700
            with lock, #6, L6720
            with wider opening, L6730
            for use with tools, #7, L6725

Microcapillary tube, A4651
   sealant, A4652

Micro-Fine
   disposable insulin syringes, up to 1 cc, per syringe, A4206
   lancets, box of 100, A4259

Microlipids, enteral nutrition, B4155

Microspirometer, S8190

Midazolam HCl, J2250

Mileage, ambulance, A0380, A0390

Milk, breast
   processing, T2101

Milrinone lactate, J2260

Milwaukee spinal orthosis, L1000

Minerva, spinal orthosis, L0700, L0710

Mini-bus, nonemergency transportation, A0120

Minimed
   3 cc syringe, A4232
   506 insulin pump, E0784
   insulin infusion set with bent needle wings, each, A4231
   Sof-Set 24" insulin infusion set, each, A4230

Minoxidil, S0139

Mitomycin, J9280-J9291

Mitoxantrone HCl, J9293

Mobilite hospital beds, E0293, E0295, E0297

Moducal, enteral nutrition, B4155

Moisture exchanger for use with invasive mechanical ventilation, A4483

Moisturizer, skin, A6250

Monarc-M, J7190

Monitor
   apnea, E0618
   blood glucose, E0607
      Accu-Check, E0607
      Tracer II, E0607
   blood pressure, A4670
   pacemaker, E0610, E0615
   ventilator, E0450

Monoclonal antibodies, J7505

Monoject disposable insulin syringes, up to 1 cc, per syringe, A4206

Monojector lancet device, A4258

Morcellator, C1782

Morphine sulfate, J2270, J2271, S0093
   sterile, preservative-free, J2275

Moulage, facial, D5911-D5912

Mouth exam, athletic, D9941

Mouthpiece (for respiratory equipment), A4617

Moxifloxacin, J2280

M-Prednisol-40, J1030
   -80, J1040

MRI
   contrast material, Q9952-Q9954
   low field, S8042

Mucoprotein, blood, P2038

Multifetal pregnancy reduction, ultrasound guidance, S8055

Multiple post collar, cervical, L0180-L0200

Multipositional patient support system, E0636

Muscular dystrophy, genetic test, S3853

Muse, J0275

Mutamycin, J9280

Mycophenolate mofetil, J7517

Mycophenolic acid, J7518

Mylotarg, J9300

Myochrysine, J1600

Myolin, J2360

Myotonic muscular dystrophy, genetic test, S3853

Myringotomy, S2225

N

Nafcillin sodium, S0032

Naglazyme, C9224

Nail trim, G0127, S0390

Nalbuphine HCl, J2300

Naloxone HCl, J2310

Nandrobolic L.A., J2321

Nandrolone
   decanoate, J2320-J2322

Narcan, J2310

Narrowing device, wheelchair, E0969

Nasahist B, J0945

Nasal
   application device (for CPAP device), A7032-A7034
   vaccine inhalation, J3530

Nasogastric tubing, B4081, B4082

Navelbine, J9390

ND Stat, J0945

Nebcin, J3260

Nebulizer, E0570-E0585
   aerosol compressor, E0571
   aerosol mask, A7015
   aerosols, E0580
      Airlife Brand Misty-Neb, E0580
      Power-Mist, E0580
      Up-Draft Neb-U-Mist, E0580
      Up-Mist hand-held nebulizer, E0580
   compressor, with, E0570
      Madamist II medication compressor/nebulizer, E0570
      Pulmo-Aide compressor/nebulizer, E0570
      Schuco Mist nebulizer system, E0570
   corrugated tubing
      disposable, A7010, A7018
      non-disposable, A7011
   distilled water, A7018
   drug dispensing fee, E0590
   filter
      disposable, A7013
      non-disposable, A7014
   heater, E1372
   large volume
      disposable, prefilled, A7008
      disposable, unfilled, A7007
   not used with oxygen
      durable glass, A7017
   pneumatic, administration set, A7003, A7005, A7006
   pneumatic, nonfiltered, A7004
   portable, E0570
   small volume, E0574
   spacer or nebulizer, S8100
      with mask, S8101
   ultrasonic, dome and mouthpiece, A7016
   ultrasonic, reservoir bottle
      non-disposable, A7009
   water, A7018
   water collection device large volume nebulizer, A7012
      distilled water, A7018

NebuPent, J2545

Needle, A4215
   with syringe, A4206-A4209
   brachytherapy, C1715
   non-coring, A4212

Negative pressure wound therapy
   dressing set, A6550
   pump, E2402

Nembutal sodium solution, J2515

Neocyten, J2360

Neo-Durabolic, J2320-J2322

Neomax knee support, L1800

Neoplasms, dental, D7410-D7465

Neoquess, J0500

Neosar, J9070-J9092

Neostigmine methylsulfate, J2710

Neo-Synephrine, J2370

NephrAmine, parenteral nutrition, B5000

Nesacaine MPF, J2400

Nesiritide, J2325

Neulasta, J2505

Neumega, J2355

Neurolysis
   foot, S2135

Neuromuscular stimulator, E0745
   ambulation of spinal cord injured, E0762

Neuro-Pulse, E0720

Neurostimulator
   functional transcutaneous, E0764
   generator, C1767
   implantable
      electrode, L8680
      pulse generator, L8685-L8688
      receiver, L8682
   lead, C1778
   patient programmer, L8681
   receiver and/or transmitter, C1816
   transmitter
      external, L8683-L8684

Neutrexin, J3305

Newington
   Legg Perthes orthosis, L1710
   mobility frame, L1500

Newport Lite hip orthosis, L1685

Nextep Contour Lower Leg Walker, L2999

Nextep Low Silhouette Lower Leg Walkers, L2999

Nicotine
   gum, S4995
   patches, S4990-S4991

Niemann-Pick disease, genetic test, S3849

Nightguard, D9940

Nipent, J9268

Nitric oxide, for hypoxic respiratory failure in neonate, S1025

Nitrogen mustard, J9230

Nitrous oxide, dental analgesia, D9230

Nonchemotherapy drug, oral, J8499

Noncovered services, A9270, G0293-G0294

Nonemergency transportation, A0080-A0210

Nonimpregnated gauze dressing, A6216, A6221, A6402, A6404

Nonintravenous conscious sedation, dental, D9248

Nonprescription drug, A9150

Paraffin, A4265
  bath unit, E0235

Paragard T 380-A, IUD, J7300

Paramagnetic contrast material, (Gadolinium), Q9952

Paramedic intercept, S0208

Paranasal sinus ultrasound, S9024

Paraplatin, J9045

Parapodium, mobility frame, L1500

Parenteral nutrition
  administration kit, B4224
  home infusion therapy, S9364-S9368
  pump, B9004, B9006
  solution, B4164-B5200
  supplies, not otherwise classified, B9999
  supply kit, B4220, B4222

Parenting class, S9444
  infant safety, S9447

Paricalcitol, J2501

Parking fee, nonemergency transport, A0170

Partial dentures
  fixed
    implant/adjustment-supported retainers, D6068-D6077
    pontic, D6210-D6252
    retainers, D6545-D6792
  removable, D5211-D5281

PASRR, T2010-T2011

Paste, conductive, A4558

Pathology and laboratory tests, miscellaneous, P9010-P9615

Patient lift, E0625, E0637, E0639, E0640

Patten Bottom, Legg Perthes orthosis, L1755

Pavlik harness, hip orthosis, L1650

Peak flow meter, S8110
  portable, S8096

Pediatric hip abduction splint
  Orthomedics, L1640
  Orthomerica, L1640

Pediculosis treatment, A9180

PEFR, peak expiratory flow rate meter, A4614

Pegademase bovine, J2504

Pegaspargase, J9266

Pegasys, S0145

Pegfilgastrim, J2505

Peg-L-asparaginase, J9266

Pelvic and breast exam, G0101

Pelvic belt/harness/boot, E0944

Pemetrexed, J9305

Penicillin G
  benzathine and penicillin G procaine, J0530-J0580
  potassium, J2540
  procaine, aqueous, J2510

Penlet II lancet device, A4258

Penlet lancet device, A4258

Pentamidine isethionate, J2545, S0080

Pentastarch, J2513

Pentazocine HCl, J3070

Pentobarbital sodium, J2515

Pentostatin, J9268

Percussor, E0480

Percutaneous
  access system, A4301

Perflexane lipid microspheres, Q9955

Perflutren lipid microsphere, Q9957

Performance Wrap (KO), L1825

Periapical service, D3410-D3470

Periodontal procedures, D4210-D4999

Periradicular/apicoectomy, D3410-D3426

Perlstein, ankle-foot orthosis, L1920

Permapen, J0560-J0580

Peroneal strap, L0980

Peroxide, A4244

Perphenazine, J3310, Q0175-Q0176

Persantine, J1245

Personal care services, T1019-T1020

Pessary, A4561-A4562

PET imaging
  any site, NOS, G0235
  breast, G0252
  cervical, G0330
  ovarian, G0331

Pfzerpen, J2540
  A.S., J2510

PGE1, J0270

Phamacologicals, dental, D9610, D9630

Pharmacy
  compounding and dispensing, S9430
  dispensing fee
    inhalation drugs
      per 30 days, Q0513
      per 90 days, Q0514
    supply fee
      imitial immunosuppressive drugs, Q0510
      oral anticancer antiemetic or immunosuppressive drug, Q0511-Q0512

Pharmaplast disposable insulin syringes, per syringe, A4206

Phelps, ankle-foot orthosis, L1920

Phenazine (25, 50), J2550

Phenergan, J2550

Phenobarbital sodium, J2560

Phentolamine mesylate, J2760

Phenylephrine HCl, J2370

Phenytoin sodium, J1165

Philadelphia tracheotomy cervical collar, L0172

Philly One-piece Extrication collar, L0150

pHisoHex solution, A4246

Photofrin, J9600

Photographs, dental, diagnostic, D0350

Phototherapy
  home visit service (Bili-Lite), S9098
  keratectomy (PKT), S0812
  light, E0202

Physical exam
  for college, S0622
  related to surgical procedure, S0260

Physical therapy, S8990
  shoulder stretch device, E1841

Physical therapy/therapist
  home health setting, G0151, S9131

Physican voluntary reporting program (PVRP)
  antibiotic prophylaxis, G8152-G8154
  antidepressant medication, G8126-G8131
  atrial fibrillation, G8183-G8184
  COPD, G8093-G8094
  coronary artery bypass graft, G8158-G8167

Physican voluntary reporting program —
  continued
  coronary artery disease, G8036-G8041, G8182
  diabetic patient, G8016-G8026
  ESRD, G8075-G8082
  fall assessment, G8054-G8056
  hearing assessment, G8057-G8059
  heart failure patient, G8027-G8032, G8183-G8184
  influenza vaccination, G8108-G8110
  mammogram, G8111-G8114
  mycardial infarction, G8006-G8011, G8033-G8035
  osteoporosis, G8051-G8053, G8099-G8100, G8103-G8104, G8106-G8107, G8185-G8186
  pneumococcal vaccination, G8115-G8117
  pneumonia, G8012-G8014
  thromboembolism prophylaxis, G8155-G8157
  urinary incontinence assessment, G8060-G8062
  warfarin therapy, G8183-G8184

Phytonadione, J3430

Pillo pump, E0182

Pillow
  abduction, E1399
  decubitus care, E0190
  positioning, E0190

Pin retention, per tooth, D2951

Pinworm examination, Q0113

Piperacillin sodium, S0081

Pit and fissure sealant, D1351

Pitocin, J2590

Planing, dental root, D0350

Plasma
  frozen, P9058-P9060
  multiple donor, pooled, frozen, P9023
  protein fraction, P9048
  single donor, fresh frozen, P9017

Plastazote, L3002, L3252, L3253, L3265, L5654-L5658

Plaster
  bandages
    Orthoflex Elastic Plaster Bandages, A4580
    Specialist Plaster Bandages, A4580
  Genmould Creamy Plaster, A4580
  Specialist J-Splint Plaster Roll Immobilizer, A4580
  Specialist Plaster Roll Immobilizer, A4580
  Specialist Plaster Splints, A4580

Platelet
  concentrate, each unit, P9019
  rich plasma, each unit, P9020

Platelets, P9032-P9040, P9052-P9053

Platform attachment
  forearm crutch, E0153
  walker, E0154

Platform, for home blood glucose monitor, A4255

Platinol, J9060, J9062

Plenaxis, J0128

Pleural catheter, A7042
  drainage bottle, A7043

Plicamycin, J9270

Plumbing, for home ESRD equipment, A4870

Pneumatic
  appliance, E0655-E0673, L4350-L4380
  compressor, E0650-E0652, E0675
  splint, L4350-L4380

Respiratory syncytial virus immune globulin, J1565

Respiratory therapy, G0237-G0238

Respite care, T1005
  in home, S9125
  not in home, H0045

Restorations, dental
  amalgam, D2140-D2161
  gold foil, D2410-D2430
  inlay/onlay, D2510-D2664, D6600-D6615
  resin-based composite, D2330-D2394

Restorative
  dental work, D2330-D2999
  injection
    face, S0196

Restorative injection, face, S0196

Restraint
  any type, E0710
  belts
    Posey, E0700
    Secure-All, E0700
  Bite disposable jaw locks, E0700
  body holders
    Houdini security suit, E0700
    Quick Release, one piece, E0700
    Secure-All, one piece, E0700
    System2 zippered, E0700
    UltraCare vest-style
      with sleeves, E0700
  hand
    Secure-All finger control mit, E0700
  limb holders
    Posey, E0700
    Quick Release, E0700
    Secure-All, E0700
  pelvic
    Secure-All, E0700

Retail therapy item, miscellaneous, T1999

Retainers, dental
  fixed partial denture, D6545-D6792
  implant/abutment supported, D6068-D6077
  orthodontic, D8680

Retinal
  device, intraoperative, C1784
  exam for diabetes, S3000
  tamponade, C1814
  telescreening, S0625

Retinoblastoma, genetic test, S3841

Retrieval device, insertable, C1773

Retrograde dental filling, D3430

Rhesonativ, J2790

Rheumatrex, J8610

RhoGAM, J2790

Rho(D) immune globulin, human, J2790, J2792
  minidose, J2788

Rib belt
  thoracic, L0210, L0220
  Don-Joy, L0210

Rice ankle splint, L1904

Richfoam convoluted & flat overlays, E0199

Ride Lite 200, Ride Lite 9000, manual wheelchair, K0004

Ridge augmentation/sinus lift, dental, D7950

Rimantadine HCl, G9020, G9036

Rimso, J1212

Ringer's lactate infusion, J7120

Ring, ostomy, A4404

Risperidone, long acting, J2794

Rituxan, J9310

Rituximab, J9310

Riveton, foot orthosis, L3140, L3150

RN services, T1002

Road Savage power wheelchair, K0011

Road Warrior power wheelchair, K0011

Robaxin, J2800

Robin-Aids, prosthesis
  hand, L6855, L6860
  partial hand, L6000-L6020

Robotic surgical system, S2900

Rocephin, J0696

Rocking bed, E0462

Rollabout chair, E1031

Root canal therapy, D3310-D3353

Root planning and scaling, dental, D4341

Root removal, dental, D7140, D7250

Root resection/amputation, dental, D3450

Ropivacaine hydrochloride, J2795

RSV immune globulin, J1565

Rubex, J9000

Rubidium RB-82, A9555

Rubramin PSC, J3420

S

Sabre power wheelchair, K0011

Sacral nerve stimulation test
  lead, each, A4290

Sacroiliac orthosis, L0622-L0624

Safe, hand prosthesis, L5972

Safety
  enclosure frame/canopy, for hospital bed, E0316
  equipment, E0700
  eyeglass frames, S0516
  vest, wheelchair, E0980

Saline, A4216-A4217
  hypertonic, J7130
  solution, J7030-J7050

Salivary gland excision, D7983

Saliva test, hormone level
  during menopause, S3650
  preterm labor risk, S3652

Samarium Sm-153 lexidronamm, A9605

Sam Brown, Legg Perthes orthosis, A4565

Sansibar Plus, E0601

Saquinavir, S0140

Sargramostim (GM-CSF), J2820

Satumomab pendetide, A4642

Scale, for dialysis, E1639

Schuco
  mist nebulizer system, E0570
  vac aspirator, E0600

Scintimammography, S8080

Scleral lens bandage, S0515

Scoliosis, L1000, L1200, L1300-L1499
  additions, L1010-L1120, L1210-L1290

Scott ankle splint, canvas, L1904

Scott-Craig, stirrup orthosis, L2260

Scottish-Rite, Legg Perthes orthosis, L1730

Screening
  cervical or vaginal, G0101
  colorectal cancer, G0104-G0107, G0120-G0122

Screening — *continued*
  cytopathology, G0123-G0124, G0141, G0143-G0148
  digital rectal, annual, S0605
  early periodic screening diagnosis and treatment (EPSDT), S0302
  glaucoma, G0117-G0118
  gynecological
    established patient, S0612
    new patient, S0610
  maternal serum quad marker, S3626
  newborn metabolic, S3620
  ophthalmological, including refraction
    established patient, S0621
    new patient, S0620
  preadmission, T2010-T2011
  proctoscopy, S0601
  program participation, T1023
  prostate
    digital, rectal, G0102
  prostate specific antigen test (PSA), G0103
  retinal telescreening, S0625

Sealant
  dental, D1351
  pulmonary, liquid, C2615
  skin, A6250
  tooth, D1351

Seat
  attachment, walker, E0156
  insert, wheelchair, E0992
  lift (patient), E0621, E0627-E0629

Seattle Carbon Copy II, foot prosthesis, L5976

Secure-All
  restraints, E0700
  universal pelvic traction belt, E0890

Sedation, dental
  deep, D9220-D9221
  intravenous, conscious, D9241-D9242
  non-intravenous, D9248

Sedative filling, dental, D2940

Selestoject, J0704

Semilente insulin, J1815

Sensitivity study, P7001

Septal defect implant system, C1817

Sequestrectomy, dental, D7550

Sermorelin acetate, Q0515

Serum clotting time tube, A4771

SEWHO, L3960-L3974

Sexa, G0130

Sheath
  introducer
    guiding, C1766, C1892, C1893
    other than guiding, C2629, C2629

Sheepskin pad, E0188, E0189

Shoes
  arch support, L3040-L3100
  for diabetics, A5500-A5508
  insert, L3000-L3030
    for diabetics, A5512-A5513
  lift, L3300-L3334
  miscellaneous additions, L3500-L3595
  orthopedic (*see* Orthopedic shoes), L3201-L3265
  positioning device, L3140-L3170
  post-operative
    Specialist Health/Post Operative Shoe, A9270
  transfer, L3600-L3649
  wedge, L3340-L3485

Shoulder
  abduction positioner, L3999
  braces, L3999
    Masterhinge Shoulder Brace 3, L3999
  disarticulation, prosthetic, L6300-L6320, L6550

TRANSPORTATION SERVICES INCLUDING AMBULANCE
A0000-A0999

This code range includes ground and air ambulance, nonemergency transportation (taxi, bus, automobile, wheelchair van), and ancillary transportation-related fees.

Ambulance Origin and Destination modifiers used with transportation service codes are single-digit modifiers used in combination in boxes 12 and 13 of CMS form 1491. The first digit indicates the transport's place of origin, and the destination is indicated by the second digit. The modifiers most commonly used are:

D   Diagnostic or therapeutic site other than 'P' or 'H'

E   Residential, domiciliary, custodial facility (nursing home, not skilled nursing facility)

G   Hospital-based dialysis facility (hospital or hospital-related)

H   Hospital

I   Site of transfer (for example, airport or helicopter pad) between types of ambulance

J   Non-hospital-based dialysis facility

N   Skilled nursing facility (SNF)

P   Physician's office (includes HMO non-hospital facility, clinic, etc.)

R   Residence

S   Scene of accident or acute event

X   Intermediate stop at physician's office enroute to the hospital (includes HMO non-hospital facility, clinic, etc.) Note: Modifier X can only be used as a designation code in the second position of a modifier.

See Q3019, Q3020, and S0215. For Medicaid, see T codes and T modifiers.

Claims for transportation services fall under the jurisdiction of the local contractor.

Ⓔ	**A0021**	**Ambulance service, outside state per mile, transport (Medicaid only)**
Ⓔ	**A0080**	**Non-emergency transportation, per mile — vehicle provided by volunteer (individual or organization), with no vested interest**
Ⓔ	**A0090**	**Non-emergency transportation, per mile — vehicle provided by individual (family member, self, neighbor) with vested interest**
Ⓔ	**A0100**	**Non-emergency transportation; taxi**
Ⓔ	**A0110**	**Non-emergency transportation and bus, intra- or interstate carrier**
Ⓔ	**A0120**	**Non-emergency transportation: mini-bus, mountain area transports, or other transportation systems**
Ⓔ	**A0130**	**Non-emergency transportation: wheelchair van**
Ⓔ	**A0140**	**Non-emergency transportation and air travel (private or commercial), intra- or interstate**
Ⓔ	**A0160**	**Non-emergency transportation: per mile — caseworker or social worker**
Ⓔ	**A0170**	**Transportation ancillary: parking fees, tolls, other**
Ⓔ	**A0180**	**Non-emergency transportation: ancillary: lodging — recipient**
Ⓔ	**A0190**	**Non-emergency transportation: ancillary: meals — recipient**
Ⓔ	**A0200**	**Non-emergency transportation: ancillary: lodging — escort**

Ⓔ	**A0210**	**Non-emergency transportation: ancillary: meals — escort**
Ⓐ	**A0225**	**Ambulance service, neonatal transport, base rate, emergency transport, one way**
Ⓐ	**A0380**	**BLS mileage (per mile)** See code(s): A0425
Ⓐ	**A0382**	**BLS routine disposable supplies**
Ⓐ	**A0384**	**BLS specialized service disposable supplies; defibrillation (used by ALS ambulances and BLS ambulances in jurisdictions where defibrillation is permitted in BLS ambulances)**
Ⓐ	**A0390**	**ALS mileage (per mile)** See code(s): A0425
Ⓐ	**A0392**	**ALS specialized service disposable supplies; defibrillation (to be used only in jurisdictions where defibrillation cannot be performed by BLS ambulances)**
Ⓐ	**A0394**	**ALS specialized service disposable supplies; IV drug therapy**
Ⓐ	**A0396**	**ALS specialized service disposable supplies; esophageal intubation**
Ⓐ	**A0398**	**ALS routine disposable supplies**

WAITING TIME TABLE

	UNITS		TIME
1	1/2	to	1 hr.
2	1	to	1 1/2 hrs.
3	1 1/2	to	2 hrs.
4	2	to	2 1/2 hrs.
5	2 1/2	to	3 hrs.
6	3	to	3 1/2 hrs.
7	3 1/2	to	4 hrs.
8	4	to	4 1/2 hrs.
9	4 1/2	to	5 hrs.
10	5	to	5 1/2 hrs.

Ⓐ	**A0420**	**Ambulance waiting time (ALS or BLS), one-half (1/2) hour increments** ⊘
Ⓐ	**A0422**	**Ambulance (ALS or BLS) oxygen and oxygen supplies, life sustaining situation** ⊘
Ⓐ	**A0424**	**Extra ambulance attendant, ground (ALS or BLS) or air (fixed or rotary winged); (requires medical review)** ⊘ Pertinent documentation to evaluate medical appropriateness should be included when this code is reported.
Ⓐ	**A0425**	**Ground mileage, per statute mile**
Ⓐ	**A0426**	**Ambulance service, advanced life support, non-emergency transport, level 1 (ALS 1)**
Ⓐ	**A0427**	**Ambulance service, advanced life support, emergency transport, level 1 (ALS 1 — emergency)**
Ⓐ	**A0428**	**Ambulance service, basic life support, non-emergency transport (BLS)**
Ⓐ	**A0429**	**Ambulance service, basic life support, emergency transport (BLS — emergency)**
Ⓐ	**A0430**	**Ambulance service, conventional air services, transport, one way (fixed wing)**
Ⓐ	**A0431**	**Ambulance service, conventional air services, transport, one way (rotary wing)**
Ⓐ	**A0432**	**Paramedic intercept (PI), rural area, transport furnished by a volunteer ambulance company which is prohibited by state law from billing third party payers**

Special Coverage Instructions   Noncovered by Medicare   Carrier Discretion   ☑ Quantity Alert   ● New Code   ○ Reinstated Code   ▲ Revised Code

2006 HCPCS   **1**-**9** ASC Groups   MED: Pub 100/NCD Reference   ⅃ DMEPOS Paid   ⊘ SNF Excluded   A Codes — 1

Medical and Surgical Supplies

A0433 — A4255

		Code	Description
Ⓐ		A0433	Advanced life support, level 2 (ALS 2)
Ⓐ		A0434	Specialty care transport (SCT)
Ⓐ		A0435	Fixed wing air mileage, per statute mile
Ⓐ		A0436	Rotary wing air mileage, per statute mile
Ⓔ		A0800	Ambulance transport provided between the hours of 7 p.m. and 7 a.m.
Ⓔ		A0888	Non-covered ambulance mileage, per mile (e.g., for miles traveled beyond closest appropriate facility) ⊘ MED: 100-2, 10, 20
● Ⓔ		A0998	Ambulance response and treatment, no transport
Ⓐ		A0999	Unlisted ambulance service ⊘ Determine if an alternative HCPCS Level II or a CPT code better describes the service being reported. This code should be used only if a more specific code is unavailable. MED: 100-2, 10, 10.1; 100-2, 10, 20

MEDICAL AND SURGICAL SUPPLIES *A4000-A8999*

This section covers a wide variety of medical, surgical, and some durable medical equipment (DME) related supplies and accessories. DME-related supplies, accessories, maintenance, and repair required to ensure the proper functioning of this equipment is generally covered by Medicare under the prosthetic devices provision.

MISCELLANEOUS SUPPLIES

These codes are to be filed with the Medicare local contractor, unless otherwise noted (if incident to a physicians' services, not separately billable) unless they represent incidental services or supplies which are referred to the DME regional contractor.

		Code	Description
Ⓔ	☑	A4206	Syringe with needle, sterile 1 cc, each ⊘ This code specifies a 1 cc syringe but is also used to report 3/10 cc or 1/2 cc syringes.
Ⓔ	☑	A4207	Syringe with needle, sterile 2 cc, each ⊘
Ⓔ	☑	A4208	Syringe with needle, sterile 3 cc, each ⊘
Ⓔ	☑	A4209	Syringe with needle, sterile 5 cc or greater, each ⊘
Ⓔ		A4210	Needle-free injection device, each ⊘ Sometimes covered by commercial payers with preauthorization and physician letter stating need (e.g., for insulin injection in young children). MED: 100-3, 280.1
Ⓑ		A4211	Supplies for self-administered injections ⊘ When a drug that is usually injected by the patient (e.g., insulin or calcitonin) is injected by the physician, it is excluded from Medicare coverage unless administered in an emergency situation (e.g., diabetic coma). MED: 100-2, 15, 50
Ⓑ		A4212	Non-coring needle or stylet with or without catheter
Ⓔ		A4213	Syringe, sterile, 20 cc or greater, each ⊘
▲ Ⓔ		A4215	Needle, sterile, any size, each ⊘
▲ Ⓐ	☑	A4216	Sterile water, saline and/or dextrose (diluent), 10 ml ♿⊘ MED: 100-2, 15, 50
Ⓐ	☑	A4217	Sterile water/saline, 500 ml ♿⊘ MED: 100-2, 15, 50
● Ⓝ		A4218	Sterile saline or water, metered dose dispenser, 10 ml
Ⓝ		A4220	Refill kit for implantable infusion pump ⊘ Implantable infusion pumps are covered by Medicare for 5-FUdR therapy for unresected liver or colorectal cancer and for opioid drug therapy for intractable pain. They are not covered by Medicare for heparin therapy for thromboembolic disease. Report drugs separately. MED: 100-3, 280.14

		Code	Description
Ⓨ		A4221	Supplies for maintenance of drug infusion catheter, per week (list drug separately) ♿⊘
Ⓨ		A4222	Infusion supplies for external drug infusion pump, per cassette or bag (list drugs separately) ♿⊘
	☑	A4223	Infusion supplies not used with external infusion pump, per cassette or bag (list drugs separately)
Ⓨ	☑	A4230	Infusion set for external insulin pump, non-needle cannula type ⊘ Covered by some commercial payers as ongoing supply to preauthorized pump. MED: 100-3, 280.14
Ⓨ	☑	A4231	Infusion set for external insulin pump, needle type ⊘ Covered by some commercial payers as ongoing supply to preauthorized pump. MED: 100-3, 280.14
Ⓨ	☑	A4232	Syringe with needle for external insulin pump, sterile, 3 cc ⊘ Covered by some commercial payers as ongoing supply to preauthorized pump. MED: 100-3, 280.14
● Ⓨ		A4233	Replacement battery, alkaline (other than J cell), for use with medically necessary home blood glucose monitor owned by patient, each
● Ⓨ		A4234	Replacement battery, alkaline, J cell, for use with medically necessary home blood glucose monitor owned by patient, each
● Ⓨ		A4235	Replacement battery, lithium, for use with medically necessary home blood glucose monitor owned by patient, each
● Ⓨ		A4236	Replacement battery, silver oxide, for use with medically necessary home blood glucose monitor owned by patient, each
Ⓔ	☑	A4244	Alcohol or peroxide, per pint ⊘
Ⓔ	☑	A4245	Alcohol wipes, per box ⊘
Ⓔ	☑	A4246	Betadine or PhisoHex solution, per pint ⊘
Ⓔ	☑	A4247	Betadine or iodine swabs/wipes, per box ⊘
Ⓝ	☑	A4248	Chlorhexidine containing antiseptic, 1 ml ⊘
Ⓔ	☑	A4250	Urine test or reagent strips or tablets (100 tablets or strips) ⊘ MED: 100-2, 15, 110

Note: Codes A4253-A4256 are for home blood glucose monitors. For supplies for End Stage Renal Disease (ESRD)/dialysis, see codes A4651-A4929. (Some codes in this range do not specify ESRD/dialysis, verify coverage with your contractor). For DME items for ESRD, see codes E1500-E1699.

		Code	Description
Ⓨ	☑	A4253	Blood glucose test or reagent strips for home blood glucose monitor, per 50 strips ♿⊘ Medicare covers glucose strips for diabetic patients using home glucose monitoring devices prescribed by their physicians. Medicare jurisdiction: DME regional contractor. MED: 100-3, 40.2
		~~A4254~~	~~Replacement battery, any type, for use with medically necessary home blood glucose monitor owned by patient, each~~ See code(s) A4233-A4236.
Ⓨ	☑	A4255	Platforms for home blood glucose monitor, 50 per box ♿⊘ Some Medicare contractors cover monitor platforms for diabetic patients using home glucose monitoring devices prescribed by their physicians. Medicare jurisdiction: DME regional contractor. Some commercial payers also provide this coverage to non-insulin dependent diabetics. MED: 100-3, 40.2

Special Coverage Instructions   Noncovered by Medicare   Carrier Discretion   ☑ Quantity Alert   ● New Code   ○ Reinstated Code   ▲ Revised Code

2 — A Codes   Ⓐ Age   Ⓜ Maternity   ♀ Female Only   ♂ Male Only   Ⓐ-Ⓨ APC Status Indicator   *2006 HCPCS*

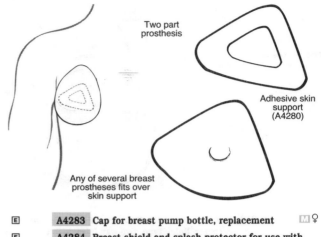

Reference chart

— pH
— Protein
— Glucose
— Ketones
— Bilirubin
— Hemoglobin

Dipstick urinalysis: The strip is dipped and color-coded squares are read at timed intervals (e.g., pH immediately; ketones at 15 sec., etc.). Results are compared against a reference chart

Tablet reagents turn specific colors when urine droplets are placed on them

Two part prosthesis

Adhesive skin support (A4280)

Any of several breast prostheses fits over skin support

Ⓨ **A4256** Normal, low, and high calibrator solution/chips ⅋⊘
Some Medicare contractors cover calibration solutions or chips for diabetic patients using home glucose monitoring devices prescribed by their physicians. Medicare jurisdiction: DME regional contractor. Some commercial payers also provide this coverage to non-insulin dependent diabetics.
MED: 100-3, 40.2

Ⓨ ☑ **A4257** Replacement lens shield cartridge for use with laser skin piercing device, each   ⅋⊘

Ⓨ ☑ **A4258** Spring-powered device for lancet, each   ⅋⊘
Some Medicare contractors cover lancing devices for diabetic patients using home glucose monitoring devices prescribed by their physicians. Medicare jurisdiction: DME regional contractor. Some commercial payers also provide this coverage to non-insulin dependent diabetics.
MED: 100-3, 40.2

Ⓨ ☑ **A4259** Lancets, per box of 100   ⅋⊘
Medicare covers lancets for diabetic patients using home glucose monitoring devices prescribed by their physicians. Medicare jurisdiction: DME regional contractor. Some commercial payers also provide this coverage to non-insulin dependent diabetics.
MED: 100-3, 40.2

~~A4260~~ ~~Levonorgestrel (contraceptive) implants system, including implants and supplies~~
See code(s) J7306.

Ⓔ **A4261** Cervical cap for contraceptive use   ♀⊘

Ⓝ ☑ **A4262** Temporary, absorbable lacrimal duct implant, each   ⊘
Always report concurrent to the implant procedure.

Ⓝ ☑ **A4263** Permanent, long-term, nondissolvable lacrimal duct implant, each
Always report concurrent to the implant procedure.

Ⓨ ☑ **A4265** Paraffin, per pound   ⅋⊘
Medicare jurisdiction: DME regional contractor.
MED: 100-3, 280.1

Ⓔ **A4266** Diaphragm for contraceptive use   ♀

Ⓔ ☑ **A4267** Contraceptive supply, condom, male, each

Ⓔ ☑ **A4268** Contraceptive supply, condom, female, each   ♀

Ⓔ ☑ **A4269** Contraceptive supply, spermicide (e.g., foam, gel), each   Ⓐ

Ⓐ ☑ **A4270** Disposable endoscope sheath, each   ⊘

Ⓐ **A4280** Adhesive skin support attachment for use with external breast prosthesis, each   Ⓐ♀⅋

Ⓔ **A4281** Tubing for breast pump, replacement   Ⓜ♀

Ⓔ **A4282** Adapter for breast pump, replacement   Ⓜ♀

Ⓔ **A4283** Cap for breast pump bottle, replacement   Ⓜ♀

Ⓔ **A4284** Breast shield and splash protector for use with breast pump, replacement   Ⓜ♀

Ⓔ **A4285** Polycarbonate bottle for use with breast pump, replacement   Ⓜ♀

Ⓔ **A4286** Locking ring for breast pump, replacement   Ⓜ♀

Ⓑ ☑ **A4290** Sacral nerve stimulation test lead, each
AHA: 1Q, '02, 9

VASCULAR CATHETERS

Ⓝ **A4300** Implantable access catheter, (e.g., venous, arterial, epidural subarachnoid, or peritoneal, etc.) external access
MED: 100-2, 15, 120

Ⓝ **A4301** Implantable access total catheter, port/reservoir (e.g., venous, arterial, epidural, subarachnoid, peritoneal, etc.)   ⊘

Ⓐ **A4305** Disposable drug delivery system, flow rate of 50 ml or greater per hour   ⊘

Ⓐ **A4306** Disposable drug delivery system, flow rate of 5 ml or less per hour   ⊘

INCONTINENCE APPLIANCES AND CARE SUPPLIES

Covered by Medicare when the medical record indicates incontinence is permanent, or of long and indefinite duration.

Medicare claims fall under the jurisdiction of the DME regional contractor for a permanent condition, and under the local contractor when provided in the physician's office for a temporary condition.

Ⓐ **A4310** Insertion tray without drainage bag and without catheter (accessories only)   ⅋
MED: 100-2, 15, 120

Ⓐ **A4311** Insertion tray without drainage bag with indwelling catheter, Foley type, two-way latex with coating (Teflon, silicone, silicone elastomer or hydrophilic, etc.)   ⅋
MED: 100-2, 15, 120

Ⓐ **A4312** Insertion tray without drainage bag with indwelling catheter, Foley type, two-way, all silicone   ⅋
MED: 100-2, 15, 120

Ⓐ **A4313** Insertion tray without drainage bag with indwelling catheter, Foley type, three-way, for continuous irrigation   ⅋
MED: 100-2, 15, 120

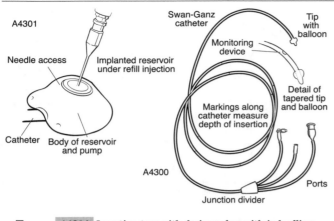

A4301 — Needle access, Implanted reservoir under refill injection, Catheter, Body of reservoir and pump

Swan-Ganz catheter, Monitoring device, Tip with balloon, Detail of tapered tip and balloon, Markings along catheter measure depth of insertion, Ports, Junction divider, A4300

Left ureter, Urachus, Peritoneum, Left ureter, Ureteral orifice, Normal anatomy anterior view, Pubic bone, Urogenital diaphragm, Side view, Urethra, Urethral sphincter, Foley-style indwelling catheter (A4344-A4346), Spongiosal muscles, Multiple port indwelling catheters allow for irrigation and drainage

Ⓐ		**A4314**	Insertion tray with drainage bag with indwelling catheter, Foley type, two-way latex with coating (Teflon, silicone, silicone elastomer or hydrophilic, etc.) MED: 100-2, 15, 120
Ⓐ		**A4315**	Insertion tray with drainage bag with indwelling catheter, Foley type, two-way, all silicone MED: 100-2, 15, 120
Ⓐ		**A4316**	Insertion tray with drainage bag with indwelling catheter, Foley type, three-way, for continuous irrigation MED: 100-2, 15, 120
Ⓐ		**A4320**	Irrigation tray with bulb or piston syringe, any purpose MED: 100-2, 15, 120
Ⓐ		**A4321**	Therapeutic agent for urinary catheter irrigation MED: 100-2, 15, 120
Ⓐ	☑	**A4322**	Irrigation syringe, bulb or piston, each MED: 100-2, 15, 120
Ⓐ	☑	**A4326**	Male external catheter specialty type with integral collection chamber, each ♂ MED: 100-2, 15, 120
Ⓐ	☑	**A4327**	Female external urinary collection device; metal cup, each ♀ MED: 100-2, 15, 120
Ⓐ	☑	**A4328**	Female external urinary collection device; pouch, each ♀ MED: 100-2, 15, 120
Ⓐ	☑	**A4330**	Perianal fecal collection pouch with adhesive, each MED: 100-2, 15, 120
Ⓐ	☑	**A4331**	Extension drainage tubing, any type, any length, with connector/adaptor, for use with urinary leg bag or urostomy pouch, each MED: 100-2, 15, 120
Ⓐ	☑	**A4332**	Lubricant, individual sterile packet, each MED: 100-2, 15, 120
Ⓐ	☑	**A4333**	Urinary catheter anchoring device, adhesive skin attachment, each MED: 100-2, 15, 120
Ⓐ	☑	**A4334**	Urinary catheter anchoring device, leg strap, each MED: 100-2, 15, 120
Ⓐ		**A4335**	Incontinence supply; miscellaneous ⊘ MED: 100-2, 15, 120

Ⓐ	☑	**A4338**	Indwelling catheter; Foley type, two-way latex with coating (Teflon, silicone, silicone elastomer, or hydrophilic, etc.), each MED: 100-2, 15, 120
Ⓐ	☑	**A4340**	Indwelling catheter; specialty type, (e.g., Coude, mushroom, wing, etc.), each MED: 100-2, 15, 120
Ⓐ	☑	**A4344**	Indwelling catheter, Foley type, two-way, all silicone, each MED: 100-2, 15, 120
Ⓐ	☑	**A4346**	Indwelling catheter; Foley type, three-way for continuous irrigation, each MED: 100-2, 15, 120
Ⓐ		**A4348**	Male external catheter with integral collection compartment, extended wear, each (e.g., 2 per month) ♂ MED: 100-2, 15, 120
	☑	**A4349**	Male external catheter, with or without adhesive, disposable, each MED: 100-2, 15, 120
Ⓐ	☑	**A4351**	Intermittent urinary catheter; straight tip, with or without coating (Teflon, silicone, silicone elastomer, or hydrophilic, etc.), each MED: 100-2, 15, 120
Ⓐ	☑	**A4352**	Intermittent urinary catheter; coude (curved) tip, with or without coating (Teflon, silicone, silicone elastomeric, or hydrophilic, etc.), each MED: 100-2, 15, 120
Ⓐ		**A4353**	Intermittent urinary catheter, with insertion supplies MED: 100-2, 15, 120
Ⓐ		**A4354**	Insertion tray with drainage bag but without catheter MED: 100-2, 15, 120
Ⓐ	☑	**A4355**	Irrigation tubing set for continuous bladder irrigation through a three-way indwelling Foley catheter, each MED: 100-2, 15, 120

EXTERNAL URINARY SUPPLIES

Medicare claims fall under the jurisdiction of the DME regional contractor for a permanent condition, and under the local contractor when provided in the physician's office for a temporary condition.

Ⓐ	☑	**A4356**	External urethral clamp or compression device (not to be used for catheter clamp), each MED: 100-2, 15, 120

Special Coverage Instructions   Noncovered by Medicare   Carrier Discretion   ☑ Quantity Alert   ● New Code   ○ Reinstated Code   ▲ Revised Code

4 — A Codes   Ⓐ Age   Ⓜ Maternity   ♀ Female Only   ♂ Male Only   Ⓐ-Ⓨ APC Status Indicator   *2006 HCPCS*

Ⓐ ☑ **A4357** Bedside drainage bag, day or night, with or without anti-reflux device, with or without tube, each ᴅ
MED: 100-2, 15, 120

Ⓐ ☑ **A4358** Urinary drainage bag, leg or abdomen, vinyl, with or without tube, with straps, each ᴅ
MED: 100-2, 15, 120

Ⓐ ☑ **A4359** Urinary suspensory without leg bag, each ᴅ
MED: 100-2, 15, 120

OSTOMY SUPPLIES

Medicare claims fall under the jurisdiction of the DME regional contractor for a permanent condition, and under the local contractor when provided in the physician's office for a temporary condition.

Ⓐ ☑ **A4361** Ostomy faceplate, each ᴅ
MED: 100-2, 15, 120

Ⓐ ☑ **A4362** Skin barrier; solid, four by four or equivalent; each ᴅ
MED: 100-2, 15, 120

○ Ⓐ **A4363** Ostomy clamp, any type, replacement only, each ᴅ

Ⓐ ☑ **A4364** Adhesive, liquid, or equal, any type, per oz. ᴅ
MED: 100-2, 15, 120

Ⓐ ☑ **A4365** Adhesive remover wipes, any type, per 50 ᴅ
MED: 100-2, 15, 120

Ⓐ ☑ **A4366** Ostomy vent, any type, each ᴅ

Ⓐ ☑ **A4367** Ostomy belt, each ᴅ
MED: 100-2, 15, 120

Ⓐ ☑ **A4368** Ostomy filter, any type, each ᴅ

Ⓐ ☑ **A4369** Ostomy skin barrier, liquid (spray, brush, etc.), per oz ᴅ
MED: 100-2, 15, 120

Ⓐ ☑ **A4371** Ostomy skin barrier, powder, per oz ᴅ
MED: 100-2, 15, 120

▲ Ⓐ ☑ **A4372** Ostomy skin barrier, solid 4x4 or equivalent, standard wear, with built-in convexity, each ᴅ
MED: 100-2, 15, 120

Ⓐ ☑ **A4373** Ostomy skin barrier, with flange (solid, flexible or accordion), with built-in convexity, any size, each ᴅ
MED: 100-2, 15, 120

Ⓐ ☑ **A4375** Ostomy pouch, drainable, with faceplate attached, plastic, each ᴅ
MED: 100-2, 15, 120

Ⓐ ☑ **A4376** Ostomy pouch, drainable, with faceplate attached, rubber, each ᴅ
MED: 100-2, 15, 120

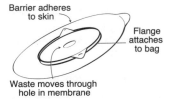

Barrier adheres to skin
Flange attaches to bag
Waste moves through hole in membrane

Faceplate flange and skin barrier combination (A4373)

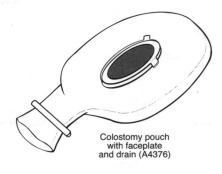

Colostomy pouch with faceplate and drain (A4376)

Ⓐ ☑ **A4377** Ostomy pouch, drainable, for use on faceplate, plastic, each ᴅ
MED: 100-2, 15, 120

Ⓐ ☑ **A4378** Ostomy pouch, drainable, for use on faceplate, rubber, each ᴅ
MED: 100-2, 15, 120

Ⓐ ☑ **A4379** Ostomy pouch, urinary, with faceplate attached, plastic, each ᴅ
MED: 100-2, 15, 120

Ⓐ ☑ **A4380** Ostomy pouch, urinary, with faceplate attached, rubber, each ᴅ⊘
MED: 100-2, 15, 120

Ⓐ ☑ **A4381** Ostomy pouch, urinary, for use on faceplate, plastic, each ᴅ
MED: 100-2, 15, 120

Ⓐ ☑ **A4382** Ostomy pouch, urinary, for use on faceplate, heavy plastic, each ᴅ
MED: 100-2, 15, 120

Ⓐ ☑ **A4383** Ostomy pouch, urinary, for use on faceplate, rubber, each ᴅ
MED: 100-2, 15, 120

Ⓐ ☑ **A4384** Ostomy faceplate equivalent, silicone ring, each ᴅ
MED: 100-2, 15, 120

Ⓐ ☑ **A4385** Ostomy skin barrier, solid 4 x 4 or equivalent, extended wear, without built-in convexity, each ᴅ
MED: 100-2, 15, 120

Ⓐ ☑ **A4387** Ostomy pouch, closed, with barrier attached, with built-in convexity (one piece), each ᴅ
MED: 100-2, 15, 120

Ⓐ ☑ **A4388** Ostomy pouch, drainable, with extended wear barrier attached, (one piece), each ᴅ
MED: 100-2, 15, 120

Ⓐ ☑ **A4389** Ostomy pouch, drainable, with barrier attached, with built-in convexity (one piece), each ᴅ
MED: 100-2, 15, 120

Ⓐ ☑ **A4390** Ostomy pouch, drainable, with extended wear barrier attached, with built-in convexity (1 piece), each ᴅ⊘
MED: 100-2, 15, 120

Ⓐ ☑ **A4391** Ostomy pouch, urinary, with extended wear barrier attached (1 piece), each ᴅ
MED: 100-2, 15, 120

Ⓐ ☑ **A4392** Ostomy pouch, urinary, with standard wear barrier attached, with built-in convexity (1 piece), each ᴅ
MED: 100-2, 15, 120

■ Special Coverage Instructions ■ Noncovered by Medicare ■ Carrier Discretion ☑ Quantity Alert ● New Code ○ Reinstated Code ▲ Revised Code

2006 HCPCS　　**❶-❾** ASC Groups　　MED: Pub 100/NCD Reference　　ᴅ DMEPOS Paid　　⊘ SNF Excluded　　**A Codes — 5**

Medical and Surgical Supplies

A4393 — A4452

A ☑ **A4393** Ostomy pouch, urinary, with extended wear barrier attached, with built-in convexity (1 piece), each ᕆ
MED: 100-2, 15, 120

A ☑ **A4394** Ostomy deodorant for use in ostomy pouch, liquid, per fluid oz. ᕆ
MED: 100-2, 15, 120

A ☑ **A4395** Ostomy deodorant for use in ostomy pouch, solid, per tablet ᕆ
MED: 100-2, 15, 120

A **A4396** Ostomy belt with peristomal hernia support ᕆ
MED: 100-2, 15, 120

A ☑ **A4397** Irrigation supply; sleeve, each ᕆ
MED: 100-2, 15, 120

A ☑ **A4398** Ostomy irrigation supply; bag, each ᕆ
MED: 100-2, 15, 120

A **A4399** Ostomy irrigation supply; cone/catheter, including brush ᕆ

A **A4400** Ostomy irrigation set ᕆ
MED: 100-2, 15, 120

A ☑ **A4402** Lubricant, per oz. ᕆ
MED: 100-2, 15, 120

A ☑ **A4404** Ostomy ring, each ᕆ
MED: 100-2, 15, 120

A ☑ **A4405** Ostomy skin barrier, non-pectin based, paste, per oz. ᕆ
MED: 100-2, 15, 120

A ☑ **A4406** Ostomy skin barrier, pectin-based, paste, per oz. ᕆ
MED: 100-2, 15, 120

A ☑ **A4407** Ostomy skin barrier, with flange (solid, flexible, or accordion), extended wear, with built-in convexity, 4 x 4 in. or smaller, each ᕆ
MED: 100-2, 15, 120

A ☑ **A4408** Ostomy skin barrier, with flange (solid, flexible or accordion), extended wear, with built-in convexity, larger than 4 x 4 in., each ᕆ
MED: 100-2, 15, 120

A ☑ **A4409** Ostomy skin barrier, with flange (solid, flexible or accordion), extended wear, without built-in convexity, 4 x 4 in. or smaller, each ᕆ
MED: 100-2, 15, 120

A ☑ **A4410** Ostomy skin barrier, with flange (solid, flexible or accordion), extended wear, without built-in convexity, larger than 4 x 4 in., each ᕆ
MED: 100-2, 15, 120

● A **A4411** Ostomy skin barrier, solid 4x4 or equivalent, extended wear, with built-in convexity, each

● A **A4412** Ostomy pouch, drainable, high output, for use on a barrier with flange (2 piece system), without filter, each
MED: 100-2, 15, 120

A ☑ **A4413** Ostomy pouch, drainable, high output, for use on a barrier with flange (2 piece system), with filter, each ᕆ
MED: 100-2, 15, 120

A ☑ **A4414** Ostomy skin barrier, with flange (solid, flexible or accordion), without built-in convexity, 4 x 4 in. or smaller, each ᕆ
MED: 100-2, 15, 120

A ☑ **A4415** Ostomy skin barrier, with flange (solid, flexible or accordion), without built-in convexity, larger than 4 x 4 in., each ᕆ
MED: 100-2, 15, 120

A ☑ **A4416** Ostomy pouch, closed, with barrier attached, with filter (one piece), each ᕆ

A ☑ **A4417** Ostomy pouch, closed, with barrier attached, with built-in convexity, with filter (one piece), each ᕆ

A ☑ **A4418** Ostomy pouch, closed; without barrier attached, with filter (one piece), each ᕆ

A ☑ **A4419** Ostomy pouch, closed; for use on barrier with non-locking flange, with filter (two piece), each ᕆ

A ☑ **A4420** Ostomy pouch, closed; for use on barrier with locking flange (two piece), each ᕆ

E **A4421** Ostomy supply; miscellaneous ⊘
Determine if an alternative HCPCS Level II or a CPT code better describes the service being reported. This code should be used only if a more specific code is unavailable.

MED: 100-2, 15, 120

A **A4422** Ostomy absorbent material (sheet/pad/crystal packet) for use in ostomy pouch to thicken liquid stomal output, each ᕆ
MED: 100-2, 15, 120

A ☑ **A4423** Ostomy pouch, closed; for use on barrier with locking flange, with filter (two piece), each ᕆ

A ☑ **A4424** Ostomy pouch, drainable, with barrier attached, with filter (one piece), each ᕆ

A ☑ **A4425** Ostomy pouch, drainable; for use on barrier with non-locking flange, with filter (two piece system), each ᕆ

A ☑ **A4426** Ostomy pouch, drainable; for use on barrier with locking flange (two piece system), each ᕆ

A ☑ **A4427** Ostomy pouch, drainable; for use on barrier with locking flange, with filter (two piece system), each ᕆ

A ☑ **A4428** Ostomy pouch, urinary, with extended wear barrier attached, with faucet-type tap with valve (one piece), each ᕆ

A ☑ **A4429** Ostomy pouch, urinary, with barrier attached, with built-in convexity, with faucet-type tap with valve (one piece), each ᕆ

A ☑ **A4430** Ostomy pouch, urinary, with extended wear barrier attached, with built-in convexity, with faucet-type tap with valve (one piece), each ᕆ

A ☑ **A4431** Ostomy pouch, urinary; with barrier attached, with faucet-type tap with valve (one piece), each ᕆ

A ☑ **A4432** Ostomy pouch, urinary; for use on barrier with non-locking flange, with faucet-type tap with valve (two piece), each ᕆ

A ☑ **A4433** Ostomy pouch, urinary; for use on barrier with locking flange (two piece), each ᕆ

A ☑ **A4434** Ostomy pouch, urinary; for use on barrier with locking flange, with faucet-type tap with valve (two piece), each ᕆ

ADDITIONAL MISCELLANEOUS SUPPLIES

A ☑ **A4450** Tape, non-waterproof, per 18 sq. in. ᕆ
See also code A4452.

MED: 100-2, 15, 120

A ☑ **A4452** Tape, waterproof, per 18 sq. in. ᕆ
See also code A4450.

MED: 100-2, 15, 120

| Special Coverage Instructions | Noncovered by Medicare | Carrier Discretion | ☑ Quantity Alert | ● New Code | ○ Reinstated Code | ▲ Revised Code |

6 — A Codes   A Age   M Maternity   ♀ Female Only   ♂ Male Only   A-Y APC Status Indicator   *2006 HCPCS*

A ☑ **A4455** Adhesive remover or solvent (for tape, cement or other adhesive), per oz. ⌨
MED: 100-2, 15, 120

E **A4458** Enema bag with tubing, reusable

A **A4462** Abdominal dressing holder, each ⌨
Dressings applied by a physician are included as part of the professional service. Surgical dressings obtained by the patient to perform homecare as prescribed by the physician are covered.
MED: 100-2, 15, 100

A **A4465** Nonelastic binder for extremity ⊘

A **A4470** Gravlee jet washer ⊘
The Gravlee jet washer is a disposable device used to detect endometrial cancer. It is covered only in patients exhibiting clinical symptoms or signs suggestive of endometrial disease. Medicare jurisdiction: local contractor.
MED: 100-2, 16, 90; 100-3, 230.5

A **A4480** VABRA aspirator ♀ ⊘
The VABRA aspirator is a disposable device used to detect endometrial cancer. It is covered only in patients exhibiting clinical symptoms or signs suggestive of endometrial disease. Medicare jurisdiction: local contractor.
MED: 100-2, 16, 90; 100-3, 230.6

A ☑ **A4481** Tracheostoma filter, any type, any size, each ⌨
MED: 100-2, 15, 120

A **A4483** Moisture exchanger, disposable, for use with invasive mechanical ventilation ⌨
Medicare jurisdiction: DME regional contractor.
MED: 100-2, 15, 120

E ☑ **A4490** Surgical stocking above knee length, each ⊘
MED: 100-2, 15, 100; 100-2, 15, 110; 100-3, 280.1

E ☑ **A4495** Surgical stocking thigh length, each ⊘
MED: 100-2, 15, 100; 100-2, 15, 110; 100-3, 280.1

E ☑ **A4500** Surgical stocking below knee length, each ⊘
MED: 100-2, 15, 100; 100-2, 15, 110; 100-3, 280.1

E ☑ **A4510** Surgical stocking full-length, each ⊘
MED: 100-2, 15, 100; 100-2, 15, 110; 100-3, 280.1

☑ **A4520** Incontinence garment, any type, (e.g., brief, diaper), each
MED: 100-3, 280.1

E ☑ **A4534** Youth-sized incontinence product, brief, each
MED: 100-3, 280.1

B **A4550** Surgical trays ⊘
Medicare jurisdiction: local contractor.

E ☑ **A4554** Disposable underpads, all sizes (e.g., Chux's) ⊘
MED: 100-2, 15, 120; 100-3, 280.1

Y ☑ **A4556** Electrodes (e.g., apnea monitor), per pair ⌨⊘

Y ☑ **A4557** Lead wires (e.g., apnea monitor), per pair ⌨⊘

Y **A4558** Conductive paste or gel ⌨

N **A4561** Pessary, rubber, any type A♀⌨
Medicare jurisdiction: DME regional contractor.

N **A4562** Pessary, non-rubber, any type A♀⌨
Medicare jurisdiction: DME regional contractor.

A **A4565** Slings
Dressings applied by a physician are included as part of the professional service. Surgical dressings obtained by the patient to perform homecare as prescribed by the physician are covered.

E **A4570** Splint ⊘
Dressings applied by a physician are included as part of the professional service.
MED: 100-2, 15, 100

E **A4575** Topical hyperbaric oxygen chamber, disposable ⊘
MED: 100-3, 20.29

E **A4580** Cast supplies (e.g., plaster) ⊘
See Q4001-Q4048.
MED: 100-2, 15, 100

E **A4590** Special casting material (e.g., fiberglass) ⊘
See Q4001-Q4048.
MED: 100-2, 15, 100

Y **A4595** Electrical stimulator supplies, 2 lead, per month, (e.g., TENS, NMES) ⌨⊘
MED: 100-3, 160.13

● Y **A4604** Tubing with integrated heating element for use with positive airway pressure device

☑ **A4605** Tracheal suction catheter, closed system, each

A **A4606** Oxygen probe for use with oximeter device, replacement

Y ☑ **A4608** Transtracheal oxygen catheter, each ⌨⊘
Medicare jurisdiction: DME regional contractor.

SUPPLIES FOR OXYGEN AND RELATED RESPIRATORY EQUIPMENT

Y **A4611** Battery, heavy duty; replacement for patient-owned ventilator ⌨⊘
Medicare jurisdiction: DME regional contractor.

Y **A4612** Battery cables; replacement for patient-owned ventilator ⌨⊘
Medicare jurisdiction: DME regional contractor.

Y **A4613** Battery charger; replacement for patient-owned ventilator ⌨⊘
Medicare jurisdiction: DME regional contractor.

A **A4614** Peak expiratory flow rate meter, hand held ⌨⊘

Y **A4615** Cannula, nasal ⊘
MED: 100-3, 160.6; 100-4, 20, 100.2

Y ☑ **A4616** Tubing (oxygen), per foot ⊘
MED: 100-3, 160.6; 100-4, 20, 100.2

Y **A4617** Mouthpiece ⊘
MED: 100-3, 160.6; 100-4, 20, 100.2

Y **A4618** Breathing circuits ⌨⊘
MED: 100-3, 160.6; 100-4, 20, 100.2

Y **A4619** Face tent ⌨⊘
MED: 100-3, 160.6; 100-4, 20, 100.2

Y **A4620** Variable concentration mask ⊘
MED: 100-3, 160.6; 100-4, 20, 100.2

A **A4623** Tracheostomy, inner cannula ⌨
MED: 100-2, 15, 120; 100-3, 20.9

Y ☑ **A4624** Tracheal suction catheter, any type other than closed system, each ⌨⊘

A **A4625** Tracheostomy care kit for new tracheostomy ⌨⊘
MED: 100-2, 15, 120

A ☑ **A4626** Tracheostomy cleaning brush, each ⌨⊘
MED: 100-2, 15, 120

E **A4627** Spacer, bag or reservoir, with or without mask, for use with metered dose inhaler ⊘
MED: 100-2, 15, 110

Medical and Surgical Supplies

A4628 — A4707

Y ☑ **A4628** Oropharyngeal suction catheter, each   🦽⊘

A **A4629** Tracheostomy care kit for established tracheostomy   🦽
MED: 100-2, 15, 120

SUPPLIES FOR OTHER DURABLE MEDICAL EQUIPMENT

▲ Y ☑ **A4630** Replacement batteries, medically necessary, transcutaneous electrical stimulator, owned by patient   🦽⊘
Medicare jurisdiction: DME regional contractor.
MED: 100-3, 160.7

Y **A4632** Replacement battery for external infusion pump, any type, each   ⊘

Y **A4633** Replacement bulb/lamp for ultraviolet light therapy system, each   🦽

A **A4634** Replacement bulb for therapeutic light box, tabletop model

Y ☑ **A4635** Underarm pad, crutch, replacement, each   🦽⊘
Medicare jurisdiction: DME regional contractor.
MED: 100-3, 280.1

Y ☑ **A4636** Replacement, handgrip, cane, crutch, or walker, each   🦽⊘
Medicare jurisdiction: DME regional contractor.
MED: 100-3, 280.1

Y ☑ **A4637** Replacement, tip, cane, crutch, walker, each   🦽⊘
Medicare jurisdiction: DME regional contractor.
MED: 100-3, 280.1

Y ☑ **A4638** Replacement battery for patient-owned ear pulse generator, each   🦽⊘

Y **A4639** Replacement pad for infrared heating pad system, each   🦽

Y **A4640** Replacement pad for use with medically necessary alternating pressure pad owned by patient   🦽⊘
Medicare jurisdiction: DME regional contractor.
MED: 100-3, 280.1; 100-8, 5, 5.1.1.2.1

SUPPLIES FOR RADIOLOGIC PROCEDURES

▲ N **A4641** Radiopharmaceutical, diagnostic, not otherwise classified
Medicare jurisdiction: local contractor.

▲ H ☑ **A4642** Indium In-111 satumomab pendetide, diagnostic, per study dose, up to 6 millicuries
Use this code for Oncoscint. Medicare jurisdiction: local contractor.
AHA: 2Q, '02, 8, 9

~~**A4643** Supply of additional high dose contrast material(s) during magnetic resonance imaging, e.g., gadoteridol injection~~
See code(s) Q9952-Q9954.

~~**A4644** Supply of low osmolar contrast material (100-199 mgs of iodine)~~
See code(s) Q9944-Q9946.

~~**A4645** Supply of low osmolar contrast material (200-299 mgs of iodine)~~
See code(s) Q9960-Q9961.

~~**A4646** Supply of low osmolar contrast material (300-399 mgs of iodine)~~
See code(s) Q9962-Q9963.

~~**A4647** Supply of paramagnetic contrast material (e.g., gadolinium)~~
See code(s) Q9952-Q9954.

A **A4649** Surgical supply; miscellaneous   ⊘
Determine if an alternative HCPCS Level II or a CPT code better describes the service being reported. This code should be used only if a more specific code is unavailable. Medicare jurisdiction: local contractor.

NOTE: Some supplies for ESRD/dialysis appear in range A4651-A4929. For glucose monitor/supplies see A4253-A4259. For DME items for ESRD see codes E1500-E1699 (Many codes found in this range no longer specify "ESRD/dialysis." Verify coverage with your contractor.)

A ☑ **A4651** Calibrated microcapillary tube, each   ⊘
MED: 100-4, 8, 130; 100-4, 8, 70; 100-4, 8, 80; 100-4, 8, 90; 100-4, 8, 90.1; 100-4, 8, 90.3.2

A **A4652** Microcapillary tube sealant   ⊘
MED: 100-4, 8, 130; 100-4, 8, 70; 100-4, 8, 80; 100-4, 8, 90; 100-4, 8, 90.1; 100-4, 8, 90.3.2

A ☑ **A4653** Peritoneal dialysis catheter anchoring device, belt, each   ⊘

~~**A4656** Needle, any size, each~~

A ☑ **A4657** Syringe, with or without needle, each   ⊘
MED: 100-4, 8, 130; 100-4, 8, 70; 100-4, 8, 80; 100-4, 8, 90; 100-4, 8, 90.1; 100-4, 8, 90.3.2

A **A4660** Sphygmomanometer/blood pressure apparatus with cuff and stethoscope   ⊘
MED: 100-4, 8, 130; 100-4, 8, 70; 100-4, 8, 80; 100-4, 8, 90; 100-4, 8, 90.1; 100-4, 8, 90.3.2

A **A4663** Blood pressure cuff only   ⊘
MED: 100-4, 8, 130; 100-4, 8, 70; 100-4, 8, 80; 100-4, 8, 90; 100-4, 8, 90.1; 100-4, 8, 90.3.2

E **A4670** Automatic blood pressure monitor   ⊘
MED: 100-3, 20.19; 100-4, 8, 130; 100-4, 8, 70; 100-4, 8, 80; 100-4, 8, 90; 100-4, 8, 90.1; 100-4, 8, 90.3.2

B ☑ **A4671** Disposable cycler set used with cycler dialysis machine, each   ⊘
MED: 100-4, 8, 130; 100-4, 8, 70; 100-4, 8, 80; 100-4, 8, 90; 100-4, 8, 90.1; 100-4, 8, 90.3.2

B ☑ **A4672** Drainage extension line, sterile, for dialysis, each ⊘
MED: 100-4, 8, 130; 100-4, 8, 70; 100-4, 8, 80; 100-4, 8, 90; 100-4, 8, 90.1; 100-4, 8, 90.3.2

B **A4673** Extension line with easy lock connectors, used with dialysis   ⊘
MED: 100-4, 8, 130; 100-4, 8, 70; 100-4, 8, 80; 100-4, 8, 90; 100-4, 8, 90.1; 100-4, 8, 90.3.2

B ☑ **A4674** Chemicals/antiseptics solution used to clean/sterilize dialysis equipment, per 8 oz   ⊘
MED: 100-4, 8, 130; 100-4, 8, 70; 100-4, 8, 80; 100-4, 8, 90; 100-4, 8, 90.1; 100-4, 8, 90.3.2

A ☑ **A4680** Activated carbon filter for hemodialysis, each   ⊘
MED: 100-3, 230.7; 100-4, 8, 130; 100-4, 8, 70; 100-4, 8, 80; 100-4, 8, 90; 100-4, 8, 90.1; 100-4, 8, 90.3.2

A ☑ **A4690** Dialyzer (artificial kidneys), all types, all sizes, for hemodialysis, each   ⊘
MED: 100-4, 8, 130; 100-4, 8, 70; 100-4, 8, 80; 100-4, 8, 90; 100-4, 8, 90.1; 100-4, 8, 90.3.2

A ☑ **A4706** Bicarbonate concentrate, solution, for hemodialysis, per gallon   ⊘
MED: 100-4, 8, 130; 100-4, 8, 70; 100-4, 8, 80; 100-4, 8, 90; 100-4, 8, 90.1; 100-4, 8, 90.3.2

A ☑ **A4707** Bicarbonate concentrate, powder, for hemodialysis, per packet   ⊘
MED: 100-4, 8, 130; 100-4, 8, 70; 100-4, 8, 80; 100-4, 8, 90; 100-4, 8, 90.1; 100-4, 8, 90.3.2

Special Coverage Instructions   Noncovered by Medicare   Carrier Discretion   ☑ Quantity Alert   ● New Code   ○ Reinstated Code   ▲ Revised Code

8 — A Codes   A Age   M Maternity   ♀ Female Only   ♂ Male Only   A-Y APC Status Indicator   ***2006 HCPCS***

Ⓐ ☑ **A4708** Acetate concentrate solution, for hemodialysis, per gallon ⊘
MED: 100-4, 8, 130; 100-4, 8, 70; 100-4, 8, 80; 100-4, 8, 90; 100-4, 8, 90.1; 100-4, 8, 90.3.2

Ⓐ ☑ **A4709** Acid concentrate, solution, for hemodialysis, per gallon ⊘
MED: 100-4, 8, 130; 100-4, 8, 70; 100-4, 8, 80; 100-4, 8, 90; 100-4, 8, 90.1; 100-4, 8, 90.3.2

Ⓐ ☑ **A4714** Treated water (deionized, distilled, or reverse osmosis) for peritoneal dialysis, per gallon ⊘
MED: 100-3, 230.7; 100-4, 8, 130; 100-4, 8, 70; 100-4, 8, 80; 100-4, 8, 90; 100-4, 8, 90.1; 100-4, 8, 90.3.2

Ⓐ **A4719** Y set tubing for peritoneal dialysis ⊘
MED: 100-4, 8, 130; 100-4, 8, 70; 100-4, 8, 80; 100-4, 8, 90; 100-4, 8, 90.1; 100-4, 8, 90.3.2

Ⓐ ☑ **A4720** Dialysate solution, any concentration of dextrose, fluid volume greater than 249 cc, but less than or equal to 999 cc, for peritoneal dialysis ⊘
MED: 100-4, 8, 130; 100-4, 8, 70; 100-4, 8, 80; 100-4, 8, 90; 100-4, 8, 90.1; 100-4, 8, 90.3.2

Ⓐ ☑ **A4721** Dialysate solution, any concentration of dextrose, fluid volume greater than 999 cc, but less than or equal to 1999 cc, for peritoneal dialysis ⊘
MED: 100-4, 8, 130; 100-4, 8, 70; 100-4, 8, 80; 100-4, 8, 90; 100-4, 8, 90.1; 100-4, 8, 90.3.2

Ⓐ ☑ **A4722** Dialysate solution, any concentration of dextrose, fluid volume greater than 1999 cc, but less than or equal to 2999 cc, for peritoneal dialysis ⊘
MED: 100-4, 8, 130; 100-4, 8, 70; 100-4, 8, 80; 100-4, 8, 90; 100-4, 8, 90.1; 100-4, 8, 90.3.2

Ⓐ ☑ **A4723** Dialysate solution, any concentration of dextrose, fluid volume greater than 2999 cc, but less than or equal to 3999 cc, for peritoneal dialysis ⊘
MED: 100-4, 8, 130; 100-4, 8, 70; 100-4, 8, 80; 100-4, 8, 90; 100-4, 8, 90.1; 100-4, 8, 90.3.2

Ⓐ ☑ **A4724** Dialysate solution, any concentration of dextrose, fluid volume greater than 3999 cc, but less than or equal to 4999 cc, for peritoneal dialysis ⊘
MED: 100-4, 8, 130; 100-4, 8, 70; 100-4, 8, 80; 100-4, 8, 90; 100-4, 8, 90.1; 100-4, 8, 90.3.2

Ⓐ ☑ **A4725** Dialysate solution, any concentration of dextrose, fluid volume greater than 4999 cc, but less than or equal to 5999 cc, for peritoneal dialysis ⊘
MED: 100-4, 8, 130; 100-4, 8, 70; 100-4, 8, 80; 100-4, 8, 90; 100-4, 8, 90.1; 100-4, 8, 90.3.2

Ⓐ ☑ **A4726** Dialysate solution, any concentration of dextrose, fluid volume greater than 5999 cc ⊘
MED: 100-4, 8, 130; 100-4, 8, 70; 100-4, 8, 80; 100-4, 8, 90; 100-4, 8, 90.1; 100-4, 8, 90.3.2

Ⓑ ☑ **A4728** Dialysate solution, non-dextrose containing, 500 ml ⊘

Ⓐ ☑ **A4730** Fistula cannulation set for hemodialysis, each ⊘
MED: 100-4, 8, 130; 100-4, 8, 70; 100-4, 8, 80; 100-4, 8, 90; 100-4, 8, 90.1; 100-4, 8, 90.3.2

Ⓐ ☑ **A4736** Topical anesthetic, for dialysis, per gm ⊘
MED: 100-4, 8, 130; 100-4, 8, 70; 100-4, 8, 80; 100-4, 8, 90; 100-4, 8, 90.1; 100-4, 8, 90.3.2

Ⓐ ☑ **A4737** Injectable anesthetic, for dialysis, per 10 ml ⊘
MED: 100-4, 8, 130; 100-4, 8, 70; 100-4, 8, 80; 100-4, 8, 90; 100-4, 8, 90.1; 100-4, 8, 90.3.2

Ⓐ **A4740** Shunt accessory, for hemodialysis, any type ⊘
Medicare jurisdiction: DME regional contractor.
MED: 100-4, 8, 130; 100-4, 8, 70; 100-4, 8, 80; 100-4, 8, 90; 100-4, 8, 90.1; 100-4, 8, 90.3.2

Ⓐ ☑ **A4750** Blood tubing, arterial or venous, for hemodialysis, each ⊘
MED: 100-4, 8, 130; 100-4, 8, 70; 100-4, 8, 80; 100-4, 8, 90; 100-4, 8, 90.1; 100-4, 8, 90.3.2

Ⓐ **A4755** Blood tubing, arterial and venous combined, for hemodialysis, each ⊘
MED: 100-4, 8, 130; 100-4, 8, 70; 100-4, 8, 80; 100-4, 8, 90; 100-4, 8, 90.1; 100-4, 8, 90.3.2

Ⓐ ☑ **A4760** Dialysate solution test kit, for peritoneal dialysis, any type, each ⊘
MED: 100-4, 8, 130; 100-4, 8, 70; 100-4, 8, 80; 100-4, 8, 90; 100-4, 8, 90.1; 100-4, 8, 90.3.2

Ⓐ ☑ **A4765** Dialysate concentrate, powder, additive for peritoneal dialysis, per packet ⊘
MED: 100-4, 8, 130; 100-4, 8, 70; 100-4, 8, 80; 100-4, 8, 90; 100-4, 8, 90.1; 100-4, 8, 90.3.2

Ⓐ **A4766** Dialysate concentrate, solution, additive for peritoneal dialysis, per 10 ml ⊘
MED: 100-4, 8, 130; 100-4, 8, 70; 100-4, 8, 80; 100-4, 8, 90; 100-4, 8, 90.1; 100-4, 8, 90.3.2

Ⓐ **A4770** Blood collection tube, vacuum, for dialysis, per 50 ⊘
MED: 100-4, 8, 130; 100-4, 8, 70; 100-4, 8, 80; 100-4, 8, 90; 100-4, 8, 90.1; 100-4, 8, 90.3.2

Ⓐ ☑ **A4771** Serum clotting time tube, for dialysis, per 50 ⊘
MED: 100-4, 8, 130; 100-4, 8, 70; 100-4, 8, 80; 100-4, 8, 90; 100-4, 8, 90.1; 100-4, 8, 90.3.2

Ⓐ ☑ **A4772** Blood glucose test strips, for dialysis, per 50 ⊘
MED: 100-4, 8, 130; 100-4, 8, 70; 100-4, 8, 80; 100-4, 8, 90; 100-4, 8, 90.1; 100-4, 8, 90.3.2

Ⓐ ☑ **A4773** Occult blood test strips, for dialysis, per 50 ⊘
MED: 100-4, 8, 130; 100-4, 8, 70; 100-4, 8, 80; 100-4, 8, 90; 100-4, 8, 90.1; 100-4, 8, 90.3.2

Ⓐ ☑ **A4774** Ammonia test strips, for dialysis, per 50 ⊘
MED: 100-4, 8, 130; 100-4, 8, 70; 100-4, 8, 80; 100-4, 8, 90; 100-4, 8, 90.1; 100-4, 8, 90.3.2

Ⓐ ☑ **A4802** Protamine sulfate, for hemodialysis, per 50 mg ⊘
MED: 100-4, 8, 130; 100-4, 8, 70; 100-4, 8, 80; 100-4, 8, 90; 100-4, 8, 90.1; 100-4, 8, 90.3.2

Ⓐ ☑ **A4860** Disposable catheter tips for peritoneal dialysis, per 10 ⊘
MED: 100-4, 8, 130; 100-4, 8, 70; 100-4, 8, 80; 100-4, 8, 90; 100-4, 8, 90.1; 100-4, 8, 90.3.2

Ⓐ **A4870** Plumbing and/or electrical work for home hemodialysis equipment ⊘
MED: 100-4, 8, 130; 100-4, 8, 70; 100-4, 8, 80; 100-4, 8, 90; 100-4, 8, 90.1; 100-4, 8, 90.3.2

Ⓐ **A4890** Contracts, repair and maintenance, for hemodialysis equipment ⊘
MED: 100-2, 15, 110.2

Ⓐ ☑ **A4911** Drain bag/bottle, for dialysis, each ⊘

Ⓐ **A4913** Miscellaneous dialysis supplies, not otherwise specified ⊘
Pertinent documentation to evaluate medical appropriateness should be included when this code is reported. Determine if an alternative HCPCS Level II or a CPT code better describes the service being reported. This code should be used only if a more specific code is unavailable.

Ⓐ ☑ **A4918** Venous pressure clamp, for hemodialysis, each ⊘

Ⓐ ☑ **A4927** Gloves, non-sterile, per 100 ⊘

Ⓐ ☑ **A4928** Surgical mask, per 20 ⊘

Ⓐ **A4929** Tourniquet for dialysis, each ⊘

Ⓐ **A4930** Gloves, sterile, per pair ⊘

Ⓐ **A4931** Oral thermometer, reusable, any type, each ⊘

Special Coverage Instructions   Noncovered by Medicare   Carrier Discretion   ☑ Quantity Alert   ● New Code   ○ Reinstated Code   ▲ Revised Code

2006 HCPCS   **1**-**9** ASC Groups   MED: Pub 100/NCD Reference   ᠪ DMEPOS Paid   ⊘ SNF Excluded   A Codes — 9

Medical and Surgical Supplies

A4932 — A5508

E   **A4932** Rectal thermometer, reusable, any type, each

ADDITIONAL OSTOMY SUPPLIES
Medicare claims fall under the jurisdiction of the DME regional contractor, unless otherwise noted.

A ☑ **A5051** Ostomy pouch, closed; with barrier attached (one piece), each
MED: 100-2, 15, 120

A ☑ **A5052** Ostomy pouch, closed; without barrier attached (one piece), each
MED: 100-2, 15, 120

A ☑ **A5053** Ostomy pouch, closed; for use on faceplate, each
MED: 100-2, 15, 120

A ☑ **A5054** Ostomy pouch, closed; for use on barrier with flange (two piece), each
MED: 100-2, 15, 120

A **A5055** Stoma cap
MED: 100-2, 15, 120

A ☑ **A5061** Ostomy pouch, drainable; with barrier attached, (one piece), each

A ☑ **A5062** Ostomy pouch, drainable; without barrier attached (one piece), each
MED: 100-2, 15, 120

A ☑ **A5063** Ostomy pouch, drainable; for use on barrier with flange (two piece system), each
MED: 100-2, 15, 120

A ☑ **A5071** Ostomy pouch, urinary; with barrier attached (one piece), each
MED: 100-2, 15, 120

A ☑ **A5072** Ostomy pouch, urinary; without barrier attached (one piece), each
MED: 100-2, 15, 120

A ☑ **A5073** Ostomy pouch, urinary; for use on barrier with flange (two piece), each
MED: 100-2, 15, 120

A **A5081** Continent device; plug for continent stoma
MED: 100-2, 15, 120

A **A5082** Continent device; catheter for continent stoma
MED: 100-2, 15, 120

A **A5093** Ostomy accessory; convex insert
Medicare jurisdiction: local contractor.
MED: 100-2, 15, 120

ADDITIONAL INCONTINENCE APPLIANCES/SUPPLIES
Medicare claims fall under the jurisdiction of the DME regional contractor, unless otherwise noted.

A ☑ **A5102** Bedside drainage bottle, with or without tubing, rigid or expandable, each
MED: 100-2, 15, 120

A **A5105** Urinary suspensory; with leg bag, with or without tube
MED: 100-2, 15, 120

A **A5112** Urinary leg bag; latex
MED: 100-2, 15, 120

A ☑ **A5113** Leg strap; latex, replacement only, per set
MED: 100-2, 15, 120

A ☑ **A5114** Leg strap; foam or fabric, replacement only, per set
MED: 100-2, 15, 120

SUPPLIES FOR EITHER INCONTINENCE OR OSTOMY APPLIANCES
For additional skin barrier codes see new codes A4405-A4415.

~~A5110 Skin barrier, wipes or swabs, per box 50~~
See code(s) A5120.

● A **A5120** Skin barrier, wipes or swabs, each
MED: 100-2, 15, 120

A ☑ **A5121** Skin barrier; solid, 6 x 6 or equivalent, each
MED: 100-2, 15, 120

A ☑ **A5122** Skin barrier; solid, 8 x 8 or equivalent, each
MED: 100-2, 15, 120

A **A5126** Adhesive or non-adhesive; disk or foam pad
MED: 100-2, 15, 120

A ☑ **A5131** Appliance cleaner, incontinence and ostomy appliances, per 16 oz
MED: 100-2, 15, 120

A **A5200** Percutaneous catheter/tube anchoring device, adhesive skin attachment
MED: 100-2, 15, 120

DIABETIC SHOES, FITTING, AND MODIFICATIONS
According to Medicare, documentation from the prescribing physician must certify the diabetic patient has one of the following conditions: peripheral neuropathy with evidence of callus formation; history of preulcerative calluses; history of ulceration; foot deformity; previous amputation; or poor circulation. The footwear must be fitted and furnished by a podiatrist, pedorthist, orthotist, or prosthetist.

Y ☑ **A5500** For diabetics only, fitting (including follow-up) custom preparation and supply of off-the-shelf depth-inlay shoe manufactured to accommodate multi-density insert(s), per shoe
MED: 100-2, 15, 140

Y ☑ **A5501** For diabetics only, fitting (including follow-up) custom preparation and supply of shoe molded from cast(s) of patient's foot (custom molded shoe), per shoe
MED: 100-2, 15, 140

Y ☑ **A5503** For diabetics only, modification (including fitting) of off-the-shelf depth-inlay shoe or custom molded shoe with roller or rigid rocker bottom, per shoe
MED: 100-2, 15, 140

Y ☑ **A5504** For diabetics only, modification (including fitting) of off-the-shelf depth-inlay shoe or custom molded shoe with wedge(s), per shoe
MED: 100-2, 15, 140

Y ☑ **A5505** For diabetics only, modification (including fitting) of off-the-shelf depth-inlay shoe or custom molded shoe with metatarsal bar, per shoe
MED: 100-2, 15, 140

Y ☑ **A5506** For diabetics only, modification (including fitting) of off-the-shelf depth-inlay shoe or custom molded shoe with off-set heel(s), per shoe
MED: 100-2, 15, 140

Y ☑ **A5507** For diabetics only, not otherwise specified modification (including fitting) of off-the-shelf depth-inlay shoe or custom molded shoe, per shoe
MED: 100-2, 15, 140

Y ☑ **A5508** For diabetics only, deluxe feature of off-the-shelf depth-inlay shoe or custom-molded shoe, per shoe
MED: 100-2, 15, 140

Special Coverage Instructions   Noncovered by Medicare   Carrier Discretion   ☑ Quantity Alert   ● New Code   ○ Reinstated Code   ▲ Revised Code

10 — A Codes   A Age   M Maternity   ♀ Female Only   ♂ Male Only   A-Y APC Status Indicator   *2006 HCPCS*

A5500 ~~For diabetics only, direct formed, molded to foot with external heat source (i.e., heat gun) multiple density insert(s), prefabricated, per shoe~~
See code(s) A5512.

E   A5510 For diabetics only, direct formed, compression molded to patient's foot without external heat source, multiple-density insert(s) prefabricated, per shoe
MED: 100-2, 15, 140

A5511 ~~For diabetics only, custom molded from model of patient's foot, multiple density insert(s), custom fabricated, per shoe~~
See code(s) A5513.

● B   A5512 For diabetics only, multiple density insert, direct formed, molded to foot after external heat source of 230 degrees Fahrenheit or higher, total contact with patient's foot, including arch, base layer minimum of 1/4 inch material of shore a 35 durometer or 3/16 inch material of shore a 40 durometer (or higher), prefabricated, each

● B   A5513 For diabetics only, multiple density insert, custom molded from model of patient's foot, total contact with patient's foot, including arch, base layer minimum of 1/4 inch material of shore a 35 durometer or 3/16 inch material of shore a 40 durometer (or higher), includes arch filler and other shaping material, custom fabricated, each

DRESSINGS

Medicare claims for A6021-A6404 fall under the jurisdiction of the local contractor if the supply or accessory is used for an implanted prosthetic device (e.g., pleural catheter) or implanted DME (e.g., infusion pump). Medicare claims for other uses of A6021-A6404 fall under the jurisdiction of the DME regional contractor. The jurisdiction for Medicare claims containing all other codes falls to the DME regional contractor, unless otherwise noted.

E   A6000 Non-contact wound warming wound cover for use with the non-contact wound warming device and warming card ⊘
MED: 100-2, 16, 20

A ☑ A6010 Collagen based wound filler, dry form, per gram of collagen ㋕
MED: 100-2, 15, 100

A ☑ A6011 Collagen based wound filler, gel/paste, per gram of collagen ㋕
MED: 100-2, 15, 100

A ☑ A6021 Collagen dressing, pad size 16 sq. in. or less, each ㋕
MED: 100-2, 15, 100

A ☑ A6022 Collagen dressing, pad size more than 16 sq. in. but less than or equal to 48 sq. in., each ㋕
MED: 100-2, 15, 100

A ☑ A6023 Collagen dressing, pad size more than 48 sq. in., each ㋕
MED: 100-2, 15, 100

A ☑ A6024 Collagen dressing wound filler, per 6 in. ㋕
MED: 100-2, 15, 100

E ☑ A6025 Gel sheet for dermal or epidermal application, (e.g., silicone, hydrogel, other), each ⊘

A ☑ A6154 Wound pouch, each ㋕
MED: 100-2, 15, 100

A ☑ A6196 Alginate or other fiber gelling dressing, wound cover, pad size 16 sq. in. or less, each dressing ㋕
MED: 100-2, 15, 100

A ☑ A6197 Alginate or other fiber gelling dressing, wound cover, pad size more than 16 sq. in. but less than or equal to 48 sq. in., each dressing
MED: 100-2, 15, 100

A ☑ A6198 Alginate or other fiber gelling dressing, wound cover, pad size more than 48 sq. in., each dressing
MED: 100-2, 15, 100

A ☑ A6199 Alginate or other fiber gelling dressing, wound filler, per 6 in. ㋕
MED: 100-2, 15, 100

A ☑ A6200 Composite dressing, pad size 16 sq. in. or less, without adhesive border, each dressing ㋕
MED: 100-2, 15, 100

A ☑ A6201 Composite dressing, pad size more than 16 sq. in. but less than or equal to 48 sq. in., without adhesive border, each dressing ㋕
MED: 100-2, 15, 100

A ☑ A6202 Composite dressing, pad size more than 48 sq. in., without adhesive border, each dressing ㋕
MED: 100-2, 15, 100

A ☑ A6203 Composite dressing, pad size 16 sq. in. or less, with any size adhesive border, each dressing ㋕
MED: 100-2, 15, 100

A ☑ A6204 Composite dressing, pad size more than 16 sq. in. but less than or equal to 48 sq. in., with any size adhesive border, each dressing ㋕
MED: 100-2, 15, 100

A ☑ A6205 Composite dressing, pad size more than 48 sq. in., with any size adhesive border, each dressing
MED: 100-2, 15, 100

A ☑ A6206 Contact layer, 16 sq. in. or less, each dressing
MED: 100-2, 15, 100

A ☑ A6207 Contact layer, more than 16 sq. in. but less than or equal to 48 sq. in., each dressing ㋕
MED: 100-2, 15, 100

A ☑ A6208 Contact layer, more than 48 sq. in., each dressing
MED: 100-2, 15, 100

A ☑ A6209 Foam dressing, wound cover, pad size 16 sq. in. or less, without adhesive border, each dressing ㋕
MED: 100-2, 15, 100

A ☑ A6210 Foam dressing, wound cover, pad size more than 16 sq. in. but less than or equal to 48 sq. in., without adhesive border, each dressing ㋕
MED: 100-2, 15, 100

A ☑ A6211 Foam dressing, wound cover, pad size more then 48 sq. in., without adhesive border, each dressing ㋕
MED: 100-2, 15, 100

A ☑ A6212 Foam dressing, wound cover, pad size 16 sq. in. or less, with any size adhesive border, each dressing ㋕
MED: 100-2, 15, 100

A ☑ A6213 Foam dressing, wound cover, pad size more than 16 sq. in. but less than or equal to 48 sq. in., with any size adhesive border, each dressing
MED: 100-2, 15, 100

A ☑ A6214 Foam dressing, wound cover, pad size more than 48 sq. in., with any size adhesive border, each dressing ㋕
MED: 100-2, 15, 100

A ☑ A6215 Foam dressing, wound filler, per gram
MED: 100-2, 15, 100

Special Coverage Instructions   Noncovered by Medicare   Carrier Discretion   ☑ Quantity Alert   ● New Code   ○ Reinstated Code   ▲ Revised Code

2006 HCPCS   1-9 ASC Groups   MED: Pub 100/NCD Reference   ㋕ DMEPOS Paid   ⊘ SNF Excluded   A Codes — 11

A ☑ **A6216** Gauze, non-impregnated, non-sterile, pad size 16 sq. in. or less, without adhesive border, each dressing
MED: 100-2, 15, 100

A ☑ **A6217** Gauze, non-impregnated, non-sterile, pad size more than 16 sq. in. but less than or equal to 48 sq. in., without adhesive border, each dressing
MED: 100-2, 15, 100

A ☑ **A6218** Gauze, non-impregnated, non-sterile, pad size more than 48 sq. in., without adhesive border, each dressing
MED: 100-2, 15, 100

A ☑ **A6219** Gauze, non-impregnated, pad size 16 sq. in. or less, with any size adhesive border, each dressing
MED: 100-2, 15, 100

A ☑ **A6220** Gauze, non-impregnated, pad size more than 16 sq. in. but less than or equal to 48 sq. in., with any size adhesive border, each dressing
MED: 100-2, 15, 100

A ☑ **A6221** Gauze, non-impregnated, pad size more than 48 sq. in., with any size adhesive border, each dressing
MED: 100-2, 15, 100

A ☑ **A6222** Gauze, impregnated with other than water, normal saline, or hydrogel, pad size 16 sq. in. or less, without adhesive border, each dressing
MED: 100-2, 15, 100

A ☑ **A6223** Gauze, impregnated with other than water, normal saline, or hydrogel, pad size more than 16 sq. in. but less than or equal to 48 sq. in., without adhesive border, each dressing
MED: 100-2, 15, 100

A ☑ **A6224** Gauze, impregnated with other than water, normal saline, or hydrogel, pad size more than 48 sq. in., without adhesive border, each dressing
MED: 100-2, 15, 100

A ☑ **A6228** Gauze, impregnated, water or normal saline, pad size 16 sq. in. or less, without adhesive border, each dressing
MED: 100-2, 15, 100

A ☑ **A6229** Gauze, impregnated, water or normal saline, pad size more than 16 sq. in. but less than or equal to 48 sq. in., without adhesive border, each dressing
MED: 100-2, 15, 100

A ☑ **A6230** Gauze, impregnated, water or normal saline, pad size more than 48 sq. in., without adhesive border, each dressing
MED: 100-2, 15, 100

A ☑ **A6231** Gauze, impregnated, hydrogel, for direct wound contact, pad size 16 sq. in. or less, each dressing
MED: 100-2, 15, 100

A ☑ **A6232** Gauze, impregnated, hydrogel, for direct wound contact, pad size greater than 16 sq. in., but less than or equal to 48 sq. in., each dressing
MED: 100-2, 15, 100

A ☑ **A6233** Gauze, impregnated, hydrogel for direct wound contact, pad size more than 48 sq. in., each dressing
MED: 100-2, 15, 100

A ☑ **A6234** Hydrocolloid dressing, wound cover, pad size 16 sq. in. or less, without adhesive border, each dressing
MED: 100-2, 15, 100

A ☑ **A6235** Hydrocolloid dressing, wound cover, pad size more than 16 sq. in. but less than or equal to 48 sq. in., without adhesive border, each dressing
MED: 100-2, 15, 100

A ☑ **A6236** Hydrocolloid dressing, wound cover, pad size more than 48 sq. in., without adhesive border, each dressing
MED: 100-2, 15, 100

A ☑ **A6237** Hydrocolloid dressing, wound cover, pad size 16 sq. in. or less, with any size adhesive border, each dressing
MED: 100-2, 15, 100

A ☑ **A6238** Hydrocolloid dressing, wound cover, pad size more than 16 sq. in. but less than or equal to 48 sq. in., with any size adhesive border, each dressing
MED: 100-2, 15, 100

A ☑ **A6239** Hydrocolloid dressing, wound cover, pad size more than 48 sq. in., with any size adhesive border, each dressing
MED: 100-2, 15, 100

A ☑ **A6240** Hydrocolloid dressing, wound filler, paste, per fluid oz.
MED: 100-2, 15, 100

A ☑ **A6241** Hydrocolloid dressing, wound filler, dry form, per gram
MED: 100-2, 15, 100

A ☑ **A6242** Hydrogel dressing, wound cover, pad size 16 sq. in. or less, without adhesive border, each dressing
MED: 100-2, 15, 100

A ☑ **A6243** Hydrogel dressing, wound cover, pad size more than 16 sq. in. but less than or equal to 48 sq. in., without adhesive border, each dressing
MED: 100-2, 15, 100

A ☑ **A6244** Hydrogel dressing, wound cover, pad size more than 48 sq. in., without adhesive border, each dressing
MED: 100-2, 15, 100

A ☑ **A6245** Hydrogel dressing, wound cover, pad size 16 sq. in. or less, with any size adhesive border, each dressing
MED: 100-2, 15, 100

A ☑ **A6246** Hydrogel dressing, wound cover, pad size more than 16 sq. in. but less than or equal to 48 sq. in., with any size adhesive border, each dressing
MED: 100-2, 15, 100

A ☑ **A6247** Hydrogel dressing, wound cover, pad size more than 48 sq. in., with any size adhesive border, each dressing
MED: 100-2, 15, 100

A ☑ **A6248** Hydrogel dressing, wound filler, gel, per fluid oz.
MED: 100-2, 15, 100

A **A6250** Skin sealants, protectants, moisturizers, ointments, any type, any size
Surgical dressings applied by a physician are included as part of the professional service. Surgical dressings obtained by the patient to perform homecare as prescribed by the physician are covered.

MED: 100-2, 15, 100

A ☑ **A6251** Specialty absorptive dressing, wound cover, pad size 16 sq. in. or less, without adhesive border, each dressing
MED: 100-2, 15, 100

Special Coverage Instructions   Noncovered by Medicare   Carrier Discretion   ☑ Quantity Alert   ● New Code   ○ Reinstated Code   ▲ Revised Code

12 — A Codes   Ⓐ Age   Ⓜ Maternity   ♀ Female Only   ♂ Male Only   Ⓐ-☑ APC Status Indicator   *2006 HCPCS*

A ☑ **A6252** Specialty absorptive dressing, wound cover, pad size more than 16 sq. in. but less than or equal to 48 sq. in., without adhesive border, each dressing ㅊ
MED: 100-2, 15, 100

A ☑ **A6253** Specialty absorptive dressing, wound cover, pad size more than 48 sq. in., without adhesive border, each dressing ㅊ
MED: 100-2, 15, 100

A ☑ **A6254** Specialty absorptive dressing, wound cover, pad size 16 sq. in. or less, with any size adhesive border, each dressing ㅊ
MED: 100-2, 15, 100

A ☑ **A6255** Specialty absorptive dressing, wound cover, pad size more than 16 sq. in. but less than or equal to 48 sq. in., with any size adhesive border, each dressing ㅊ
MED: 100-2, 15, 100

A ☑ **A6256** Specialty absorptive dressing, wound cover, pad size more than 48 sq. in., with any size adhesive border, each dressing
MED: 100-2, 15, 100

A ☑ **A6257** Transparent film, 16 sq. in. or less, each dressing ㅊ
Surgical dressings applied by a physician are included as part of the professional service. Surgical dressings obtained by the patient to perform homecare as prescribed by the physician are covered. Use this code for Polyskin, Tegaderm, and Tegaderm HP.

MED: 100-2, 15, 100

A ☑ **A6258** Transparent film, more than 16 sq. in. but less than or equal to 48 sq. in., each dressing ㅊ
Surgical dressings applied by a physician are included as part of the professional service. Surgical dressings obtained by the patient to perform homecare as prescribed by the physician are covered.

MED: 100-2, 15, 100

A ☑ **A6259** Transparent film, more than 48 sq. in., each dressing ㅊ
Surgical dressings applied by a physician are included as part of the professional service. Surgical dressings obtained by the patient to perform homecare as prescribed by the physician are covered.

MED: 100-2, 15, 100

A **A6260** Wound cleansers, any type, any size ⊘
Surgical dressings applied by a physician are included as part of the professional service. Surgical dressings obtained by the patient to perform homecare as prescribed by the physician are covered.

MED: 100-2, 15, 100

A ☑ **A6261** Wound filler, gel/paste, per fluid oz., not elsewhere classified
Surgical dressings applied by a physician are included as part of the professional service. Surgical dressings obtained by the patient to perform homecare as prescribed by the physician are covered.

MED: 100-2, 15, 100

A ☑ **A6262** Wound filler, dry form, per gram, not elsewhere classified
MED: 100-2, 15, 100

A ☑ **A6266** Gauze, impregnated, other than water, normal saline, or zinc paste, any width, per linear yard ㅊ
Surgical dressings applied by a physician are included as part of the professional service. Surgical dressings obtained by the patient to perform homecare as prescribed by the physician are covered.

MED: 100-2, 15, 100

A ☑ **A6402** Gauze, non-impregnated, sterile, pad size 16 sq. in. or less, without adhesive border, each dressing ㅊ
Surgical dressings applied by a physician are included as part of the professional service. Surgical dressings obtained by the patient to perform homecare as prescribed by the physician are covered.

MED: 100-2, 15, 100

A ☑ **A6403** Gauze, non-impregnated, sterile, pad size more than 16 sq. in. but less than or equal to 48 sq. in., without adhesive border, each dressing ㅊ
Surgical dressings applied by a physician are included as part of the professional service. Surgical dressings obtained by the patient to perform homecare as prescribed by the physician are covered.

MED: 100-2, 15, 100

A ☑ **A6404** Gauze, non-impregnated, sterile, pad size more than 48 sq. in., without adhesive border, each dressing
MED: 100-2, 15, 100

☑ **A6407** Packing strips, non-impregnated, up to two in. in width, per linear yard ㅊ

A ☑ **A6410** Eye pad, sterile, each ㅊ
MED: 100-2, 15, 100

A ☑ **A6411** Eye pad, non-sterile, each ㅊ
MED: 100-2, 15, 100

E ☑ **A6412** Eye patch, occlusive, each

A ☑ **A6441** Padding bandage, non-elastic, non-woven/ non-knitted, width greater than or equal to 3 in. and less than 5 in., per yard ㅊ

A ☑ **A6442** Conforming bandage, non-elastic, knitted/woven, non-sterile, width less than 3 in., per yard ㅊ

A ☑ **A6443** Conforming bandage, non-elastic, knitted/woven, non-sterile, width greater than or equal to 3 in. and less than 5 in., per yard ㅊ

A ☑ **A6444** Conforming bandage, non-elastic, knitted/woven, non-sterile, width greater than or equal to 5 in., per yard ㅊ

A ☑ **A6445** Conforming bandage, non-elastic, knitted/woven, sterile, width less than 3 in., per yard ㅊ

A ☑ **A6446** Conforming bandage, non-elastic, knitted/woven, sterile, width greater than or equal to 3 in. and less than 5 in., per yard ㅊ

A ☑ **A6447** Conforming bandage, non-elastic, knitted/woven, sterile, width greater than or equal to 5 in., per yard ㅊ

A ☑ **A6448** Light compression bandage, elastic, knitted/woven, width less than 3 in., per yard ㅊ

A ☑ **A6449** Light compression bandage, elastic, knitted/woven, width greater than or equal to 3 in. and less than 5 in., per yard ㅊ

A ☑ **A6450** Light compression bandage, elastic, knitted/woven, width greater than or equal to 5 in., per yard ㅊ

A ☑ **A6451** Moderate compression bandage, elastic, knitted/woven, load resistance of 1.25 to 1.34 foot pounds at 50 percent maximum stretch, width greater than or equal to 3 in. and less than 5 in., per yard ㅊ

A ☑ **A6452** High compression bandage, elastic, knitted/woven, load resistance greater than or equal to 1.35 foot pounds at 50 percent maximum stretch, width greater than or equal to 3 in. and less than five in., per yard ㅊ

A ☑ **A6453** Self-adherent bandage, elastic, non-knitted/non-woven, width less than 3 in., per yard ㅊ

| Special Coverage Instructions | Noncovered by Medicare | Carrier Discretion | ☑ Quantity Alert | ● New Code | ○ Reinstated Code | ▲ Revised Code |

2006 HCPCS   **1-9** ASC Groups   MED: Pub 100/NCD Reference   ㅊ DMEPOS Paid   ⊘ SNF Excluded   **A Codes — 13**

Medical and Surgical Supplies

A6454 — A7006

A ☑ **A6454** Self-adherent bandage, elastic, non-knitted/non-woven, width greater than or equal to 3 in. and less than 5 in., per yard ♿

A ☑ **A6455** Self-adherent bandage, elastic, non-knitted/non-woven, width greater than or equal to 5 in., per yard ♿

A ☑ **A6456** Zinc paste impregnated bandage, non-elastic, knitted/woven, width greater than or equal to 3 in. and less than 5 in., per yard ♿

● A **A6457** Tubular dressing with or without elastic, any width, per linear yard

A **A6501** Compression burn garment, bodysuit (head to foot), custom fabricated ♿
MED: 100-2, 15, 100

A **A6502** Compression burn garment, chin strap, custom fabricated ♿
MED: 100-2, 15, 100

A **A6503** Compression burn garment, facial hood, custom fabricated ♿
MED: 100-2, 15, 100

A **A6504** Compression burn garment, glove to wrist, custom fabricated ♿
MED: 100-2, 15, 100

A **A6505** Compression burn garment, glove to elbow, custom fabricated ♿
MED: 100-2, 15, 100

A **A6506** Compression burn garment, glove to axilla, custom fabricated ♿
MED: 100-2, 15, 100

A **A6507** Compression burn garment, foot to knee length, custom fabricated ♿
MED: 100-2, 15, 100

A **A6508** Compression burn garment, foot to thigh length, custom fabricated ♿
MED: 100-2, 15, 100

A **A6509** Compression burn garment, upper trunk to waist including arm openings (vest), custom fabricated ♿
MED: 100-2, 15, 100

A **A6510** Compression burn garment, trunk, including arms down to leg openings (leotard), custom fabricated ♿
MED: 100-2, 15, 100

A **A6511** Compression burn garment, lower trunk including leg openings (panty), custom fabricated ♿
MED: 100-2, 15, 100

A **A6512** Compression burn garment, not otherwise classified
MED: 100-2, 15, 100

● B **A6513** Compression burn mask, face and/or neck, plastic or equal, custom fabricated

● E **A6530** Gradient compression stocking, below knee, 18-30 mm Hg, each
MED: 100-3, 280.1

● A **A6531** Gradient compression stocking, below knee, 30-40 mm Hg, each
MED: 100-2, 15, 100

● A **A6532** Gradient compression stocking, below knee, 40-50 mm Hg, each
MED: 100-2, 15, 100

● E **A6533** Gradient compression stocking, thigh length, 18-30 mm Hg, each
MED: 100-2, 15, 130; 100-3, 280.1

● E **A6534** Gradient compression stocking, thigh length, 30-40 mm Hg, each
MED: 100-2, 15, 130; 100-3, 280.1

● E **A6535** Gradient compression stocking, thigh length, 40-50 mm Hg, each
MED: 100-2, 15, 130; 100-3, 280.1

● E **A6536** Gradient compression stocking, full length/chap style, 18-30 mm Hg, each
MED: 100-2, 15, 130; 100-3, 280.1

● E **A6537** Gradient compression stocking, full length/chap style, 30-40 mm Hg, each
MED: 100-2, 15, 130; 100-3, 280.1

● E **A6538** Gradient compression stocking, full length/chap style, 40-50 mm Hg, each
MED: 100-2, 15, 130; 100-3, 280.1

● E **A6539** Gradient compression stocking, waist length, 18-30 mm Hg, each
MED: 100-2, 15, 130; 100-3, 280.1

● E **A6540** Gradient compression stocking, waist length, 30-40 mm Hg, each
MED: 100-2, 15, 130; 100-3, 280.1

● E **A6541** Gradient compression stocking, waist length, 40-50 mm Hg, each
MED: 100-2, 15, 130; 100-3, 280.1

● E **A6542** Gradient compression stocking, custom made
MED: 100-2, 15, 130; 100-3, 280.1

● E **A6543** Gradient compression stocking, lymphedema
MED: 100-2, 15, 130; 100-3, 280.1

● E **A6544** Gradient compression stocking, garter belt
MED: 100-2, 15, 130; 100-3, 280.1

● E **A6549** Gradient compression stocking, not otherwise specified
MED: 100-2, 15, 130; 100-3, 280.1

▲ Y ☑ **A6550** Wound care set, for negative pressure wound therapy electrical pump, includes all supplies and accessories ♿

~~A6551~~ ~~Canister set for negative pressure wound therapy electrical pump, stationary or portable, each~~

Y ☑ **A7000** Canister, disposable, used with suction pump, each ♿⊘
Medicare jurisdiction: DME regional contractor.

Y ☑ **A7001** Canister, non-disposable, used with suction pump, each ♿⊘
Medicare jurisdiction: DME regional contractor.

Y **A7002** Tubing, used with suction pump, each ♿⊘
Medicare jurisdiction: DME regional contractor.

Y **A7003** Administration set, with small volume nonfiltered pneumatic nebulizer, disposable ♿⊘
Medicare jurisdiction: DME regional contractor.

Y **A7004** Small volume nonfiltered pneumatic nebulizer, disposable ♿⊘
Medicare jurisdiction: DME regional contractor.

Y **A7005** Administration set, with small volume nonfiltered pneumatic nebulizer, non-disposable ♿⊘
Medicare jurisdiction: DME regional contractor.

Y **A7006** Administration set, with small volume filtered pneumatic nebulizer ♿⊘
Medicare jurisdiction: DME regional contractor.

▬ Special Coverage Instructions   ▬ Noncovered by Medicare   ▬ Carrier Discretion   ☑ Quantity Alert   ● New Code   ○ Reinstated Code   ▲ Revised Code

14 — A Codes   A Age   M Maternity   ♀ Female Only   ♂ Male Only   A-Y APC Status Indicator   **2006 HCPCS**

Ⓨ   A7007   **Large volume nebulizer, disposable, unfilled, used with aerosol compressor**   ⅓⊘
Medicare jurisdiction: DME regional contractor.

Ⓨ   A7008   **Large volume nebulizer, disposable, prefilled, used with aerosol compressor**   ⅓⊘
Medicare jurisdiction: DME regional contractor.

Ⓨ   A7009   **Reservoir bottle, non-disposable, used with large volume ultrasonic nebulizer**   ⅓⊘

Ⓨ ☑ A7010   **Corrugated tubing, disposable, used with large volume nebulizer, 100 feet**   ⅓⊘
Medicare jurisdiction: DME regional contractor.

Ⓨ ☑ A7011   **Corrugated tubing, non-disposable, used with large volume nebulizer, 10 feet**   ⊘

Ⓨ   A7012   **Water collection device, used with large volume nebulizer**   ⅓⊘
Medicare jurisdiction: DME regional contractor.

Ⓨ   A7013   **Filter, disposable, used with aerosol compressor** ⅓⊘
Medicare jurisdiction: DME regional contractor.

Ⓨ   A7014   **Filter, non-disposable, used with aerosol compressor or ultrasonic generator**   ⅓⊘
Medicare jurisdiction: DME regional contractor.

Ⓨ   A7015   **Aerosol mask, used with DME nebulizer**   ⅓⊘
Medicare jurisdiction: DME regional contractor.

Ⓨ   A7016   **Dome and mouthpiece, used with small volume ultrasonic nebulizer**   ⅓⊘

Ⓨ   A7017   **Nebulizer, durable, glass or autoclavable plastic, bottle type, not used with oxygen**   ⅓⊘
Medicare jurisdiction: DME regional contractor.
MED: 100-3, 280.1

Ⓨ ☑ A7018   **Water, distilled, used with large volume nebulizer, 1000 ml**   ⅓⊘
Medicare jurisdiction: DME regional contractor.

Ⓨ ☑ A7025   **High frequency chest wall oscillation system vest, replacement for use with patient owned equipment, each**   ⅓

Ⓨ ☑ A7026   **High frequency chest wall oscillation system hose, replacement for use with patient owned equipment, each**   ⅓

Ⓨ ☑ A7030   **Full face mask used with positive airway pressure device, each**   ⅓

Ⓨ ☑ A7031   **Face mask interface, replacement for full face mask, each**   ⅓

▲ Ⓨ ☑ A7032   **Cushion for use on nasal mask interface, replacement only, each**   ⅓

▲ Ⓨ   A7033   **Pillow for use on nasal cannula type interface, replacement only, pair**   ⅓

Ⓨ   A7034   **Nasal interface (mask or cannula type) used with positive airway pressure device, with or without head strap**

Ⓨ   A7035   **Headgear used with positive airway pressure device**   ⅓

Ⓨ   A7036   **Chinstrap used with positive airway pressure device**   ⅓

Ⓨ   A7037   **Tubing used with positive airway pressure device** ⅓

Ⓨ   A7038   **Filter, disposable, used with positive airway pressure device**   ⅓

Ⓨ   A7039   **Filter, non disposable, used with positive airway pressure device**   ⅓

Ⓐ   A7040   **One way chest drain valve**

Ⓐ   A7041   **Water seal drainage container and tubing for use with implanted chest tube**

Ⓐ   A7042   **Implanted pleural catheter, each**   ⅓

Ⓐ   A7043   **Vacuum drainage bottle and tubing for use with implanted catheter**   ⅓

Ⓨ   A7044   **Oral interface used with positive airway pressure device, each**   ⅓

    A7045   **Exhalation port with or without swivel used with accessories for positive airway devices, replacement only**
MED: 100-3, 230.17

Ⓨ ☑ A7046   **Water chamber for humidifier, used with positive airway pressure device, replacement, each**   ⅓⊘
MED: 100-3, 230.17

Ⓐ ☑ A7501   **Tracheostoma valve, including diaphragm, each** ⅓⊘
Medicare jurisdiction: DME regional contractor.
MED: 100-2, 15, 120

Ⓐ ☑ A7502   **Replacement diaphragm/faceplate for tracheostoma valve, each**   ⅓
Medicare jurisdiction: DME regional contractor.
MED: 100-2, 15, 120

Ⓐ ☑ A7503   **Filter holder or filter cap, reusable, for use in a tracheostoma heat and moisture exchange system, each**   ⅓
Medicare jurisdiction: DME regional contractor.
MED: 100-2, 15, 120

Ⓐ ☑ A7504   **Filter for use in a tracheostoma heat and moisture exchange system, each**   ⅓
MED: 100-2, 15, 120

Ⓐ ☑ A7505   **Housing, reusable without adhesive, for use in a heat and moisture exchange system and/or with a tracheostoma valve, each**   ⅓
MED: 100-2, 15, 120

Ⓐ ☑ A7506   **Adhesive disc for use in a heat and moisture exchange system and/or with tracheostoma valve, any type each**   ⅓
MED: 100-2, 15, 120

Ⓐ ☑ A7507   **Filter holder and integrated filter without adhesive, for use in a tracheostoma heat and moisture exchange system, each**   ⅓
Medicare jurisdiction: DME regional contractor.
MED: 100-2, 15, 120

Ⓐ ☑ A7508   **Housing and integrated adhesive, for use in a tracheostoma heat and moisture exchange system and/or with a tracheostoma valve, each**   ⅓
Medicare jurisdiction: DME regional contractor.
MED: 100-2, 15, 120

Ⓐ ☑ A7509   **Filter holder and integrated filter housing, and adhesive, for use as a tracheostoma heat and moisture exchange system, each**   ⅓
Medicare jurisdiction: DME regional contractor.
MED: 100-2, 15, 120

Ⓐ ☑ A7520   **Tracheostomy/laryngectomy tube, non-cuffed, polyvinylchloride (PVC), silicone or equal, each** ⅓

Ⓐ ☑ A7521   **Tracheostomy/laryngectomy tube, cuffed, polyvinylchloride (PVC), silicone or equal, each** ⅓

Ⓐ ☑ A7522   **Tracheostomy/laryngectomy tube, stainless steel or equal (sterilizable and reusable), each**   ⅓

Ⓐ ☑ A7523   **Tracheostoma shower protector, each**

| Special Coverage Instructions | Noncovered by Medicare | Carrier Discretion | ☑ Quantity Alert | ● New Code | ○ Reinstated Code | ▲ Revised Code |

2006 HCPCS   1-9 ASC Groups   MED: Pub 100/NCD Reference   ⅓ DMEPOS Paid   ⊘ SNF Excluded   **A Codes — 15**

Ⓐ ☑ **A7524** Tracheostoma stent/stud/button, each   ♿

Ⓐ ☑ **A7525** Tracheostomy mask, each   ♿

Ⓐ ☑ **A7526** Tracheostomy tube collar/holder, each   ♿

☑ **A7527** Tracheostomy/laryngectomy tube plug/stop, each

ADMINISTRATIVE, MISCELLANEOUS & INVESTIGATIONAL *A9000-A9999*

This section of codes reports items such as nonprescription drugs, noncovered items/services, exercise equipment and, most notably, radiopharmaceutical diagnostic imaging agents.

Ⓑ **A9150** Nonprescription drug   ⊘
     Medicare jurisdiction: local contractor.

☑ **A9152** Single vitamin/mineral/trace element, oral, per dose, not otherwise specified

☑ **A9153** Multiple vitamins, with or without minerals and trace elements, oral, per dose, not otherwise specified

A9180 Pediculosis (lice infestation) treatment, topical, for administration by patient/caretaker

Ⓔ **A9270** Noncovered item or service   ⊘
     Medicare jurisdiction: local or DME regional contractor.
     MED: 100-2, 16, 20

● Ⓔ **A9275** Home glucose disposable monitor, includes test strips

Ⓔ **A9280** Alert or alarm device, not otherwise classified   ⊘

● Ⓔ **A9281** Reaching/grabbing device, any type, any length, each

● Ⓔ **A9282** Wig, any type, each

Ⓔ **A9300** Exercise equipment   ⊘
     MED: 100-2, 15, 110.1; 100-3, 280.1

▲ Ⓗ ☑ **A9500** Technetium Tc-99m sestamibi, diagnostic, per study dose, up to 40 millicuries
     Use this code for Cardiolite.
     MED: 100-4, 12, 70; 100-4, 13, 20; 100-4, 13, 90

▲ Ⓗ ☑ **A9502** Technetium Tc-99m tetrofosmin, diagnostic, per study dose, up to 40 millicuries
     Use this code for Myoview.
     MED: 100-4, 12, 70; 100-4, 13, 20; 100-4, 13, 90

▲ Ⓝ ☑ **A9503** Technetium Tc-99m medronate, diagnostic, per study dose, up to 30 millicuries
     MED: 100-4, 12, 70; 100-4, 13, 20; 100-4, 13, 90
     AHA: 2Q, '02, 9

▲ Ⓗ **A9504** Technetium Tc-99m apcitide, diagnostic, per study dose, up to 20 millicuries
     Use this code for Acutect.
     MED: 100-4, 12, 70; 100-4, 13, 20; 100-4, 13, 90
     AHA: 2Q, '02, 9; 4Q, '01, 5

▲ Ⓗ ☑ **A9505** Thallium Tl-201 thallous chloride, diagnostic, per millicurie
     Use this code for Thallous Chloride USP.
     MED: 100-4, 12, 70; 100-4, 13, 20; 100-4, 13, 90
     AHA: 2Q, '02, 9

▲ Ⓗ ☑ **A9507** Indium In-111 capromab pendetide, diagnostic, per study dose, up to 10 millicuries
     Use this code for Prostascint.
     MED: 100-4, 12, 70; 100-4, 13, 20; 100-4, 13, 90

▲ Ⓗ ☑ **A9508** Iodine I-131 iobenguane sulfate, diagnostic, per 0.5 millicurie
     Use this code for MIBG.
     AHA: 2Q, '02, 9

▲ Ⓗ ☑ **A9510** Technetium Tc-99m disofenin, diagnostic, per study dose, up to 15 millicuries

~~A9511~~ ~~Supply of radiopharmaceutical diagnostic imaging agent, technetium Tc-99m, Depreotide, per millicurie~~
     See code(s) A9536.

▲ Ⓝ ☑ **A9512** Technetium Tc-99m pertechnetate, diagnostic, per millicurie
     Use this code for TechneScan.

~~A9513~~ ~~Supply of radiopharmaceutical diagnostic imaging agent, technetium Tc-99m mebrofenin, per mCi~~
     See code(s) A9537.

~~A9514~~ ~~Supply of radiopharmaceutical diagnostic imaging agent, technetium Tc-99m pyrophosphate, per mCi~~
     See code(s) A9538.

~~A9515~~ ~~Supply of radiopharmaceutical diagnostic imaging agent, technetium Tc-99m pentetate, per mCi~~
     See code(s) A9539.

▲ Ⓗ ☑ **A9516** Iodine I-123 sodium iodide capsule(s), diagnostic, per 100 microcuries

▲ Ⓗ ☑ **A9517** Iodine I-131 sodium iodide capsule(s), therapeutic, per millicurie   ⊘

~~A9518~~ ~~Supply of radiopharmaceutical diagnostic imaging agent, technetium Tc-99m macroaggregated albumin, per mCi~~
     See code(s) A9540.

~~A9520~~ ~~Supply of radiopharmaceutical diagnostic imaging agent, technetium Tc-99m sulfur colloid, per mCi~~
     See code(s) A9541.

▲ Ⓗ ☑ **A9521** Technetium Tc-99m exametazime, diagnostic, per study dose, up to 25 millicuries
     Use this code for Ceretec.

~~A9522~~ ~~Supply of radiopharmaceutical diagnostic imaging agent, Indium-111 ibritumomab tiuxetan, per mCi~~
     See code(s) A9542.

~~A9523~~ ~~Supply of radiopharmaceutical therapeutic imaging agent, yttrium-90 ibritumomab tiuxetan, per mCi~~
     See code(s) A9543.

▲ Ⓗ ☑ **A9524** Iodine I-131 iodinated serum albumin, diagnostic, per 5 microcuries
     MED: 100-4, 12, 70; 100-4, 13, 20; 100-4, 13, 90

~~A9525~~ ~~Supply of low or iso-osmolar contrast material, 10 mg of iodine~~
     See code(s) Q9945-Q9951.

▲ Ⓗ ☑ **A9526** Nitrogen N-13 ammonia, diagnostic, per study dose, up to 40 millicuries
     MED: 100-3, 220.6

▲ Ⓗ ☑ **A9528** Iodine I-131 sodium iodide capsule(s), diagnostic, per millicurie

▲ Ⓗ ☑ **A9529** Iodine I-131 sodium iodide solution, diagnostic, per millicurie

▲ Ⓗ ☑ **A9530** Iodine I-131 sodium iodide solution, therapeutic, per millicurie

▲ Ⓗ ☑ **A9531** Iodine I-131 sodium iodide, diagnostic, per microcurie (up to 100 microcuries)

| Special Coverage Instructions | Noncovered by Medicare | Carrier Discretion | ☑ Quantity Alert | ● New Code | ○ Reinstated Code | ▲ Revised Code |

16 — A Codes   Ⓐ Age   Ⓜ Maternity   ♀ Female Only   ♂ Male Only   Ⓐ-Ⓨ APC Status Indicator   *2006 HCPCS*

▲ Ⓗ ☑ **A9532** Iodine I-125 serum albumin, diagnostic, per 5 microcuries

~~A9533 Supply of radiopharmaceutical diagnostic imaging agent, I-131 tositumomab, per millicurie~~
See code(s) A9544.

~~A9534 Supply of radiopharmaceutical therapeutic imaging agent, I-131 tositumomab, per millicurie~~
See code(s) A9545.

● Ⓚ **A9535** Injection, methylene blue, 1 ml

● Ⓗ **A9536** Technetium Tc-99m depreotide, diagnostic, per study dose, up to 35 millicuries

● Ⓝ **A9537** Technetium Tc-99m mebrofenin, diagnostic, per study dose, up to 15 millicuries

● Ⓝ **A9538** Technetium Tc-99m pyrophosphate, diagnostic, per study dose, up to 25 millicuries

● Ⓝ **A9539** Technetium Tc-99m pentetate, diagnostic, per study dose, up to 25 millicuries

● Ⓝ **A9540** Technetium Tc-99m macroaggregated albumin, diagnostic, per study dose, up to 10 millicuries

● Ⓝ **A9541** Technetium Tc-99m sulfur colloid, diagnostic, per study dose, up to 20 millicuries

● Ⓗ **A9542** Indium In-111 ibritumomab tiuxetan, diagnostic, per study dose, up to 5 millicuries

● Ⓗ **A9543** Yttrium Y-90 ibritumomab tiuxetan, therapeutic, per treatment dose, up to 40 millicuries

● Ⓗ **A9544** Iodine I-131 tositumomab, diagnostic, per study dose

● Ⓗ **A9545** Iodine I-131 tositumomab, therapeutic, per treatment dose

● Ⓝ **A9546** Cobalt Co-57/58, cyanocobalamin, diagnostic, per study dose, up to 1 microcurie

● Ⓗ **A9547** Indium In-111 oxyquinoline, diagnostic, per 0.5 millicurie

● Ⓗ **A9548** Indium In-111 pentetate, diagnostic, per 0.5 millicurie

● Ⓗ **A9549** Technetium Tc-99m arcitumomab, diagnostic, per study dose, up to 25 millicuries

● Ⓗ **A9550** Technetium Tc-99m sodium gluceptate, diagnostic, per study dose, up to 25 millicurie

● Ⓗ **A9551** Technetium Tc-99m succimer, diagnostic, per study dose, up to 10 millicuries

● Ⓗ **A9552** Fluorodeoxyglucose F-18 FDG, diagnostic, per study dose, up to 45 millicuries

● Ⓗ **A9553** Chromium Cr-51 sodium chromate, diagnostic, per study dose, up to 250 microcuries

● Ⓗ **A9554** Iodine I-125 sodium iothalamate, diagnostic, per study dose, up to 10 microcuries

● Ⓗ **A9555** Rubidium Rb-82, diagnostic, per study dose, up to 60 millicuries
Use this code for Cardiogen 82.

● Ⓗ **A9556** Gallium Ga-67 citrate, diagnostic, per millicurie

● Ⓗ **A9557** Technetium Tc-99m bicisate, diagnostic, per study dose, up to 25 millicuries
Use this code for Neurolite.

● Ⓝ **A9558** Xenon Xe-133 gas, diagnostic, per 10 millicuries

● Ⓝ **A9559** Cobalt Co-57 cyanocobalamin, oral, diagnostic, per study dose, up to 1 microcurie
Use this code for Cobatope 57, Rubratope 57.

● Ⓗ **A9560** Technetium Tc-99m labeled red blood cells, diagnostic, per study dose, up to 30 millicuries

● Ⓝ **A9561** Technetium Tc-99m oxidronate, diagnostic, per study dose, up to 30 millicuries

● Ⓗ **A9562** Technetium Tc-99m mertiatide, diagnostic, per study dose, up to 15 millicuries
Use this code for MAG-3.

● Ⓗ **A9563** Sodium phosphate P-32, therapeutic, per millicurie

● Ⓗ **A9564** Chromic phosphate P-32 suspension, therapeutic, per millicurie
Use this code for Phosphocol (P32).

● Ⓗ **A9565** Indium In-111 pentetreotide, diagnostic, per millicurie
Use this code for Octreoscan.

● Ⓗ **A9566** Technetium Tc-99m fanolesomab, diagnostic, per study dose, up to 25 millicuries

● Ⓗ **A9567** Technetium Tc-99m pentetate, diagnostic, aerosol, per study dose, up to 75 millicuries

▲ Ⓗ ☑ **A9600** Strontium Sr-89 chloride, therapeutic, per millicurie
Medicare jurisdiction: local contractor.
AHA: 2Q, '02, 9

▲ Ⓗ ☑ **A9605** Samarium Sm-153 lexidronamm, therapeutic, per 50 millicuries
Use this code for Quadramet. Medicare jurisdiction: DME regional contractor.
AHA: 2Q, '02, 9

● Ⓝ **A9698** Nonradioactive contrast imaging material, not otherwise classified, per study
MED: 100-4, 12, 70; 100-4, 13, 20; 100-4, 13, 90

▲ Ⓝ **A9699** Radiopharmaceutical, therapeutic, not otherwise classified

Ⓔ **A9700** Supply of injectable contrast material for use in echocardiography, per study
MED: 100-4, 12, 30.4
AHA: 4Q, '01, 5

Ⓐ **A9900** Miscellaneous DME supply, accessory, and/or service component of another HCPCS code ⊘
Medicare jurisdiction: local contractor if implanted DME; if other, regional contractor.

Ⓐ **A9901** DME delivery, set up, and/or dispensing service component of another HCPCS code ⊘
Medicare jurisdiction: local contractor if implanted DME; if other, regional contractor.

Ⓨ **A9999** Miscellaneous DME supply or accessory, not otherwise specified ⊘

Special Coverage Instructions   Noncovered by Medicare   Carrier Discretion   ☑ Quantity Alert   ● New Code   ○ Reinstated Code   ▲ Revised Code

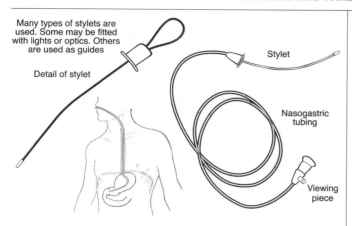

Detail of stylet

Many types of stylets are used. Some may be fitted with lights or optics. Others are used as guides

Stylet

Nasogastric tubing

Viewing piece

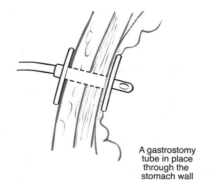

A gastrostomy tube in place through the stomach wall

ENTERAL AND PARENTERAL THERAPY *B4000-B9999*

This section includes codes for supplies, formulae, nutritional solutions, and infusion pumps.

ENTERAL FORMULAE AND ENTERAL MEDICAL SUPPLIES

Certification of medical necessity is required for coverage. Submit a revision to the certification of medical necessity if the patient's daily volume changes by more than one liter; if there is a change in infusion method; or if there is a change from premix to home mix or parenteral to enteral therapy.

Ⓐ **B4034** Enteral feeding supply kit; syringe, per day ⊘
MED: 100-2, 15, 120; 100-3, 180.2; 100-4, 20, 100.2.2; 100-4, 20, 100.2.2.3

Ⓐ **B4035** Enteral feeding supply kit; pump fed, per day ⊘
MED: 100-2, 15, 120; 100-3, 180.2; 100-4, 20, 100.2.2; 100-4, 20, 100.2.2.3

Ⓐ **B4036** Enteral feeding supply kit; gravity fed, per day ⊘
MED: 100-2, 15, 120; 100-3, 180.2; 100-4, 20, 100.2.2; 100-4, 20, 100.2.2.3

Ⓐ **B4081** Nasogastric tubing with stylet ⊘
MED: 100-2, 15, 120; 100-3, 180.2; 100-4, 20, 100.2.2; 100-4, 20, 100.2.2.3

Ⓐ **B4082** Nasogastric tubing without stylet ⊘
MED: 100-2, 15, 120; 100-3, 180.2; 100-4, 20, 100.2.2; 100-4, 20, 100.2.2.3

Ⓐ **B4083** Stomach tube — Levine type ⊘
MED: 100-2, 15, 120; 100-3, 180.2; 100-4, 20, 100.2.2; 100-4, 20, 100.2.2.3

Ⓐ **B4086** Gastrostomy/jejunostomy tube, any material, any type, (standard or low profile), each ⊘

Ⓔ **B4100** Food thickener, administered orally, per oz.

☑ **B4102** Enteral formula, for adults, used to replace fluids and electrolytes (e.g., clear liquids), 500 ml = 1 unit
MED: 100-3, 180.2

☑ **B4103** Enteral formula, for pediatrics, used to replace fluids and electrolytes (e.g., clear liquids), 500 ml = 1 unit
MED: 100-3, 180.2

☑ **B4104** Additive for enteral formula (e.g., fiber)
MED: 100-3, 180.2

▲ ☑ **B4149** Enteral formula, manufactured blenderized natural foods with intact nutrients, includes proteins, fats, carbohydrates, vitamins and minerals, may include fiber, administered through an enteral feeding tube, 100 calories = 1 unit
MED: 100-2, 15, 120; 100-3, 180.2; 100-4, 20, 100.2.2; 100-4, 20, 100.2.2.3

Ⓐ **B4150** Enteral formula, nutritionally complete with intact nutrients, includes proteins, fats, carbohydrates, vitamins and minerals, may include fiber, administered through an enteral feeding tube, 100 calories = 1 unit ⊘
Use this code for Enrich, Ensure, Ensure HN, Ensure Powder, Isocal, Lonalac Powder, Meritene, Meritene Powder, Osmolite, Osmolite HN, Portagen Powder, Sustacal, Renu, Sustagen Powder, Travasorb.

MED: 100-2, 15, 120; 100-3, 180.2; 100-4, 20, 100.2.2; 100-4, 20, 100.2.2.3

Ⓐ **B4152** Enteral formula, nutritionally complete, calorically dense (equal to or greater than 1.5 kcal/ml) with intact nutrients, includes proteins, fats, carbohydrates, vitamins and minerals, may include fiber, administered through an enteral feeding tube, 100 calories = 1 unit ⊘
Use this code for Magnacal, Isocal HCN, Sustacal HC, Ensure Plus, Ensure Plus HN.

MED: 100-2, 15, 120; 100-3, 180.2; 100-4, 20, 100.2.2; 100-4, 20, 100.2.2.3

Ⓐ **B4153** Enteral formula, nutritionally complete, hydrolyzed proteins (amino acids and peptide chain), includes fats, carbohydrates, vitamins and minerals, may include fiber, administered through an enteral feeding tube, 100 calories = 1 unit ⊘
Use this code for Criticare HN, Vivonex t.e.n. (Total Enteral Nutrition), Vivonex HN, Vital (Vital HN), Travasorb HN, Isotein HN, Precision HN, Precision Isotonic.

MED: 100-2, 15, 120; 100-3, 180.2; 100-4, 20, 100.2.2; 100-4, 20, 100.2.2.3

Ⓐ **B4154** Enteral formula, nutritionally complete, for special metabolic needs, excludes inherited disease of metabolism, includes altered composition of proteins, fats, carbohydrates, vitamins and/or minerals, may include fiber, administered through an enteral feeding tube, 100 calories = 1 unit ⊘
Use this code for Hepatic-aid, Travasorb Hepatic, Travasorb MCT, Travasorb Renal, Traum-aid, Tramacal, Aminaid.

MED: 100-2, 15, 120; 100-3, 180.2; 100-4, 20, 100.2.2; 100-4, 20, 100.2.2.3

Ⓐ **B4155** Enteral formula, nutritionally incomplete/modular nutrients, includes specific nutrients, carbohydrates (e.g., glucose polymers), proteins/amino acids (e.g., glutamine, arginine), fat (e.g., medium chain triglycerides) or combination, administered through an enteral feeding tube, 100 calories = 1 unit ⊘
Use this code for Propac, Gerval Protein, Promix, Casec, Moducal, Controlyte, Polycose Liquid or Powder, Sumacal, Microlipids, MCT Oil, Nutri-source.

MED: 100-2, 15, 120; 100-3, 180.2; 100-4, 20, 100.2.2; 100-4, 20, 100.2.2.3

B4034—B4155

Special Coverage Instructions   Noncovered by Medicare   Carrier Discretion   ☑ Quantity Alert   ● New Code   ○ Reinstated Code   ▲ Revised Code

2006 HCPCS   **1**-**9** ASC Groups   MED: Pub 100/NCD Reference   ⅃ DMEPOS Paid   ⊘ SNF Excluded   **B Codes — 19**

Enteral and Parenteral Therapy

B4157— B5100

☑ **B4157** Enteral formula, nutritionally complete, for special metabolic needs for inherited disease of metabolism, includes proteins, fats, carbohydrates, vitamins and minerals, may include fiber, administered through an enteral feeding tube, 100 calories = 1 unit
MED: 100-3, 180.2

☑ **B4158** Enteral formula, for pediatrics, nutritionally complete with intact nutrients, includes proteins, fats, carbohydrates, vitamins and minerals, may include fiber and/or iron, administered through an enteral feeding tube, 100 calories = 1 unit
MED: 100-3, 180.2

☑ **B4159** Enteral formula, for pediatrics, nutritionally complete soy based with intact nutrients, includes proteins, fats, carbohydrates, vitamins and minerals, may include fiber and/or iron, administered through an enteral feeding tube, 100 calories = 1 unit
MED: 100-3, 180.2

☑ **B4160** Enteral formula, for pediatrics, nutritionally complete calorically dense (equal to or greater than 0.7 kcal/ml) with intact nutrients, includes proteins, fats, carbohydrates, vitamins and minerals, may include fiber, administered through an enteral feeding tube, 100 calories = 1 unit
MED: 100-3, 180.2

☑ **B4161** Enteral formula, for pediatrics, hydrolyzed/amino acids and peptide chain proteins, includes fats, carbohydrates, vitamins and minerals, may include fiber, administered through an enteral feeding tube, 100 calories = 1 unit
MED: 100-3, 180.2

☑ **B4162** Enteral formula, for pediatrics, special metabolic needs for inherited disease of metabolism, includes proteins, fats, carbohydrates, vitamins and minerals, may include fiber, administered through an enteral feeding tube, 100 calories = 1 unit
MED: 100-3, 180.2

PARENTERAL NUTRITION SOLUTIONS AND SUPPLIES

Ⓐ **B4164** Parenteral nutrition solution; carbohydrates (dextrose), 50% or less (500 ml = 1 unit) — home mix ⊘
MED: 100-2, 15, 120; 100-3, 180.2; 100-4, 20, 100.2.2; 100-4, 20, 100.2.2.3

Ⓐ **B4168** Parenteral nutrition solution; amino acid, 3.5%, (500 ml = 1 unit) — home mix ⊘
MED: 100-2, 15, 120; 100-3, 180.2; 100-4, 20, 100.2.2; 100-4, 20, 100.2.2.3

Ⓐ **B4172** Parenteral nutrition solution; amino acid, 5.5% through 7%, (500 ml = 1 unit) — home mix ⊘
MED: 100-2, 15, 120; 100-3, 180.2; 100-4, 20, 100.2.2; 100-4, 20, 100.2.2.3

Ⓐ **B4176** Parenteral nutrition solution; amino acid, 7% through 8.5%, (500 ml = 1 unit) — home mix ⊘
MED: 100-2, 15, 120; 100-3, 180.2; 100-4, 20, 100.2.2; 100-4, 20, 100.2.2.3

Ⓐ **B4178** Parenteral nutrition solution; amino acid, greater than 8.5% (500 ml = 1 unit) — home mix ⊘
MED: 100-2, 15, 120; 100-3, 180.2; 100-4, 20, 100.2.2; 100-4, 20, 100.2.2.3

Ⓐ **B4180** Parenteral nutrition solution; carbohydrates (dextrose), greater than 50% (500 ml = 1 unit) — home mix ⊘
MED: 100-2, 15, 120; 100-3, 180.2; 100-4, 20, 100.2.2; 100-4, 20, 100.2.2.3

~~**B4184** Parenteral nutrition solution; lipids, 10% with administration set (500 ml = 1 unit)~~

● Ⓑ **B4185** Parenteral nutrition solution, per 10 grams lipids

~~**B4186** Parenteral nutrition solution; lipids, 20% with administration set (500 ml = 1 unit)~~

Ⓐ ☑ **B4189** Parenteral nutrition solution; compounded amino acid and carbohydrates with electrolytes, trace elements, and vitamins, including preparation, any strength, 10 to 51 grams of protein — premix ⊘
MED: 100-2, 15, 120; 100-3, 180.2; 100-4, 20, 100.2.2; 100-4, 20, 100.2.2.3

Ⓐ ☑ **B4193** Parenteral nutrition solution; compounded amino acid and carbohydrates with electrolytes, trace elements, and vitamins, including preparation, any strength, 52 to 73 grams of protein — premix ⊘
MED: 100-2, 15, 120; 100-3, 180.2; 100-4, 20, 100.2.2; 100-4, 20, 100.2.2.3

Ⓐ ☑ **B4197** Parenteral nutrition solution; compounded amino acid and carbohydrates with electrolytes, trace elements and vitamins, including preparation, any strength, 74 to 100 grams of protein — premix ⊘
MED: 100-2, 15, 120; 100-3, 180.2; 100-4, 20, 100.2.2; 100-4, 20, 100.2.2.3

Ⓐ ☑ **B4199** Parenteral nutrition solution; compounded amino acid and carbohydrates with electrolytes, trace elements and vitamins, including preparation, any strength, over 100 grams of protein — premix ⊘
MED: 100-2, 15, 120; 100-3, 180.2; 100-4, 20, 100.2.2; 100-4, 20, 100.2.2.3

Ⓐ **B4216** Parenteral nutrition; additives (vitamins, trace elements, heparin, electrolytes) — home mix, per day ⊘
MED: 100-2, 15, 120; 100-3, 180.2; 100-4, 20, 100.2.2; 100-4, 20, 100.2.2.3

Ⓐ **B4220** Parenteral nutrition supply kit; premix, per day ⊘
MED: 100-2, 15, 120; 100-3, 180.2; 100-4, 20, 100.2.2; 100-4, 20, 100.2.2.3

Ⓐ **B4222** Parenteral nutrition supply kit; home mix, per day ⊘
MED: 100-2, 15, 120; 100-3, 180.2; 100-4, 20, 100.2.2; 100-4, 20, 100.2.2.3

Ⓐ **B4224** Parenteral nutrition administration kit, per day ⊘
MED: 100-2, 15, 120; 100-3, 180.2; 100-4, 20, 100.2.2; 100-4, 20, 100.2.2.3

Ⓐ **B5000** Parenteral nutrition solution; compounded amino acid and carbohydrates with electrolytes, trace elements, and vitamins, including preparation, any strength, renal — Amirosyn RF, NephrAmine, RenAmine — premix ⊘
Use this code for Amirosyn-RF, NephrAmine, RenAmin.
MED: 100-2, 15, 120; 100-3, 180.2; 100-4, 20, 100.2.2; 100-4, 20, 100.2.2.3

Ⓐ **B5100** Parenteral nutrition solution; compounded amino acid and carbohydrates with electrolytes, trace elements, and vitamins, including preparation, any strength, hepatic — FreAmine HBC, HepatAmine — premix ⊘
Use this code for FreAmine HBC, HepatAmine.
MED: 100-2, 15, 120; 100-3, 180.2; 100-4, 20, 100.2.2; 100-4, 20, 100.2.2.3

Special Coverage Instructions   Noncovered by Medicare   Carrier Discretion   ☑ Quantity Alert   ● New Code   ○ Reinstated Code   ▲ Revised Code

20 — B Codes   Ⓐ Age   Ⓜ Maternity   ♀ Female Only   ♂ Male Only   Ⓐ-Ⓨ APC Status Indicator   *2006 HCPCS*

Ⓐ   **B5200**   Parenteral nutrition solution; compounded amino acid and carbohydrates with electrolytes, trace elements, and vitamins, including preparation, any strength, stress — branch chain amino acids — premix ⊘
MED: 100-2, 15, 120; 100-3, 180.2; 100-4, 20, 100.2.2; 100-4, 20, 100.2.2.3

ENTERAL AND PARENTERAL PUMPS

Submit documentation of the need for the infusion pump. Medicare will reimburse for the simplest model that meets the patient's needs.

Ⓐ   **B9000**   Enteral nutrition infusion pump — without alarm ⊘
MED: 100-2, 15, 120; 100-3, 180.2; 100-4, 20, 100.2.2; 100-4, 20, 100.2.2.3

Ⓐ   **B9002**   Enteral nutrition infusion pump — with alarm ⊘
MED: 100-2, 15, 120; 100-3, 180.2; 100-4, 20, 100.2.2; 100-4, 20, 100.2.2.3

Ⓐ   **B9004**   Parenteral nutrition infusion pump, portable ⊘
MED: 100-2, 15, 120; 100-3, 180.2; 100-4, 20, 100.2.2; 100-4, 20, 100.2.2.3

Ⓐ   **B9006**   Parenteral nutrition infusion pump, stationary ⊘
MED: 100-2, 15, 120; 100-3, 180.2; 100-4, 20, 100.2.2; 100-4, 20, 100.2.2.3

Ⓐ   **B9998**   NOC for enteral supplies ⊘
MED: 100-2, 15, 120; 100-3, 180.2; 100-4, 20, 100.2.2; 100-4, 20, 100.2.2.3

Ⓐ   **B9999**   NOC for parenteral supplies ⊘
Determine if an alternative HCPCS Level II or a CPT code better describes the service being reported. This code should be used only if a more specific code is unavailable.

MED: 100-2, 15, 120; 100-3, 180.2; 100-4, 20, 100.2.2; 100-4, 20, 100.2.2.3

Special Coverage Instructions   Noncovered by Medicare   Carrier Discretion   ☑ Quantity Alert   ● New Code   ○ Reinstated Code   ▲ Revised Code

2006 HCPCS   **1**-**9** ASC Groups   MED: Pub 100/NCD Reference   ⅗ DMEPOS Paid   ⊘ SNF Excluded   **B Codes — 21**

OUTPATIENT PPS *C1000-C9999*

This section reports drugs, biologicals, and devices eligible for transitional pass-through payments for hospitals, and for items classified in new-technology ambulatory payment classifications (APCs) under the outpatient prospective payment system. These supplies can be billed in addition to the APC for ambulatory surgery center services when billing APCs to Medicare. Similar to all reimbursement requirements, Medicare makes transitional pass-through payments for a device only in conjunction with a procedure for its implantation or insertion. Consequently, a device will be considered medically necessary and eligible for a transitional pass-through payment only if the associated procedure is also medically necessary and payable under the outpatient prospective payment system.

CMS established categories for determining transitional pass-through payment devices, effective April 1, 2001, to meet the requirements of the Medicare, Medicaid, and SCHIP Benefits Improvement and Protection Act (BIPA). These new codes are also in the C series of HCPCS and are exclusively for use in billing for transitional pass-through payments. The introduction of categories does not affect payment methods. The transitional pass-through payment for a device will continue to be based on the charge on the individual bill, reduced to cost, and subject to a deduction that represents the cost of similar devices already included in the APC payment rate.

Each item previously determined to qualify fits in one of these categories. Other items may be billed using the category codes, even though CMS has not qualified them on an item-specific basis, as long as they:

- Meet the definition of a device that qualifies for transitional pass-through payments and other requirements and definitions

- Are described by the long descriptor associated with an active category code assigned by CMS

- Correlate with the definitions of terms and other general explanations issued by CMS to accompany coding assignments in this or subsequent instructions

- Have been approved by the Food and Drug Administration, if required. Some investigational devices have received an FDA investigational device exemption and may qualify

- Are considered reasonable and necessary for the diagnosis or treatment of an illness or injury

- Are an integral part of the procedure

- Are used for one patient only, are single use, come in contact with human tissue, and are surgically implanted or inserted. They may or may not remain with the patient when the patient is released from the hospital

- Cannot be taken as a depreciation, such as equipment, instruments, apparatuses, or implements

- Are not supplies used during the service or procedure, other than radiological site markers

- Are not materials such as biological or synthetics that are used to replace human skin

Future program memorandums will announce any new categories CMS develops. Keep in mind that the qualification of a device for transitional pass-through payments is temporary.

C1070 ~~Supply of radiopharmaceutical diagnostic imaging agent, cyanocobalamin Co 57/58, per 0.5 mCi~~
See code(s) A9546.

C1080 ~~Supply of radiopharmaceutical diagnostic imaging agent, I 131 tositumomab, per dose~~
See code(s) A9544.

C1081 ~~Supply of radiopharmaceutical therapeutic imaging agent, I 131 tositumomab, per dose~~
See code(s) A9545.

C1082 ~~Supply of radiopharmaceutical diagnostic imaging agent, Indium 111 ibritumomab tiuxetan, per dose~~
See code(s) A9542.

C1083 ~~Supply of radiopharmaceutical therapeutic imaging agent, yttrium 90 ibritumomab tiuxetan, per dose~~
See code(s) A9543.

C1001 ~~Supply of radiopharmaceutical diagnostic imaging agent, Indium 111 oxyquinoline, per 0.5 mCi~~
See code(s) A9547.

C1002 ~~Supply of radiopharmaceutical diagnostic imaging agent, Indium 111 pentetate, per 0.5 mCi~~
See code(s) A9548.

C1003 ~~Supply of radiopharmaceutical diagnostic imaging agent, technetium Tc 99m fanolesomab, per dose (10-20 mCi)~~
See code(s) A9566.

C1122 ~~Supply of radiopharmaceutical diagnostic imaging agent, technetium Tc 99m arcitumomab, per vial~~
See code(s) A9549.

[K] ☑ **C1178 Injection, busulfan, per 6 mg** ⊘
Use this code for Busulfex.

C1200 ~~Supply of radiopharmaceutical diagnostic imaging agent, technetium Tc 99m sodium glucoheptonate, per vial~~
See code(s) A9550.

C1201 ~~Supply of radiopharmaceutical diagnostic imaging agent, technetium Tc 99m succimer, per vial~~
See code(s) A9551.

[S] **C1300 Hyperbaric oxygen under pressure, full body chamber, per 30 minute interval** ⊘

C1305 ~~Graftskin, per 44 square centimeters~~
See code(s) J7340.

[N] **C1713 Anchor/screw for opposing bone-to-bone or soft tissue-to-bone (implantable)**
AHA: 1Q, '01, 5; 3Q, '02, 5

[N] **C1714 Catheter, transluminal atherectomy, directional**
AHA: 1Q, '01, 5; 3Q, '02, 5; 4Q, '03, 8

[N] **C1715 Brachytherapy needle**
AHA: 1Q, '01, 5; 3Q, '02, 5

[H] **C1716 Brachytherapy source, gold 198, per source** ⊘
AHA: 1Q, '01, 5; 3Q, '02, 5

[H] **C1717 Brachytherapy source, high dose rate iridium 192, per source**
AHA: 1Q, '01, 5; 3Q, '02, 5

[H] **C1718 Brachytherapy source, iodine 125, per source** ⊘
AHA: 1Q, '01, 5; 3Q, '02, 5; 1Q, '04, 2

[H] **C1719 Brachytherapy source, non-high dose rate iridium 192, per source** ⊘
AHA: 1Q, '01, 5; 3Q, '02, 5

[H] **C1720 Brachytherapy source, palladium 103, per source** ⊘
AHA: 1Q, '01, 5; 3Q, '02, 5; 1Q, '04, 2

[N] **C1721 Cardioverter-defibrillator, dual chamber (implantable)**
AHA: 1Q, '01, 5; 3Q, '02, 5

[N] **C1722 Cardioverter-defibrillator, single chamber (implantable)**
AHA: 1Q, '01, 5; 3Q, '02, 5

[N] **C1724 Catheter, transluminal atherectomy, rotational**
AHA: 1Q, '01, 5; 3Q, '02, 5; 4Q, '03, 8

Special Coverage Instructions | Noncovered by Medicare | Carrier Discretion | ☑ Quantity Alert | ● New Code | ○ Reinstated Code | ▲ Revised Code

2006 HCPCS | ■-🖵 ASC Groups | MED: Pub 100/NCD Reference | ⅃ DMEPOS Paid | ⊘ SNF Excluded | C Codes — 23

Outpatient PPS

C1725 — C1814

N   **C1725** Catheter, transluminal angioplasty, non-laser (may include guidance, infusion/perfusion capability)
AHA: 1Q, '01, 5; 3Q, '02, 5; 4Q, '03, 8

N   **C1726** Catheter, balloon dilatation, non-vascular
AHA: 1Q, '01, 5; 3Q, '02, 5

N   **C1727** Catheter, balloon tissue dissector, non-vascular (insertable)
AHA: 1Q, '01, 5; 3Q, '02, 5

N   **C1728** Catheter, brachytherapy seed administration
AHA: 1Q, '01, 5; 3Q, '02, 5

N   **C1729** Catheter, drainage
AHA: 1Q, '01, 5; 3Q, '02, 5

N   **C1730** Catheter, electrophysiology, diagnostic, other than 3D mapping (19 or fewer electrodes)
AHA: 1Q, '01, 5; 3Q, '01, 4, 5; 3Q, '02, 5

N   **C1731** Catheter, electrophysiology, diagnostic, other than 3D mapping (20 or more electrodes)
AHA: 1Q, '01, 5; 3Q, '02, 5

N   **C1732** Catheter, electrophysiology, diagnostic/ablation, 3D or vector mapping
AHA: 1Q, '01, 5; 3Q, '01, 53Q, '02, 5

N   **C1733** Catheter, electrophysiology, diagnostic/ablation, other than 3D or vector mapping, other than cool-tip
AHA: 3Q, '01, 4, 5; 1Q, '01, 5; 3Q, '02, 5

N   **C1750** Catheter, hemodialysis, long-term
AHA: 1Q, '01, 5; 3Q, '02, 5; 4Q, '03, 8

N   **C1751** Catheter, infusion, inserted peripherally, centrally or midline (other than hemodialysis)
AHA: 1Q, '01, 4, 5; 3Q, '01, 5; 3Q, '02, 5; 4Q, '03, 8

N   **C1752** Catheter, hemodialysis, short-term
AHA: 1Q, '01, 5; 3Q, '02, 5; 4Q, '03, 8

N   **C1753** Catheter, intravascular ultrasound
AHA: 1Q, '01, 5; 3Q, '02, 5; 4Q, '03, 8

N   **C1754** Catheter, intradiscal
AHA: 1Q, '01, 5; 3Q, '02, 5; 4Q, '03, 8

N   **C1755** Catheter, intraspinal
AHA: 1Q, '01, 5; 3Q, '02, 5; 4Q, '03, 8

N   **C1756** Catheter, pacing, transesophageal
AHA: 1Q, '01, 5; 3Q, '02, 5; 4Q, '03, 8

N   **C1757** Catheter, thrombectomy/embolectomy
AHA: 1Q, '01, 5; 3Q, '02, 5; 4Q, '03, 8

N   **C1758** Catheter, ureteral
AHA: 1Q, '01, 6; 3Q, '02, 5; 4Q, '03, 8

N   **C1759** Catheter, intracardiac echocardiography
AHA: 1Q, '01, 5; 3Q, '01, 4; 3Q, '02, 5; 4Q, '03, 8

N   **C1760** Closure device, vascular (implantable/insertable)
AHA: 1Q, '01, 6; 3Q, '02, 5; 4Q, '03, 8

N   **C1762** Connective tissue, human (includes fascia lata)
AHA: 1Q, '01, 6; 3Q, '02, 5; 3Q, '03, 12; 4Q, '03, 8

N   **C1763** Connective tissue, non-human (includes synthetic)
AHA: 1Q, '01, 6; 3Q, '02, 5; 3Q, '03, 12; 4Q, '03, 8

N   **C1764** Event recorder, cardiac (implantable)
AHA: 1Q, '01, 6; 3Q, '02, 5; 4Q, '03, 8

N   **C1765** Adhesion barrier   ⊘

N   **C1766** Introducer/sheath, guiding, intracardiac electrophysiological, steerable, other than peel-away
AHA: 3Q, '01, 5; 3Q, '02, 5

N   **C1767** Generator, neurostimulator (implantable)
AHA: 1Q, '01, 4, 6; 1Q, '02, 9; 3Q, '02, 5; 4Q, '03, 8

N   **C1768** Graft, vascular
AHA: 1Q, '01, 6; 3Q, '02, 5; 4Q, '03, 8

N   **C1769** Guide wire
AHA: 1Q, '01, 6; 3Q, '01, 4; 3Q, '02, 5; 4Q, '03, 8

N   **C1770** Imaging coil, magnetic resonance (insertable)
AHA: 1Q, '01, 6; 3Q, '02, 5; 4Q, '03, 8

N   **C1771** Repair device, urinary, incontinence, with sling graft
AHA: 1Q, '01, 6; 3Q, '01, 4, 5; 3Q, '02, 5; 4Q, '03, 8

N   **C1772** Infusion pump, programmable (implantable)
AHA: 1Q, '01, 6; 3Q, '02, 5

N   **C1773** Retrieval device, insertable (used to retrieve fractured medical devices)
AHA: 1Q, '01, 6; 3Q, '02, 5; 4Q, '03, 8

~~C1775 Supply of radiopharmaceutical diagnostic imaging agent, fluorodeoxyglucose f18 (2-deoxy-2 [18f] fluoro-d-glucose), per dose (4-40 mci/ml)~~
See code(s) A9552.

N   **C1776** Joint device (implantable)
AHA: 1Q, '01, 6; 3Q, '01, 5; 3Q, '02, 5

N   **C1777** Lead, cardioverter-defibrillator, endocardial single coil (implantable)
AHA: 1Q, '01, 6; 3Q, '02, 5

N   **C1778** Lead, neurostimulator (implantable)
AHA: 1Q, '01, 4, 6; 3Q, '02, 5; 1Q, '02, 9

N   **C1779** Lead, pacemaker, transvenous VDD single pass
AHA: 1Q, '01, 6; 3Q, '02, 5

N   **C1780** Lens, intraocular (new technology)
AHA: 1Q, '01, 6; 3Q, '02, 5

N   **C1781** Mesh (implantable)
AHA: 1Q, '01, 6; 3Q, '02, 5

N   **C1782** Morcellator
AHA: 1Q, '01, 6; 3Q, '02, 5

H   **C1783** Ocular implant, aqueous drainage assist device   ⊘

N   **C1784** Ocular device, intraoperative, detached retina
AHA: 1Q, '01, 6; 3Q, '02, 5

N   **C1785** Pacemaker, dual chamber, rate-responsive (implantable)
AHA: 1Q, '01, 6; 3Q, '02, 5; 4Q, '03, 8

N   **C1786** Pacemaker, single chamber, rate-responsive (implantable)
AHA: 1Q, '01, 6; 3Q, '02, 5; 4Q, '03, 8

N   **C1787** Patient programmer, neurostimulator
AHA: 1Q, '01, 6; 3Q, '02, 5; 4Q, '03, 8

N   **C1788** Port, indwelling (implantable)
AHA: 1Q, '01, 6; 3Q, '01, 4; 3Q, '02, 5; 4Q, '03, 8

N   **C1789** Prosthesis, breast (implantable)
AHA: 1Q, '01, 6; 3Q, '02, 5; 4Q, '03, 8

N   **C1813** Prosthesis, penile, inflatable
AHA: 1Q, '01, 6; 3Q, '02, 5; 4Q, '03, 8

H   **C1814** Retinal tamponade device, silicone oil   ⊘

Special Coverage Instructions   Noncovered by Medicare   Carrier Discretion   ☑ Quantity Alert   ● New Code   ○ Reinstated Code   ▲ Revised Code

24 — C Codes   A Age   M Maternity   ♀ Female Only   ♂ Male Only   A-Y APC Status Indicator   **2006 HCPCS**

Ⓝ　　**C1815** Prosthesis, urinary sphincter (implantable)
AHA: 1Q, '01, 6; 3Q, '02, 5; 4Q, '03, 8

Ⓝ　　**C1816** Receiver and/or transmitter, neurostimulator (implantable)
AHA: 1Q, '01, 6; 3Q, '02, 5; 4Q, '03, 8

Ⓝ　　**C1817** Septal defect implant system, intracardiac
AHA: 1Q, '01, 6; 3Q, '02, 5; 4Q, '03, 8

Ⓗ　　**C1818** Integrated keratoprosthesis　　⊘
AHA: 4Q, '03, 4

Ⓗ　　**C1819** Surgical tissue localization and excision device (implantable)
This code has been added, effective January 1, 2004.

Ⓝ　　**C1874** Stent, coated/covered, with delivery system
AHA: 1Q, '01, 6; 3Q, '01, 4, 5; 3Q, '02, 5, 9; 4Q, '03, 8

Ⓝ　　**C1875** Stent, coated/covered, without delivery system
AHA: 1Q, '01, 6; 3Q, '02, 5, 9; 4Q, '03, 8

Ⓝ　　**C1876** Stent, non-coated/non-covered, with delivery system
AHA: 1Q, '01, 6; 3Q, '01, 4, 5; 3Q, '01, 4; 3Q, '02, 5; 4Q, '03, 8

Ⓝ　　**C1877** Stent, non-coated/non-covered, without delivery system
AHA: 1Q, '01, 6; 3Q, '01, 4; 3Q, '02, 5; 4Q, '03, 8

Ⓝ　　**C1878** Material for vocal cord medialization, synthetic (implantable)
AHA: 1Q, '01, 6; 3Q, '02, 5

Ⓝ　　**C1879** Tissue marker (implantable)
AHA: 1Q, '01, 6; 3Q, '02, 5; 4Q, '03, 8

Ⓝ　　**C1880** Vena cava filter
AHA: 1Q, '01, 6; 3Q, '02, 5; 4Q, '03, 8

Ⓝ　　**C1881** Dialysis access system (implantable)
AHA: 1Q, '01, 6; 3Q, '02, 5; 4Q, '03, 8

Ⓝ　　**C1882** Cardioverter-defibrillator, other than single or dual chamber (implantable)
AHA: 1Q, '01, 5; 3Q, '02, 5

Ⓝ　　**C1883** Adaptor/extension, pacing lead or neurostimulator lead (implantable)
AHA: 1Q, '01, 5; 1Q, '02, 9; 3Q, '02, 5

Ⓗ　　**C1884** Embolization protective system　　⊘

Ⓝ　　**C1885** Catheter, transluminal angioplasty, laser
AHA: 1Q, '01, 5; 3Q, '02, 5; 4Q, '03, 8

Ⓝ　　**C1887** Catheter, guiding (may include infusion/perfusion capability)
AHA: 1Q, '01, 5; 3Q, '01, 4, 5; 3Q, '02, 5

Ⓗ　　**C1888** Catheter, ablation, non-cardiac, endovascular (implantable)　　⊘

Ⓝ　　**C1891** Infusion pump, non-programmable, permanent (implantable)
AHA: 1Q, '01, 6; 3Q, '02, 5; 4Q, '03, 8

Ⓝ　　**C1892** Introducer/sheath, guiding, intracardiac electrophysiological, fixed-curve, peel-away
AHA: 1Q, '01, 6; 3Q, '02, 5

Ⓝ　　**C1893** Introducer/sheath, guiding, intracardiac electrophysiological, fixed-curve, other than peel-away
AHA: 1Q, '01, 6; 3Q, '01, 4; 3Q, '02, 5

Ⓝ　　**C1894** Introducer/sheath, othe than guiding, intracardiac electrophysiological, non-laser
AHA: 1Q, '01, 4, 6; 3Q, '02, 5

Ⓝ　　**C1895** Lead, cardioverter-defibrillator, endocardial dual coil (implantable)
AHA: 1Q, '01, 6; 3Q, '02, 5

Ⓝ　　**C1896** Lead, cardioverter-defibrillator, other than endocardial single or dual coil (implantable)
AHA: 1Q, '01, 6; 3Q, '02, 5

Ⓝ　　**C1897** Lead, neurostimulator test kit (implantable)
AHA: 1Q, '01, 6; 1Q, '02, 9; 3Q, '02, 5

Ⓝ　　**C1898** Lead, pacemaker, other than transvenous VDD single pass
AHA: 1Q, '01, 6; 3Q, '01, 4; 3Q, '02, 5, 8

Ⓝ　　**C1899** Lead, pacemaker/cardioverter-defibrillator combination (implantable)
AHA: 1Q, '01, 6; 3Q, '02, 5

Ⓗ　　**C1900** Lead, left ventricular coronary venous system　　⊘

Ⓗ　　**C2614** Probe, percutaneous lumbar discectomy　　⊘

Ⓝ　　**C2615** Sealant, pulmonary, liquid
AHA: 1Q, '01, 6; 3Q, '02, 5

Ⓗ　　**C2616** Brachytherapy source, yttrium 90, per source　　⊘
AHA: 3Q, '02, 5; 3Q, '03, 11

Ⓝ　　**C2617** Stent, non-coronary, temporary, without delivery system
AHA: 1Q, '01, 6; 3Q, '02, 5; 4Q, '03, 8

Ⓝ　　**C2618** Probe, cryoablation　　⊘
AHA: 1Q, '01, 6; 3Q, '02, 5; 4Q, '03, 8

Ⓝ　　**C2619** Pacemaker, dual chamber, non-rate-responsive (implantable)
AHA: 1Q, '01, 6; 3Q, '01, 4; 3Q, '02, 5

Ⓝ　　**C2620** Pacemaker, single chamber, non-rate-responsive (implantabe)
AHA: 1Q, '01, 6; 3Q, '02, 5; 4Q, '03, 8

Ⓝ　　**C2621** Pacemaker, other than single or dual chamber (implantable)
AHA: 1Q, '01, 6; 3Q, '02, 5, 8; 4Q, '03, 8

Ⓝ　　**C2622** Prosthesis, penile, non-inflatable
AHA: 1Q, '01, 6; 3Q, '02, 5; 4Q, '03, 8

Ⓝ　　**C2625** Stent, non-coronary, temporary, with delivery system
AHA: 1Q, '01, 6; 3Q, '02, 5; 4Q, '03, 8

Ⓝ　　**C2626** Infusion pump, non-programmable, temporary (implantable)
AHA: 1Q, '01, 6; 3Q, '02, 5

Ⓝ　　**C2627** Catheter, suprapubic/cystoscopic
AHA: 1Q, '01, 5; 3Q, '02, 5; 4Q, '03, 8

Ⓝ　　**C2628** Catheter, occlusion
AHA: 1Q, '01, 5; 3Q, '02, 5; 4Q, '03, 8

Ⓝ　　**C2629** Introducer/sheath, other than guiding, intracardiac electrophysiological, laser
AHA: 1Q, '01, 6; 3Q, '02, 5

Ⓝ　　**C2630** Catheter, electrophysiology, diagnostic/ablation, other than 3D or vector mapping, cool-tip
AHA: 1Q, '01, 5; 3Q, '02, 5

Ⓝ　　**C2631** Repair device, urinary, incontinence, without sling graft
AHA: 1Q, '01, 6; 3Q, '02, 5; 4Q, '03, 8

Ⓗ　☑　**C2632** Brachytherapy solution, iodine 125, per mci　　⊘

Ⓗ　　**C2633** Brachytherapy source, cesium 131, per sources

Special Coverage Instructions　　Noncovered by Medicare　　Carrier Discretion　　☑ Quantity Alert　　● New Code　　○ Reinstated Code　　▲ Revised Code

2006 HCPCS　　🔢-🔢 ASC Groups　　MED: Pub 100/NCD Reference　　♿ DMEPOS Paid　　⊘ SNF Excluded　　**C Codes — 25**

Outpatient PPS

C2634 — C9202

▲ Ⓗ **C2634** Brachytherapy source, high-activity, Iodine-125, greater than 1.01 mCi (NIST), per source
AHA: 2Q, '05, 8

▲ Ⓗ **C2635** Brachytherapy source, high-activity, Paladium-103, greater than 2.2 mCi (NIST), per source
AHA: 2Q, '05, 8

Ⓗ **C2636** Brachytherapy linear source, palladium 103, per 1 mm

● Ⓗ **C2637** Brachytherapy source, ytterbium-169, per source
AHA: 3Q, '05, 7

Ⓢ **C8900** Magnetic resonance angiography with contrast, abdomen

Ⓢ **C8901** Magnetic resonance angiography without contrast, abdomen

Ⓢ **C8902** Magnetic resonance angiography without contrast followed by with contrast, abdomen

Ⓢ **C8903** Magnetic resonance imaging with contrast, breast; unilateral

Ⓢ **C8904** Magnetic resonance imaging without contrast, breast; unilateral

Ⓢ **C8905** Magnetic resonance imaging without contrast followed by with contrast, breast; unilateral

Ⓢ **C8906** Magnetic resonance imaging with contrast, breast; bilateral

Ⓢ **C8907** Magnetic resonance imaging without contrast, breast; bilateral

Ⓢ **C8908** Magnetic resonance imaging without contrast followed by with contrast, breast; bilateral

Ⓢ **C8909** Magnetic resonance angiography with contrast, chest (excluding myocardium)

Ⓢ **C8910** Magnetic resonance angiography without contrast, chest (excluding myocardium)

Ⓢ **C8911** Magnetic resonance angiography without contrast followed by with contrast, chest (excluding myocardium)

Ⓢ **C8912** Magnetic resonance angiography with contrast, lower extremity

Ⓢ **C8913** Magnetic resonance angiography without contrast, lower extremity

Ⓢ **C8914** Magnetic resonance angiography without contrast followed by with contrast, lower extremity

Ⓢ **C8918** Magnetic resonance angiography with contrast, pelvis
AHA: 4Q, '03, 4

Ⓢ **C8919** Magnetic resonance angiography without contrast, pelvis
AHA: 4Q, '03, 4

Ⓢ **C8920** Magnetic resonance angiography without contrast followed by with contrast, pelvis
AHA: 4Q, '03, 4

● Ⓢ **C8950** Intravenous infusion for therapy/diagnosis; up to 1 hour

● Ⓝ **C8951** Intravenous infusion for therapy/diagnosis; each additional hour (List separately in addition to C8950

● Ⓧ **C8952** Therapeutic, prophylactic or diagnostic injection; intravenous push

● Ⓢ **C8953** Chemotherapy administration, intravenous; push technique

● Ⓢ **C8954** Chemotherapy administration, intravenous; infusion technique, up to one hour

● Ⓝ **C8955** Chemotherapy administration, intravenous; infusion technique, each additional hour (List separately in addition to C8954)

● Ⓣ **C8956** Refilling and maintenance of portable or implantable pump or reservoir for drug delivery for therapy/diagnosis, systemic (e.g. intravenous, intra-arterial)

● Ⓢ **C8957** Intravenous infusion for therapy/diagnosis; initiation of prolonged infusion (more than 8 hours), requiring the use of portable or implantable pump

~~C9000~~ ~~Injection, sodium chromate Cr 51, per 0.25 millicurie~~
See code(s) A9553.

Ⓚ **C9003** Palivizumab-RSV-igM, per 50 mg ⊘
Use this code for Palivizumab, Synagis.

~~C9007~~ ~~Baclofen intrathecal screening kit (1 amp)~~
See code(s) J0476.

~~C9008~~ ~~Baclofen intrathecal refill kit, per 500 mcg~~
See code(s) J0475.

~~C9000~~ ~~Baclofen intrathecal refill kit, per 2000 mcg~~
See code(s) J0475.

~~C9013~~ ~~Supply of Co 57 cobaltous chloride, radiopharmaceutical diagnostic imaging agent~~
See code(s) A9559.

~~C9102~~ ~~Supply of radiopharmaceutical diagnostic imaging agent, 51 sodium chromate, per 50 mCi~~
See code(s) A9553.

~~C9103~~ ~~Supply of radiopharmaceutical diagnostic imaging agent, sodium iothalamate I 125 injection, per 10 μCi~~
See code(s) A9554.

~~C9105~~ ~~Injection, hepatitis B immune globulin, per 1 ml~~
See code(s) 90371.

~~C9112~~ ~~Injection, perflutren lipid microsphere, per 2 ml vial~~
See code(s) Q9957.

Ⓖ **C9113** Injection, pantoprazole sodium, per vial ⊘
Use this code for Protonix.

Ⓖ **C9121** Injection, argatroban, per 5 mg ⊘
Use this code for Acova.

~~C9123~~ ~~Human fibroblast derived temporary skin substitute, per 247 sq. cm~~
See code(s) J7342.

~~C9126~~ ~~Injection natalizumab per 5 mg~~

~~C9127~~ ~~Injection, paclitaxel protein-bound particles, per 1 mg~~
See code(s) J9264.

~~C9128~~ ~~Injection, pegaptanib dodium, per 0.3 mg~~
See code(s) J2503.

~~C9129~~ ~~Injection, clofarabine, per 1 mg~~
See code(s) J9027.

~~C9200~~ ~~Bilayered cellular matrix, per 36 sq. cm.~~
See code(s) J7340.

~~C9201~~ ~~Dermagraft, per 37.5 sq. cm.~~
See code(s) J7342.

~~C9202~~ ~~Injection, suspension of microspheres of human serum albumin with octafluoropropane, per 3 ml~~
See code(s) Q9956.

~~C9203 Injection, perflexane lipid microspheres, per 10 ml vial~~
See code(s) Q9955.

~~C9205 Injection, oxaliplatin, per 5 mg~~
See code(s) J9263.

~~C9206 Collagen glycosaminoglycan bilayer matrix, per cm2~~
See code(s) J7343.

~~C9211 Injection, alefacept, for intravenous use, per 7.5 mg~~
See code(s) J0215.

~~C9212 Injection, alefacept, for intramuscular use, per 7.5 mg~~
See code(s) J0215.

~~C9218 Injection, azacitidine, per 1 mg~~
See code(s) J9025.

C9220 Sodium hyaluronate per 30 mg dose, for intra-articular injection
Use this code for Hyalgan, Orthovisc, Supartz.

C9221 Acellular dermal tissue matrix, per 16 cm²
Use this code for Graftjacket Regular Matrix.

C9222 Decellularized soft tissue scaffold, per 1 cc
Use this code for Graftjacket Soft Tissue Matrix.

~~C9223 Injection adenosine for diagnostic or therapeutic use, 6 mg (not to be used to report any adenosine phosphate compounds, instead use A9270)~~
See code(s) J0150, J0152.

● K C9224 Injection, galsulfase, per 5 mg
Use this code for Naglazyme.
AHA: 3Q, '05, 7

● G C9225 Injection, fluocinolone acetonide intravitreal implant, per 0.59 mg
Use this code for Retisert.
AHA: 3Q, '05, 7

~~C9226 Injection, ziconotide for intrathecal infusion, per 5 mcg~~
See code(s) J2278.

A C9399 Unclassified drugs or biologicals

~~C9400 Supply of radiopharmaceutical diagnostic imaging agent, thallous chloride Tl 201, per mCi, brand name~~
See code(s) A9505.

~~C9401 Supply of therapeutic radiopharmaceutical, strontium 89 chloride, brand name, per mCi~~
See code(s) A9600.

~~C9402 Supply of radiopharmaceutical therapeutic imaging agent, I 131 sodium iodide capsule, per mCi, brand name~~
See code(s) A9517.

~~C9403 Supply of radiopharmaceutical diagnostic agent, I-131 sodium iodide capsule, per mCi~~
See code(s) A9528.

~~C9404 Supply of radiopharmaceutical diagnostic agent, I-131 sodium iodide solution, per mCi, brand name~~
See code(s) A9529.

~~C9405 Supply of radiopharmaceutical therapeutic agent, I-131 sodium iodide solution, per mCi, brand name~~
See code(s) A9530.

~~C9410 Injection, dexrazoxane HCl, per 250 mg, brand name~~
See code(s) J1190.

~~C9411 Injection, pamidronate disodium, per 30 mg, brand name~~
See code(s) J2430.

~~C9413 Sodium hyaluronate, per 20 to 25 mg dose for intra-articular injection, brand name~~
See code(s) J7317.

~~C9414 Etoposide, oral, 50 mg, brand name~~
See code(s) J8560.

~~C9415 Doxorubicin HCl, 10 mg, brand name~~
See code(s) J9000.

~~C9417 Bleomycin sulfate, 15 units, brand name~~
See code(s) J9040.

~~C9418 Cisplatin, powder or solution, per 10 mg, brand name~~
See code(s) J9060.

~~C9419 Injection, cladribine, per 1 mg, brand name~~
See code(s) J9065.

~~C9420 Cyclophosphamide, 100 mg, brand name~~
See code(s) J9070.

~~C9421 Cyclophosphamide, lyophilized, 100 mg, brand name~~
See code(s) J9093.

~~C9422 Cytarabine, 100 mg, brand name~~
See code(s) J9100.

~~C9423 Dacarbazine, 100 mg, brand name~~
See code(s) J9130.

~~C9424 Daunorubicin, 10 mg~~
See code(s) J9150.

~~C9425 Etoposide, 10 mg, brand name~~
See code(s) J9181.

~~C9426 Floxuridine, 500 mg, brand name~~
See code(s) J9200.

~~C9427 Ifosfamide, 1 gm, brand name~~
See code(s) J9208.

~~C9428 Mesna, 200 mg, brand name~~
See code(s) J9209.

~~C9429 Idarubicin HCl, 5 mg, brand name~~
See code(s) J9211.

~~C9430 Leuprolide acetate, per 1 mg, brand name~~
See code(s) J9218.

~~C9431 Paclitaxel, 30 mg, brand name~~
See code(s) J9265.

~~C9432 Mitomycin, 5 mg, brand name~~
See code(s) J9280.

~~C9433 Thiotepa, 15 mg, brand name~~
See code(s) J9340.

~~C9435 Injection, gonadorelin HCl, brand name, per 100 mcg~~
See code(s) J1620.

~~C9436 Azathioprine, parenteral, brand name, per 100 mg~~
See code(s) J7501.

~~C9437 Carmustine, brand name, 100 mg~~
See code(s) J9050.

~~C9438 Cyclosporine, oral, 100 mg, brand name~~
See code(s) J7502.

~~C9439 Diethylstilbestrol diphosphate, brand name, 250 mg~~
See code(s) J9165.

Special Coverage Instructions   Noncovered by Medicare   Carrier Discretion   ☑ Quantity Alert   ● New Code   ○ Reinstated Code   ▲ Revised Code

2006 HCPCS   1-9 ASC Groups   MED: Pub 100/NCD Reference   ⅃ DMEPOS Paid   ⊘ SNF Excluded   C Codes — 27

~~C9440　Vinorelbine tartrate, brand name, per 10 mg~~
　　　See code(s) J9390.

~~C9704　Injection or insertion of inert substance for submucosal/intramuscular injection(s) into the upper gastrointestinal tract, under fluoroscopic guidance~~
　　　See code(s) 0133T.

~~C9713　Noncontact laser vaporization of prostate, including coagulation control of intraoperative and postoperative bleeding~~
　　　See code(s) 52648.

[S]　C9716　Creations of thermal anal lesions by radiofrequency energy

~~C9718　Kyphoplasty, one vertebral body, unilateral or bilateral injection~~
　　　See code(s) 22523.

~~C9719　Kyphoplasty, one vertebral body, unilateral or bilateral injection; each additional vertebral body (list separately in addition to code for primary procedure)~~
　　　See code(s) 22525.

~~C9720　High energy (greater than 0.22mj/mm2) extracorporeal shock wave (ESW) treatment for chronic lateral epicondylitis (tennis elbow)~~
　　　See code(s) 0102T.

~~C9721　High energy (greater than 0.22mj/mm2) extracorporeal shock wave (ESW) treatment for chronic plantar fasciitis~~
　　　See code(s) 28890.

~~C9722　Stereoscopic kilovolt x ray imaging with infrared tracking for localization of target volume (do not report C9722 in conjunction with G0173, G0243, G0251, G0339 or G0340)~~
　　　See code(s) 77421.

●　[S]　C9723　Dynamic infrared blood perfusion imaging (DIRI)

●　[T]　C9724　Endoscopic full-thickness plication in the gastric cardia using endoscopic plication system (EPS); includes endoscopy

●　[S]　C9725　Placement of endorectal intracavitary applicator for high intensity brachytherapy
　　　AHA: 3Q, '05, 7

Special Coverage Instructions　　　Noncovered by Medicare　　　Carrier Discretion　　　☑ Quantity Alert　● New Code　○ Reinstated Code　▲ Revised Code

28 — C Codes　　　Ⓐ Age　　　Ⓜ Maternity　　　♀ Female Only　　　♂ Male Only　　　Ⓐ-Ⓨ APC Status Indicator　　　2006 HCPCS

DENTAL PROCEDURES *D0000-D9999*

The D, or dental, codes are a separate category of national codes. The Current Dental Terminology (CDT-2005) code set is copyrighted by the American Dental Association (ADA). CDT-2005 is included in HCPCS Level II. Decisions regarding the modification, deletion, or addition of CDT-2005 codes are made by the ADA and not the national panel responsible for the administration of HCPCS.

The Department of Health and Human Services has an agreement with the AMA pertaining to the use of the CPT codes for physician services; it also has an agreement with the ADA to include CDT-2005 as a set of HCPCS Level II codes for use in billing for dental services.

DIAGNOSTIC D0100-D0999

CLINICAL ORAL EVALUATION

All dental codes fall under the jurisdiction of the Medicare local contractor.

E   **D0120** Periodic oral examination
This procedure is covered if its purpose is to identify a patient's existing infections prior to kidney transplantation.

E   **D0140** Limited oral evaluation — problem focused

S   **D0150** Comprehensive oral evaluation — new or established patient
This procedure is covered if its purpose is to identify a patient's existing infections prior to kidney transplantation.
MED: 100-2, 15, 150; 100-2, 16, 140; 100-3, 260.6

E   **D0160** Detailed and extensive oral evaluation — problem focused, by report
Pertinent documentation to evaluate medical appropriateness should be included when this code is reported.

E   **D0170** Re-evaluation — limited, problem focused (established patient; not postoperative visit)

E   **D0180** Comprehensive periodontal evaluation — new or established patient
See also equivalent CPT E&M codes.

RADIOGRAPHS

E   **D0210** Intraoral — complete series (including bitewings)
See code(s): 70320

E ☑ **D0220** Intraoral — periapical, first film
See code(s): 70300

E ☑ **D0230** Intraoral — periapical, each additional film
See code(s): 70310

S   **D0240** Intraoral — occlusal film
MED: 100-2, 15, 150; 100-2, 16, 140

S ☑ **D0250** Extraoral — first film
MED: 100-2, 15, 150; 100-2, 16, 140

S ☑ **D0260** Extraoral — each additional film
MED: 100-2, 15, 150; 100-2, 16, 140

S ☑ **D0270** Bitewing — single film
MED: 100-2, 15, 150; 100-2, 16, 140

S ☑ **D0272** Bitewings — two films
MED: 100-2, 15, 150; 100-2, 16, 140

S ☑ **D0274** Bitewings — four films
MED: 100-2, 15, 150; 100-2, 16, 140

S ☑ **D0277** Vertical bitewings — 7 to 8 films
MED: 100-2, 15, 150; 100-2, 16, 140

E   **D0290** Posterior-anterior or lateral skull and facial bone survey film
See code(s): 70150

E   **D0310** Sialography
See code(s): 70390

E   **D0320** Temporomandibular joint arthrogram, including injection
See code(s): 70332

E   **D0321** Other temporomandibular joint films, by report
See code(s): 76499

E   **D0322** Tomographic survey
MED: 100-3, 260.6

E   **D0330** Panoramic film
See code(s): 70320

E   **D0340** Cephalometric film
See code(s): 70350

E   **D0350** Oral/facial photographic images
This code excludes conventional radiographs.

TEST AND LABORATORY EXAMINATIONS

E   **D0415** Collection of microorganisms for culture and sensitivity
This procedure is covered if its purpose is to identify a patient's existing infections prior to kidney transplantation.
See code(s): D0410

D0416 Viral culture

D0421 Genetic test for susceptibility to oral diseases

E   **D0425** Caries susceptibility tests
This procedure is covered by Medicare if its purpose is to identify a patient's existing infections prior to kidney transplantation.
See code(s): D0420

D0431 Adjunctive pre-diagnostic test that aids in detection of mucosal abnormalities including premalignant and malignant lesions, not to include cytology or biopsy procedures

S   **D0460** Pulp vitality tests
This procedure is covered by Medicare if its purpose is to identify a patient's existing infections prior to kidney transplantation.
MED: 100-2, 15, 150; 100-2, 16, 140; 100-3, 260.6

E   **D0470** Diagnostic casts

S   **D0472** Accession of tissue, gross examination, preparation and transmission of written report
MED: 100-2, 15, 150; 100-2, 16, 140; 100-3, 260.6

S   **D0473** Accession of tissue, gross and microscopic examination, preparation and transmission of written report
MED: 100-2, 15, 150; 100-2, 16, 140; 100-3, 260.6

S   **D0474** Accession of tissue, gross and microscopic examination, including assessment of surgical margins for presence of disease, preparation and transmission of written report
MED: 100-2, 15, 150; 100-2, 16, 140; 100-3, 260.6

D0475 Decalcification procedure

D0476 Special stains for microorganisms

D0477 Special stains, not for microorganisms

D0478 Immunohistochemical stains

D0479 Tissue in-situ hybridization, including interpretation

Special Coverage Instructions   Noncovered by Medicare   Carrier Discretion   ☑ Quantity Alert   ● New Code   ○ Reinstated Code   ▲ Revised Code

2006 HCPCS   ❶-❾ ASC Groups   MED: Pub 100/NCD Reference   ♿ DMEPOS Paid   ⊘ SNF Excluded   **D Codes — 29**

Dental Procedures

D0120 — D0479

Dental Procedures

D0480 — D2722

S D0480 Processing and interpretation of exfoliative cytologic smears, including the preparation and transmission of written report
MED: 100-2, 15, 150; 100-2, 16, 140; 100-3, 260.6

D0481 Electron microscopy — diagnostic

D0482 Direct immunofluorescence

D0483 Indirect immunofluorescence

D0484 Consultation on slides prepared elsewhere

D0485 Consultation, including preparation of slides from biopsy material supplied by referring source

S D0502 Other oral pathology procedures, by report
Pertinent documentation to evaluate medical appropriateness should be included when this code is reported. This procedure is covered by Medicare if its purpose is to identify a patient's existing infections prior to kidney transplantation.
MED: 100-2, 15, 150; 100-2, 16, 140; 100-3, 260.6

S D0999 Unspecified diagnostic procedure, by report
Determine if an alternative HCPCS Level II or a CPT code better describes the service being reported. This code should be used only if a more specific code is unavailable.
MED: 100-2, 15, 150; 100-2, 16, 140; 100-3, 260.6

PREVENTIVE D1000-D1999

DENTAL PROPHYLAXIS

E D1110 Prophylaxis — adult A

E D1120 Prophylaxis — child A

TOPICAL FLUORIDE TREATMENT (OFFICE PROCEDURE)

E D1201 Topical application of fluoride (including prophylaxis) — child A

E D1203 Topical application of fluoride (prophylaxis not included) — child A

E D1204 Topical application of fluoride (prophylaxis not included) — adult A

E D1205 Topical application of fluoride (including prophylaxis) — adult A
See code(s): D1202

OTHER PREVENTIVE SERVICES

E D1310 Nutritional counseling for control of dental disease
MED: 100-2, 16, 10

E D1320 Tobacco counseling for the control and prevention of oral disease
MED: 100-2, 16, 10

E D1330 Oral hygiene instructions
MED: 100-2, 16, 10

E ☑ D1351 Sealant — per tooth

SPACE MAINTENANCE (PASSIVE APPLIANCES)

S D1510 Space maintainer — fixed-unilateral
MED: 100-2, 16, 140

S D1515 Space maintainer — fixed-bilateral
MED: 100-2, 15, 150; 100-2, 16, 140

S D1520 Space maintainer — removable-unilateral
MED: 100-2, 15, 150; 100-2, 16, 140

S D1525 Space maintainer — removable-bilateral
MED: 100-2, 15, 150; 100-2, 16, 140

S D1550 Recementation of space maintainer
MED: 100-2, 15, 150; 100-2, 16, 140

E ☑ D2140 Amalgam — one surface, primary or permanent

E ☑ D2150 Amalgam — two surfaces, primary or permanent

E ☑ D2160 Amalgam — three surfaces, primary or permanent

E ☑ D2161 Amalgam — four or more surfaces, primary or permanent

RESIN RESTORATIONS

E ☑ D2330 Resin-based composite — one surface, anterior

E ☑ D2331 Resin-based composite — two surfaces, anterior

E ☑ D2332 Resin-based composite — three surfaces, anterior

E ☑ D2335 Resin-based composite — four or more surfaces or involving incisal angle (anterior)

E D2390 Resin-based composite crown, anterior

E D2391 Resin-based composite — one surface, posterior

E D2392 Resin-based composite — two surfaces, posterior

E D2393 Resin-based composite — three surfaces, posterior

E D2394 Resin-based composite — four or more surfaces, posterior

GOLD FOIL RESTORATIONS

E ☑ D2410 Gold foil — one surface

E ☑ D2420 Gold foil — two surfaces

E ☑ D2430 Gold foil — three surfaces

INLAY/ONLAY RESTORATIONS

E ☑ D2510 Inlay — metallic — one surface

E ☑ D2520 Inlay — metallic — two surfaces

E ☑ D2530 Inlay — metallic — three or more surfaces

E ☑ D2542 Onlay — metallic — two surfaces

E ☑ D2543 Onlay — metallic — three surfaces

E ☑ D2544 Onlay — metallic — four or more surfaces

E ☑ D2610 Inlay — porcelain/ceramic — one surface

E ☑ D2620 Inlay — porcelain/ceramic — two surfaces

E ☑ D2630 Inlay — porcelain/ceramic — three or more surfaces

E ☑ D2642 Onlay — porcelain/ceramic — two surfaces

E ☑ D2643 Onlay — porcelain/ceramic — three surfaces

E ☑ D2644 Onlay — porcelain/ceramic — four or more surfaces

E ☑ D2650 Inlay — resin-based composite composite/resin — one surface

E ☑ D2651 Inlay — resin-based composite composite/resin — two surfaces

E ☑ D2652 Inlay — resin-based composite composite/resin — three or more surfaces

E ☑ D2662 Onlay — resin-based composite composite/resin — two surfaces

E ☑ D2663 Onlay — resin-based composite composite/resin — three surfaces

E ☑ D2664 Onlay — resin-based composite composite/resin — four or more surfaces

CROWNS — SINGLE RESTORATION ONLY

E D2710 Crown — resin-based composite (indirect)

D2712 Crown — 3/4 resin-based composite (indirect)

E D2720 Crown — resin with high noble metal

E D2721 Crown — resin with predominantly base metal

E D2722 Crown — resin with noble metal

Special Coverage Instructions | Noncovered by Medicare | Carrier Discretion | ☑ Quantity Alert | ● New Code | ○ Reinstated Code | ▲ Revised Code

30 — D Codes | A Age | M Maternity | ♀ Female Only | ♂ Male Only | A-Y APC Status Indicator | **2006 HCPCS**

E	D2740	Crown — porcelain/ceramic substrate
E	D2750	Crown — porcelain fused to high noble metal
E	D2751	Crown — porcelain fused to predominantly base metal
E	D2752	Crown — porcelain fused to noble metal
E	D2780	Crown — 3/4 cast high noble metal
E	D2781	Crown — 3/4 cast predominately base metal
E	D2782	Crown — 3/4 cast noble metal
E	D2783	Crown — 3/4 porcelain/ceramic
E	D2790	Crown — full cast high noble metal
E	D2791	Crown — full cast predominantly base metal
E	D2792	Crown — full cast noble metal
	D2794	Crown — titanium
E	D2799	Provisional crown

Do not use this code to report a temporary crown for routine prosthetic restoration.

OTHER RESTORATIVE SERVICES

E	D2910	Recement inlay, onlay or partial coverage restoration
	D2915	Recement cast or prefabricated post and core
E	D2920	Recement crown
E	D2930	Prefabricated stainless steel crown — primary tooth
E	D2931	Prefabricated stainless steel crown — permanent tooth
E	D2932	Prefabricated resin crown
E	D2933	Prefabricated stainless steel crown with resin window
	D2934	Prefabricated esthetic coated stainless steel crown — primary tooth
E	D2940	Sedative filling
E	D2950	Core buildup, including any pins
E	D2951	Pin retention — per tooth, in addition to restoration
E	D2952	Cast post and core in addition to crown
E	D2953	Each additional cast post — same tooth

Report in addition to code D2952.

E	D2954	Prefabricated post and core in addition to crown
E	D2955	Post removal (not in conjunction with endodontic therapy)
E	D2957	Each additional prefabricated post — same tooth

Report in addition to code D2954.

E	D2960	Labial veneer (resin laminate) — chairside
E	D2961	Labial veneer (resin laminate) — laboratory
E	D2962	Labial veneer (porcelain laminate) — laboratory
	D2971	Additional procedures to construct new crown under existing partial denture framework
	D2975	Coping
E	D2980	Crown repair, by report

Pertinent documentation to evaluate medical appropriateness should be included when this code is reported.

S	D2999	Unspecified restorative procedure, by report

Determine if an alternative HCPCS Level II or a CPT code better describes the service being reported. This code should be used only if a more specific code is unavailable.

MED: 100-2, 15, 150; 100-2, 16, 140

ENDODONTICS D3000-D3999

PULP CAPPING

E	D3110	Pulp cap — direct (excluding final restoration)
E	D3120	Pulp cap — indirect (excluding final restoration)

PULPOTOMY

E	D3220	Therapeutic pulpotomy (excluding final restoration) — removal of pulp coronal to the dentinocemental junction and application of medicament

Do not use this code to report the first stage of root canal therapy.

E	D3221	Pulpal debridement, primary and permanent teeth

PULPAL THERAPY ON PRIMARY TEETH (INCLUDES PRIMARY TEETH WITH SUCCEDANEOUS TEETH AND PLACEMENT OF RESORBABLE FILLING)

E	D3230	Pulpal therapy (resorbable filling) — anterior, primary tooth (excluding final restoration)
E	D3240	Pulpal therapy (resorbable filling) — posterior, primary tooth (excluding final restoration)

ROOT CANAL THERAPY (INCLUDING TREATMENT PLAN, CLINICAL PROCEDURES, AND FOLLOW-UP CARE, INCLUDES PRIMARY TEETH WITHOUT SUCCEDANEOUS TEETH AND PERMANENT TEETH)

E	D3310	Anterior (excluding final restoration)
E	D3320	Bicuspid (excluding final restoration)
E	D3330	Molar (excluding final restoration)
E	D3331	Treatment of root canal obstruction; non-surgical access
E	D3332	Incomplete endodontic therapy; inoperable, unrestorable or fractured tooth
E	D3333	Internal root repair of perforation defects
E	D3346	Retreatment of previous root canal therapy — anterior
E	D3347	Retreatment of previous root canal therapy — bicuspid
E	D3348	Retreatment of previous root canal therapy — molar
E	D3351	Apexification/recalcification — initial visit (apical closure/calcific repair of perforations, root resorption, etc.)
E	D3352	Apexification/recalcification — interim medication replacement (apical closure/calcific repair of perforations, root resorption, etc.)
E	D3353	Apexification/recalcification — final visit (includes completed root canal therapy — apical closure/calcific repair of perforations, root resorption, etc.)

APICOECTOMY/PERIRADICULAR SERVICES

E		D3410	Apicoectomy/periradicular surgery — anterior
E		D3421	Apicoectomy/periradicular surgery — bicuspid (first root)
E		D3425	Apicoectomy/periradicular surgery — molar (first root)
E	☑	D3426	Apicoectomy/periradicular surgery (each additional root)
E	☑	D3430	Retrograde filling — per root
E	☑	D3450	Root amputation — per root

Special Coverage Instructions   Noncovered by Medicare   Carrier Discretion   ☑ Quantity Alert   ● New Code   ○ Reinstated Code   ▲ Revised Code

2006 HCPCS   ⬛-⑨ ASC Groups   MED: Pub 100/NCD Reference   ♿ DMEPOS Paid   ⊘ SNF Excluded   **D Codes — 31**

Dental Procedures

D3460 — D5140

D3460 Endodontic endosseous implant
MED: 100-2, 15, 150; 100-2, 16, 140

D3470 Intentional reimplantation (including necessary splinting)

OTHER ENDODONTIC PROCEDURES

D3910 Surgical procedure for isolation of tooth with rubber dam

D3920 Hemisection (including any root removal), not including root canal therapy

D3950 Canal preparation and fitting of preformed dowel or post

⒮ D3999 Unspecified endodontic procedure, by report
Determine if an alternative HCPCS Level II or a CPT code better describes the service being reported. This code should be used only if a more specific code is unavailable.
MED: 100-2, 15, 150; 100-2, 16, 140

PERIODONTICS D4000-D4999

SURGICAL SERVICES (INCLUDING USUAL POSTOPERATIVE SERVICES)

Ⓔ ☑ D4210 Gingivectomy or gingivoplasty — four or more contiguous teeth or bounded teeth spaces per quadrant
See code(s): 41820

Ⓔ ☑ D4211 Gingivectomy or gingivoplasty — one to three contiguous teeth or bounded teeth spaces per quadrant
See also CPT code (64400-64530).

Ⓔ ☑ D4240 Gingival flap procedure, including root planing — four or more contiguous teeth or bounded teeth spaces per quadrant

Ⓔ D4241 Gingival flap procedure, including root planing — one to three contiguous teeth or bounded teeth spaces per quadrant
See also D4240.

Ⓔ D4245 Apically positioned flap

Ⓔ D4249 Clinical crown lengthening — hard tissue

⒮ ☑ D4260 Osseous surgery (including flap entry and closure) — four or more contiguous teeth or bounded teeth spaces per quadrant
MED: 100-2, 15, 150; 100-2, 16, 140

Ⓔ D4261 Osseous surgery (including flap entry and closure) — one to three contiguous teeth or bounded teeth spaces per quadrant
See CPT code 41823.

⒮ ☑ D4263 Bone replacement graft — first site in quadrant
MED: 100-2, 15, 150; 100-2, 16, 140; 100-3, 260.6

⒮ ☑ D4264 Bone replacement graft — each additional site in quadrant (use if performed on same date of service as D4263)
MED: 100-2, 15, 150; 100-2, 16, 140; 100-3, 260.6

Ⓔ D4265 Biologic materials to aid in soft and osseous tissue regeneration

Ⓔ ☑ D4266 Guided tissue regeneration — resorbable barrier, per site

Ⓔ ☑ D4267 Guided tissue regeneration — nonresorbable barrier, per site (includes membrane removal)

⒮ ☑ D4268 Surgical revision procedure, per tooth
MED: 100-2, 15, 150; 100-2, 16, 140

⒮ D4270 Pedicle soft tissue graft procedure
MED: 100-2, 15, 150; 100-2, 16, 140

⒮ D4271 Free soft tissue graft procedure (including donor site surgery)
MED: 100-2, 15, 150; 100-2, 16, 140

⒮ D4273 Subepithelial connective tissue graft procedures, per tooth
For tissue grafts, see CPT 15000 and related codes.
MED: 100-2, 15, 150; 100-2, 16, 140; 100-3, 260.6

Ⓔ D4274 Distal or proximal wedge procedure (when not performed in conjunction with surgical procedures in the same anatomical area)

Ⓔ D4275 Soft tissue allograft
For tissue grafts, see CPT 15000 and related codes.

Ⓔ D4276 Combined connective tissue and double pedicle graft, per tooth
For tissue/pedicle grafts see CPT 15000 and related codes.

ADJUNCTIVE PERIODONTAL SERVICES

Ⓔ D4320 Provisional splinting — intracoronal

Ⓔ D4321 Provisional splinting — extracoronal

Ⓔ ☑ D4341 Periodontal scaling and root planing — four or more teeth per quadrant

Ⓔ D4342 Periodontal scaling and root planing — one to three teeth, per quadrant

⒮ D4355 Full mouth debridement to enable comprehensive evaluation and diagnosis
This procedure is covered by Medicare if its purpose is to identify a patient's existing infections prior to kidney transplantation. For debridement see CPT 11000 and related codes.
MED: 100-2, 15, 150; 100-2, 16, 140; 100-3, 260.6

⒮ D4381 Localized delivery of antimicrobial agents via a controlled release vehicle into diseased crevicular tissue, per tooth, by report
Pertinent documentation to evaluate medical appropriateness should be included when this code is reported.
MED: 100-2, 15, 150; 100-2, 16, 140; 100-3, 260.6

OTHER PERIODONTAL SERVICES

Ⓔ D4910 Periodontal maintenance

Ⓔ D4920 Unscheduled dressing change (by someone other than treating dentist)

Ⓔ D4999 Unspecified periodontal procedure, by report
Determine if an alternative HCPCS Level II or a CPT code better describes the service being reported. This code should be used only if a more specific code is unavailable.

PROSTHODONTICS (REMOVABLE) D5000-D5899

COMPLETE DENTURES (INCLUDING ROUTINE POST DELIVERY CARE)

Ⓔ D5110 Complete denture — maxillary

Ⓔ D5120 Complete denture — mandibular

Ⓔ D5130 Immediate denture — maxillary

Ⓔ D5140 Immediate denture — mandibular

PARTIAL DENTURES (INCLUDING ROUTINE POST DELIVERY CARE)

E   **D5211**   Maxillary partial denture — resin base (including any conventional clasps, rests and teeth)

E   **D5212**   Mandibular partial denture — resin base (including any conventional clasps, rests and teeth)

E   **D5213**   Maxillary partial denture — cast metal framework with resin denture bases (including any conventional clasps, rests and teeth)

E   **D5214**   Mandibular partial denture — cast metal framework with resin denture bases (including any conventional clasps, rests and teeth)

  D5225   Maxillary partial denture — flexible base (including any clasps, rests and teeth)

  D5226   Mandibular partial denture — flexible base (including any clasps, rests and teeth)

E   **D5281**   Removable unilateral partial denture — one piece cast metal (including clasps and teeth)

ADJUSTMENTS TO REMOVABLE PROSTHESES

E   **D5410**   Adjust complete denture — maxillary

E   **D5411**   Adjust complete denture — mandibular

E   **D5421**   Adjust partial denture — maxillary

E   **D5422**   Adjust partial denture — mandibular

REPAIRS TO COMPLETE DENTURES

E   **D5510**   Repair broken complete denture base

E   **D5520**   Replace missing or broken teeth — complete denture (each tooth)

REPAIRS TO PARTIAL DENTURES

E   **D5610**   Repair resin denture base

E   **D5620**   Repair cast framework

E   **D5630**   Repair or replace broken clasp

E ☑   **D5640**   Replace broken teeth — per tooth

E   **D5650**   Add tooth to existing partial denture

E   **D5660**   Add clasp to existing partial denture

E   **D5670**   Replace all teeth and acrylic on cast metal framework (maxillary)

E   **D5671**   Replace all teeth and acrylic on cast metal framework (mandibular)

DENTURE REBASE PROCEDURES

E   **D5710**   Rebase complete maxillary denture

E   **D5711**   Rebase complete mandibular denture

E   **D5720**   Rebase maxillary partial denture

E   **D5721**   Rebase mandibular partial denture

DENTURE RELINE PROCEDURES

E   **D5730**   Reline complete maxillary denture (chairside)

E   **D5731**   Reline complete mandibular denture (chairside)

E   **D5740**   Reline maxillary partial denture (chairside)

E   **D5741**   Reline mandibular partial denture (chairside)

E   **D5750**   Reline complete maxillary denture (laboratory)

E   **D5751**   Reline complete mandibular denture (laboratory)

E   **D5760**   Reline maxillary partial denture (laboratory)

E   **D5761**   Reline mandibular partial denture (laboratory)

OTHER REMOVABLE PROSTHETIC SERVICES

E   **D5810**   Interim complete denture (maxillary)

E   **D5811**   Interim complete denture (mandibular)

E   **D5820**   Interim partial denture (maxillary)

E   **D5821**   Interim partial denture (mandibular)

E   **D5850**   Tissue conditioning, maxillary

E   **D5851**   Tissue conditioning, mandibular

E   **D5860**   Overdenture — complete, by report
Pertinent documentation to evaluate medical appropriateness should be included when this code is reported.

E   **D5861**   Overdenture — partial, by report
Pertinent documentation to evaluate medical appropriateness should be included when this code is reported.

E   **D5862**   Precision attachment, by report
Pertinent documentation to evaluate medical appropriateness should be included when this code is reported.

E   **D5867**   Replacement of replaceable part of semi-precision or precision attachment (male or female component)

E   **D5875**   Modification of removable prosthesis following implant surgery

E   **D5899**   Unspecified removable prosthodontic procedure, by report
Determine if an alternative HCPCS Level II or a CPT code better describes the service being reported. This code should be used only if a more specific code is unavailable.

MAXILLOFACIAL PROSTHETICS D5900-D5999

S   **D5911**   Facial moulage (sectional)
MED: 100-2, 15, 120; 100-2, 15, 150

S   **D5912**   Facial moulage (complete)
MED: 100-2, 15, 120

E   **D5913**   Nasal prosthesis
See code(s): 21087

E   **D5914**   Auricular prosthesis
See code(s): 21086

E   **D5915**   Orbital prosthesis
See code(s): L8611

E   **D5916**   Ocular prosthesis
See also CPT code (21077, 65770, 66982-66985, 92330-92335, 92358, 92393).
See code(s): V2623, V2629

E   **D5919**   Facial prosthesis
See code(s): 21088

E   **D5922**   Nasal septal prosthesis
See code(s): 30220

E   **D5923**   Ocular prosthesis, interim
See code(s): 92330

E   **D5924**   Cranial prosthesis
See code(s): 62143

E   **D5925**   Facial augmentation implant prosthesis
See code(s): 21208

E   **D5926**   Nasal prosthesis, replacement
See code(s): 21087

E   **D5927**   Auricular prosthesis, replacement
See code(s): 21086

E   **D5928**   Orbital prosthesis, replacement
See code(s): 67550

Special Coverage Instructions   Noncovered by Medicare   Carrier Discretion   ☑ Quantity Alert   ● New Code   ○ Reinstated Code   ▲ Revised Code

2006 HCPCS   1-9 ASC Groups   MED: Pub 100/NCD Reference   ↳ DMEPOS Paid   ⊘ SNF Excluded   **D Codes — 33**

Dental Procedures

D5929 — D6071

E   **D5929** Facial prosthesis, replacement
See code(s): 21088

E   **D5931** Obturator prosthesis, surgical
See code(s): 21079

E   **D5932** Obturator prosthesis, definitive
See code(s): 21080

E   **D5933** Obturator prosthesis, modification
See code(s): 21080

E   **D5934** Mandibular resection prosthesis with guide flange
See code(s): 21081

E   **D5935** Mandibular resection prosthesis without guide flange
See code(s): 21081

E   **D5936** Obturator/prosthesis, interim
See code(s): 21079

E   **D5937** Trismus appliance (not for TMD treatment)
MED: 100-2, 15, 120

E   **D5951** Feeding aid
MED: 100-2, 15, 120; 100-2, 16, 140

E   **D5952** Speech aid prosthesis, pediatric
See code(s): 21084

E   **D5953** Speech aid prosthesis, adult
See code(s): 21084

E   **D5954** Palatal augmentation prosthesis
See code(s): 21082

E   **D5955** Palatal lift prosthesis, definitive
See code(s): 21083

E   **D5958** Palatal lift prosthesis, interim
See code(s): 21083

E   **D5959** Palatal lift prosthesis, modification
See code(s): 21083

E   **D5960** Speech aid prosthesis, modification
See code(s): 21084

E   **D5982** Surgical stent
For oral surgical stent see CPT code. Surgical stent. Periodontal stent, skin graft stent, columellar stent.

See code(s): 21085

S   **D5983** Radiation carrier
MED: 100-2, 15, 150; 100-2, 16, 140

S   **D5984** Radiation shield
MED: 100-2, 15, 150; 100-2, 16, 140

S   **D5985** Radiation cone locator
MED: 100-2, 15, 150; 100-2, 16, 140

E   **D5986** Fluoride gel carrier

S   **D5987** Commissure splint
MED: 100-2, 15, 150; 100-2, 16, 140

E   **D5988** Surgical splint. See also CPT.
See also CPT code (21085)

E   **D5999** Unspecified maxillofacial prosthesis, by report
Determine if an alternative HCPCS Level II or a CPT code better describes the service being reported. This code should be used only if a more specific code is unavailable.

IMPLANT SERVICES D6000-D6199

E   **D6010** Surgical placement of implant body: endosteal implant
See code(s): 21248

E   **D6040** Surgical placement: eposteal implant
See code(s): 21245

E   **D6050** Surgical placement: transosteal implant
See code(s): 21244

E   **D6053** Implant/abutment supported removable denture for completely edentulous arch
MED: 100-2, 15, 150

E   **D6054** Implant/abutment supported removable denture for partially edentulous arch
MED: 100-2, 15, 150

E   **D6055** Dental implant supported connecting bar
MED: 100-2, 15, 150

E   **D6056** Prefabricated abutment — includes placement
MED: 100-2, 15, 150

E   **D6057** Custom abutment — includes placement
MED: 100-2, 15, 150

E   **D6058** Abutment supported porcelain/ceramic crown
MED: 100-2, 15, 150

E   **D6059** Abutment supported porcelain fused to metal crown (high noble metal)
MED: 100-2, 15, 150

E   **D6060** Abutment supported porcelain fused to metal crown (predominantly base metal)
MED: 100-2, 15, 150

E   **D6061** Abutment supported porcelain fused to metal crown (noble metal)
MED: 100-2, 15, 150

E   **D6062** Abutment supported cast metal crown (high noble metal)
MED: 100-2, 15, 150

E   **D6063** Abutment supported cast metal crown (predominantly base metal)
MED: 100-2, 15, 150

E   **D6064** Abutment supported cast metal crown (noble metal)
MED: 100-2, 15, 150

E   **D6065** Implant supported porcelain/ceramic crown
MED: 100-2, 15, 150

E   **D6066** Implant supported porcelain fused to metal crown (titanium, titanium alloy, high noble metal)
MED: 100-2, 15, 150

E   **D6067** Implant supported metal crown (titanium, titanium alloy, high noble metal)
MED: 100-2, 15, 150

E   **D6068** Abutment supported retainer for porcelain/ceramic FPD
MED: 100-2, 15, 150

E   **D6069** Abutment supported retainer for porcelain fused to metal FPD (high noble metal)
MED: 100-2, 15, 150

E   **D6070** Abutment supported retainer for porcelain fused to metal FPD (predominately base metal)
MED: 100-2, 15, 150

E   **D6071** Abutment supported retainer for porcelain fused to metal FPD (noble metal)
MED: 100-2, 15, 150

Special Coverage Instructions   Noncovered by Medicare   Carrier Discretion   ☑ Quantity Alert   ● New Code   ○ Reinstated Code   ▲ Revised Code

34 — D Codes   A Age   M Maternity   ♀ Female Only   ♂ Male Only   A-Y APC Status Indicator   *2006 HCPCS*

E   **D6072**   Abutment supported retainer for cast metal FPD (high noble metal)
MED: 100-2, 15, 150

E   **D6073**   Abutment supported retainer for cast metal FPD (predominately base metal)
MED: 100-2, 15, 150

E   **D6074**   Abutment supported retainer for cast metal FPD (noble metal)
MED: 100-2, 15, 150

E   **D6075**   Implant supported retainer for ceramic FPD
MED: 100-2, 15, 150

E   **D6076**   Implant supported retainer for porcelain fused to metal FPD (titanium, titanium alloy, or high noble metal)
MED: 100-2, 15, 150

E   **D6077**   Implant supported retainer for cast metal FPD (titanium, titanium alloy, or high noble metal)
MED: 100-2, 15, 150

E   **D6078**   Implant/abutment supported fixed denture for completely edentulous arch
MED: 100-2, 15, 150

E   **D6079**   Implant/abutment supported fixed denture for partially edentulous arch
MED: 100-2, 15, 150

E   **D6080**   Implant maintenance procedures, including removal of prosthesis, cleansing of prosthesis and abutments, reinsertion of prosthesis
MED: 100-2, 15, 150

E   **D6090**   Repair implant supported prosthesis, by report
Pertinent documentation to evaluate medical appropriateness should be included when this code is reported.

See code(s): 21299

     D6094   Abutment supported crown — (titanium)

E   **D6095**   Repair implant abutment, by report
Pertinent documentation to evaluate medical appropriateness should be included when this code is reported.

See code(s): 21299

E   **D6100**   Implant removal, by report
Pertinent documentation to evaluate medical appropriateness should be included when this code is reported.

See code(s): 21299

     D6190   Radiographic/surgical implant index, by report

     D6194   Abutment supported retainer crown for FPD — (titanium)

E   **D6199**   Unspecified implant procedure, by report
See code(s): 21299

     D6205   Pontic — indirect resin based composite

PROSTHODONTICS (FIXED) D6200–D6999

FIXED PARTIAL DENTURE PONTICS

E   **D6210**   Pontic — cast high noble metal
Each abutment and each pontic constitute a unit in a prosthesis. An alloy of at least 60 percent gold (Au), palladium (Pd), or platinum (Pt) is considered a high noble metal.

E   **D6211**   Pontic — cast predominantly base metal
Each abutment and each pontic constitute a unit in a prosthesis. An alloy of less than 25 percent gold (Au), palladium (Pd), or platinum (Pt) is considered a high noble metal.

E   **D6212**   Pontic — cast noble metal
Each abutment and each pontic constitute a unit in a prosthesis. An alloy of at least 25 percent gold (Au), palladium (Pd), or platinum (Pt) is considered a high noble metal.

     D6214   Pontic — titanium

E   **D6240**   Pontic — porcelain fused to high noble metal
Each abutment and each pontic constitute a unit in a prosthesis. An alloy of at least 60 percent gold (Au), palladium (Pd), or platinum (Pt) is considered a high noble metal.

E   **D6241**   Pontic — porcelain fused to predominantly base metal
Each abutment and each pontic constitute a unit in a prosthesis. An alloy of less than 25 percent gold (Au), palladium (Pd), or platinum (Pt) is considered a high noble metal.

E   **D6242**   Pontic — porcelain fused to noble metal
Each abutment and each pontic constitute a unit in a prosthesis. An alloy of at least 60 percent gold (Au), palladium (Pd), or platinum (Pt) is considered a high noble metal.

E   **D6245**   Pontic — porcelain/ceramic
MED: 100-2, 15, 150

E   **D6250**   Pontic — resin with high noble metal
Each abutment and each pontic constitute a unit in a prosthesis. An alloy of at least 60 percent gold (Au), palladium (Pd), or platinum (Pt) is considered a high noble metal.

E   **D6251**   Pontic — resin with predominantly base metal
Each abutment and each pontic constitute a unit in a prosthesis. An alloy of less than 25 percent gold (Au), palladium (Pd), or platinum (Pt) is considered a high noble metal.

E   **D6252**   Pontic — resin with noble metal
Each abutment and each pontic constitute a unit in a prosthesis. An alloy of at least 25 percent gold (Au), palladium (Pd), or platinum (Pt) is considered a high noble metal.

E   **D6253**   Provisional pontic

E   **D6545**   Retainer — cast metal for resin bonded fixed prosthesis

E   **D6548**   Retainer — porcelain/ceramic for resin bonded fixed prosthesis
MED: 100-2, 15, 150

E   **D6600**   Inlay — porcelain/ceramic, two surfaces
MED: 100-2, 15, 150

E   **D6601**   Inlay — porcelain/ceramic, three or more surfaces
MED: 100-2, 15, 150

E   **D6602**   Inlay — cast high noble metal, two surfaces
MED: 100-2, 15, 150

E   **D6603**   Inlay — cast high noble metal, three or more surfaces
MED: 100-2, 15, 150

E   **D6604**   Inlay — cast predominantly base metal, two surfaces
MED: 100-2, 15, 150

E   **D6605**   Inlay — cast predominantly base metal, three or more surfaces
MED: 100-2, 15, 150

E   **D6606**   Inlay — cast noble metal, two surfaces
MED: 100-2, 15, 150

E   **D6607**   Inlay — cast noble metal, three or more surfaces
MED: 100-2, 15, 150

E   **D6608**   Onlay — porcelain/ceramic, two surfaces
MED: 100-2, 15, 150

Dental Procedures

D6609 — D7241

E   **D6609** Onlay — porcelain/ceramic, three or more surfaces
MED: 100-2, 15, 150

E   **D6610** Onlay — cast high noble metal, two surfaces
MED: 100-2, 15, 150

E   **D6611** Onlay — cast high noble metal, three or more surfaces
MED: 100-2, 15, 150

E   **D6612** Onlay — cast predominantly base metal, two surfaces
MED: 100-2, 15, 150

E   **D6613** Onlay — cast predominantly base metal, three or more surfaces
MED: 100-2, 15, 150

E   **D6614** Onlay — cast noble metal, two surfaces
MED: 100-2, 15, 150

E   **D6615** Onlay — cast noble metal, three or more surfaces
MED: 100-2, 15, 150

  D6624 Inlay — titanium

  D6634 Onlay — titanium

  D6710 Crown — indirect resin based composite

FIXED PARTIAL DENTURE RETAINERS — CROWNS

E   **D6720** Crown — resin with high noble metal
An alloy of at least 60 percent gold (Au), palladium (Pd), or platinum (Pt) is considered a high noble metal.

E   **D6721** Crown — resin with predominantly base metal
An alloy of less than 25 percent gold (Au), palladium (Pd), or platinum (Pt) is considered a base metal.

E   **D6722** Crown — resin with noble metal
An alloy of at least 25 percent gold (Au), palladium (Pd), or platinum (Pt) is considered a noble metal.

E   **D6740** Crown — porcelain/ceramic
MED: 100-2, 15, 150

E   **D6750** Crown — porcelain fused to high noble metal
An alloy of at least 60 percent gold (Au), palladium (Pd), or platinum (Pt) is considered a high noble metal.

E   **D6751** Crown — porcelain fused to predominantly base metal
An alloy of less than 25 percent gold (Au), palladium (Pd), or platinum (Pt) is considered a base metal.

E   **D6752** Crown — porcelain fused to noble metal
An alloy of at least 25 percent gold (Au), palladium (Pd), or platinum (Pt) is considered a noble metal.

E   **D6780** Crown — 3/4 cast high noble metal
An alloy of at least 60 percent gold (Au), palladium (Pd), or platinum (Pt) is considered a high noble metal.

E   **D6781** Crown — 3/4 cast predominately base metal
An alloy of less than 25 percent gold (Au), palladium (Pd), or platinum (Pt) is considered a base metal.
MED: 100-2, 15, 150

E   **D6782** Crown — 3/4 cast noble metal
An alloy of at least 25 percent gold (Au), palladium (Pd), or platinum (Pt) is considered a noble metal.
MED: 100-2, 15, 150

E   **D6783** Crown — 3/4 porcelain/ceramic
MED: 100-2, 15, 150

E   **D6790** Crown — full cast high noble metal
An alloy of at least 60 percent gold (Au), palladium (Pd), or platinum (Pt) is considered a high noble metal.

E   **D6791** Crown — full cast predominantly base metal
An alloy of less than 25 percent gold (Au), palladium (Pd), or platinum (Pt) is considered a base metal.

E   **D6792** Crown — full cast noble metal
An alloy of at least 25 percent gold (Au), palladium (Pd), or platinum (Pt) is considered a noble metal.

E   **D6793** Provisional retainer crown

  D6794 Crown — titanium

OTHER FIXED PARTIAL DENTURE SERVICES

S   **D6920** Connector bar
MED: 100-2, 15, 150; 100-2, 16, 140; 100-3, 260.6

E   **D6930** Recement fixed partial denture

E   **D6940** Stress breaker

E   **D6950** Precision attachment

E   **D6970** Cast post and core in addition to fixed partial denture retainer

E   **D6971** Cast post as part of fixed partial denture retainer

E   **D6972** Prefabricated post and core in addition to fixed partial denture retainer

E   **D6973** Core build up for retainer, including any pins

E   **D6975** Coping — metal

E   **D6976** Each additional cast post — same tooth
Report this code in addition to codes D6970 or D6971.
MED: 100-2, 15, 150

E   **D6977** Each additional prefabricated post — same tooth
Report this code in addition to code D6972.
MED: 100-2, 15, 150

E   **D6980** Fixed partial denture repair, by report
Pertinent documentation to evaluate medical appropriateness should be included when this code is reported.

E   **D6985** Pediatric partial denture, fixed   A

E   **D6999** Unspecified, fixed prosthodontic procedure, by report
Determine if an alternative HCPCS Level II or a CPT code better describes the service being reported. This code should be used only if a more specific code is unavailable.

S   **D7111** Extraction, coronal remnants — deciduous tooth
MED: 100-2, 16, 140

S   **D7140** Extraction, erupted tooth or exposed root (elevation and/or forceps removal)
MED: 100-2, 16, 140

SURGICAL EXTRACTIONS (INCLUDES LOCAL ANESTHESIA AND ROUTINE POSTOPERATIVE CARE)

S   **D7210** Surgical removal of erupted tooth requiring elevation of mucoperiosteal flap and removal of bone and/or section of tooth
MED: 100-2, 15, 150; 100-2, 16, 140

S   **D7220** Removal of impacted tooth — soft tissue
MED: 100-2, 15, 150; 100-2, 16, 140

S   **D7230** Removal of impacted tooth — partially bony
MED: 100-2, 15, 150; 100-2, 16, 140

S   **D7240** Removal of impacted tooth — completely bony
MED: 100-2, 15, 150; 100-2, 16, 140

S   **D7241** Removal of impacted tooth — completely bony, with unusual surgical complications
MED: 100-2, 15, 150; 100-2, 16, 140

Special Coverage Instructions   Noncovered by Medicare   Carrier Discretion   ☑ Quantity Alert   ● New Code   ○ Reinstated Code   ▲ Revised Code

36 — D Codes   A Age   M Maternity   ♀ Female Only   ♂ Male Only   A-Y APC Status Indicator   *2006 HCPCS*

⑤	**D7250**	Surgical removal of residual tooth roots (cutting procedure) MED: 100-2, 15, 150; 100-2, 16, 140

OTHER SURGICAL PROCEDURES

⑤	**D7260**	Orolantral fistula closure MED: 100-2, 15, 150; 100-2, 16, 140
⑤	**D7261**	Primary closure of a sinus perforation See equivalent CPT code for repair of mucous membranes. MED: 100-2, 16, 140
E	**D7270**	Tooth reimplantation and/or stabilization of accidentally evulsed or displaced tooth
E	**D7272**	Tooth transplantation (includes reimplantation from one site to another and splinting and/or stabilization)
E	**D7280**	Surgical access of an unerupted tooth
E	**D7282**	Mobilization of erupted or malpositioned tooth to aid eruption
	D7283	Placement of device to facilitate eruption of impacted tooth
E	**D7285**	Biopsy of oral tissue — hard (bone, tooth) See code(s): 20220, 20225, 20240, 20245
E	**D7286**	Biopsy of oral tissue — soft See code(s): 40808
E	**D7287**	Exfoliative cytological sample collection
	D7288	Brush biopsy — transepithelial sample collection
E	**D7290**	Surgical repositioning of teeth
⑤	**D7291**	Transseptal fiberotomy/supra crestal fiberotomy, by report Pertinent documentation to evaluate medical appropriateness should be included when this code is reported. MED: 100-2, 15, 150; 100-2, 16, 140

ALVEOLOPLASTY — SURGICAL PREPARATION OF RIDGE FOR DENTURES

E	☑	**D7310**	Alveoloplasty in conjunction with extractions — per quadrant See code(s): 41874
	☑	**D7311**	Alveoloplasty in conjunction with extractions — one to three teeth or tooth spaces, per quadrant
E	☑	**D7320**	Alveoloplasty not in conjunction with extractions — per quadrant See code(s): 41870
	☑	**D7321**	Alveoloplasty not in conjunction with extractions — one to three teeth or tooth spaces, per quadrant

VESTIBULOPLASTY

E	**D7340**	Vestibuloplasty — ridge extension (second epithelialization) See code(s): 40840, 40842, 40843, 40844
E	**D7350**	Vestibuloplasty — ridge extension (including soft tissue grafts, muscle reattachments, revision of soft tissue attachment and management of hypertrophied and hyperplastic tissue) See code(s): 40845

SURGICAL EXCISION OF REACTIVE INFLAMMATORY LESIONS (SCAR TISSUE OR LOCALIZED CONGENITAL LESIONS)

E	☑	**D7410**	Excision of benign lesion up to 1.25 cm
E		**D7411**	Excision of benign lesion greater than 1.25 cm See CPT codes in the surgical section (11440 & 40520)
E		**D7412**	Excision of benign lesion, complicated See CPT code in the surgical section (10000 & 40000)
E		**D7413**	Excision of malignant lesion up to 1.25 cm See CPT code in the surgical section (11442)
E		**D7414**	Excision of malignant lesion greater than 1.25 cm See CPT codes in the surgical section (11442-11446)
E		**D7415**	Excision of malignant lesion, complicated See CPT codes in the surgical section (11440-11446 with modifier 22 for complicated)
E	☑	**D7440**	Excision of malignant tumor — lesion diameter up to 1.25 cm
E	☑	**D7441**	Excision of malignant tumor — lesion diameter greater than 1.25 cm
E	☑	**D7450**	Removal of benign odontogenic cyst or tumor — lesion diameter up to 1.25 cm
E	☑	**D7451**	Removal of benign odontogenic cyst or tumor — lesion diameter greater than 1.25 cm
E	☑	**D7460**	Removal of benign nonodontogenic cyst or tumor — lesion diameter up to 1.25 cm
E	☑	**D7461**	Removal of benign nonodontogenic cyst or tumor — lesion diameter greater than 1.25 cm
E		**D7465**	Destruction of lesion(s) by physical or chemical method, by report Pertinent documentation to evaluate medical appropriateness should be included when this code is reported. See code(s): 41850
E	☑	**D7471**	Removal of lateral exostosis (maxilla or mandible) See code(s): 21031, 21032
E		**D7472**	Removal of torus palatinus See CPT code in the surgical section (21029, 21030, 21031)
E		**D7473**	Removal of torus mandibularis
E		**D7485**	Surgical reduction of osseous tuberosity
E		**D7490**	Radical resection of maxilla or mandible See code(s): 21045

SURGICAL INCISION

E	**D7510**	Incision and drainage of abscess — intraoral soft tissue See code(s): 41800
	D7511	Incision and drainage of abscess — intraoral soft tissue — complicated (includes drainage of multiple fascial spaces)
E	**D7520**	Incision and drainage of abscess — extraoral soft tissue See code(s): 40800
	D7521	Incision and drainage of abscess — extraoral soft tissue — complicated (includes drainage of multiple fascial spaces)
E	**D7530**	Removal of foreign body from mucosa, skin, or subcutaneous alveolar tissue See code(s): 41805, 41828
E	**D7540**	Removal of reaction-producing foreign bodies, musculoskeletal system See code(s): 20520, 41800, 41806

Dental Procedures

D7550 — D7941

E **D7550** Partial ostectomy/sequestrectomy for removal of non-vital bone
See code(s): 20999

E **D7560** Maxillary sinusotomy for removal of tooth fragment or foreign body
See code(s): 31020

TREATMENT OF FRACTURES — SIMPLE

E **D7610** Maxilla — open reduction (teeth immobilized, if present
See code(s): 21422

E **D7620** Maxilla — closed reduction (teeth immobilized, if present)

E **D7630** Mandible — open reduction (teeth immobilized, if present)

E **D7640** Mandible — closed reduction (teeth immobilized, if present)

E **D7650** Malar and/or zygomatic arch — open reduction

E **D7660** Malar and/or zygomatic arch — closed reduction

E **D7670** Alveolus — closed reduction, may include stabilization of teeth

E **D7671** Alveolus — open reduction, may include stabilization of teeth

E **D7680** Facial bones — complicated reduction with fixation and multiple surgical approaches

TREATMENT OF FRACTURES — COMPOUND

E **D7710** Maxilla — open reduction
See code(s): 21346

E **D7720** Maxilla — closed reduction
See code(s): 21345

E **D7730** Mandible — open reduction
See code(s): 21461, 21462

E **D7740** Mandible — closed reduction
See code(s): 21455

E **D7750** Malar and/or zygomatic arch — open reduction
See code(s): 21360, 21365

E **D7760** Malar and/or zygomatic arch — closed reduction
See code(s): 21355

E **D7770** Alveolus — open reduction stabilization of teeth
See code(s): 21422

E **D7771** Alveolus, closed reduction stabilization of teeth
See CPT code in the surgical section (21421)

E **D7780** Facial bones — complicated reduction with fixation and multiple surgical approaches
See code(s): 21433, 21435

REDUCTION OF DISLOCATION AND MANAGEMENT OF OTHER TEMPOROMANDIBULAR JOINT DYSFUNCTIONS

Procedures which are an integral part of a primary procedure should not be reported separately.

E **D7810** Open reduction of dislocation
See code(s): 21490

E **D7820** Closed reduction of dislocation
See code(s): 21480

E **D7830** Manipulation under anesthesia

E **D7840** Condylectomy

E **D7850** Surgical discectomy, with/without implant
See code(s): 21060

E **D7852** Disc repair
See code(s): 21299

E **D7854** Synovectomy
See code(s): 21299

E **D7856** Myotomy
See code(s): 21299

E **D7858** Joint reconstruction
See code(s): 21242, 21243

E **D7860** Arthrotomy
MED: 100-2, 15, 150; 100-2, 16, 140

E **D7865** Arthroplasty
See code(s): 21240

E **D7870** Arthrocentesis
See code(s): 21060

E **D7871** Non-arthroscopic lysis and lavage

E **D7872** Arthroscopy — diagnosis, with or without biopsy
See code(s): 29800

E **D7873** Arthroscopy — surgical: lavage and lysis of adhesions
See code(s): 29804

E **D7874** Arthroscopy — surgical: disc repositioning and stabilization
See code(s): 29804

E **D7875** Arthroscopy — surgical: synovectomy
See code(s): 29804

E **D7876** Arthroscopy — surgical: discectomy
See code(s): 29804

E **D7877** Arthroscopy — surgical: debridement
See code(s): 29804

E **D7880** Occlusal orthotic device, by report
See code(s): 21499

E **D7899** Unspecified TMD therapy, by report
Determine if an alternative HCPCS Level II or a CPT code better describes the service being reported. This code should be used only if a more specific code is unavailable.
See code(s): 21499

REPAIR OF TRAUMATIC WOUNDS

E ☑ **D7910** Suture of recent small wounds up to 5 cm
See code(s): 12011, 12013

COMPLICATED SUTURING (RECONSTRUCTION REQUIRING DELICATE HANDLING OF TISSUES AND WIDE UNDERMINING FOR METICULOUS CLOSURE)

E **D7911** Complicated suture — up to 5 cm
See code(s): 12051, 12052

E **D7912** Complicated suture — greater than 5 cm
See code(s): 13132

OTHER REPAIR PROCEDURES

E **D7920** Skin graft (identify defect covered, location and type of graft)

S **D7940** Osteoplasty — for orthognathic deformities
MED: 100-2, 15, 150; 100-2, 16, 140

E **D7941** Osteotomy — mandibular rami
See code(s): 21193, 21195, 21196

Special Coverage Instructions | Noncovered by Medicare | Carrier Discretion | ☑ Quantity Alert | ● New Code | ○ Reinstated Code | ▲ Revised Code

38 — D Codes   Ⓐ Age   Ⓜ Maternity   ♀ Female Only   ♂ Male Only   Ⓐ-Ⓨ APC Status Indicator   *2006 HCPCS*

E   D7943 Osteotomy — mandibular rami with bone graft; includes obtaining the graft
See code(s): 21194

E ☑ D7944 Osteotomy — segmented or subapical — per sextant or quadrant
See code(s): 21198, 21206

E   D7945 Osteotomy — body of mandible
See code(s): 21193, 21194, 21195, 21196

E   D7946 LeFort I (maxilla — total)
See code(s): 21147

E   D7947 LeFort I (maxilla — segmented)
See code(s): 21145, 21146

E   D7948 LeFort II or LeFort III (osteoplasty of facial bones for midface hypoplasia or retrusion) — without bone graft
See code(s): 21150

E   D7949 LeFort II or LeFort III — with bone graft

E   D7950 Osseous, osteoperiosteal, or cartilage graft of the mandible or facial bones — autogenous or nonautogenous, by report
Pertinent documentation to evaluate medical appropriateness should be included when this code is reported.
See code(s): 21247

☑ D7953 Bone replacement graft for ridge preservation — per site

E   D7955 Repair of maxillofacial soft and/or hard tissue defect
See code(s): 21299

E   D7960 Frenulectomy (frenectomy or frenotomy) — separate procedure
See code(s): 40819, 41010, 41115

D7963 Frenuloplasty

E ☑ D7970 Excision of hyperplastic tissue — per arch

E   D7971 Excision of pericoronal gingiva
See code(s): 41821

E   D7972 Surgical reduction of fibrous tuberosity

E   D7980 Sialolithotomy
See code(s): 42330, 42335, 42340

E   D7981 Excision of salivary gland, by report
Pertinent documentation to evaluate medical appropriateness should be included when this code is reported.
See code(s): 42408

E   D7982 Sialodochoplasty
See code(s): 42500

E   D7983 Closure of salivary fistula
See code(s): 42600

E   D7990 Emergency tracheotomy
See code(s): 31605

E   D7991 Coronoidectomy
See code(s): 21070

E   D7995 Synthetic graft — mandible or facial bones, by report
Pertinent documentation to evaluate medical appropriateness should be included when this code is reported.
See code(s): 21299

E   D7996 Implant — mandible for augmentation purposes (excluding alveolar ridge), by report
Pertinent documentation to evaluate medical appropriateness should be included when this code is reported.
See code(s): 21299

E   D7997 Appliance removal (not by dentist who placed appliance), includes removal of archbar

E   D7999 Unspecified oral surgery procedure, by report
Determine if an alternative HCPCS Level II or a CPT code better describes the service being reported. This code should be used only if a more specific code is unavailable.
See code(s): 21299

ORTHODONTICS D8000–D8999

E   D8010 Limited orthodontic treatment of the primary dentition Ⓐ

E   D8020 Limited orthodontic treatment of the transitional dentition

E   D8030 Limited orthodontic treatment of the adolescent dentition Ⓐ

E   D8040 Limited orthodontic treatment of the adult dentition Ⓐ

E   D8050 Interceptive orthodontic treatment of the primary dentition Ⓐ

E   D8060 Interceptive orthodontic treatment of the transitional dentition

E   D8070 Comprehensive orthodontic treatment of the transitional dentition

E   D8080 Comprehensive orthodontic treatment of the adolescent dentition Ⓐ

E   D8090 Comprehensive orthodontic treatment of the adult dentition Ⓐ

MINOR TREATMENT TO CONTROL HARMFUL HABITS

E   D8210 Removable appliance therapy

E   D8220 Fixed appliance therapy

OTHER ORTHODONTIC SERVICES

E   D8660 Pre-orthodontic treatment visit

E   D8670 Periodic orthodontic treatment visit (as part of contract)

E   D8680 Orthodontic retention (removal of appliances, construction and placement of retainer(s))

E   D8690 Orthodontic treatment (alternative billing to a contract fee)

E   D8691 Repair of orthodontic appliance

E   D8692 Replacement of lost or broken retainer

E   D8999 Unspecified orthodontic procedure, by report
Determine if an alternative HCPCS Level II or a CPT code better describes the service being reported. This code should be used only if a more specific code is unavailable.

ADJUNCTIVE GENERAL SERVICES D9110–D9999

UNCLASSIFIED TREATMENT

N   D9110 Palliative (emergency) treatment of dental pain — minor procedure
MED: 100-2, 15, 150; 100-2, 16, 140

| Special Coverage Instructions | Noncovered by Medicare | Carrier Discretion | ☑ Quantity Alert | ● New Code | ○ Reinstated Code | ▲ Revised Code |

2006 HCPCS   1-9 ASC Groups   MED: Pub 100/NCD Reference   ♿ DMEPOS Paid   ⊘ SNF Excluded   **D Codes — 39**

D7943 — D9110

Dental Procedures

D9210 — D9999

ANESTHESIA

E   **D9210** Local anesthesia not in conjunction with operative or surgical procedures
See code(s): 90784

E   **D9211** Regional block anesthesia

E   **D9212** Trigeminal division block anesthesia
See code(s): 64400

E   **D9215** Local anesthesia
See code(s): 90784

E ☑   **D9220** Deep sedation/general anesthesia — first 30 minutes
See also CPT code 00172-00176.

E ☑   **D9221** Deep sedation/general anesthesia — each additional 15 minutes
MED: 100-2, 15, 150; 100-2, 16, 140

N   **D9230** Analgesia, anxiolysis, inhalation of nitrous oxide
MED: 100-2, 15, 150; 100-2, 16, 140

E ☑   **D9241** Intravenous conscious sedation/analgesia — first 30 minutes
See also CPT code 90784, 99141.

See code(s): 90784

E ☑   **D9242** Intravenous conscious sedation/analgesia — each additional 15 minutes
See also CPT code 90784, 99141.

See code(s): 90784

N   **D9248** Non-intravenous conscious sedation

PROFESSIONAL CONSULTATION

E   **D9310** Consultation (diagnostic service provided by dentist or physician other than practitioner providing treatment)

PROFESSIONAL VISITS

E   **D9410** House/extended care facility call

E   **D9420** Hospital call
See also CPT E & M codes

E   **D9430** Office visit for observation (during regularly scheduled hours) — no other services performed
See also CPT E & M codes

E   **D9440** Office visit — after regularly scheduled hours
See code(s): 99050

E   **D9450** Case presentation, detailed and extensive treatment planning

DRUGS

E   **D9610** Therapeutic drug injection, by report
Pertinent documentation to evaluate medical appropriateness should be included when this code is reported.

See code(s): 90788, 90784

S   **D9630** Other drugs and/or medicaments, by report
Determine if an alternative HCPCS Level II or a CPT code better describes the service being reported. This code should be used only if a more specific code is unavailable.

MED: 100-2, 15, 150; 100-2, 16, 140

MISCELLANEOUS SERVICES

E   **D9910** Application of desensitizing medicament

E ☑   **D9911** Application of desensitizing resin for cervical and/or root surface, per tooth

E   **D9920** Behavior management, by report
Pertinent documentation to evaluate medical appropriateness should be included when this code is reported.

S   **D9930** Treatment of complications (postsurgical) — unusual circumstances, by report
MED: 100-2, 15, 150; 100-2, 16, 140

S   **D9940** Occlusal guard, by report
Pertinent documentation to evaluate medical appropriateness should be included when this code is reported.

MED: 100-2, 15, 150; 100-2, 16, 140

E   **D9941** Fabrication of athletic mouthguard
See code(s): 21089

     D9942 Repair and/or reline of occlusal guard

S   **D9950** Occlusion analysis — mounted case
MED: 100-2, 15, 150; 100-2, 16, 140

S   **D9951** Occlusal adjustment — limited
MED: 100-2, 15, 150; 100-2, 16, 140

S   **D9952** Occlusal adjustment — complete
MED: 100-2, 15, 150; 100-2, 16, 140

E   **D9970** Enamel microabrasion

E ☑   **D9971** Odontoplasty 1-2 teeth; includes removal of enamel projections

E ☑   **D9972** External bleaching — per arch

E ☑   **D9973** External bleaching — per tooth

E ☑   **D9974** Internal bleaching — per tooth

E   **D9999** Unspecified adjunctive procedure, by report
Determine if an alternative HCPCS Level II or a CPT code better describes the service being reported. This code should be used only if a more specific code is unavailable.

See code(s): 21499

Special Coverage Instructions   Noncovered by Medicare   Carrier Discretion   ☑ Quantity Alert   ● New Code   ○ Reinstated Code   ▲ Revised Code

40 — D Codes   A Age   M Maternity   ♀ Female Only   ♂ Male Only   A-Y APC Status Indicator   *2006 HCPCS*

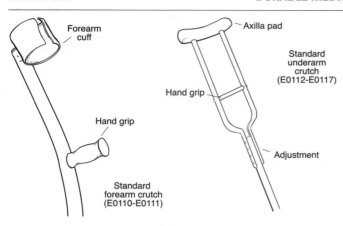

Forearm cuff

Hand grip

Hand grip

Standard forearm crutch (E0110-E0111)

Axilla pad

Standard underarm crutch (E0112-E0117)

Hand grip

Adjustment

DURABLE MEDICAL EQUIPMENT *E0100-E9999*

E codes include durable medical equipment such as canes, crutches, walkers, commodes, decubitus care, bath and toilet aids, hospital beds, oxygen and related respiratory equipment, monitoring equipment, pacemakers, patient lifts, safety equipment, restraints, traction equipment, fracture frames, wheelchairs, and artificial kidney machines.

CANES

E0100 Cane, includes canes of all materials, adjustable or fixed, with tip
White canes for the blind are not covered under Medicare.
MED: 100-2, 15, 110.1; 100-3, 280.1; 100-3, 280.2

E0105 Cane, quad or three-prong, includes canes of all materials, adjustable or fixed, with tips
MED: 100-2, 15, 110.1; 100-3, 280.1; 100-3, 280.5

CRUTCHES

E0110 Crutches, forearm, includes crutches of various materials, adjustable or fixed, pair, complete with tips and handgrips
MED: 100-2, 15, 110.1; 100-3, 280.1

E0111 Crutch, forearm, includes crutches of various materials, adjustable or fixed, each, with tip and handgrip
MED: 100-2, 15, 110.1; 100-3, 280.1

E0112 Crutches, underarm, wood, adjustable or fixed, pair, with pads, tips and handgrips
MED: 100-2, 15, 110.1; 100-3, 280.1

E0113 Crutch, underarm, wood, adjustable or fixed, each, with pad, tip and handgrip
MED: 100-2, 15, 110.1; 100-3, 280.1

E0114 Crutches, underarm, other than wood, adjustable or fixed, pair, with pads, tips and handgrips
MED: 100-2, 15, 110.1; 100-3, 280.1

▲ **E0116** Crutch, underarm, other than wood, adjustable or fixed, with PAD, tip, handgrip, with or without shock absorber, each
MED: 100-2, 15, 110.1; 100-3, 280.1

E0117 Crutch, underarm, articulating, spring assisted, each
MED: 100-2, 15, 110.1

E0118 Crutch substitute, lower leg platform, with or without wheels, each

WALKERS

E0130 Walker, rigid (pickup), adjustable or fixed height
Medicare covers walkers if patient's ambulation is impaired.
MED: 100-2, 15, 110.1; 100-3, 280.1

E0135 Walker, folding (pickup), adjustable or fixed height
Medicare covers walkers if patient's ambulation is impaired.
MED: 100-2, 15, 110.1; 100-3, 280.1

E0140 Walker, with trunk support, adjustable or fixed height, any type
MED: 100-2, 15, 110.1; 100-3, 280.1

E0141 Walker, rigid, wheeled, adjustable or fixed height
Medicare covers walkers if patient's ambulation is impaired.
MED: 100-2, 15, 110.1; 100-3, 280.1

E0143 Walker, folding, wheeled, adjustable or fixed height
Medicare covers walkers if patient's ambulation is impaired.
MED: 100-2, 15, 110.1; 100-3, 280.1

E0144 Walker, enclosed, four sided framed, rigid or folding, wheeled with posterior seat
MED: 100-2, 15, 110.1; 100-3, 280.1

E0147 Walker, heavy duty, multiple braking system, variable wheel resistance
Medicare covers safety roller walkers only in patients in severe neurological disorders or restricted use of one hand. In some cases, coverage will be extended to patients with a weight exceeding the limits of a standard wheeled walker.
MED: 100-2, 15, 110.1; 100-3, 280.5

E0148 Walker, heavy duty, without wheels, rigid or folding, any type, each

E0149 Walker, heavy duty, wheeled, rigid or folding, any type

E0153 Platform attachment, forearm crutch, each

E0154 Platform attachment, walker, each

E0155 Wheel attachment, rigid pick-up walker, per pair seat attachment, walker

ATTACHMENTS

E0156 Seat attachment, walker

E0157 Crutch attachment, walker, each

E0158 Leg extensions for walker, per set of four (4)

E0159 Brake attachment for wheeled walker, replacement, each

COMMODES

E0160 Sitz type bath or equipment, portable, used with or without commode
Medicare covers sitz baths if medical record indicates that the patient has an infection or injury of the perineal area and the sitz bath is prescribed by the physician.
MED: 100-3, 280.1

E0161 Sitz type bath or equipment, portable, used with or without commode, with faucet attachment(s)
Medicare covers sitz baths if medical record indicates that the patient has an infection or injury of the perineal area and the sitz bath is prescribed by the physician.
MED: 100-3, 280.1

Durable Medical Equipment

E0162 — E0200

Y **E0162** **Sitz bath chair**   ⅙⊘
Medicare covers sitz baths if medical record indicates that the patient has an infection or injury of the perineal area and the sitz bath is prescribed by the physician.
MED: 100-3, 280.1

Y **E0163** **Commode chair, stationary, with fixed arms**   ⅙⊘
Medicare covers commodes for patients confined to their beds or rooms, for patients without indoor bathroom facilities, and to patients who cannot climb or descend the stairs necessary to reach the bathrooms in their homes.
MED: 100-2, 15, 110.1; 100-3, 280.1

Y **E0164** **Commode chair, mobile, with fixed arms**   ⅙⊘
Medicare covers commodes for patients confined to their beds or rooms, for patients without indoor bathroom facilities, and to patients who cannot climb or descend the stairs necessary to reach the bathrooms in their homes.
MED: 100-2, 15, 110.1; 100-3, 280.1

Y **E0165** **Commode chair, stationary, with detachable arms**   ⅙⊘
Medicare covers commodes for patients confined to their beds or rooms, for patients without indoor bathroom facilities, and to patients who cannot climb or descend the stairs necessary to reach the bathrooms in their homes.
MED: 100-2, 15, 110.1; 100-3, 280.1

Y **E0166** **Commode chair, mobile, with detachable arms** ⅙⊘
Medicare covers commodes for patients confined to their beds or rooms, for patients without indoor bathroom facilities, and to patients who cannot climb or descend the stairs necessary to reach the bathrooms in their homes.
MED: 100-2, 15, 110.1; 100-3, 280.1

Y **E0167** **Pail or pan for use with commode chair**   ⅙⊘
Medicare covers commodes for patients confined to their beds or rooms, for patients without indoor bathroom facilities, and to patients who cannot climb or descend the stairs necessary to reach the bathrooms in their homes.
MED: 100-3, 280.1

Y **E0168** **Commode chair, extra wide and/or heavy duty, stationary or mobile, with or without arms, any type, each**   ⅙⊘

~~E0169~~ ~~Commode chair with seat lift mechanism~~
See code(s) E0170, E0171.

● Y **E0170** **Commode chair with integrated seat lift mechanism, electric, any type**

● Y **E0171** **Commode chair with integrated seat lift mechanism, non-electric, any type**

● E **E0172** **Seat lift mechanism placed over or on top of toilet, any type**

Y ☑ **E0175** **Foot rest, for use with commode chair, each**   ⅙⊘

DECUBITUS CARE EQUIPMENT

Y **E0180** **Pressure pad, alternating with pump**   ⅙⊘
Medicare covers pads if physicians supervise their use in patients who have decubitus ulcers or susceptibility to them. Prior authorization is required by Medicare for this item.
MED: 100-3, 280.1; 100-8, 5, 5.1.1.2.1

Y **E0181** **Pressure pad, alternating with pump, heavy duty**   ⅙⊘
Medicare covers pads if physicians supervise their use in patients who have decubitus ulcers or susceptibility to them. Prior authorization is required by Medicare for this item.
MED: 100-3, 280.1; 100-8, 5, 5.1.1.2.1

Y **E0182** **Pump for alternating pressure pad**   ⅙⊘
Medicare covers pads if physicians supervise their use in patients who have decubitus ulcers or susceptibility to them. Prior authorization is required by Medicare for this item.
MED: 100-3, 280.1; 100-8, 5, 5.1.1.2.1

Y **E0184** **Dry pressure mattress**   ⅙⊘
Medicare covers pads if physicians supervise their use in patients who have decubitus ulcers or susceptibility to them. Prior authorization is required by Medicare for this item.
MED: 100-3, 280.1; 100-8, 5, 5.1.1.2.1

Y **E0185** **Gel or gel-like pressure pad for mattress, standard mattress length and width**   ⅙⊘
Medicare covers pads if physicians supervise their use in patients who have decubitus ulcers or susceptibility to them. Prior authorization is required by Medicare for this item.
MED: 100-3, 280.1; 100-8, 5, 5.1.1.2.1

Y **E0186** **Air pressure mattress**   ⅙⊘
Medicare covers pads if physicians supervise their use in patients who have decubitus ulcers or susceptibility to them.
MED: 100-3, 280.1

Y **E0187** **Water pressure mattress**   ⅙⊘
Medicare covers pads if physicians supervise their use in patients who have decubitus ulcers or susceptibility to them.
MED: 100-3, 280.1

Y **E0188** **Synthetic sheepskin pad**   ⅙⊘
Medicare covers pads if physicians supervise their use in patients who have decubitus ulcers or susceptibility to them. Prior authorization is required by Medicare for this item.
MED: 100-3, 280.1; 100-8, 5, 5.1.1.2.1

Y **E0189** **Lambswool sheepskin pad, any size**   ⅙⊘
Medicare covers pads if physicians supervise their use in patients who have decubitus ulcers or susceptibility to them. Prior authorization is required by Medicare for this item.
MED: 100-3, 280.1; 100-8, 5, 5.1.1.2.1

E **E0190** **Positioning cushion/pillow/wedge, any shape or size**
MED: 100-2, 15, 110.1

Y ☑ **E0191** **Heel or elbow protector, each**   ⅙⊘

Y **E0193** **Powered air flotation bed (low air loss therapy)** ⅙⊘

Y **E0194** **Air fluidized bed**   ⅙⊘
An air fluidized bed is covered by Medicare if the patient has a stage 3 or stage 4 pressure sore and, without the bed, would require institutionalization. A physician's prescription is required.
MED: 100-3, 280.8

Y **E0196** **Gel pressure mattress**   ⅙⊘
Medicare covers pads if physicians supervise their use in patients who have decubitus ulcers or susceptibility to them.
MED: 100-3, 280.1

Y **E0197** **Air pressure pad for mattress, standard mattress length and width**   ⅙⊘
Medicare covers pads if physicians supervise their use in patients who have decubitus ulcers or susceptibility to them.
MED: 100-3, 280.1

Y **E0198** **Water pressure pad for mattress, standard mattress length and width**   ⅙⊘
Medicare covers pads if physicians supervise their use in patients who have decubitus ulcers or susceptibility to them.
MED: 100-3, 280.1

Y **E0199** **Dry pressure pad for mattress, standard mattress length and width**   ⅙⊘
Medicare covers pads if physicians supervise their use in patients who have decubitus ulcers or susceptibility to them.
MED: 100-3, 280.1

HEAT/COLD APPLICATION

Y **E0200** **Heat lamp, without stand (table model), includes bulb, or infrared element**   ⅙⊘
MED: 100-2, 15, 110.1; 100-3, 280.1

Special Coverage Instructions   Noncovered by Medicare   Carrier Discretion   ☑ Quantity Alert   ● New Code   ○ Reinstated Code   ▲ Revised Code

42 — E Codes   A Age   M Maternity   ♀ Female Only   ♂ Male Only   A-Y APC Status Indicator   **2006 HCPCS**

Y	**E0202**	Phototherapy (bilirubin) light with photometer	♿⊘
A	**E0203**	Therapeutic lightbox, minimum 10,000 lux, table top model	
Y	**E0205**	Heat lamp, with stand, includes bulb, or infrared element MED: 100-2, 15, 110.1; 100-3, 280.1	♿⊘
Y	**E0210**	Electric heat pad, standard MED: 100-3, 280.1	♿⊘
Y	**E0215**	Electric heat pad, moist MED: 100-3, 280.1	♿⊘
Y	**E0217**	Water circulating heat pad with pump MED: 100-3, 280.1	♿⊘
Y	**E0218**	Water circulating cold pad with pump MED: 100-3, 280.1	&#x2298;
Y	**E0220**	Hot water bottle	♿⊘
Y ☑	**E0221**	Infrared heating pad system MED: 100-3, 270.2	♿⊘
Y	**E0225**	Hydrocollator unit, includes pads MED: 100-2, 15, 230; 100-3, 280.1	♿⊘
Y	**E0230**	Ice cap or collar	♿⊘
E	**E0231**	Non-contact wound warming device (temperature control unit, AC adapter and power cord) for use with warming card and wound cover MED: 100-2, 16, 20	&#x2298;
E	**E0232**	Warming card for use with the non-contact wound warming device and non-contact wound warming wound cover MED: 100-2, 16, 20	&#x2298;
Y	**E0235**	Paraffin bath unit, portable (see medical supply code A4265 for paraffin) MED: 100-2, 15, 230; 100-3, 280.1	♿⊘
Y	**E0236**	Pump for water circulating pad MED: 100-3, 280.1	♿⊘
Y	**E0238**	Nonelectric heat pad, moist MED: 100-3, 280.1	♿⊘
Y	**E0239**	Hydrocollator unit, portable MED: 100-2, 15, 230; 100-3, 280.1	♿⊘

BATH AND TOILET AIDS

E	**E0240**	Bath/shower chair, with or without wheels, any size MED: 100-3, 280.1	&#x2298;
E ☑	**E0241**	Bathtub wall rail, each MED: 100-2, 15, 110.1; 100-3, 280.1	&#x2298;
E	**E0242**	Bathtub rail, floor base MED: 100-2, 15, 110.1; 100-3, 280.1	&#x2298;
E ☑	**E0243**	Toilet rail, each MED: 100-2, 15, 110.1; 100-3, 280.1	&#x2298;
E	**E0244**	Raised toilet seat MED: 100-3, 280.1	&#x2298;
E	**E0245**	Tub stool or bench MED: 100-3, 280.1	&#x2298;
E	**E0246**	Transfer tub rail attachment	&#x2298;
E	**E0247**	Transfer bench for tub or toilet with or without commode opening MED: 100-3, 280.1	&#x2298;

E	**E0248**	Transfer bench, heavy duty, for tub or toilet with or without commode opening MED: 100-3, 280.1	&#x2298;
Y	**E0249**	Pad for water circulating heat unit MED: 100-3, 280.1	♿⊘

HOSPITAL BEDS AND ACCESSORIES

Y	**E0250**	Hospital bed, fixed height, with any type side rails, with mattress MED: 100-2, 15, 110.1; 100-3, 280.7	♿⊘
Y	**E0251**	Hospital bed, fixed height, with any type side rails, without mattress MED: 100-2, 15, 110.1; 100-3, 280.7	♿⊘
Y	**E0255**	Hospital bed, variable height, hi-lo, with any type side rails, with mattress MED: 100-2, 15, 110.1; 100-3, 280.7	♿⊘
Y	**E0256**	Hospital bed, variable height, hi-lo, with any type side rails, without mattress MED: 100-2, 15, 110.1; 100-3, 280.7	♿⊘
Y	**E0260**	Hospital bed, semi-electric (head and foot adjustment), with any type side rails, with mattress MED: 100-2, 15, 110.1; 100-3, 280.7	♿⊘
Y	**E0261**	Hospital bed, semi-electric (head and foot adjustment), with any type side rails, without mattress MED: 100-2, 15, 110.1; 100-3, 280.7	♿⊘
Y	**E0265**	Hospital bed, total electric (head, foot, and height adjustments), with any type side rails, with mattress MED: 100-2, 15, 110.1; 100-3, 280.7	♿⊘
Y	**E0266**	Hospital bed, total electric (head, foot, and height adjustments), with any type side rails, without mattress MED: 100-2, 15, 110.1; 100-3, 280.7	♿⊘
E	**E0270**	Hospital bed, institutional type includes: oscillating, circulating and Stryker frame, with mattress MED: 100-3, 280.1	&#x2298;
Y	**E0271**	Mattress, inner spring MED: 100-3, 280.1; 100-3, 280.7	♿⊘
Y	**E0272**	Mattress, foam rubber MED: 100-3, 280.1; 100-3, 280.7	♿⊘
E	**E0273**	Bed board MED: 100-3, 280.1	&#x2298;
E	**E0274**	Over-bed table MED: 100-3, 280.1	&#x2298;
Y	**E0275**	Bed pan, standard, metal or plastic Reusable, autoclavable bedpans are covered by Medicare for bed-confined patients. MED: 100-3, 280.1	♿⊘
Y	**E0276**	Bed pan, fracture, metal or plastic Reusable, autoclavable bedpans are covered by Medicare for bed-confined patients. MED: 100-3, 280.1	♿⊘
Y	**E0277**	Powered pressure-reducing air mattress MED: 100-3, 280.1	♿⊘
Y	**E0280**	Bed cradle, any type	♿⊘
Y	**E0290**	Hospital bed, fixed height, without side rails, with mattress MED: 100-2, 15, 110.1; 100-3, 280.7	♿⊘

Special Coverage Instructions	Noncovered by Medicare	Carrier Discretion

☑ Quantity Alert   ● New Code   ○ Reinstated Code   ▲ Revised Code

♿ DMEPOS Paid   ⊘ SNF Excluded

Durable Medical Equipment

E0291 — E0441

Y   **E0291** Hospital bed, fixed height, without side rails, without mattress   🦽⊘
MED: 100-2, 15, 110.1; 100-3, 280.7

Y   **E0292** Hospital bed, variable height, hi-lo, without side rails, with mattress   🦽⊘
MED: 100-2, 15, 110.1; 100-3, 280.7

Y   **E0293** Hospital bed, variable height, hi-lo, without side rails, without mattress   🦽⊘
MED: 100-2, 15, 110.1; 100-3, 280.7

Y   **E0294** Hospital bed, semi-electric (head and foot adjustment), without side rails, with mattress 🦽⊘
MED: 100-2, 15, 110.1; 100-3, 280.7

Y   **E0295** Hospital bed, semi-electric (head and foot adjustment), without side rails, without mattress   🦽⊘
MED: 100-2, 15, 110.1; 100-3, 280.7

Y   **E0296** Hospital bed, total electric (head, foot, and height adjustments), without side rails, with mattress   🦽⊘
MED: 100-2, 15, 110.1; 100-3, 280.7

Y   **E0297** Hospital bed, total electric (head, foot, and height adjustments), without side rails, without mattress   🦽⊘
MED: 100-2, 15, 110.1; 100-3, 280.7

Y   **E0300** Pediatric crib, hospital grade, fully enclosed   🦽⊘

Y   **E0301** Hospital bed, heavy duty, extra wide, with weight capacity greater than 350 pounds, but less than or equal to 600 pounds, with any type side rails, without mattress   🦽⊘
MED: 100-3, 280.7

Y   **E0302** Hospital bed, extra heavy duty, extra wide, with weight capacity greater than 600 pounds, with any type side rails, without mattress   🦽⊘
MED: 100-3, 280.7

Y   **E0303** Hospital bed, heavy duty, extra wide, with weight capacity greater than 350 pounds, but less than or equal to 600 pounds, with any type side rails, with mattress   🦽⊘
MED: 100-3, 280.7

Y   **E0304** Hospital bed, extra heavy duty, extra wide, with weight capacity greater than 600 pounds, with any type side rails, with mattress   🦽⊘
MED: 100-3, 280.7

Y   **E0305** Bedside rails, half-length   🦽⊘
MED: 100-3, 280.7

Y   **E0310** Bedside rails, full-length   🦽⊘
MED: 100-3, 280.7

E   **E0315** Bed accessory: board, table, or support device, any type   ⊘
MED: 100-3, 280.1

Y   **E0316** Safety enclosure frame/canopy for use with hospital bed, any type   🦽⊘

Y   **E0325** Urinal; male, jug-type, any material   ♂🦽⊘
MED: 100-3, 280.1

Y   **E0326** Urinal; female, jug-type, any material   ♀🦽⊘
MED: 100-3, 280.1

E   **E0350** Control unit for electronic bowel irrigation/evacuation system   ⊘

E   **E0352** Disposable pack (water reservoir bag, speculum, valving mechanism and collection bag/box) for use with the electronic bowel irrigation/evacuation system   ⊘

E   **E0370** Air pressure elevator for heel   ⊘

Y   **E0371** Nonpowered advanced pressure reducing overlay for mattress, standard mattress length and width 🦽⊘

Y   **E0372** Powered air overlay for mattress, standard mattress length and width   🦽⊘

Y   **E0373** Nonpowered advanced pressure reducing mattress   🦽⊘

OXYGEN AND RELATED RESPIRATORY EQUIPMENT

Y   **E0424** Stationary compressed gaseous oxygen system, rental; includes container, contents, regulator, flowmeter, humidifier, nebulizer, cannula or mask, and tubing   🦽⊘
For the first claim filed for home oxygen equipment or therapy, submit a certificate of medical necessity that includes the oxygen flow rate, anticipated frequency and duration of oxygen therapy, and physician signature. Medicare accepts oxygen therapy as medically necessary in cases documenting any of the following: erythocythemia with a hematocrit greater than 56 percent; a P pulmonale on EKG; or dependent edema consistent with congestive heart failure.

MED: 100-3, 240.2

E   **E0425** Stationary compressed gas system, purchase; includes regulator, flowmeter, humidifier, nebulizer, cannula or mask, and tubing   ⊘
MED: 100-3, 240.2

E   **E0430** Portable gaseous oxygen system, purchase; includes regulator, flowmeter, humidifier, cannula or mask, and tubing   ⊘
MED: 100-3, 240.2

Y   **E0431** Portable gaseous oxygen system, rental; includes portable container, regulator, flowmeter, humidifier, cannula or mask, and tubing   🦽⊘
MED: 100-3, 240.2

Y   **E0434** Portable liquid oxygen system, rental; includes portable container, supply reservoir, humidifier, flowmeter, refill adaptor, contents gauge, cannula or mask, and tubing   🦽⊘
MED: 100-3, 240.2

E   **E0435** Portable liquid oxygen system, purchase; includes portable container, supply reservoir, flowmeter, humidifier, contents gauge, cannula or mask, tubing, and refill adapter   ⊘
MED: 100-3, 240.2

Y   **E0439** Stationary liquid oxygen system, rental; includes container, contents, regulator, flowmeter, humidifier, nebulizer, cannula or mask, and tubing   🦽⊘
MED: 100-3, 240.2

E   **E0440** Stationary liquid oxygen system, purchase; includes use of reservoir, contents indicator, regulator, flowmeter, humidifier, nebulizer, cannula or mask, and tubing   ⊘
MED: 100-3, 240.2

Y ☑   **E0441** Oxygen contents, gaseous (for use with owned gaseous stationary systems or when both a stationary and portable gaseous system are owned), one month's supply = 1 unit   🦽⊘
MED: 100-3, 240.2

| Special Coverage Instructions | Noncovered by Medicare | Carrier Discretion | ☑ Quantity Alert | ● New Code | ○ Reinstated Code | ▲ Revised Code |

44 — E Codes   A Age   M Maternity   ♀ Female Only   ♂ Male Only   A-Y APC Status Indicator   **2006 HCPCS**

E0442 Oxygen contents, liquid (for use with owned liquid stationary systems or when both a stationary and portable liquid system are owned), one month's supply = 1 unit
MED: 100-3, 240.2

E0443 Portable oxygen contents, gaseous (for use only with portable gaseous systems when no stationary gas or liquid system is used), one month's supply = 1 unit
MED: 100-3, 240.2

E0444 Portable oxygen contents, liquid (for use only with portable liquid systems when no stationary gas or liquid system is used), one month's supply = 1 unit
MED: 100-3, 240.2

E0445 Oximeter device for measuring blood oxygen levels non-invasively

E0450 Volume control ventilator, without pressure support mode, may include pressure control mode, used with invasive interface (e.g., tracheostomy tube)
MED: 100-3, 280.1

E0455 Oxygen tent, excluding croup or pediatric tents
MED: 100-3, 240.2

E0457 Chest shell (cuirass)

E0459 Chest wrap

E0460 Negative pressure ventilator; portable or stationary
MED: 100-3, 280.1

E0461 Volume control ventilator, without pressure support mode, may include pressure control mode, used with non-invasive interface (e.g., mask)
MED: 100-3, 280.1

E0462 Rocking bed, with or without side rails

E0463 Pressure support ventilator with volume control mode, may include pressure control mode, used with invasive interface (e.g., tracheostomy tube)

E0464 Pressure support ventilator with volume control mode, may include pressure control mode, used with non-invasive interface (e.g., mask)

E0470 Respiratory assist device, bi-level pressure capability, without backup rate feature, used with noninvasive interface, e.g., nasal or facial mask (intermittent assist device with continuous positive airway pressure device)
MED: 100-3, 280.1

E0471 Respiratory assist device, bi-level pressure capability, with back-up rate feature, used with noninvasive interface, e.g., nasal or facial mask (intermittent assist device with continuous positive airway pressure device)
MED: 100-3, 280.1

E0472 Respiratory assist device, bi-level pressure capability, with backup rate feature, used with invasive interface, e.g., tracheostomy tube (intermittent assist device with continuous positive airway pressure device)
MED: 100-3, 280.1

E0480 Percussor, electric or pneumatic, home model
MED: 100-3, 280.1

E0481 Intrapulmonary percussive ventilation system and related accessories
MED: 100-3, 240.5

E0482 Cough stimulating device, alternating positive and negative airway pressure

E0483 High frequency chest wall oscillation air-pulse generator system, (includes hoses and vest), each

E0484 Oscillatory positive expiratory pressure device, non-electric, any type, each

E0485 Oral device/appliance used to reduce upper airway collapsibility, adjustable or non-adjustable, prefabricated, includes fitting and adjustment

E0486 Oral device/appliance used to reduce upper airway collapsibility, adjustable or non-adjustable, custom fabricated, includes fitting and adjustment

IPPB MACHINES

E0500 IPPB machine, all types, with built-in nebulization; manual or automatic valves; internal or external power source
MED: 100-3, 280.1

HUMIDIFIERS/COMPRESSORS/NEBULIZERS FOR USE WITH OXYGEN IPPB EQUIPMENT

E0550 Humidifier, durable for extensive supplemental humidification during IPPB treatments or oxygen delivery
MED: 100-3, 280.1

E0555 Humidifier, durable, glass or autoclavable plastic bottle type, for use with regulator or flowmeter
MED: 100-3, 280.1

E0560 Humidifier, durable for supplemental humidification during IPPB treatment or oxygen delivery
MED: 100-3, 280.1

E0561 Humidifier, non-heated, used with positive airway pressure device

E0562 Humidifier, heated, used with positive airway pressure device

E0565 Compressor, air power source for equipment which is not self-contained or cylinder driven

E0570 Nebulizer, with compressor
MED: 100-3, 280.1

E0571 Aerosol compressor, battery powered, for use with small volume nebulizer
MED: 100-3, 280.1

E0572 Aerosol compressor, adjustable pressure, light duty for intermittent use

E0574 Ultrasonic/electronic aerosol generator with small volume nebulizer

Battery pack and controls
Nebulizer
IPPB unit in use
Nebulizer reservoir
Oxygen supply tube
Intermittent Positive Pressure Breathing (IPPB) devices

Ⓨ   **E0575** Nebulizer, ultrasonic, large volume   ♿⊘
MED: 100-3, 280.1

Ⓨ   **E0580** Nebulizer, durable, glass or autoclavable plastic, bottle type, for use with regulator or flowmeter ♿⊘
MED: 100-3, 280.1

Ⓨ   **E0585** Nebulizer, with compressor and heater   ♿⊘
MED: 100-3, 280.1

~~E0590~~ ~~Dispensing fee covered drug administered through DME nebulizer suction pump, home model, portable~~

SUCTION PUMP/ROOM VAPORIZERS

Ⓨ   **E0600** Respiratory suction pump, home model, portable or stationary, electric   ♿⊘
MED: 100-3, 280.1

Ⓨ   **E0601** Continuous airway pressure (CPAP) device   ♿⊘
MED: 100-3, 240.4

Ⓨ   **E0602** Breast pump, manual, any type   Ⓜ♀♿⊘

Ⓐ   **E0603** Breast pump, electric (AC and/or DC), any type   Ⓜ♀⊘

Ⓐ   **E0604** Breast pump, heavy duty, hospital grade, piston operated, pulsatile vacuum suction/release cycles, vacuum regulator, supplies, transformer, electric (AC and/or DC)   Ⓜ♀⊘

Ⓨ   **E0605** Vaporizer, room type   ♿⊘
MED: 100-3, 280.1

Ⓨ   **E0606** Postural drainage board   ♿⊘
MED: 100-3, 280.1

MONITORING EQUIPMENT

Ⓨ   **E0607** Home blood glucose monitor   ♿⊘

Medicare covers home blood testing devices for diabetic patients when the devices are prescribed by the patients' physicians. Many commercial payers provide this coverage to non-insulin dependent diabetics as well.

MED: 100-3, 230.16

PACEMAKER MONITOR

Ⓨ   **E0610** Pacemaker monitor, self-contained, checks battery depletion, includes audible and visible check systems   ♿⊘
MED: 100-3, 20.8; 100-3, 20.8; 100-3, 20.8.1; 100-3, 20.8.1; 100-3, 20.8.2

Ⓨ   **E0615** Pacemaker monitor, self-contained, checks battery depletion and other pacemaker components, includes digital/visible check systems   ♿⊘
MED: 100-3, 20.8; 100-3, 20.8; 100-3, 20.8.1; 100-3, 20.8.1; 100-3, 20.8.2

Ⓝ   **E0616** Implantable cardiac event recorder with memory, activator and programmer   ⊘

Ⓨ   **E0617** External defibrillator with integrated electrocardiogram analysis   ♿⊘

Ⓐ   **E0618** Apnea monitor, without recording feature   ♿

Ⓐ   **E0619** Apnea monitor, with recording feature   ♿

Ⓨ   **E0620** Skin piercing device for collection of capillary blood, laser, each   ♿⊘

PATIENT LIFTS

Ⓨ   **E0621** Sling or seat, patient lift, canvas or nylon   ♿⊘
MED: 100-3, 280.1

Ⓔ   **E0625** Patient lift, bathroom or toilet, not otherwise classified   ⊘
MED: 100-3, 280.1

Ⓨ   **E0627** Seat lift mechanism incorporated into a combination lift-chair mechanism   ♿⊘
MED: 100-3, 280.4; 100-4, 20, 100; 100-4, 20, 130.2; 100-4, 20, 130.3; 100-4, 20, 130.4; 100-4, 20, 130.5
See code(s): Q0080

Ⓨ   **E0628** Separate seat lift mechanism for use with patient owned furniture — electric   ♿⊘
MED: 100-3, 280.4; 100-4, 20, 100; 100-4, 20, 130.2; 100-4, 20, 130.3; 100-4, 20, 130.4; 100-4, 20, 130.5
See code(s): Q0078

Ⓨ   **E0629** Separate seat lift mechanism for use with patient owned furniture — nonelectric   ♿⊘
MED: 100-4, 20, 100; 100-4, 20, 130.2; 100-4, 20, 130.3; 100-4, 20, 130.4; 100-4, 20, 130.5
See code(s): Q0079

Ⓨ   **E0630** Patient lift, hydraulic, with seat or sling   ♿⊘
MED: 100-3, 280.1

Ⓨ   **E0635** Patient lift, electric, with seat or sling   ♿⊘
MED: 100-3, 280.1

Ⓨ   **E0636** Multipositional patient support system, with integrated lift, patient accessible controls   ♿

▲ Ⓔ   **E0637** Combination sit to stand system, any size including pediatric, with seatlift feature, with or without wheels   ♿⊘
MED: 100-3, 280.1

▲ Ⓔ   **E0638** Standing frame system, one position (e.g., upright, supine or prone stander), any size including pediatric, with or without wheels   ♿⊘
MED: 100-3, 280.1

   E0639 Patient lift, moveable from room to room with disassembly and reassembly, includes all components/accessories

   E0640 Patient lift, fixed system, includes all components/accessories

● Ⓔ   **E0641** Standing frame system, multi-position (e.g., three-way stander), any size including pediatric, with or without wheels   ♿⊘
MED: 100-3, 280.1

● Ⓔ   **E0642** Standing frame system, mobile (dynamic stander), any size including pediatric   ♿⊘
MED: 100-3, 280.1

PNEUMATIC COMPRESSOR AND APPLIANCES

Ⓨ   **E0650** Pneumatic compressor, nonsegmental home model   ♿⊘
MED: 100-3, 280.6

Ⓨ   **E0651** Pneumatic compressor, segmental home model without calibrated gradient pressure   ♿⊘
MED: 100-3, 280.6

Ⓨ   **E0652** Pneumatic compressor, segmental home model with calibrated gradient pressure   ♿⊘
MED: 100-3, 280.6

Ⓨ   **E0655** Nonsegmental pneumatic appliance for use with pneumatic compressor, half arm   ♿⊘
MED: 100-3, 280.6

Ⓨ   **E0660** Nonsegmental pneumatic appliance for use with pneumatic compressor, full leg   ♿⊘
MED: 100-3, 280.6

▭ Special Coverage Instructions   ▭ Noncovered by Medicare   ▭ Carrier Discretion   ☑ Quantity Alert   ● New Code   ○ Reinstated Code   ▲ Revised Code

46 — E Codes   ⒶAge   ⓂMaternity   ♀ Female Only   ♂ Male Only   Ⓐ-Ⓨ APC Status Indicator   *2006 HCPCS*

☑ **E0665** Nonsegmental pneumatic appliance for use with pneumatic compressor, full arm ᵬ⊘
MED: 100-3, 280.6

☑ **E0666** Nonsegmental pneumatic appliance for use with pneumatic compressor, half leg ᵬ⊘
MED: 100-3, 280.6

☑ **E0667** Segmental pneumatic appliance for use with pneumatic compressor, full leg ᵬ⊘
MED: 100-3, 280.6

☑ **E0668** Segmental pneumatic appliance for use with pneumatic compressor, full arm ᵬ⊘
MED: 100-3, 280.6

☑ **E0669** Segmental pneumatic appliance for use with pneumatic compressor, half leg ᵬ⊘
MED: 100-3, 280.6

☑ **E0671** Segmental gradient pressure pneumatic appliance, full leg ᵬ⊘
MED: 100-3, 280.6

☑ **E0672** Segmental gradient pressure pneumatic appliance, full arm ᵬ⊘
MED: 100-3, 280.6

☑ **E0673** Segmental gradient pressure pneumatic appliance, half leg ᵬ⊘
MED: 100-3, 280.6

☑ **E0675** Pneumatic compression device, high pressure, rapid inflation/deflation cycle, for arterial insufficiency (unilateral or bilateral system) ᵬ⊘

☑ **E0691** Ultraviolet light therapy system panel, includes bulbs/lamps, timer and eye protection; treatment area two sq. feet or less ᵬ

☑ **E0692** Ultraviolet light therapy system panel, includes bulbs/lamps, timer and eye protection, four foot panel ᵬ

☑ **E0693** Ultraviolet light therapy system panel, includes bulbs/lamps, timer and eye protection, six foot panel ᵬ

☑ **E0694** Ultraviolet multidirectional light therapy system in six foot cabinet, includes bulbs/lamps, timer and eye protection ᵬ

SAFETY EQUIPMENT

Ⓔ **E0700** Safety equipment (e.g., belt, harness or vest) ⊘

☑ **E0701** Helmet with face guard and soft interface material, prefabricated ᵬ

● Ⓑ **E0705** Transfer board or device, any type, each

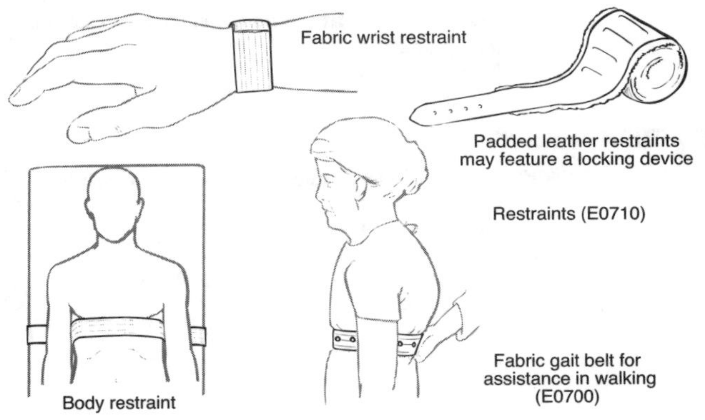

Fabric wrist restraint

Padded leather restraints may feature a locking device

Restraints (E0710)

Fabric gait belt for assistance in walking (E0700)

Body restraint

RESTRAINTS

Ⓔ **E0710** Restraint, any type (body, chest, wrist or ankle) ⊘

TRANSCUTANEOUS AND/OR NEUROMUSCULAR ELECTRICAL NERVE STIMULATORS — TENS

☑ **E0720** TENS, two lead, localized stimulation ᵬ⊘
While TENS is covered when employed to control chronic pain, it is not covered for experimental treatment, as in motor function disorders like MS. Prior authorization is required by Medicare for this item.

MED: 100-3, 130.5; 100-3, 130.5; 100-3, 130.6; 100-3, 130.6; 100-3, 160.2; 100-3, 160.2; 100-3, 160.2; 100-3, 160.7.1; 100-3, 230.1; 100-3, 230.1; 100-3, 40.5; 100-3, 40.5; 100-3, 40.5; 100-3, 40.5; 100-3, 40.5; 100-3, 40.5; 100-3, 40.5; 100-3, 40.5; 100-3, 40.5; 100-3, 40.5; 100-3, 40.5; 100-3, 40.5; 100-3, 40.5; 100-3, 40.5; 100-3, 40.5; 100-3, 40.5; 100-8, 5, 5.1.1.2.1

☑ **E0730** TENS, four or more leads, for multiple nerve stimulation ᵬ⊘
While TENS is covered when employed to control chronic pain, it is not covered for experimental treatment, as in motor function disorders like MS. Prior authorization is required by Medicare for this item.

MED: 100-3, 130.5; 100-3, 130.5; 100-3, 130.6; 100-3, 130.6; 100-3, 130.6; 100-3, 160.2; 100-3, 160.2; 100-3, 160.2; 100-3, 160.7.1; 100-3, 230.1; 100-3, 230.1; 100-3, 40.5; 100-3, 40.5; 100-3, 40.5; 100-3, 40.5; 100-3, 40.5; 100-3, 40.5; 100-3, 40.5; 100-3, 40.5; 100-3, 40.5; 100-3, 40.5; 100-3, 40.5; 100-3, 40.5; 100-3, 40.5; 100-3, 40.5; 100-3, 40.5; 100-8, 5, 5.1.1.2.1

☑ **E0731** Form-fitting conductive garment for delivery of TENS or NMES (with conductive fibers separated from the patient's skin by layers of fabric) ᵬ⊘
MED: 100-3, 160.13

☑ **E0740** Incontinence treatment system, pelvic floor stimulator, monitor, sensor and/or trainer ᵬ⊘
MED: 100-3, 230.8

☑ **E0744** Neuromuscular stimulator for scoliosis ᵬ⊘

☑ **E0745** Neuromuscular stimulator, electronic shock unit ᵬ⊘
MED: 100-3, 160.12

Ⓔ **E0746** Electromyography (EMG), biofeedback device ⊘
Biofeedback therapy is covered by Medicare only for re-education of specific muscles or for treatment of incapacitating muscle spasm or weakness. Medicare jurisdiction: local contractor.

MED: 100-3, 30.1; 100-3, 30.1.1

☑ **E0747** Osteogenesis stimulator, electrical, noninvasive, other than spinal applications ᵬ⊘
Medicare covers noninvasive osteogenic stimulation for nonunion of long bone fractures, failed fusion, or congenital pseudoarthroses.

MED: 100-3, 150.2

☑ **E0748** Osteogenesis stimulator, electrical, noninvasive, spinal applications ᵬ⊘
Medicare covers noninvasive osteogenic stimulation as an adjunct to spinal fusion surgery for patients at high risk of pseudoarthroses due to previously failed spinal fusion, or for those undergoing fusion of three or more vertebrae.

MED: 100-3, 150.2

Ⓝ **E0749** Osteogenesis stimulator, electrical, surgically implanted ᵬ⊘
Medicare covers invasive osteogenic stimulation for nonunion of long bone fractures or as an adjunct to spinal fusion surgery for patients at high risk of pseudoarthroses due to previously failed spinal fusion, or for those undergoing fusion of three or more vertebrae.

MED: 100-3, 150.2

Special Coverage Instructions   Noncovered by Medicare   Carrier Discretion   ☑ Quantity Alert   ● New Code   ○ Reinstated Code   ▲ Revised Code

2006 HCPCS   ❶-❾ ASC Groups   MED: Pub 100/NCD Reference   ᵬ DMEPOS Paid   ⊘ SNF Excluded   **E Codes — 47**

Durable Medical Equipment

E0752 — E0900

~~E0752~~ ~~Implantable neurostimulator electrode, each~~
See code(s) L8680.

~~E0754~~ ~~Patient programmer (external) for use with implantable programmable neurostimulator pulse generator~~
See code(s) L8681.

E   **E0755** Electronic salivary reflex stimulator (intraoral/noninvasive)   ⊘

~~E0756~~ ~~Implantable neurostimulator pulse generator~~
See code(s) L8685-L8688.

~~E0757~~ ~~Implantable neurostimulator radiofrequency receiver~~
See code(s) L8682.

~~E0758~~ ~~Radiofrequency transmitter (external) for use with implantable neurostimulator radiofrequency receiver~~
See code(s) L8683.

~~E0759~~ ~~Radiofrequency transmitter (external) for use with implantable sacral root neurostimulator receiver for bowel and bladder management, replacement~~
See code(s) L8684.

Y   **E0760** Osteogenesis stimulator, low intensity ultrasound, non-invasive   ዻ⊘
MED: 100-3, 150.2

E   **E0761** Non-thermal pulsed high frequency radiowaves, high peak power electromagnetic energy treatment device

● B   **E0762** Transcutaneous electrical joint stimulation device system, includes all accessories

● Y   **E0764** Functional neuromuscular stimulator, transcutaneous stimulation of muscles of ambulation with computer control, used for walking by spinal cord injured, entire system, after completion of training program
MED: 100-3, 160.12

Y   **E0765** FDA approved nerve stimulator, with replaceable batteries, for treatment of nausea and vomiting ዻ⊘

E0769 Electrical stimulation or electromagnetic wound treatment device, not otherwise classified
MED: 100-4, 32, 11.1

INFUSION SUPPLIES

Y   **E0776** IV pole   ዻ⊘

Y   **E0779** Ambulatory infusion pump, mechanical, reusable, for infusion 8 hours or greater   ዻ⊘

Y   **E0780** Ambulatory infusion pump, mechanical, reusable, for infusion less than 8 hours   ዻ⊘

Y   **E0781** Ambulatory infusion pump, single or multiple channels, electric or battery operated, with administrative equipment, worn by patient   ዻ⊘
Medicare jurisdiction: DME local or regional contractor. Bill Medicare claims for regional contractor when the infusion is initiated in the physician's office but the patient does not return during the same day of business.
MED: 100-3, 280.14

N   **E0782** Infusion pump, implantable, non-programmable (includes all components, e.g., pump, catheter, connectors, etc.)   ዻ⊘
Medicare jurisdiction: local contractor.
MED: 100-3, 280.14

N   **E0783** Infusion pump system, implantable, programmable (includes all components, e.g., pump, catheter, connectors, etc.)   ዻ⊘
Medicare jurisdiction: local contractor.
MED: 100-3, 280.14

Y   **E0784** External ambulatory infusion pump, insulin   ዻ⊘
Covered by some commercial payers with preauthorization.
MED: 100-3, 280.14

N   **E0785** Implantable intraspinal (epidural/intrathecal) catheter used with implantable infusion pump, replacement   ዻ⊘
Medicare jurisdiction: local contractor.
MED: 100-3, 280.14

N   **E0786** Implantable programmable infusion pump, replacement (excludes implantable intraspinal catheter)   ዻ⊘
Medicare jurisdiction: local contractor.
MED: 100-3, 280.14

Y   **E0791** Parenteral infusion pump, stationary, single or multichannel   ዻ⊘
MED: 100-2, 15, 120; 100-3, 180.2; 100-4, 20, 100.2.2; 100-4, 20, 100.2.2.3

TRACTION — ALL TYPES

N   **E0830** Ambulatory traction device, all types, each   ⊘
MED: 100-3, 280.1

TRACTION — CERVICAL

Y   **E0840** Traction frame, attached to headboard, cervical traction   ዻ⊘
MED: 100-3, 280.1

E0849 Traction equipment, cervical, free-standing stand/frame, pneumatic, applying traction force to other than mandible

Y   **E0850** Traction stand, freestanding, cervical traction ዻ⊘
MED: 100-3, 280.1

Y   **E0855** Cervical traction equipment not requiring additional stand or frame   ዻ⊘

TRACTION — OVERDOOR

Y   **E0860** Traction equipment, overdoor, cervical   ዻ⊘
MED: 100-3, 280.1

TRACTION — EXTREMITY

Y   **E0870** Traction frame, attached to footboard, extremity traction (e.g., Buck's)   ዻ⊘
MED: 100-3, 280.1

Y   **E0880** Traction stand, freestanding, extremity traction (e.g., Buck's)   ዻ⊘
MED: 100-3, 280.1

TRACTION — PELVIC

Y   **E0890** Traction frame, attached to footboard, pelvic traction   ዻ⊘
MED: 100-3, 280.1

Y   **E0900** Traction stand, freestanding, pelvic traction (e.g., Buck's)   ዻ⊘
MED: 100-3, 280.1

TRAPEZE EQUIPMENT, FRACTURE FRAME, AND OTHER ORTHOPEDIC DEVICES

Ⓨ		**E0910**	Trapeze bars, also known as Patient Helper, attached to bed, with grab bar ♿⊘ MED: 100-3, 280.1
● Ⓨ		**E0911**	Trapeze bar, heavy duty, for patient weight capacity greater than 250 pounds, attached to bed, with grab bar ·MED: 100-3, 280.1
● Ⓨ		**E0912**	Trapeze bar, heavy duty, for patient weight capacity greater than 250 pounds, free standing, complete with grab bar MED: 100-3, 280.1
Ⓨ		**E0920**	Fracture frame, attached to bed, includes weights ♿⊘ MED: 100-3, 280.1
Ⓨ		**E0930**	Fracture frame, freestanding, includes weights ♿⊘ MED: 100-3, 280.1
▲ Ⓨ		**E0935**	Continuous passive motion exercise device for use on knee only ♿⊘ MED: 100-3, 280.1
Ⓨ		**E0940**	Trapeze bar, freestanding, complete with grab bar ♿⊘ MED: 100-3, 280.1
Ⓨ		**E0941**	Gravity assisted traction device, any type ♿⊘ MED: 100-3, 280.1
Ⓨ		**E0942**	Cervical head harness/halter ♿⊘
Ⓨ		**E0944**	Pelvic belt/harness/boot ♿⊘
Ⓨ		**E0945**	Extremity belt/harness ♿⊘
Ⓨ		**E0946**	Fracture frame, dual with cross bars, attached to bed (e.g., Balken, Four Poster) ♿⊘ MED: 100-3, 280.1
Ⓨ		**E0947**	Fracture frame, attachments for complex pelvic traction ♿⊘ MED: 100-3, 280.1
Ⓨ		**E0948**	Fracture frame, attachments for complex cervical traction ♿⊘ MED: 100-3, 280.1
Ⓔ		**E0950**	Wheelchair accessory, tray, each ♿⊘ MED: 100-3, 280.1
Ⓔ		**E0951**	Heel loop/holder, any type, with or without ankle strap, each
Ⓔ		**E0952**	Toe loop/holder, any type, each MED: 100-3, 280.1
		~~E0953~~	~~Pneumatic tire, each~~ See code(s) E2211.
		~~E0954~~	~~Semi pneumatic caster, each~~ See code(s) E2219.
Ⓨ	☑	**E0955**	Wheelchair accessory, headrest, cushioned, any type, including fixed mounting hardware, each ♿⊘
Ⓨ	☑	**E0956**	Wheelchair accessory, lateral trunk or hip support, any type, including fixed mounting hardware, each ♿⊘
Ⓨ	☑	**E0957**	Wheelchair accessory, medial thigh support, any type, including fixed mounting hardware, each ♿⊘
Ⓐ		**E0958**	Manual wheelchair accessory, one-arm drive attachment, each ♿⊘ MED: 100-3, 280.1

Ⓑ		**E0959**	Manual wheelchair accessory, adapter for amputee, each ♿⊘ MED: 100-3, 280.1
Ⓨ		**E0960**	Wheelchair accessory, shoulder harness/straps or chest strap, including any type mounting hardware ♿⊘
Ⓑ		**E0961**	Manual wheelchair accessory, wheel lock brake extension (handle), each ♿⊘ MED: 100-3, 280.1
Ⓑ		**E0966**	Manual wheelchair accessory, headrest extension, each ♿⊘ MED: 100-3, 280.1
Ⓨ ☑		**E0967**	Manual wheelchair accessory, hand rim with projections, any type, replacement only, each ♿⊘ MED: 100-3, 280.1
Ⓨ		**E0968**	Commode seat, wheelchair ♿⊘ MED: 100-3, 280.1
Ⓨ		**E0969**	Narrowing device, wheelchair ♿⊘ MED: 100-3, 280.1
Ⓑ		**E0970**	No. 2 footplates, except for elevating legrest ⊘ MED: 100-3, 280.1 See code(s): K0037, K0042
▲ Ⓑ ☑		**E0971**	Manual wheelchair accessory, anti-tipping device, each ♿⊘ DME fee schedule reflects a base billing unit of each. MED: 100-3, 280.1
		~~E0972~~	~~Wheelchair accessory, transfer board or device, each~~ See code(s) E0705.
Ⓑ		**E0973**	Wheelchair accessory, adjustable height, detachable armrest, complete assembly, each ♿⊘ MED: 100-3, 280.1
Ⓑ		**E0974**	Manual wheelchair accessory, anti-rollback device, each ♿⊘ MED: 100-3, 280.1
Ⓨ		**E0977**	Wedge cushion, wheelchair ♿⊘
Ⓑ		**E0978**	Wheelchair accessory, positioning belt/safety belt/pelvic strap, each ♿⊘
Ⓨ		**E0980**	Safety vest, wheelchair ♿⊘
Ⓨ ☑		**E0981**	Wheelchair accessory, seat upholstery, replacement only, each ♿⊘
Ⓨ ☑		**E0982**	Wheelchair accessory, back upholstery, replacement only, each ♿⊘
Ⓨ		**E0983**	Manual wheelchair accessory, power add-on to convert manual wheelchair to motorized wheelchair, joystick control ♿⊘
Ⓨ		**E0984**	Manual wheelchair accessory, power add-on to convert manual wheelchair to motorized wheelchair, tiller control ♿⊘
Ⓨ		**E0985**	Wheelchair accessory, seat lift mechanism ♿⊘
Ⓨ ☑		**E0986**	Manual wheelchair accessory, push activated power assist, each ♿⊘
Ⓑ		**E0990**	Wheelchair accessory, elevating leg rest, complete assembly, each ♿⊘ MED: 100-3, 280.1
Ⓑ		**E0992**	Manual wheelchair accessory, solid seat insert ♿⊘
Ⓨ ☑		**E0994**	Armrest, each ♿⊘ MED: 100-3, 280.1
Ⓑ		**E0995**	Wheelchair accessory, calf rest/pad, each ♿⊘ MED: 100-3, 280.1

Durable Medical Equipment

E0996 — E1087

~~E0996~~   ~~Tire, solid, each~~
See code(s) E2220.

☑   **E0997**   Caster with fork
MED: 100-3, 280.1

☑   **E0998**   Caster without fork
MED: 100-3, 280.1

☑   **E0999**   Pneumatic tire with wheel
MED: 100-3, 280.1

~~E1000~~   ~~Tire, pneumatic caster~~
See code(s) E2214.

~~E1001~~   ~~Wheel, single~~
See code(s) E2224.

☑   **E1002**   Wheelchair accessory, power seating system, tilt only

☑   **E1003**   Wheelchair accessory, power seating system, recline only, without shear reduction

☑   **E1004**   Wheelchair accessory, power seating system, recline only, with mechanical shear reduction

☑   **E1005**   Wheelchair accessory, power seating system, recline only, with power shear reduction

☑   **E1006**   Wheelchair accessory, power seating system, combination tilt and recline, without shear reduction

☑   **E1007**   Wheelchair accessory, power seating system, combination tilt and recline, with mechanical shear reduction

☑   **E1008**   Wheelchair accessory, power seating system, combination tilt and recline, with power shear reduction

☑ ☑   **E1009**   Wheelchair accessory, addition to power seating system, mechanically linked leg elevation system, including pushrod and leg rest, each

☑ ☑   **E1010**   Wheelchair accessory, addition to power seating system, power leg elevation system, including leg rest, pair

☑   **E1011**   Modification to pediatric size wheelchair, width adjustment package (not to be dispensed with initial chair)
MED: 100-3, 280.1

☑   **E1014**   Reclining back, addition to pediatric size wheelchair
MED: 100-3, 280.1

☑   **E1015**   Shock absorber for manual wheelchair, each
MED: 100-3, 280.1

☑   **E1016**   Shock absorber for power wheelchair, each
MED: 100-3, 280.1

☑   **E1017**   Heavy duty shock absorber for heavy duty or extra heavy duty manual wheelchair, each
MED: 100-3, 280.1

☑   **E1018**   Heavy duty shock absorber for heavy duty or extra heavy duty power wheelchair, each
MED: 100-3, 280.1

~~E1019~~   ~~Wheelchair accessory, power seating system, heavy duty feature, patient weight capacity greater than 250 pounds and less than or equal to 400 pounds~~

☑   **E1020**   Residual limb support system for wheelchair
MED: 100-3, 280.3

~~E1021~~   ~~Wheelchair accessory, power seating system, extra heavy duty feature, weight capacity greater than 400 pounds~~

~~E1025~~   ~~Lateral thoracic support, non-contoured, for pediatric wheelchair, each (includes hardware)~~

~~E1026~~   ~~Lateral thoracic support, contoured, for pediatric wheelchair, each (includes hardware)~~

~~E1027~~   ~~Lateral/anterior support, for pediatric wheelchair, each (includes hardware)~~

☑   **E1028**   Wheelchair accessory, manual swingaway, retractable or removable mounting hardware for joystick, other control interface or positioning accessory

☑   **E1029**   Wheelchair accessory, ventilator tray, fixed

☑   **E1030**   Wheelchair accessory, ventilator tray, gimbaled

ROLLABOUT CHAIR

☑   **E1031**   Rollabout chair, any and all types with casters five in. or greater
MED: 100-3, 280.1

☑   **E1035**   Multi-positional patient transfer system, with integrated seat, operated by care giver
MED: 100-2, 15, 110

☑   **E1037**   Transport chair, pediatric size
MED: 100-3, 280.1

▲ ☑   **E1038**   Transport chair, adult size, patient weight capacity up to and including 300 pounds
MED: 100-3, 280.1

▲ ☑   **E1039**   Transport chair, adult size, heavy duty, patient weight capacity greater than 300 pounds

WHEELCHAIRS — FULLY RECLINING

Ⓐ   **E1050**   Fully reclining wheelchair; fixed full-length arms, swing-away, detachable, elevating legrests
MED: 100-3, 280.1

Ⓐ   **E1060**   Fully reclining wheelchair; detachable arms, desk or full-length, swing-away, detachable, elevating legrests
MED: 100-3, 280.1

Ⓐ   **E1070**   Fully reclining wheelchair; detachable arms, desk or full-length, swing-away, detachable footrests
MED: 100-3, 280.1

Ⓐ   **E1083**   Hemi-wheelchair; fixed full-length arms, swing-away, detachable, elevating legrests
MED: 100-3, 280.1

Ⓐ   **E1084**   Hemi-wheelchair; detachable arms, desk or full-length, swing-away, detachable, elevating legrests
MED: 100-3, 280.1

Ⓐ   **E1085**   Hemi-wheelchair; fixed full-length arms, swing-away, detachable footrests
MED: 100-3, 280.1

See code(s): K0002

Ⓐ   **E1086**   Hemi-wheelchair; detachable arms, desk or full-length, swing-away, detachable footrests
MED: 100-3, 280.1

See code(s): K0002

Ⓐ   **E1087**   High-strength lightweight wheelchair; fixed full-length arms, swing-away, detachable, elevating legrests
MED: 100-3, 280.1

| Special Coverage Instructions | Noncovered by Medicare | Carrier Discretion | ☑ Quantity Alert | ● New Code | ○ Reinstated Code | ▲ Revised Code |

50 — E Codes   Ⓐ Age   Ⓜ Maternity   ♀ Female Only   ♂ Male Only   Ⓐ-Ⓨ APC Status Indicator   **2006 HCPCS**

Ⓐ **E1088** High-strength lightweight wheelchair; detachable arms, desk or full-length, swing-away, detachable elevating legrests   ♿⃠
MED: 100-3, 280.1

Ⓐ **E1089** High-strength lightweight wheelchair; fixed-length arms, swing-away, detachable footrests   ⃠
MED: 100-3, 280.1
See code(s): K0004

Ⓐ **E1090** High-strength lightweight wheelchair; detachable arms, desk or full-length, swing-away, detachable footrests   ⃠
MED: 100-3, 280.1
See code(s): K0004

Ⓐ **E1092** Wide, heavy-duty wheelchair; detachable arms, desk or full-length, swing-away, detachable elevating legrests   ♿⃠
MED: 100-3, 280.1

Ⓐ **E1093** Wide, heavy-duty wheelchair; detachable arms, desk or full-length arms, swing-away, detachable footrests   ♿⃠
MED: 100-3, 280.1

WHEELCHAIR — SEMI-RECLINING

Ⓐ **E1100** Semi-reclining wheelchair; fixed full-length arms, swing-away, detachable, elevating legrests   ♿⃠
MED: 100-3, 280.1

Ⓐ **E1110** Semi-reclining wheelchair; detachable arms, desk or full-length, elevating legrest   ♿⃠
MED: 100-3, 280.1

WHEELCHAIR — STANDARD

Ⓐ **E1130** Standard wheelchair; fixed full-length arms, fixed or swing-away, detachable footrests   ⃠
MED: 100-3, 280.1
See code(s): K0001

Ⓐ **E1140** Wheelchair; detachable arms, desk or full-length, swing-away, detachable footrests   ⃠
MED: 100-3, 280.1
See code(s): K0001

Ⓨ **E1150** Wheelchair; detachable arms, desk or full-length, swing-away, detachable, elevating legrests   ♿⃠
MED: 100-3, 280.1

Ⓐ **E1160** Wheelchair; fixed full-length arms, swing-away, detachable, elevating legrests   ♿⃠
MED: 100-3, 280.1

Ⓐ **E1161** Manual adult size wheelchair, includes tilt in space   ♿

WHEELCHAIR — AMPUTEE

Ⓐ **E1170** Amputee wheelchair; fixed full-length arms, swing-away, detachable, elevating legrests   ♿⃠
MED: 100-3, 280.1

Ⓐ **E1171** Amputee wheelchair; fixed full-length arms, without footrests or legrests   ♿⃠
MED: 100-3, 280.1

Ⓐ **E1172** Amputee wheelchair; detachable arms, desk or full-length, without footrests or legrests   ♿⃠
MED: 100-3, 280.1

Ⓐ **E1180** Amputee wheelchair; detachable arms, desk or full-length, swing-away, detachable footrests   ♿⃠
MED: 100-3, 280.1

Ⓐ **E1190** Amputee wheelchair; detachable arms, desk or full-length, swing-away, detachable, elevating legrests   ♿⃠
MED: 100-3, 280.1

Ⓐ **E1195** Heavy duty wheelchair; fixed full-length arms, swing-away, detachable, elevating legrests   ♿⃠
MED: 100-3, 280.1

Ⓐ **E1200** Amputee wheelchair; fixed full-length arms, swing-away, detachable footrests   ♿⃠
MED: 100-3, 280.1

WHEELCHAIR — POWER

~~**E1210** Motorized wheelchair; fixed full length arms, swing-away, detachable, elevating legrests~~

~~**E1211** Motorized wheelchair; detachable arms, desk or full-length, swing-away, detachable, elevating legrests~~

~~**E1212** Motorized wheelchair; fixed full length arms, swing-away, detachable footrests~~
See code(s) K0010.

~~**E1213** Motorized wheelchair; detachable arms, desk or full-length, swing-away, detachable footrests~~
See code(s) K0010.

WHEELCHAIR — SPECIAL SIZE

Ⓐ **E1220** Wheelchair; specially sized or constructed (indicate brand name, model number, if any, and justification)   ⃠
MED: 100-3, 280.3

Ⓐ **E1221** Wheelchair with fixed arm, footrests   ♿⃠
MED: 100-3, 280.3

Ⓐ **E1222** Wheelchair with fixed arm, elevating legrests   ♿⃠
MED: 100-3, 280.3

Ⓐ **E1223** Wheelchair with detachable arms, footrests   ♿⃠
MED: 100-3, 280.3

Ⓐ **E1224** Wheelchair with detachable arms, elevating legrests   ♿⃠
MED: 100-3, 280.3

Ⓨ **E1225** Wheelchair accessory, manual semi-reclining back, (recline greater than 15 degrees, but less than 80 degrees), each   ♿⃠
MED: 100-3, 280.3

Ⓑ **E1226** Wheelchair accessory, manual fully reclining back, (recline greater than 80 degrees), each   ♿⃠
See also K0028
MED: 100-3, 280.1

Ⓨ **E1227** Special height arms for wheelchair   ♿⃠
MED: 100-3, 280.3

Ⓨ **E1228** Special back height for wheelchair   ♿⃠
MED: 100-3, 280.3

E1229 Wheelchair, pediatric size, not otherwise specified

Ⓨ **E1230** Power operated vehicle (three- or four-wheel nonhighway), specify brand name and model number   ♿⃠
Prior authorization is required by Medicare for this item.
MED: 100-3, 280.9; 100-8, 5, 5.1.1.2.1

Ⓨ **E1231** Wheelchair, pediatric size, tilt-in-space, rigid, adjustable, with seating system   ♿
MED: 100-3, 280.1

Durable Medical Equipment

E1232 — E1540

Y   E1232   Wheelchair, pediatric size, tilt-in-space, folding, adjustable, with seating system   ♿
MED: 100-3, 280.1

Y   E1233   Wheelchair, pediatric size, tilt-in-space, rigid, adjustable, without seating system   ♿
MED: 100-3, 280.1

Y   E1234   Wheelchair, pediatric size, tilt-in-space, folding, adjustable, without seating system   ♿
MED: 100-3, 280.1

Y   E1235   Wheelchair, pediatric size, rigid, adjustable, with seating system   ♿
MED: 100-3, 280.1

Y   E1236   Wheelchair, pediatric size, folding, adjustable, with seating system   ♿
MED: 100-3, 280.1

Y   E1237   Wheelchair, pediatric size, rigid, adjustable, without seating system   ♿
MED: 100-3, 280.1

Y   E1238   Wheelchair, pediatric size, folding, adjustable, without seating system   ♿
MED: 100-3, 280.1

E1239   Power wheelchair, pediatric size, not otherwise specified

WHEELCHAIR — LIGHTWEIGHT

A   E1240   Lightweight wheelchair; detachable arms, desk or full-length, swing-away, detachable, elevating legrest   ♿⊘
MED: 100-3, 280.1

A   E1250   Lightweight wheelchair; fixed full-length arms, swing-away, detachable footrests   ⊘
MED: 100-3, 280.1
See code(s): K0003

A   E1260   Lightweight wheelchair; detachable arms, desk or full-length, swing-away, detachable footrests   ⊘
MED: 100-3, 280.1
See code(s): K0003

A   E1270   Lightweight wheelchair; fixed full-length arms, swing-away, detachable elevating legrests   ♿⊘
MED: 100-3, 280.1

WHEELCHAIR — HEAVY-DUTY

A   E1280   Heavy-duty wheelchair; detachable arms, desk or full-length, elevating legrests   ♿⊘
MED: 100-3, 280.1

A   E1285   Heavy-duty wheelchair; fixed full-length arms, swing-away, detachable footrests   ⊘
MED: 100-3, 280.1
See code(s): K0006

A   E1290   Heavy-duty wheelchair; detachable arms, desk or full-length, swing-away, detachable footrests   ⊘
MED: 100-3, 280.1
See code(s): K0006

A   E1295   Heavy-duty wheelchair; fixed full-length arms, elevating legrests   ♿⊘
MED: 100-3, 280.1

Y   E1296   Special wheelchair seat height from floor   ♿⊘
MED: 100-3, 280.3

Y   E1297   Special wheelchair seat depth, by upholstery   ♿⊘
MED: 100-3, 280.3

Y   E1298   Special wheelchair seat depth and/or width, by construction   ♿⊘
MED: 100-3, 280.3

WHIRLPOOL — EQUIPMENT

E   E1300   Whirlpool, portable (overtub type)   ⊘
MED: 100-3, 280.1

Y   E1310   Whirlpool, nonportable (built-in type)   ♿⊘
MED: 100-3, 280.1

REPAIRS AND REPLACEMENT SUPPLIES

Y   ☑   E1340   Repair or nonroutine service for durable medical equipment requiring the skill of a technician, labor component, per 15 minutes   ⊘
Medicare jurisdiction: local contractor if repair or implanted DME.

MED: 100-2, 15, 110.2

ADDITIONAL OXYGEN RELATED EQUIPMENT

Y   E1353   Regulator   ⊘
MED: 100-3, 240.2

Y   E1355   Stand/rack   ⊘
MED: 100-3, 240.2

Y   E1372   Immersion external heater for nebulizer   ♿⊘
MED: 100-3, 240.2

Y   E1390   Oxygen concentrator, single delivery port, capable of delivering 85 percent or greater oxygen concentration at the prescribed flow rate   ♿⊘
MED: 100-3, 240.2

Y   ☑   E1391   Oxygen concentrator, dual delivery port, capable of delivering 85 percent or greater oxygen concentration at the prescribed flow rate, each ♿⊘
MED: 100-3, 240.2

●   E1392   Portable oxygen concentrator, rental   ♿
MED: 100-3, 240.2

N   E1399   Durable medical equipment, miscellaneous   ⊘
Determine if an alternative HCPCS Level II or a CPT code better describes the service being reported. This code should be used only if a more specific code is unavailable. Medicare jurisdiction: local contractor if repair or implanted DME.

Y   E1405   Oxygen and water vapor enriching system with heated delivery   ♿⊘
MED: 100-3, 240.2; 100-4, 20, 20; 100-4, 20, 20.4

Y   E1406   Oxygen and water vapor enriching system without heated delivery   ♿⊘
MED: 100-3, 240.2; 100-4, 20, 20; 100-4, 20, 20.4

ARTIFICIAL KIDNEY MACHINES AND ACCESSORIES

For glucose monitors, see A4253-A4256. For supplies for ESRD, see procedure codes A4651-A4929.

A   E1500   Centrifuge, for dialysis   ⊘

A   E1510   Kidney, dialysate delivery system kidney machine, pump recirculating, air removal system, flowrate meter, power off, heater and temp control with alarm, IV poles, pressure gauge, concentrate container   ⊘

A   E1520   Heparin infusion pump for hemodialysis   ⊘

A   E1530   Air bubble detector for hemodialysis, each, replacement   ⊘

A   E1540   Pressure alarm for hemodialysis, each, replacement   ⊘

Special Coverage Instructions   Noncovered by Medicare   Carrier Discretion   ☑ Quantity Alert   ● New Code   ○ Reinstated Code   ▲ Revised Code

52 — E Codes   A Age   M Maternity   ♀ Female Only   ♂ Male Only   A-Y APC Status Indicator   *2006 HCPCS*

Ⓐ		**E1550**	Bath conductivity meter for hemodialysis, each ⊘
Ⓐ		**E1560**	Blood leak detector for hemodialysis, each, replacement ⊘
Ⓐ		**E1570**	Adjustable chair, for ESRD patients ⊘
Ⓐ	☑	**E1575**	Transducer protectors/fluid barriers, for hemodialysis, any size, per 10 ⊘
Ⓐ		**E1580**	Unipuncture control system for hemodialysis ⊘
Ⓐ		**E1590**	Hemodialysis machine ⊘
Ⓐ		**E1592**	Automatic intermittent peritoneal dialysis system ⊘
Ⓐ		**E1594**	Cycler dialysis machine for peritoneal dialysis ⊘
Ⓐ		**E1600**	Delivery and/or installation charges for hemodialysis equipment ⊘
Ⓐ		**E1610**	Reverse osmosis water purification system, for hemodialysis ⊘ MED: 100-3, 230.7
Ⓐ		**E1615**	Deionizer water purification system, for hemodialysis ⊘ MED: 100-3, 230.7
Ⓐ		**E1620**	Blood pump for hemodialysis, replacement ⊘
Ⓐ		**E1625**	Water softening system, for hemodialysis ⊘ MED: 100-3, 230.7
Ⓐ		**E1630**	Reciprocating peritoneal dialysis system ⊘
Ⓐ		**E1632**	Wearable artificial kidney, each ⊘
Ⓑ	☑	**E1634**	Peritoneal dialysis clamps, each ⊘ MED: 100-4, 8, 130; 100-4, 8, 70; 100-4, 8, 80; 100-4, 8, 90; 100-4, 8, 90.1; 100-4, 8, 90.3.2
Ⓐ		**E1635**	Compact (portable) travel hemodialyzer system ⊘
Ⓐ	☑	**E1636**	Sorbent cartridges, for hemodialysis, per 10 ⊘
Ⓐ	☑	**E1637**	Hemostats, each ⊘
Ⓐ	☑	**E1639**	Scale, each ⊘
Ⓐ		**E1699**	Dialysis equipment, not otherwise specified ⊘ Determine if an alternative HCPCS Level II or a CPT code better describes the service being reported. This code should be used only if a more specific code is unavailable. Pertinent documentation to evaluate medical appropriateness should be included when this code is reported.

JAW MOTION REHABILITATION SYSTEM AND ACCESSORIES

Ⓨ		**E1700**	Jaw motion rehabilitation system ⅋⊘ Medicare jurisdiction: local contractor.
Ⓨ	☑	**E1701**	Replacement cushions for jaw motion rehabilitation system, package of six ⅋⊘ Medicare jurisdiction: local contractor.
Ⓨ	☑	**E1702**	Replacement measuring scales for jaw motion rehabilitation system, package of 200 ⅋⊘ Medicare jurisdiction: local contractor.

OTHER ORTHOPEDIC DEVICES

Ⓨ		**E1800**	Dynamic adjustable elbow extension/flexion device, includes soft interface material ⅋⊘
Ⓨ		**E1801**	Bi-directional static progressive stretch elbow device with range of motion adjustment, includes cuffs ⅋⊘
Ⓨ		**E1802**	Dynamic adjustable forearm pronation/supination device, includes soft interface material ⅋
Ⓨ		**E1805**	Dynamic adjustable wrist extension/flexion device, includes soft interface material ⅋⊘
Ⓨ		**E1806**	Bi-directional static progressive stretch wrist device with range of motion adjustment, includes cuffs ⅋⊘

Ⓨ		**E1810**	Dynamic adjustable knee extension/flexion device, includes soft interface material ⅋⊘
Ⓨ		**E1811**	Bi-directional progressive stretch knee device with range of motion adjustment, includes cuffs ⅋⊘
● Ⓨ		**E1812**	Dynamic knee, extension/flexion device with active resistance control
Ⓨ		**E1815**	Dynamic adjustable ankle extension/flexion, includes soft interface material ⅋⊘
Ⓨ		**E1816**	Bi-directional static progressive stretch ankle device with range of motion adjustment, includes cuffs ⅋⊘
Ⓨ		**E1818**	Bi-directional static progressive stretch forearm pronation/supination device with range of motion adjustment, includes cuffs ⅋
Ⓨ		**E1820**	Replacement soft interface material, dynamic adjustable extension/flexion device ⅋⊘
Ⓨ		**E1821**	Replacement soft interface material/cuffs for bi-directional static progressive stretch device ⅋⊘
Ⓨ		**E1825**	Dynamic adjustable finger extension/flexion device, includes soft interface material ⅋⊘
Ⓨ		**E1830**	Dynamic adjustable toe extension/flexion device, includes soft interface material ⅋⊘
Ⓨ		**E1840**	Dynamic adjustable shoulder flexion/abduction/rotation device, includes soft interface material ⅋⊘
		E1841	Multi-directional static progressive stretch shoulder device, with range of motion adjustability, includes cuffs
Ⓐ		**E1902**	Communication board, non-electronic augmentative or alternative communication device ⊘
		E2000	Gastric suction pump, home model, portable or stationary, electric ⅋⊘
		E2100	Blood glucose monitor with integrated voice synthesizer ⅋ MED: 100-3, 230.16
		E2101	Blood glucose monitor with integrated lancing/blood sample ⅋⊘ MED: 100-3, 230.16
Ⓨ		**E2120**	Pulse generator system for tympanic treatment of inner ear endolymphatic fluid ⅋⊘
Ⓨ	☑	**E2201**	Manual wheelchair accessory, nonstandard seat frame, width greater than or equal to 20 in. and less than 24 in. ⅋⊘
Ⓨ	☑	**E2202**	Manual wheelchair accessory, nonstandard seat frame width, 24-27 in. ⅋⊘
Ⓨ	☑	**E2203**	Manual wheelchair accessory, nonstandard seat frame depth, 20 to less than 22 in. ⅋⊘
Ⓨ	☑	**E2204**	Manual wheelchair accessory, nonstandard seat frame depth, 22 to 25 in. ⅋⊘
		E2205	Manual wheelchair accessory, handrim without projections, any type, replacement only, each
		E2206	Manual wheelchair accessory, wheel lock assembly, complete, each
● Ⓨ		**E2207**	Wheelchair accessory, crutch and cane holder, each
● Ⓨ		**E2208**	Wheelchair accessory, cylinder tank carrier, each
● Ⓨ		**E2209**	Wheelchair accessory, arm trough, each
● Ⓨ		**E2210**	Wheelchair accessory, bearings, any type, replacement only, each
● Ⓨ		**E2211**	Manual wheelchair accessory, pneumatic propulsion tire, any size, each

Durable Medical Equipment

E2212 — E2366

● ☑ **E2212** Manual wheelchair accessory, tube for pneumatic propulsion tire, any size, each

● ☑ **E2213** Manual wheelchair accessory, insert for pneumatic propulsion tire (removable), any type, any size, each

● ☑ **E2214** Manual wheelchair accessory, pneumatic caster tire, any size, each

● ☑ **E2215** Manual wheelchair accessory, tube for pneumatic caster tire, any size, each

● ☑ **E2216** Manual wheelchair accessory, foam filled propulsion tire, any size, each

● ☑ **E2217** Manual wheelchair accessory, foam filled caster tire, any size, each

● ☑ **E2218** Manual wheelchair accessory, foam propulsion tire, any size, each

● ☑ **E2219** Manual wheelchair accessory, foam caster tire, any size, each

● ☑ **E2220** Manual wheelchair accessory, solid (rubber/plastic) propulsion tire, any size, each

● ☑ **E2221** Manual wheelchair accessory, solid (rubber/plastic) caster tire (removable), any size, each

● ☑ **E2222** Manual wheelchair accessory, solid (rubber/plastic) caster tire with integrated wheel, any size, each

● ☑ **E2223** Manual wheelchair accessory, valve, any type, replacement only, each

● ☑ **E2224** Manual wheelchair accessory, propulsion wheel excludes tire, any size, each

● ☑ **E2225** Manual wheelchair accessory, caster wheel excludes tire, any size, replacement only, each

● ☑ **E2226** Manual wheelchair accessory, caster fork, any size, replacement only, each

E2291 Back, planar, for pediatric size wheelchair including fixed attaching hardware

E2292 Seat, planar, for pediatric size wheelchair including fixed attaching hardware

E2293 Back, contoured, for pediatric size wheelchair including fixed attaching hardware

E2294 Seat, contoured, for pediatric size wheelchair including fixed attaching hardware

☑ **E2300** Power wheelchair accessory, power seat elevation system ⊘

☑ **E2301** Power wheelchair accessory, power standing system ⊘

☑ **E2310** Power wheelchair accessory, electronic connection between wheelchair controller and one power seating system motor, including all related electronics, indicator feature, mechanical function selection switch, and fixed mounting hardware ৬⊘

☑ **E2311** Power wheelchair accessory, electronic connection between wheelchair controller and two or more power seating system motors, including all related electronics, indicator feature, mechanical function selection switch, and fixed mounting hardware ৬⊘

☑ **E2320** Power wheelchair accessory, hand or chin control interface, remote joystick or touchpad, proportional, including all related electronics, and fixed mounting hardware ৬⊘

☑ **E2321** Power wheelchair accessory, hand control interface, remote joystick, nonproportional, including all related electronics, mechanical stop switch, and fixed mounting hardware ৬⊘

☑ **E2322** Power wheelchair accessory, hand control interface, multiple mechanical switches, nonproportional, including all related electronics, mechanical stop switch, and fixed mounting hardware ৬⊘

☑ **E2323** Power wheelchair accessory, specialty joystick handle for hand control interface, prefabricated ৬⊘

☑ **E2324** Power wheelchair accessory, chin cup for chin control interface ৬⊘

☑ **E2325** Power wheelchair accessory, sip and puff interface, nonproportional, including all related electronics, mechanical stop switch, and manual swingaway mounting hardware ৬⊘

☑ **E2326** Power wheelchair accessory, breath tube kit for sip and puff interface ৬⊘

☑ **E2327** Power wheelchair accessory, head control interface, mechanical, proportional, including all related electronics, mechanical direction change switch, and fixed mounting hardware ৬⊘

☑ **E2328** Power wheelchair accessory, head control or extremity control interface, electronic, proportional, including all related electronics and fixed mounting hardware ৬⊘

☑ **E2329** Power wheelchair accessory, head control interface, contact switch mechanism, nonproportional, including all related electronics, mechanical stop switch, mechanical direction change switch, head array, and fixed mounting hardware ৬⊘

☑ **E2330** Power wheelchair accessory, head control interface, proximity switch mechanism, nonproportional, including all related electronics, mechanical stop switch, mechanical direction change switch, head array, and fixed mounting hardware ৬⊘

☑ **E2331** Power wheelchair accessory, attendant control, proportional, including all related electronics and fixed mounting hardware ⊘

☑ ☑ **E2340** Power wheelchair accessory, nonstandard seat frame width, 20-23 in. ৬⊘

☑ ☑ **E2341** Power wheelchair accessory, nonstandard seat frame width, 24-27 in. ৬⊘

☑ ☑ **E2342** Power wheelchair accessory, nonstandard seat frame depth, 20 or 21 in. ৬⊘

☑ ☑ **E2343** Power wheelchair accessory, nonstandard seat frame depth, 22-25 in. ৬⊘

☑ **E2351** Power wheelchair accessory, electronic interface to operate speech generating device using power wheelchair control interface ৬⊘

☑ ☑ **E2360** Power wheelchair accessory, 22 NF non-sealed lead acid battery, each ৬⊘

☑ **E2361** Power wheelchair accessory, 22 NF sealed lead acid battery, each, (e.g., gel cell, absorbed glassmat) ৬⊘

☑ ☑ **E2362** Power wheelchair accessory, group 24 non-sealed lead acid battery, each ৬⊘

☑ ☑ **E2363** Power wheelchair accessory, group 24 sealed lead acid battery, each (e.g., gel cell, absorbed glassmat) ৬⊘

☑ ☑ **E2364** Power wheelchair accessory, U-1 non-sealed lead acid battery, each ৬⊘

☑ ☑ **E2365** Power wheelchair accessory, U-1 sealed lead acid battery, each (e.g., gel cell, absorbed glassmat) ৬⊘

☑ ☑ **E2366** Power wheelchair accessory, battery charger, single mode, for use with only one battery type, sealed or non-sealed, each ৬⊘

Special Coverage Instructions   Noncovered by Medicare   Carrier Discretion   ☑ Quantity Alert   ● New Code   ○ Reinstated Code   ▲ Revised Code

54 — E Codes   Ⓐ Age   Ⓜ Maternity   ♀ Female Only   ♂ Male Only   Ⓐ-Ⓨ APC Status Indicator   *2006 HCPCS*

☑ ☑ **E2367** Power wheelchair accessory, battery charger, dual mode, for use with either battery type, sealed or non-sealed, each   ♿⊘

E2368 Power wheelchair component, motor, replacement only

E2369 Power wheelchair component, gear box, replacement only

E2370 Power wheelchair component, motor and gear box combination, replacement only

● ☑ **E2371** Power wheelchair accessory, group 27 sealed lead acid battery, (e.g., gel cell, absorbed glassmat), each

● ☑ **E2372** Power wheelchair accessory, group 27 nonsealed lead acid battery, each

☑ **E2399** Power wheelchair accessory, not otherwise classified interface, including all related electronics and any type mounting hardware   ⊘

☑ **E2402** Negative pressure wound therapy electrical pump, stationary or portable   ♿⊘

☑ ☑ **E2500** Speech generating device, digitized speech, using pre-recorded messages, less than or equal to 8 minutes recording time   ♿⊘
MED: 100-3, 50.1

☑ ☑ **E2502** Speech generating device, digitized speech, using pre-recorded messages, greater than 8 minutes but less than or equal to 20 minutes recording time ♿⊘
MED: 100-3, 50.1

☑ ☑ **E2504** Speech generating device, digitized speech, using pre-recorded messages, greater than 20 minutes but less than or equal to 40 minutes recording time ♿⊘
MED: 100-3, 50.1

☑ ☑ **E2506** Speech generating device, digitized speech, using pre-recorded messages, greater than 40 minutes recording time   ♿⊘
MED: 100-3, 50.1

☑ **E2508** Speech generating device, synthesized speech, requiring message formulation by spelling and access by physical contact with the device   ♿⊘
MED: 100-3, 50.1

☑ **E2510** Speech generating device, synthesized speech, permitting multiple methods of message formulation and multiple methods of device access   ♿⊘
MED: 100-3, 50.1

☑ **E2511** Speech generating software program, for personal computer or personal digital assistant   ♿⊘
MED: 100-3, 50.1

☑ **E2512** Accessory for speech generating device, mounting system   ♿⊘
MED: 100-3, 50.1

☑ **E2599** Accessory for speech generating device, not otherwise classified   ⊘
MED: 100-3, 50.1

E2601 General use wheelchair seat cushion, width less than 22 in., any depth

E2602 General use wheelchair seat cushion, width 22 in. or greater, any depth

E2603 Skin protection wheelchair seat cushion, width less than 22 in., any depth

E2604 Skin protection wheelchair seat cushion, width 22 in. or greater, any depth

E2605 Positioning wheelchair seat cushion, width less than 22 in., any depth

E2606 Positioning wheelchair seat cushion, width 22 in. or greater, any depth

E2607 Skin protection and positioning wheelchair seat cushion, width less than 22 in., any depth

E2608 Skin protection and positioning wheelchair seat cushion, width 22 in. or greater, any depth

E2609 Custom fabricated wheelchair seat cushion, any size

E2610 Wheelchair seat cushion, powered

E2611 General use wheelchair back cushion, width less than 22 in., any height, including any type mounting hardware

E2612 General use wheelchair back cushion, width 22 in. or greater, any height, including any type mounting hardware

E2613 Positioning wheelchair back cushion, posterior, width less than 22 in., any height, including any type mounting hardware

E2614 Positioning wheelchair back cushion, posterior, width 22 in. or greater, any height, including any type mounting hardware

E2615 Positioning wheelchair back cushion, posterior-lateral, width less than 22 in., any height, including any type mounting hardware

E2616 Positioning wheelchair back cushion, posterior-lateral, width 22 in. or greater, any height, including any type mounting hardware

E2617 Custom fabricated wheelchair back cushion, any size, including any type mounting hardware

E2618 Wheelchair accessory, solid seat support base (replaces sling seat), for use with manual wheelchair or lightweight power wheelchair, includes any type mounting hardware

E2619 Replacement cover for wheelchair seat cushion or back cushion, each

E2620 Positioning wheelchair back cushion, planar back with lateral supports, width less than 22 in., any height, including any type mounting hardware

E2621 Positioning wheelchair back cushion, planar back with lateral supports, width 22 in. or greater, any height, including any type mounting hardware

E8000 Gait trainer, pediatric size, posterior support, includes all accessories and components

E8001 Gait trainer, pediatric size, upright support, includes all accessories and components

E8002 Gait trainer, pediatric size, anterior support, includes all accessories and components

Special Coverage Instructions   Noncovered by Medicare   Carrier Discretion   ☑ Quantity Alert   ● New Code   ○ Reinstated Code   ▲ Revised Code

2006 HCPCS   🔟-🔟 ASC Groups   **MED:** Pub 100/NCD Reference   ♿ DMEPOS Paid   ⊘ SNF Excluded   **E Codes — 55**

PROCEDURES/PROFESSIONAL SERVICES (TEMPORARY)
G0000-G9999

The G codes are used to identify professional health care procedures and services that would otherwise be coded in CPT but for which there are no CPT codes.

G codes fall under the jurisdiction of the local contractor.

L   **G0008** Administration of influenza virus vaccine when no physician fee schedule service on the same day

L   **G0009** Administration of pneumococcal vaccine when no physician fee schedule service on the same day

K   **G0010** Administration of hepatitis B vaccine when no physician fee schedule service on the same day

A   **G0027** Semen analysis; presence and/or motility of sperm excluding Huhner   ⊘

PET scan codes G0030-G0047, G0125, G0210-G0218, G0220-G0234, G0253-G0254, and G0296 have been deleted. To report use CPT codes 78811-78813.

~~G0030 PET myocardial perfusion imaging, (following previous PET, G0030-G0047); single study, rest or stress (exercise and/or pharmacologic)~~

~~G0031 PET myocardial perfusion imaging, (following previous PET, G0030-G0047); multiple studies, rest or stress (exercise and/or pharmacologic)~~

~~G0032 PET myocardial perfusion imaging, (following rest SPECT, 78464); single study, rest or stress (exercise and/or pharmacologic)~~

~~G0033 PET myocardial perfusion imaging, (following rest SPECT, 78464); multiple studies, rest or stress (exercise and/or pharmacologic)~~

~~G0034 PET myocardial perfusion imaging, (following stress SPECT, 78465); single study, rest or stress (exercise and/or pharmacologic)~~

~~G0035 PET myocardial perfusion imaging, (following stress SPECT, 78465); multiple studies, rest or stress (exercise and/or pharmacologic)~~

~~G0036 PET myocardial perfusion imaging, (following coronary angiography, 93510-93520); single study, rest or stress (exercise and/or pharmacologic)~~

~~G0037 PET myocardial perfusion imaging, (following coronary angiography, 93510-93520); multiple studies, rest or stress (exercise and/or pharmacologic)~~

~~G0038 PET myocardial perfusion imaging, (following stress planar myocardial perfusion, 78460); single study, rest or stress (exercise and/or pharmacologic)~~

~~G0039 PET myocardial perfusion imaging, (following stress planar myocardial perfusion, 78460); multiple studies, rest or stress (exercise and/or pharmacologic)~~

~~G0040 PET myocardial perfusion imaging, (following stress echocardiogram, 93350); single study, rest or stress (exercise and/or pharmacologic)~~

~~G0041 PET myocardial perfusion imaging, (following stress echocardiogram, 93350); multiple studies, rest or stress (exercise and/or pharmacologic)~~

~~G0042 PET myocardial perfusion imaging, (following stress nuclear ventriculogram, 78481 or 78483); single study, rest or stress (exercise and/or pharmacologic)~~

~~G0043 PET myocardial perfusion imaging, (following stress nuclear ventriculogram, 78481 or 78483); multiple studies, rest or stress (exercise and/or pharmacologic)~~

~~G0044 PET myocardial perfusion imaging, (following rest ECG, 93000); single study, rest or stress (exercise and/or pharmacologic)~~

~~G0045 PET myocardial perfusion imaging, (following rest ECG, 93000); multiple studies, rest or stress (exercise and/or pharmacologic)~~

~~G0046 PET myocardial perfusion imaging, (following stress ECG, 93015); single study, rest or stress (exercise and/or pharmacologic)~~

~~G0047 PET myocardial perfusion imaging, (following stress ECG, 93015); multiple studies, rest or stress (exercise and/or pharmacologic)~~

V   **G0101** Cervical or vaginal cancer screening; pelvic and clinical breast examination   ♀
G0101 can be reported with an E/M code when a separately identifiable E/M service was provided.

AHA: 3Q, '01, 6; 4Q, '02, 8

N   **G0102** Prostate cancer screening; digital rectal examination   ♂
MED: 100-3, 210.1; 100-4, 18, 50

A   **G0103** Prostate cancer screening; prostate specific antigen test (PSA), total   ♂
MED: 100-3, 210.1; 100-4, 18, 50

S   **G0104** Colorectal cancer screening; flexible sigmoidoscopy   ⊘
Medicare covers colorectal screening for cancer via flexible sigmoidoscopy once every four years for patients 50 years or older.

T   **G0105** Colorectal cancer screening; colonoscopy on individual at high risk   2⊘
An individual with ulcerative enteritis or a history of a malignant neoplasm of the lower gastrointestinal tract is considered at high-risk for colorectal cancer, as defined by CMS.

AHA: 3Q, '01, 6

S   **G0106** Colorectal cancer screening; alternative to G0104, screening sigmoidoscopy, barium enema

A   **G0107** Colorectal cancer screening; fecal-occult blood test, 1-3 simultaneous determinations
Medicare covers colorectal screening for cancer via fecal-occult blood test once every year for patients 50 years or older.

A   **G0108** Diabetes outpatient self-management training services, individual, per 30 minutes   ⊘

A   **G0109** Diabetes self-management training services, group session (2 or more), per 30 minutes   ⊘

~~G0110 NETT pulmonary rehabilitation; education/skills training, individual~~

~~G0111 NETT pulmonary rehabilitation; education/skills, group~~

~~G0112 NETT pulmonary rehabilitation; nutritional guidance, initial~~

~~G0113 NETT pulmonary rehabilitation; nutritional guidance, subsequent~~

~~G0114 NETT pulmonary rehabilitation; psychosocial consultation~~

~~G0115 NETT pulmonary rehabilitation; psychological testing~~

~~G0116 NETT pulmonary rehabilitation; psychosocial counselling~~

S   **G0117** Glaucoma screening for high risk patients furnished by an optometrist or ophthalmologist
AHA: 3Q, '01, 12; 1Q, '02, 4

Special Coverage Instructions   Noncovered by Medicare   Carrier Discretion   ☑ Quantity Alert   ● New Code   ○ Reinstated Code   ▲ Revised Code

2006 HCPCS   1-9 ASC Groups   MED: Pub 100/NCD Reference   ⅄ DMEPOS Paid   ⊘ SNF Excluded   **G Codes — 57**

Procedures/Professional Services (Temporary)

G0118 — G0181

S   **G0118** Glaucoma screening for high risk patient furnished under the direct supervision of an optometrist or ophthalmologist
AHA: 3Q, '01, 12; 1Q, '02, 4

S   **G0120** Colorectal cancer screening; alternative to G0105, screening colonoscopy, barium enema

T   **G0121** Colorectal cancer screening; colonoscopy on individual not meeting criteria for high risk ☑⊘
AHA: 3Q, '01, 12; 1Q, '02, 4

E   **G0122** Colorectal cancer screening; barium enema ⊘

A   **G0123** Screening cytopathology, cervical or vaginal (any reporting system), collected in preservative fluid, automated thin layer preparation, screening by cytotechnologist under physician supervision ♀
See also P3000-P3001.

MED: 100-3, 190.2

A   **G0124** Screening cytopathology, cervical or vaginal (any reporting system), collected in preservative fluid, automated thin layer preparation, requiring interpretation by physician ♀
See also P3000-P3001.

MED: 100-3, 190.2

~~**G0125** PET imaging regional or whole body; single pulmonary nodule~~

T   **G0127** Trimming of dystrophic nails, any number ⊘
MED: 100-2, 15, 290; 100-2, 15, 290

B   **G0128** Direct (face-to-face with patient) skilled nursing services of a registered nurse provided in a comprehensive outpatient rehabilitation facility, each 10 minutes beyond the first 5 minutes ⊘

P   **G0129** Occupational therapy requiring the skills of a qualified occupational therapist, furnished as a component of a partial hospitalization treatment program, per day ⊘

X   **G0130** Single energy x-ray absorptiometry (SEXA) bone density study, one or more sites; appendicular skeleton (peripheral) (e.g., radius, wrist, heel)
MED: 100-3, 150.3

E   **G0141** Screening cytopathology smears, cervical or vaginal, performed by automated system, with manual rescreening, requiring interpretation by physician ♀

A   **G0143** Screening cytopathology, cervical or vaginal (any reporting system), collected in preservative fluid, automated thin layer preparation, with manual screening and rescreening by cytotechnologist under physician supervision ♀

A   **G0144** Screening cytopathology, cervical or vaginal (any reporting system), collected in preservative fluid, automated thin layer preparation, with screening by automated system, under physician supervision ♀

A   **G0145** Screening cytopathology, cervical or vaginal (any reporting system), collected in preservative fluid, automated thin layer preparation, with screening by automated system and manual rescreening under physician supervision ♀

A   **G0147** Screening cytopathology smears, cervical or vaginal, performed by automated system under physician supervision ♀

A   **G0148** Screening cytopathology smears, cervical or vaginal, performed by automated system with manual rescreening ♀

B   **G0151** Services of physical therapist in home health setting, each 15 minutes ⊘

B   **G0152** Services of occupational therapist in home health setting, each 15 minutes ⊘

B   **G0153** Services of speech and language pathologist in home health setting, each 15 minutes ⊘

B   **G0154** Services of skilled nurse in home health setting, each 15 minutes ⊘

B   **G0155** Services of clinical social worker in home health setting, each 15 minutes ⊘

B   **G0156** Services of home health aide in home health setting, each 15 minutes ⊘

T   **G0166** External counterpulsation, per treatment session ⊘
MED: 100-3, 20.20

N   **G0168** Wound closure utilizing tissue adhesive(s) only ⊘
AHA: 3Q, '01, 13; 4Q, '01, 12

S   **G0173** Linear accelerator based stereotactic radiosurgery, complete course of therapy in one session

V   **G0175** Scheduled interdisciplinary team conference (minimum of three exclusive of patient care nursing staff) with patient present ⊘

P   **G0176** Activity therapy, such as music, dance, art or play therapies not for recreation, related to the care and treatment of patient's disabling mental health problems, per session (45 minutes or more) ⊘

P   **G0177** Training and educational services related to the care and treatment of patient's disabling mental health problems per session (45 minutes or more) ⊘

E   **G0179** Physician re-certification for Medicare-covered home health services under a home health plan of care (patient not present), including contacts with home health agency and review of reports of patient status required by physicians to affirm the initial implementation of the plan of care that meets patient's needs, per re-certification period ⊘

E   **G0180** Physician certification for Medicare-covered home health services under a home health plan of care (patient not present), including contacts with home health agency and review of reports of patient status required by physicians to affirm the initial implementation of the plan of care that meets patient's needs, per certification period ⊘

E   **G0181** Physician supervision of a patient receiving Medicare-covered services provided by a participating home health agency (patient not present) requiring complex and multidisciplinary care modalities involving regular physician development and/or revision of care plans, review of subsequent reports of patient status, review of laboratory and other studies, communication (including telephone calls) with other health care professionals involved in the patient's care, integration of new information into the medical treatment plan and/or adjustment of medical therapy, within a calendar month, 30 minutes or more ⊘

▬ Special Coverage Instructions   ▬ Noncovered by Medicare   ▬ Carrier Discretion   ☑ Quantity Alert   ● New Code   ○ Reinstated Code   ▲ Revised Code

58 — G Codes   **A** Age   **M** Maternity   ♀ Female Only   ♂ Male Only   **A-Y** APC Status Indicator   *2006 HCPCS*

E **G0182** Physician supervision of a patient under a Medicare-approved hospice (patient not present) requiring complex and multidisciplinary care modalities involving regular physician development and/or revision of care plans, review of subsequent reports of patient status, review of laboratory and other studies, communication (including telephone calls) with other health care professionals involved in the patient's care, integration of new information into the medical treatment plan and/or adjustment of medical therapy, within a calendar month, 30 minutes or more ⊘

T **G0186** Destruction of localized lesion of choroid (for example, choroidal neovascularization); photocoagulation, feeder vessel technique (one or more sessions) ⊘

A **G0202** Screening mammography, producing direct digital image, bilateral, all views
AHA: 1Q, '02, 3; 1Q, '03, 7, 10

S **G0204** Diagnostic mammography, producing direct digital image, bilateral, all views
AHA: 1Q, '03, 7

S **G0206** Diagnostic mammography, producing direct digital image, unilateral, all views
AHA: 1Q, '03, 7

~~G0210~~ ~~PET imaging whole body; diagnosis; lung cancer, nonsmall cell~~

~~G0211~~ ~~PET imaging whole body; initial staging; lung cancer; nonsmall cell~~

~~G0212~~ ~~PET imaging whole body; restaging; lung cancer; nonsmall~~

~~G0213~~ ~~PET imaging whole body; diagnosis; colorectal~~

~~G0214~~ ~~PET imaging whole body; initial staging; colorectal~~

~~G0215~~ ~~PET imaging whole body; restaging; colorectal cancer This code has been deleted~~

~~G0216~~ ~~PET imaging whole body; diagnosis; melanoma~~

~~G0217~~ ~~PET imaging whole body; initial staging; melanoma~~

~~G0218~~ ~~PET imaging whole body; restaging; melanoma~~

E **G0219** PET imaging whole body; melanoma for non-covered indications
MED: 100-3, 220.6; 100-4, 13, 60

AHA: 1Q, '02, 10

~~G0220~~ ~~PET imaging whole body; diagnosis; lymphoma~~

~~G0221~~ ~~PET imaging whole body; initial staging; lymphoma~~

~~G0222~~ ~~PET imaging whole body; restaging; lymphoma~~

~~G0223~~ ~~PET imaging whole body or regional; diagnosis; head and neck cancer; excluding thyroid and CNS cancers~~

~~G0224~~ ~~PET imaging whole body or regional; initial staging; head and neck cancer; excluding thyroid and CNS cancers~~

~~G0225~~ ~~PET imaging whole body or regional; restaging; head and neck cancer, excluding thyroid and CNS cancers~~

~~G0226~~ ~~PET imaging whole body; diagnosis; esophageal cancer~~

~~G0227~~ ~~PET imaging whole body; initial staging; esophageal cancer~~

~~G0228~~ ~~PET imaging whole body; restaging; esophageal cancer~~

~~G0229~~ ~~PET imaging; metabolic brain imaging for presurgical evaluation of refractory seizures~~

~~G0230~~ ~~PET imaging; metabolic assessment for myocardial viability following inconclusive SPECT study~~

~~G0231~~ ~~PET, whole body, for recurrence of colorectal or colorectal metastatic cancer; gamma cameras only~~

~~G0232~~ ~~PET, whole body, for recurrence of lymphoma; gamma cameras only~~

~~G0233~~ ~~PET, whole body, for recurrence of melanoma; gamma cameras only~~

~~G0234~~ ~~PET, regional or whole body, for solitary pulmonary nodule following CT or for initial staging of pathologically diagnosed nonsmall cell lung cancer; gamma cameras only~~

● E **G0235** PET imaging, any site, not otherwise specified
MED: 100-4, 13, 60.14

S **G0237** Therapeutic procedures to increase strength or endurance of respiratory muscles, face-to-face, one-on-one, each 15 minutes (includes monitoring) ⊘

S **G0238** Therapeutic procedures to improve respiratory function, other than described by G0237, one-on-one, face-to-face, per 15 minutes (includes monitoring) ⊘
Medicare covers colorectal screening for cancer via fecal-occult blood test once every year for patients 50 years or older.

S **G0239** Therapeutic procedures to improve respiratory function or increase strength or endurance of respiratory muscles, two or more individuals (includes monitoring) ⊘

~~G0242~~ ~~Multisource photon stereotactic radiosurgery (cobalt 60 multisource converging beams) plan, including dose volume histograms for target and critical structure tolerances, plan optimization performed for highly conformal distributions, plan positional accuracy and dose verification, all lesions treated, per course of treatment~~
See code(s) 77261-77370.

S **G0243** Multi-source photon stereotactic radiosurgery, delivery including collimator changes and custom plugging, complete course of treatment, all lesions

~~G0244~~ ~~Observation care provided by a facility to a patient with CHF, chest pain, or asthma, minimum eight hours~~
See code(s) G0378.

V **G0245** Initial physician evaluation and management of a diabetic patient with diabetic sensory neuropathy resulting in a loss of protective sensation (LOPS) which must include: (1) the diagnosis of LOPS, (2) a patient history, (3) a physical examination that consists of at least the following elements: (a) visual inspection of the forefoot, hindfoot and toe web spaces, (b) evaluation of a protective sensation, (c) evaluation of foot structure and biomechanics, (d) evaluation of vascular status and skin integrity, and (e) evaluation and recommendation of footwear and (4) patient education
MED: 100-3, 70.2.1

AHA: 4Q, '02, 9

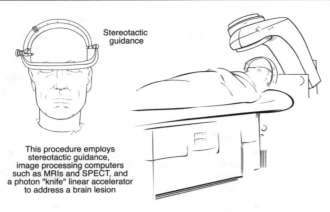

Stereotactic guidance

This procedure employs stereotactic guidance, image processing computers such as MRIs and SPECT, and a photon "knife" linear accelerator to address a brain lesion

Ⓥ **G0246** Follow-up physician evaluation and management of a diabetic patient with diabetic sensory neuropathy resulting in a loss of protective sensation (LOPS) to include at least the following: (1) a patient history, (2) a physical examination that includes: (a) visual inspection of the forefoot, hindfoot and toe web spaces, (b) evaluation of protective sensation, (c) evaluation of foot structure and biomechanics, (d) evaluation of vascular status and skin integrity, and (e) evaluation and recommendation of footwear, and (3) patient education
MED: 100-3, 70.2.1

AHA: 4Q, '02, 9

Ⓣ **G0247** Routine foot care by a physician of a diabetic patient with diabetic sensory neuropathy resulting in a loss of protective sensation (LOPS) to include, the local care of superficial wounds (i.e., superficial to muscle and fascia) and at least the following if present: (1) local care of superficial wounds, (2) debridement of corns and calluses, and (3) trimming and debridement of nails   ⊘
MED: 100-3, 70.2.1

AHA: 4Q, '02, 9

Ⓢ **G0248** Demonstration, at initial use, of home INR monitoring for patient with mechanical heart valve(s) who meets Medicare coverage criteria, under the direction of a physician; includes: demonstrating use and care of the INR monitor, obtaining at least one blood sample, provision of instructions for reporting home INR test results, and documentation of patient ability to perform testing   ⊘
MED: 100-3, 210.1

AHA: 4Q, '02, 9

Ⓢ **G0249** Provision of test materials and equipment for home INR monitoring to patient with mechanical heart valve(s) who meets Medicare coverage criteria; includes provision of materials for use in the home and reporting of test results to physician; per four tests   ⊘
MED: 100-3, 210.1

AHA: 4Q, '02, 9

Ⓔ **G0250** Physician review, interpretation and patient management of home INR testing for a patient with mechanical heart valve(s) who meets other coverage criteria; per four tests (does not require face-to-face service)   ⊘
MED: 100-3, 210.1

AHA: 4Q, '02, 9

Ⓢ **G0251** Linear accelerator based stereotactic radiosurgery, delivery including collimator changes and custom plugging, fractionated treatment, all lesions, per session, maximum five sessions per course of treatment   ⊘

Ⓔ **G0252** PET imaging, full and partial-ring PET scanners only, for initial diagnosis of breast cancer and/or surgical planning for breast cancer (e.g., initial staging of axillary lymph nodes)   ⊘

~~G0253 PET imaging for breast cancer, full and partial ring PET scanners only, staging/restaging of local regional recurrence or distant metastases (i.e., staging/restaging after or prior to course of treatment)~~

~~G0254 PET imaging for breast cancer, full and partial ring PET scanners only, evaluation of response to treatment, performed during course of treatment~~

Ⓔ **G0255** Current perception threshold/sensory nerve conduction test, (SNCT) per limb, any nerve   ⊘
MED: 100-3, 160.23

AHA: 4Q, '02, 9

Ⓢ **G0257** Unscheduled or emergency dialysis treatment for an ESRD patient in a hospital outpatient department that is not certified as an ESRD facility   ⊘
AHA: 4Q, '02, 9; 1Q, '03, 9

~~G0258 Intravenous infusion during separately payable observation stay, per observation stay (must be reported with G0244)~~

Ⓝ **G0259** Injection procedure for sacroiliac joint; arthrography   ⊘
AHA: 4Q, '02, 9

Ⓣ **G0260** Injection procedure for sacroiliac joint; provision of anesthetic, steroid and/or other therapeutic agent, with or without arthrography   ❶⊘
AHA: 4Q, '02, 9

~~G0263 Direct admission of patient with diagnosis of congestive heart failure, chest pain or asthma for observation services that meet all criteria for G0244~~
See code(s) G0379.

~~G0264 Initial nursing assessment of patient directly admitted to observation with diagnosis other than CHF, chest pain or asthma or patient directly admitted to observation with diagnosis of CHF, chest pain or asthma when the observation stay does not qualify for G0244~~

Ⓐ **G0265** Cryopreservation, freezing and storage of cells for therapeutic use, each cell line

Ⓐ **G0266** Thawing and expansion of frozen cells for therapeutic use, each aliquot

Ⓢ **G0267** Bone marrow or peripheral stem cell harvest, modification or treatment to eliminate cell type(s) (e.g., T-cells, metastatic carcinoma)

Ⓧ **G0268** Removal of impacted cerumen (one or both ears) by physician on same date of service as audiologic function testing
AHA: 1Q, '03, 12

Ⓝ **G0269** Placement of occlusive device into either a venous or arterial access site, post surgical or interventional procedure (e.g., angioseal plug, vascular plug)

Special Coverage Instructions   Noncovered by Medicare   Carrier Discretion   ☑ Quantity Alert   ● New Code   ○ Reinstated Code   ▲ Revised Code

60 — G Codes   Ⓐ Age   Ⓜ Maternity   ♀ Female Only   ♂ Male Only   Ⓐ-Ⓨ APC Status Indicator   *2006 HCPCS*

A   G0270 Medical nutrition therapy; reassessment and subsequent intervention(s) following second referral in same year for change in diagnosis, medical condition or treatment regimen (including additional hours needed for renal disease), individual, face to face with the patient, each 15 minutes ⊘

A   G0271 Medical nutrition therapy, reassessment and subsequent intervention(s) following second referral in same year for change in diagnosis, medical condition, or treatment regimen (including additional hours needed for renal disease), group (2 or more individuals), each 30 minutes ⊘

N   G0275 Renal artery angiography (unilateral or bilateral) performed at the time of cardiac catheterization, includes catheter placement, injection of dye, flush aortogram and radiologic supervision and interpretation and production of images (list separately in addition to primary procedure)

N   G0278 Iliac artery angiography performed at the same time of cardiac catheterization, includes catheter placement, injection of dye, radiologic supervision and interpretation and production of images (list separately in addition to primary procedure) ⊘

G0279 Extracorporeal shock wave therapy; involving elbow epicondylitis

G0280 Extracorporeal shock wave therapy; involving other than elbow epicondylitis or plantar fasciitis

A   G0281 Electrical stimulation, (unattended), to one or more areas, for chronic Stage III and Stage IV pressure ulcers, arterial ulcers, diabetic ulcers, and venous stasis ulcers not demonstrating measurable signs of healing after 30 days of conventional care, as part of a therapy plan of care
AHA: 1Q, '03, 7; 2Q, '03, 7

E   G0282 Electrical stimulation, (unattended), to one or more areas, for wound care other than described in G0281 ⊘
MED: 100-3, 270.1; 100-3, 270.1; 100-3, 270.1; 100-3, 270.1
AHA: 1Q, '03, 7; 2Q, '03, 7

A   G0283 Electrical stimulation (unattended), to one or more areas for indication(s) other than wound care, as part of a therapy plan of care
AHA: 1Q, '03, 7; 2Q, '03, 7

T   G0288 Reconstruction, computed tomographic angiography of aorta for surgical planning for vascular surgery

N   G0289 Arthroscopy, knee, surgical, for removal of loose body, foreign body, debridement/shaving of articular cartilage (chondroplasty) at the time of other surgical knee arthroscopy in a different compartment of the same knee ⊘

T   G0290 Transcatheter placement of a drug eluting intracoronary stent(s), percutaneous, with or without other therapeutic intervention, any method; single vessel ⊘
AHA: 4Q, '02, 9; 3Q, '03, 11; 4Q, '03, 7

T   G0291 Transcatheter placement of a drug eluting intracoronary stent(s), percutaneous, with or without other therapeutic intervention, any method; each additional vessel ⊘
AHA: 4Q, '02, 9; 3Q, '03, 11; 4Q, '03, 7

S   G0293 Noncovered surgical procedure(s) using conscious sedation, regional, general or spinal anesthesia in a Medicare qualifying clinical trial, per day ⊘
AHA: 4Q, '02, 9

S   G0294 Noncovered procedure(s) using either no anesthesia or local anesthesia only, in a Medicare qualifying clinical trial, per day ⊘
AHA: 4Q, '02, 9

E   G0295 Electromagnetic therapy, to one or more areas, for wound care other than described in G0329 or for other uses
MED: 100-3, 270.1; 100-3, 270.1; 100-3, 270.1; 100-3, 270.1
AHA: 1Q, '03, 7

G0296 PET imaging, full and partial ring PET scanner only, for restaging of previously-treated thyroid cancer of follicular cell origin following negative I-131 whole body scan

T   G0297 Insertion of single chamber pacing cardioverter defibrillator pulse generator ⊘
AHA: 4Q, '03, 4, 7

T   G0298 Insertion of dual chamber pacing cardioverter defibrillator pulse generator ⊘
AHA: 4Q, '03, 4, 7

T   G0299 Insertion or repositioning of electrode lead for single chamber pacing cardioverter defibrillator and insertion of pulse generator ⊘
AHA: 4Q, '03, 4, 7

T   G0300 Insertion or repositioning of electrode lead(s) for dual chamber pacing cardioverter defibrillator and insertion of pulse generator ⊘
AHA: 4Q, '03, 4, 7

S   ☑   G0302 Preoperative pulmonary surgery services for preparation for LVRS, complete course of services, to include a minimum of 16 days of services ⊘

S   ☑   G0303 Preoperative pulmonary surgery services for preparation for LVRS, 10 to 15 days of services ⊘

S   ☑   G0304 Preoperative pulmonary surgery services for preparation for LVRS, 1 to 9 days of services ⊘

S   ☑   G0305 Postdischarge pulmonary surgery services after LVRS, minimum of 6 days of services ⊘

A   G0306 Complete CBC, automated (HgB, HCT, RBC, WBC, without platelet count) and automated WBC differential count

A   G0307 Complete CBC, automated (HgB, HCT, RBC, WBC; without platelet count)

A   G0308 ESRD related services during the course of treatment, for patients under 2 years of age to include monitoring for the adequacy of nutrition, assessment of growth and development, and counseling of parents; with 4 or more face-to-face physician visits per month   A ⊘
MED: 100-2, 11, 130.1

A   G0309 ESRD related services during the course of treatment, for patients under 2 years of age to include monitoring for the adequacy of nutrition, assessment of growth and development, and counseling of parents; with 2 or 3 face-to-face physician visits per month   A
MED: 100-2, 11, 130.1

A   G0310 ESRD related services during the course of treatment, for patients under 2 years of age to include monitoring for the adequacy of nutrition, assessment of growth and development, and counseling of parents; with 1 face-to-face physician visit per month   A
MED: 100-2, 11, 130.1

Special Coverage Instructions   Noncovered by Medicare   Carrier Discretion   ☑ Quantity Alert   ● New Code   ○ Reinstated Code   ▲ Revised Code

2006 HCPCS   1–9 ASC Groups   MED: Pub 100/NCD Reference   ᕙ DMEPOS Paid   ⊘ SNF Excluded   **G Codes — 61**

Ⓐ   **G0311** ESRD related services during the course of treatment, for patients between 2 and 11 years of age to include monitoring for the adequacy of nutrition, assessment of growth and development, and counseling of parents; with 4 or more face-to-face physician visits per month Ⓐ⊘
MED: 100-2, 11, 130.1

Ⓐ   **G0312** ESRD related services during the course of treatment, for patients between 2 and 11 years of age to include monitoring for the adequacy of nutrition, assessment of growth and development, and counseling of parents; with 2 or 3 face-to-face physician visits per month Ⓐ⊘
MED: 100-2, 11, 130.1

Ⓐ   **G0313** ESRD related services during the course of treatment, for patients between 2 and 11 years of age to include monitoring for the adequacy of nutrition, assessment of growth and development, and counseling of parents; with 1 face-to-face physician visit per month Ⓐ⊘
MED: 100-2, 11, 130.1

Ⓐ   **G0314** ESRD related services during the course of treatment, for patients between 12 and 19 years of age to include monitoring for the adequacy of nutrition, assessment of growth and development, and counseling of parents; with 4 or more face-to-face physician visits per month Ⓐ⊘
MED: 100-2, 11, 130.1

Ⓐ   **G0315** ESRD related services during the course of treatment, for patients between 12 and 19 years of age to include monitoring for the adequacy of nutrition, assessment of growth and development, and counseling of parents; with 2 or 3 face-to-face physician visits per month Ⓐ⊘
MED: 100-2, 11, 130.1

Ⓐ   **G0316** ESRD related services during the course of treatment, for patients between 12 and 19 years of age to include monitoring for the adequacy of nutrition, assessment of growth and development, and counseling of parents; with 1 face-to-face physician visit per month Ⓐ⊘
MED: 100-2, 11, 130.1

Ⓐ   **G0317** ESRD related services during the course of treatment, for patients 20 years of age and over; with 4 or more face-to-face physician visits per month Ⓐ⊘
MED: 100-2, 11, 130.1

Ⓐ   **G0318** ESRD related services during the course of treatment, for patients 20 years of age and over; with 2 or 3 face-to-face physician visits per month Ⓐ⊘
MED: 100-2, 11, 130.1

Ⓐ   **G0319** ESRD related services during the course of treatment, for patients 20 years of age and over; with 1 face-to-face physician visit per month Ⓐ⊘
MED: 100-2, 11, 130.1

Ⓐ   **G0320** ESRD related services for home dialysis patients per full month; for patients under 2 years of age to include monitoring for adequacy of nutrition, assessment of growth and development, and counseling of parents Ⓐ⊘
MED: 100-2, 11, 130.1

Ⓐ   **G0321** ESRD related services for home dialysis patients per full month; for patients 2 to 11 years of age to include monitoring for adequacy of nutrition, assessment of growth and development, and counseling of parents Ⓐ⊘
MED: 100-2, 11, 130.1

Ⓐ   **G0322** ESRD related services for home dialysis patients per full month; for patients 12 to 19 years of age to include monitoring for adequacy of nutrition, assessment of growth and development, and counseling of parents Ⓐ⊘
MED: 100-2, 11, 130.1

Ⓐ   **G0323** ESRD related services for home dialysis patients per full month; for patients 20 years of age and older Ⓐ⊘
MED: 100-2, 11, 130.1

Ⓐ   **G0324** End stage renal disease (ESRD) related services less than full month, per day; for patients under two years of age Ⓐ⊘
MED: 100-2, 11, 130.1

Ⓐ   **G0325** End stage renal disease (ESRD) related services less than full month, per day; for patients between two and eleven years of age Ⓐ⊘
MED: 100-2, 11, 130.1

Ⓐ   **G0326** End stage renal disease (ESRD) related services less than full month, per day; for patients between twelve and nineteen years of age Ⓐ⊘
MED: 100-2, 11, 130.1

Ⓐ   **G0327** End stage renal disease (ESRD) related services less than full month, per day; for patients twenty years of age and over Ⓐ⊘
MED: 100-2, 11, 130.1

Ⓐ   **G0328** Colorectal cancer screening; fecal-occult blood test, immunoassay, 1-3 simultaneous determinations

Ⓐ   **G0329** Electromagnetic therapy, to one or more areas for chronic Stage III and Stage IV pressure ulcers, arterial ulcers, diabetic ulcers and venous stasis ulcers not demonstrating measurable signs of healing after 30 days of conventional care as part of a therapy plan of care

G0330 PET imaging initial diagnosis cervical

G0331 PET imaging restaging ovarian

● Ⓢ   **G0332** Preadministration-related services for intravenous infusion of immunoglobulin, per infusion encounter

● Ⓜ   **G0333** Pharmacy dispensing fee for inhalation drug(s); initial 30-day supply as a beneficiary

~~**G0336** PET imaging, brain imaging for the differential diagnosis of Alzheimer's disease with aberrant features vs. fronto-temporal dementia~~

G0337 Hospice evaluation and counseling services, pre-election

~~**G0338** Linear accelerator based stereotactic radiosurgery plan, including does volume histograms for target and critical structure tolerances, plan optimization performed for highly conformal distributions, plan positional accuracy and does verification, all lesions treated, per course of treatment~~
See code(s) 77261-77370.

Ⓢ   **G0339** Image guided robotic linear accelerator base stereotactic radiosurgery, complete course of therapy in one session, or first session of fractionated treatment

---

▨ Special Coverage Instructions   ▨ Noncovered by Medicare   ▨ Carrier Discretion   ☑ Quantity Alert   ● New Code   ○ Reinstated Code   ▲ Revised Code

62 — G Codes   Ⓐ Age   Ⓜ Maternity   ♀ Female Only   ♂ Male Only   Ⓐ-Ⓨ APC Status Indicator   *2006 HCPCS*

S   **G0340** Image guided robotic linear accelerator based stereotactic radiosurgery, delivery including collimator changes and custom plugging, fractionated treatment, all lesions, per session, second through fifth sessions, maximum five sessions per course of treatment

C   **G0341** Percutaneous islet cell transplant, includes portal vein catheterization and infusion
MED: 100-3, 260.3

C   **G0342** Laparoscopy for islet cell transplant, includes portal vein catheterization and infusion
MED: 100-3, 260.3

C   **G0343** Laparotomy for islet cell transplant, includes portal vein catheterization and infusion
MED: 100-3, 260.3

G0344 Initial preventive physical examination; face-to-face visit, services limited to new beneficiary during the first six months of Medicare enrollment
Exam must be performed within six months of the beneficiary's initial coverage date.

~~**G0345** Intravenous infusion, hydration; initial, up to one hour~~
See code(s) 90760.

~~**G0346** Each additional hour, up to eight hours (list separately In addition to code for primary procedure)~~
See code(s) 90761.

~~**G0347** Intravenous infusion, for therapeutic/diagnostic (specify substance or drug); initial, up to one hour~~
See code(s) 90765.

~~**G0348** Each additional hour, up to eight hours (list separately In addition to code for primary procedure and report in conjunction with G0347)~~
See code(s) 90766.

~~**G0349** Additional sequential infusion, up to one hour (list separately in addition to code for primary procedure)~~
See code(s) 90767.

~~**G0350** Concurrent infusion (list separately in addition to code for primary procedure) report only once per substance/drug regardless of duration, report G0350 in conjunction with G0345~~
See code(s) 90768.

~~**G0351** Therapeutic or diagnostic injection (specify substance or drug); subcutaneous or intramuscular~~
See code(s) 90772.

~~**G0353** Intravenous push, single or initial substance/drug~~
See code(s) 90774.

~~**G0354** Each additional sequential intravenous push (list separately in addition to code for primary procedure)~~
See code(s) 90775.

~~**G0355** Chemotherapy administration, subcutaneous or intramuscular nonhormonal antineoplastic~~
See code(s) 96401.

~~**G0356** Hormonal antineoplastic~~
See code(s) 96402.

~~**G0357** Intravenous, push technique, single or initial substance/drug~~
See code(s) 96409.

~~**G0358** Intravenous, push technique, each additional substance/drug (list separately in addition to code for primary procedure)~~
See code(s) 96411.

~~**G0359** Chemotherapy administration, intravenous infusion technique; up to one hour, single or initial substance/drug~~
See code(s) 96413.

~~**G0360** Each additional hour, one to eight hours (list separately in addition to code for primary procedure) use G0360 in conjunction with G0359~~
See code(s) 96415.

~~**G0361** Initiation of prolonged chemotherapy infusion (more than eight hours), requiring use of a portable or implantable pump~~
See code(s) 96416.

~~**G0362** Each additional sequential infusion (different substance/drug), up to one hour (use with G0359)~~
See code(s) 96417.

~~**G0363** Irrigation of implanted venous access device for drug delivery systems (do not report G0363 if an injection or infusion is provided on the same day)~~

G0364 Bone marrow aspiration performed with bone marrow biopsy through the same incision on the same date of service

G0365 Vessel mapping of vessels for hemodialysis access (services for preoperative vessel mapping prior to creation of hemodialysis access using an autogenous hemodialysis conduit, including arterial inflow and venous outflow)

G0366 Electrocardiogram, routine ECG with at least 12 leads; with interpretation and report, performed as a component of the initial preventive physical examination

G0367 Tracing only, without interpretation and report, performed as a component of the initial preventive physical examination

G0368 Interpretation and report only, performed as a component of the initial preventive physical examination

~~**G0369** Pharmacy supply fee for initial immunosuppressive drugs first month following transplant.~~
See code(s) Q0510.

~~**G0370** Pharmacy supply fee for oral anticancer oral antiemetic or immunosuppressive drugs~~
See code(s) Q0511, Q0512.

~~**G0371** Pharmacy dispensing fee for inhalation drugs; per 30 days~~
See code(s) Q0513.

● M   **G0372** Physician service required to establish and document the need for a power mobility device (use in addition to primary evaluation and management code)

~~**G0374** Pharmacy dispensing fee for inhalation drug(s); per 90 days~~

● S   **G0375** Smoking and tobacco use cessation counseling visit; intermediate, greater than 3 minutes up to 10 minutes
Medicare will cover G0375 and G0376 for a combined total of eight sessions per 12 month period.

AHA: 3Q, '05, 9

Special Coverage Instructions   Noncovered by Medicare   Carrier Discretion   ☑ Quantity Alert   ● New Code   ○ Reinstated Code   ▲ Revised Code

2006 HCPCS   **1**-**9** ASC Groups   MED: Pub 100/NCD Reference   Ⅎ DMEPOS Paid   ⊘ SNF Excluded   **G Codes — 63**

● Ⓢ **G0376** Smoking and tobacco use cessation counseling visit; intensive, greater than 10 minutes
Medicare will cover G0375 and G0376 for a combined total of eight sessions per 12 month period.

AHA: 3Q, '05, 9

● **G0378** Hospital observation service, per hour

● **G0379** Direct admission of patient for hospital observation care

Ⓢ ☑ **G3001** Administration and supply of tositumomab, 450 mg

PHYSICIAN'S VOLUNTARY REPORTING PROGRAM CODES

HCPCS codes G8006-G8186 are to be used for the physician's voluntary reporting program in which CMS seeks to analyze the quality of care provided to Medicare beneficiaries. Reporting of these codes is voluntary. Physicians should not charge for these codes. Unless otherwise indicated, report these codes in addition to office visit, home visit, nursing facility, and domiciliary evaluation and management codes. For additional information, please visit the following website: http://www.cms.hhs.gov/providers/p4p/

● Ⓜ **G8006** Acute myocardial infarction: patient documented to have received aspirin at arrival

● Ⓜ **G8007** Acute myocardial infarction: patient not documented to have received aspirin at arrival

● Ⓜ **G8008** Clinician documented that acute myocardial infarction patient was not an eligible candidate to receive aspirin at arrival measure

● Ⓜ **G8009** Acute myocardial infarction: patient documented to have received beta-blocker at arrival

● Ⓜ **G8010** Acute myocardial infarction: patient not documented to have received beta-blocker at arrival

● Ⓜ **G8011** Clinician documented that acute myocardial infarction patient was not an eligible candidate for beta-blocker at arrival measure

● Ⓜ **G8012** Pneumonia: patient documented to have received antibiotic within 4 hours of presentation

● Ⓜ **G8013** Pneumonia: patient not documented to have received antibiotic within 4 hours of presentation

● Ⓜ **G8014** Clinician documented that pneumonia patient was not an eligible candidate for antibiotic within 4 hours of presentation measure

● Ⓜ **G8015** Diabetic patient with most recent hemoglobin A1c level (within the last 6 months) documented as greater than 9%
Report this code in addition to office visit; office consult; home visit; nursing facility; or initial preventive physical exam evaluation and management codes.

● Ⓜ **G8016** Diabetic patient with most recent hemoglobin A1c level (within the last 6 months) documented as less than or equal to 9%
Report this code in addition to office visit; home visit; nursing facility; domiciliary; or initial preventive physical exam evaluation and management codes.

● Ⓜ **G8017** Clinician documented that diabetic patient was not eligible candidate for hemoglobin A1c measure
Report this code in addition to office visit; home visit; nursing facility; domiciliary; or initial preventive physical exam evaluation and management codes.

● Ⓜ **G8018** Clinician has not provided care for the diabetic patient for the required time for hemoglobin A1c measure (6 months)
Report this code in addition to office visit; home visit; nursing facility; domiciliary; or initial preventive physical exam evaluation and management codes.

● Ⓜ **G8019** Diabetic patient with most recent low-density lipoprotein (within the last 12 months) documented as greater than or equal to 100 mg/dl

● Ⓜ **G8020** Diabetic patient with most recent low-density lipoprotein (within the last 12 months) documented as less than 100 mg/dl

● Ⓜ **G8021** Clinician documented that diabetic patient was not eligible candidate for low-density lipoprotein measure

● Ⓜ **G8022** Clinician has not provided care for the diabetic patient for the required time for low-density lipoprotein measure (12 months)

● Ⓜ **G8023** Diabetic patient with most recent blood pressure (within the last 6 months) documented as equal to or greater than 140 systolic or equal to or greater than 80 mm Hg diastolic

● Ⓜ **G8024** Diabetic patient with most recent blood pressure (within the last 6 months) documented less than 140 systolic and less than 80 diastolic

● Ⓜ **G8025** Clinician documented that the diabetic patient was not eligible candidate for blood pressure measure (within the last 6 months)

● Ⓜ **G8026** Clinician has not provided care for the diabetic patient for the required time for blood measure (within the last 6 months)

● Ⓜ **G8027** Heart failure patient with left ventricular systolic dysfunction (LVSD) documented to be on either angiotensin-converting enzyme-inhibitor or angiotensin-receptor blocker (ACE-1 or ARB) therapy

● Ⓜ **G8028** Heart failure patient with left ventricular systolic dysfunction (LVSD) not documented to be on either angiotensin-converting enzyme-inhibitor or angiotensin-receptor blocker (ACE-1 or ARB) therapy
Patients with LVEF < 40% or with moderately or severely depressed left ventricular systolic function.

● Ⓜ **G8029** Clinician documented that heart failure patient was not an eligible candidate for either angiotensin-converting enzyme-inhibitor or angiotensin-receptor blocker (ACE-I or ARB) therapy measure
Patients with LVEF < 40% or with moderately or severely depressed left ventricular systolic function.

● Ⓜ **G8030** Heart failure patient with left ventricular systolic dysfunction (LVSD) documented to be on beta-blocker therapy
Patients with LVEF < 40% or with moderately or severely depressed left ventricular systolic function.

● Ⓜ **G8031** Heart failure patient with left ventricular systolic dysfunction (LVSD) not documented to be on beta-blocker therapy
Patients with LVEF < 40% or with moderately or severely depressed left ventricular systolic function.

● Ⓜ **G8032** Clinician documented that heart failure patient was not eligible candidate for beta-blocker therapy measure
Patients with LVEF < 40% or with moderately or severely depressed left ventricular systolic function.

● Ⓜ **G8033** Prior myocardial infarction — coronary artery disease patient documented to be on beta-blocker therapy

● Ⓜ **G8034** Prior myocardial infarction — coronary artery disease patient not documented to be on beta-blocker therapy

● Ⓜ **G8035** Clinician documented that prior myocardial infarction — coronary artery disease patient was not eligible candidate for beta-blocker therapy measure

░ Special Coverage Instructions   ░ Noncovered by Medicare   ░ Carrier Discretion   ☑ Quantity Alert   ● New Code   ○ Reinstated Code   ▲ Revised Code

64 — G Codes   Ⓐ Age   Ⓜ Maternity   ♀ Female Only   ♂ Male Only   Ⓐ-Ⓨ APC Status Indicator   *2006 HCPCS*

● Ⓜ **G8036** Coronary artery disease patient documented to be on antiplatelet therapy

● Ⓜ **G8037** Coronary artery disease patient not documented to be on antiplatelet therapy

● Ⓜ **G8038** Clinician documented that coronary artery disease patient was not eligible candidate for antiplatelet therapy measure

● Ⓜ **G8039** Coronary artery disease — patient with low-density lipoprotein documented to be greater than 100 mg/dl

● Ⓜ **G8040** Coronary artery disease — patient with low-density lipoprotein documented to be less than or equal to 100 mg/dl

● Ⓜ **G8041** Clinician documented that coronary artery disease patient was not eligible candidate for low-density lipoprotein measure

● Ⓜ **G8051** Patient (female) documented to have been assessed for osteoporosis
This code is for female patients age 75 years or older.

● Ⓜ **G8052** Patient (female) not documented to have been assessed for osteoporosis
This code is for female patients age 75 years or older.

● Ⓜ **G8053** Clinician documented that (female) patient was not an eligible candidate for osteoporosis assessment measure
This code is for female patients age 75 years or older.

● **G8054** Patient not documented for the assessment of falls within last 12 months
Report this code in addition to office visit; office consult; home visit; nursing facility; or initial preventive physical exam evaluation and management code. This code is for patients age 75 years or older.

● Ⓜ **G8055** Patient documented for the assessment of falls within last 12 months
Report this code in addition to office visit; office consult; home visit; nursing facility; or initial preventive physical exam evaluation and management code. This code is for patients age 75 years or older.

● Ⓜ **G8056** Clinician documented that patient was not an eligible candidate for the falls assessment measure within the last 12 months
Report this code in addition to office visit; office consult; home visit; nursing facility; or initial preventive physical exam evaluation and management code. This code is for patients age 75 years or older.

● Ⓜ **G8057** Patient documented to have received hearing assessment
Report this code in addition to office visit; office consult; home visit; nursing facility; or initial preventive physical exam evaluation and management code. This code is for patients age 75 years or older.

● Ⓜ **G8058** Patient not documented to have received hearing assessment
Report this code in addition to office visit; office consult; home visit; nursing facility; or initial preventive physical exam evaluation and management code. This code is for patients age 75 years or older.

● Ⓜ **G8059** Clinician documented that patient was not an eligible candidate for hearing assessment measure
Report this code in addition to office visit; office consult; home visit; nursing facility; or initial preventive physical exam evaluation and management code. This code is for patients age 75 years or older.

● Ⓜ **G8060** Patient documented for the assessment of urinary incontinence
Report this code in addition to office visit; office consult; home visit; nursing facility; or initial preventive physical exam evaluation and management code. This code is for patients age 75 years or older.

● Ⓜ **G8061** Patient not documented for the assessment of urinary incontinence
Report this code in addition to office visit; office consult; home visit; nursing facility; or initial preventive physical exam evaluation and management code. This code is for patients age 75 years or older.

● Ⓜ **G8062** Clinician documented that patient was not an eligible candidate for urinary incontinence assessment measure
Report this code in addition to office visit; office consult; home visit; nursing facility; or initial preventive physical exam evaluation and management code. This code is for patients age 75 years or older.

● Ⓜ **G8075** End-stage renal disease patient with documented dialysis dose of URR greater than or equal to 65% (or Kt/V greater than or equal to 1.2)
Use with codes G0308-G0327, 90945, 90947.

● Ⓜ **G8076** End-stage renal disease patient with documented dialysis dose of URR less than 65% (or Kt/V less than 1.2)
Use with codes G0308-G0327, 90945, 90947.

● Ⓜ **G8077** Clinician documented that end-stage renal disease patient was not eligible candidate for URR or Kt/V measure
Use with codes G0308-G0327, 90945, 90947.

● Ⓜ **G8078** End-stage renal disease patient with documented hematocrit greater than or equal to 33 (or hemoglobin greater than or equal to 11)
Use with codes G0308-G0327, 90945, 90947.

● Ⓜ **G8079** End-stage renal disease patient with documented hematocrit less than 33 (or hemoglobin less than 11)
Use with codes G0308-G0327, 90945, 90947.

● Ⓜ **G8080** Clinician documented that end-stage renal disease patient was not eligible candidate for hematocrit (hemoglobin) measure
Use with codes G0308-G0327, 90945, 90947.

● Ⓜ **G8081** End-stage renal disease patient requiring hemodialysis vascular access documented to have received autogenous AV fistula
Use with codes G0308-G0327, 90945, 90947, 36818-36812, 36825.

● Ⓜ **G8082** End-stage renal disease patient requiring hemodialysis documented to have received vascular access other than autogenous AV fistula
Use with codes G0308-G0327, 90945, 90947, 36818-36812, 36825.

● Ⓜ **G8093** Newly diagnosed chronic obstructive pulmonary disease (COPD) patient documented to have received smoking cessation intervention, within 3 months of diagnosis
Report this code in addition to office visit; office consult; home visit; nursing facility; evaluation and management codes and smoking and tobacco use cessation counseling codes.

● Ⓜ **G8094** Newly diagnosed chronic obstructive pulmonary disease (COPD) patient not documented to have received smoking cessation intervention, within 3 months of diagnosis
Report this code in addition to office visit; office consult; home visit; nursing facility; evaluation and management codes and smoking and toba

---

| Special Coverage Instructions | Noncovered by Medicare | Carrier Discretion | ☑ Quantity Alert | ● New Code | ○ Reinstated Code | ▲ Revised Code |

Procedures/Professional Services (Temporary)

G8099 — G8153

● Ⓜ **G8099** Osteoporosis patient documented to have been prescribed calcium and vitamin D supplements

● Ⓜ **G8100** Clinician documented that osteoporosis patient was not eligible candidate for calcium and vitamin D supplement measure

● Ⓜ **G8103** Newly diagnosed osteoporosis patient documented to have been treated with antiresorptive therapy and/or parathyroid hormone treatment measure within 3 months of diagnosis

● Ⓜ **G8104** Clinician documented that newly diagnosed osteoporosis patient was not an eligible candidate for antiresorptive therapy and/or parathyroid hormone treatment measure within 3 months of diagnosis

● Ⓜ **G8106** Within 6 months of suffering a nontraumatic fracture, female patient 65 years of age or older documented to have undergone bone mineral density testing or to have been prescribed a drug to treat or prevent osteoporosis

● Ⓜ **G8107** Clinician documented that female patient 65 years of age or older who suffered a nontraumatic fracture within the last 6 months was not an eligible candidate for measure to test bone mineral density or drug to treat or prevent osteoporosis

● Ⓜ **G8108** Patient documented to have received influenza vaccination during influenza season
Use this code for patients age 50 years and older.

● Ⓜ **G8109** Patient not documented to have received influenza vaccination during influenza season
Report this code in addition to office visit; office consult; nursing facility; domiciliary evaluation and management codes and influenza vaccine administration code. Use this code for patients age 50 years and older.

● Ⓜ **G8110** Clinician documented that patient was not an eligible candidate for influenza vaccination measure
Report this code in addition to office visit; office consult; nursing facility; domiciliary evaluation and management codes and influenza vaccine administration code. Use this code for patients age 50 years and older.

● Ⓜ **G8111** Patient (female) documented to have received a mammogram during the measurement year or prior year to the measurement year
Report this code in addition to office visit; office consult; home visit; nursing facility; domiciliary or initial preventive physical exam evaluation and management codes. Use this code for patients age 40 years and older.

● Ⓜ **G8112** Patient (female) not documented to have received a mammogram during the measurement year or prior year to the measurement year
Report this code in addition to office visit; office consult; home visit; nursing facility; domiciliary or initial preventive physical exam evaluation and management codes. Use this code for patients age 40 years and older.

● Ⓜ **G8113** Clinician documented that female patient was not an eligible candidate for mammography measure
Report this code in addition to office visit; office consult; home visit; nursing facility; domiciliary or initial preventive physical exam evaluation and management codes. Use this code for patients age 40 years and older.

● Ⓜ **G8114** Clinician did not provide care to patient for the required time of mammography measure (i.e., measurement year or prior year)
Report this code in addition to office visit; office consult; home visit; nursing facility; domiciliary or initial preventive physical exam evaluation and management codes. Use this code for patients age 40 years and older.

● Ⓜ **G8115** Patient documented to have received pneumococcal vaccination
Report this code in addition to office visit; office consult; home visit; nursing facility; domiciliary or initial preventive physical exam evaluation and management codes, and pneumococcal vaccination administraction codes. Use this code for patients age 65 years and over.

● Ⓜ **G8116** Patient not documented to have received pneumococcal vaccination
Report this code in addition to office visit; office consult; home visit; nursing facility; domiciliary or initial preventive physical exam evaluation and management codes, and pneumococcal vaccination administraction codes. Use this code for patients age 65 years and over.

● Ⓜ **G8117** Clinician documented that patient was not eligible candidate for pneumococcal vaccination measure
Report this code in addition to office visit; office consult; home visit; nursing facility; domiciliary or initial preventive physical exam evaluation and management codes, and pneumococcal vaccination administration codes. Use this code for patients age 65 years and over.

● Ⓜ **G8126** Patient documented as being treated with antidepressant medication during the entire 12 week acute treatment phase
Report this code in addition to office visit and psychiatry evaluation and management codes. Use this code for patients age 18 and older.

● Ⓜ **G8127** Patient not documented as being treated with antidepressant medication during the entire 12 week acute treatment phase
Report this code in addition to office visit and psychiatry evaluation and management codes. Use this code for patients age 18 and older.

● Ⓜ **G8128** Clinician documented that patient was not eligible candidate for antidepressant medication during the entire 12 week acute treatment phase measure
Report this code in addition to office visit and psychiatry evaluation and management codes. Use this code for patients age 18 and older.

● Ⓜ **G8129** Patient documented as being treated with antidepressant medication for at least 6 months continuous treatment phase
Report this code in addition to office visit and psychiatry evaluation and management codes. Use this code for patients age 18 and older.

● Ⓜ **G8130** Patient not documented as being treated with antidepressant medication for at least 6 months continuous treatment phase
Report this code in addition to office visit and psychiatry evaluation and management codes. Use this code for patients age 18 and older.

● Ⓜ **G8131** Clinician documented that patient was not an eligible candidate for antidepressant medication for continuous treatment phase
Report this code in addition to office visit and psychiatry evaluation and management codes. Use this code for patients age 18 and older.

● **G8135** Patient not documented to have received antibiotic prophylaxis one hour prior to incision time (two hours for vancomycin)

● Ⓜ **G8152** Patient documented to have received antibiotic prophylaxis one hour prior to incision time (two hours for vancomycin)

● Ⓜ **G8153** Patient not documented to have received antibiotic prophylaxis one hour prior to incision time (two hours for vancomycin)

▨ Special Coverage Instructions   ▨ Noncovered by Medicare   ▨ Carrier Discretion   ☑ Quantity Alert   ● New Code   ○ Reinstated Code   ▲ Revised Code

66 — G Codes   Ⓐ Age   Ⓜ Maternity   ♀ Female Only   ♂ Male Only   Ⓐ-Ⓨ APC Status Indicator   *2006 HCPCS*

● Ⓜ   **G8154**   Clinician documented that patient was not an eligible candidate for antibiotic prophylaxis one hour prior to incision time (two hours for vancomycin) measure

● Ⓜ   **G8155**   Patient with documented receipt of thromboembolism prophylaxis

● Ⓜ   **G8156**   Patient without documented receipt of thromboembolism prophylaxis

● Ⓜ   **G8157**   Clinician documented that patient was not an eligible candidate for thromboembolism prophylaxis measure

● Ⓜ   **G8158**   Patient documented to have received coronary artery bypass graft with use of internal mammary artery
Report this code in addition to CPT codes 33533-33536.

● Ⓜ   **G8159**   Patient documented to have received coronary artery bypass graft without use of internal mammary artery
Report this code in addition to CPT codes 33533-33536.

● Ⓜ   **G8160**   Clinician documented that patient was not an eligible candidate for coronary artery bypass graft with use of internal mammary artery measure
Report this code in addition to CPT codes 33533-33536.

● Ⓜ   **G8161**   Patient with isolated coronary artery bypass graft documented to have received pre-operative beta-blockade
Report this code in addition to CPT codes 33510-33514, 33516, and 33533-33536.

● Ⓜ   **G8162**   Patient with isolated coronary artery bypass graft not documented to have received pre-operative beta-blockade
Report this code in addition to CPT codes 33510-33514, 33516, and 33533-33536.

● Ⓜ   **G8163**   Clinician documented that patient with isolated coronary artery bypass graft was not an eligible candidate for pre-operative beta-blockade measure
Report this code in addition to CPT codes 33510-33514, 33516, and 33533-33536.

● Ⓜ   **G8164**   Patient with isolated coronary artery bypass graft documented to have prolonged intubation
Report this code in addition to CPT codes 33510-33514, 33516, and 33533-33536.

● Ⓜ   **G8165**   Patient with isolated coronary artery bypass graft not documented to have prolonged intubation
Report this code in addition to CPT codes 33510-33514, 33516, and 33533-33536.

● Ⓜ   **G8166**   Patient with isolated coronary artery bypass graft documented to have required surgical re-exploration
Report this code in addition to CPT codes 33510-33514, 33516, and 33533-33536.

● Ⓜ   **G8167**   Patient with isolated coronary artery bypass graft did not require surgical re-exploration
Report this code in addition to CPT codes 33510-33514, 33516, and 33533-33536.

● Ⓜ   **G8170**   Patient with isolated coronary artery bypass graft documented to have been discharged on aspirin or clopidogrel

● Ⓜ   **G8171**   Patient with isolated coronary artery bypass graft not documented to have been discharged on aspirin or clopidogrel

● Ⓜ   **G8172**   Clinician documented that patient with isolated coronary artery bypass graft was not an eligible cadidate for antiplatelet therapy at discharge measure

● Ⓜ   **G8182**   Clinician has not provided care for the cardiac patient for the required time for low-density lipoprotein measure (6 months)

● Ⓜ   **G8183**   Patient with heart failure and atrial fibrillation documented to be on Warfarin therapy

● Ⓜ   **G8184**   Clinician documented that patient with heart failure and atrial fibrillation was not an eligible candidate for Wafarin therapy measure

● Ⓜ   **G8185**   Patient diagnosed with symptomatic osteoarthritis with documented annual assessment of function and pain

● Ⓜ   **G8186**   Clinician documented that symptomatic osteoarthritis patient was not an eligible candidate for annual assessment of function and pain measure

Ⓑ   **G9001**   Coordinated care fee, initial rate   ⊘

Ⓑ   **G9002**   Coordinated care fee, maintenance rate   ⊘

Ⓑ   **G9003**   Coordinated care fee, risk adjusted high, initial   ⊘

Ⓑ   **G9004**   Coordinated care fee, risk adjusted low, initial   ⊘

Ⓑ   **G9005**   Coordinated care fee, risk adjusted maintenance ⊘

Ⓑ   **G9006**   Coordinated care fee, home monitoring   ⊘

Ⓑ   **G9007**   Coordinated care fee, schedule team conference ⊘

Ⓑ   **G9008**   Coordinated care fee, physician coordinated care oversight services   ⊘

Ⓔ   **G9009**   Coordinated care fee, risk adjusted maintenance, Level 3

Ⓔ   **G9010**   Coordinated care fee, risk adjusted maintenance, Level 4   ⊘

Ⓔ   **G9011**   Coordinated care fee, risk adjusted maintenance, Level 5   ⊘

Ⓔ   **G9012**   Coordinated care fee, risk adjusted maintenance, other specified care management   ⊘

Ⓔ   **G9013**   ESRD demo basic bundle Level 1

Ⓔ   **G9014**   ESRD demo expanded bundle including venous access and related services

Ⓔ   **G9016**   Smoking cessation counseling, individual, in the absence of or in addition to any other evaluation and management service, per session (6-10 minutes) [demonstration project code only]   ⊘

Ⓐ   **G9017**   Amantadine hydrochloride, oral, generic name, 100 mg (for use in a Medicare-approved demonstration project)

Ⓐ   **G9018**   Zanamivir, inhalation powder administration through inhaler, generic, per 10 mg (for use as a Medicare-approved demonstration project)
This code was developed in anticipation of a generic drug.

Ⓐ   **G9019**   Oseltamivir phosphate, oral, generic, 75 mg (for use in a Medicare-approved demonstration project)
This code was developed in anticipation of a generic drug.

Ⓐ   **G9020**   Rimantadine hydrochloride, oral, generic, 100 mg (for use in a Medicare-approved demonstration project)

~~G9021~~   ~~Chemotherapy assessment for nausea and/or vomiting, patient reported, performed at the time of chemotherapy administration; assessment Level 1; not at all (for use in a Medicare-approved demonstration project)~~

~~G9022~~   ~~Chemotherapy assessment for nausea and/or vomiting, patient reported, performed at the time of chemotherapy administration; assessment Level 2; a little (for use in a Medicare-approved demonstration project)~~

| Special Coverage Instructions | Noncovered by Medicare | Carrier Discretion | ☑ Quantity Alert | ● New Code | ○ Reinstated Code | ▲ Revised Code |

2006 HCPCS   ❶-❾ ASC Groups   MED: Pub 100/NCD Reference   ॐ DMEPOS Paid   ⊘ SNF Excluded   **G Codes — 67**

G9023 ~~Chemotherapy assessment for nausea and/or vomiting, patient reported, performed at the time of chemotherapy administration; assessment Level 3: quite a bit (for use in a Medicare approved demonstration project)~~

G9024 ~~Chemotherapy assessment for nausea and/or vomiting, patient reported, performed at the time of chemotherapy administration; assessment Level 4: very much (for use in a Medicare approved demonstration project)~~

G9025 ~~Chemotherapy assessment for pain, patient reported, performed at the time of chemotherapy administration, assessment Level 1: not at all (for use in a Medicare approved demonstration project)~~

G9026 ~~Chemotherapy assessment for pain, patient reported, performed at the time of chemotherapy administration, assessment Level 2: a little (for use in a Medicare approved demonstration project)~~

G9027 ~~Chemotherapy assessment for pain, patient reported, performed at the time of chemotherapy administration assessment Level 3: quite a bit (for use in a Medicare approved demonstration project)~~

G9028 ~~Chemotherapy assessment for pain, patient reported, performed at the time of the chemotherapy administration, assessment Level 4: very much (for use in a Medicare approved demonstration project)~~

G9029 ~~Chemotherapy assessment for lack of energy (fatigue), patient reported, performed at the time of chemotherapy administration, assessment Level 1: not at all (for use in a Medicare approved demonstration project)~~

G9030 ~~Chemotherapy assessment for lack of energy (fatigue), patient reported, performed at the time of chemotherapy administration, assessment Level 2: a little (for use in a Medicare approved demonstration project)~~

G9031 ~~Chemotherapy assessment for lack of energy (fatigue), patient reported, performed at the time of chemotherapy administration, assessment Level 3: quite a bit (for use in a Medicare approved demonstration project)~~

G9032 ~~Chemotherapy assessment for lack of energy (fatigue), patient reported, performed at the time of chemotherapy administration, assessment Level 4: very much (for use in a Medicare approved demonstration project)~~

Ⓐ   G9033   Amantadine hydrochloride, oral, brand name, 100 mg (for use in a Medicare-approved demonstration project)

Ⓐ   G9034   Zanamivir, inhalation powder, administered through inhaler, brand name, 10 mg (for use in a Medicare-approved demonstration project)

Ⓐ   G9035   Oseltamivir phosphate, oral, brand name, 75 mg (for use in a Medicare-approved demonstration project)

Ⓐ   G9036   Rimantadine hydrochloride, oral, brand name, 100 mg (for use in a Medicare-approved demonstration project)

▲ Ⓑ   G9041   Sensory integrative techniques to enhance sensory processing and promote adaptive responses to environmental demands, self care/home management training (e.g. activities of daily living (ADL) and compensatory training, meal preparation, safety procedures, and instructions in use of assistive technology devices/adaptive equipment), community/work reintegration training (e.g. shopping, transportation, money management, avocational activities and/or work environment modification analysis, work task analysis), direct one-on-one contact by the provider, each 15 minutes

▲ Ⓑ   G9042   Sensory integrative techniques to enhance sensory processing and promote adaptive responses to environmental demands, self care/home management training (e.g. activities of daily living (ADL) and compensatory training, meal preparation, safety procedures, and instructions in use of assistive technology devices/adaptive equipment), community/work reintegration training (e.g. shopping, transportation, money management, avocational activities and/or work environment modification analysis, work task analysis), direct one-on-one contact by the provider, each 15 minutes

▲ Ⓑ   G9043   Sensory integrative techniques to enhance sensory processing and promote adaptive responses to environmental demands, self care/home management training (e.g. activities of daily living (ADL) and compensatory training, meal preparation, safety procedures, and instructions in use of assistive technology devices/adaptive equipment), community/work reintegration training (e.g. shopping, transportation, money management, avocational activities and/or work environment modification analysis, work task anaylsis), direct one-on-one contact by the provider, each 15 minutes

▲ Ⓑ   G9044   Sensory integrative techniques to enhance sensory processing and promote adaptive responses to environmental demands, self care/home management training (e.g. activities of daily living (ADL) and compensatory training, meal preparation, safety procedures, and instructions in use of assistive technology devices/adaptive equipment), community/work reintegration training (e.g. shopping, transportation, money management, avocational activities and/or work environment modification analysis, work task analysis), direct one-on-one contact by the provider, each 15 minutes

●   G9050   Oncology; primary focus of visit; work-up, evaluation, or staging at the time of cancer diagnosis or recurrence (for use in a Medicare-approved demonstration project)

●   G9051   Oncology; primary focus of visit; treatment decision-making after disease is staged or restaged, discussion of treatment options, supervising/coordinating active cancer directed therapy or managing consequences of cancer directed therapy (for use in a Medicare-approved demonstration project)

●   G9052   Oncology; primary focus of visit; surveillance for disease recurrence for patient who has completed definitive cancer-directed therapy and currently lacks evidence of recurrent disease; cancer directed therapy might be considered in the future (for use in a Medicare-approved demonstration project)

● **G9053** Oncology; primary focus of visit; expectant management of patient with evidence of cancer for whom no cancer directed therapy is being administered or arranged at present; cancer directed therapy might be considered in the future (for use in a Medicare-approved demonstration project)

● **G9054** Oncology; primary focus of visit; supervising, coordinating or managing care of patient with terminal cancer or for whom other medical illness prevents further cancer treatment; includes symptom management, end-of-life care planning, management of palliative therapies (for use in a Medicare-approved demonstration project)

● **G9055** Oncology; primary focus of visit; other, unspecified service not otherwise listed (for use in a Medicare-approved demonstration project)

● **G9056** Oncology; practice guidelines; management adheres to guidelines (for use in a Medicare-approved demonstration project)

● **G9057** Oncology; practice guidelines; management differs from guidelines as a result of patient enrollment in an institutional review board approved clinical trial (for use in a Medicare-approved demonstration project)

● **G9058** Oncology; practice guidelines; management differs from guidelines because the treating physician disagrees with guideline recommendations (for use in a Medicare-approved demonstration project)

● **G9059** Oncology; practice guidelines; management differs from guidelines because the patient, after being offered treatment consistent with guidelines, has opted for alternative treatment or management, including no treatment (for use in a Medicare-approved demonstration project)

● **G9060** Oncology; practice guidelines; management differs from guidelines for reason(s) associated with patient comorbid illness or performance status not factored into guidelines (for use in a Medicare-approved demonstration project)

● **G9061** Oncology; practice guidelines; patient's condition not addressed by available guidelines (for use in a Medicare-approved demonstration project)

● **G9062** Oncology; practice guidelines; management differs from guidelines for other reason(s) not listed (for use in a Medicare-approved demonstration project)

● **G9063** Oncology; disease status; limited to non-small cell lung cancer; extent of disease initially established as stage I (prior to neo-adjuvant therapy, if any) with no evidence of disease progression, recurrence, or metastases (for use in a Medicare-approved demonstration project)

● **G9064** Oncology; disease status; limited to non-small cell lung cancer; extent of disease initially established as stage II (prior to neo-adjuvant therapy, if any) with no evidence of disease progression, recurrence, or metastases (for use in a Medicare-approved demonstration project)

● **G9065** Oncology; disease status; limited to non-small cell lung cancer; extent of disease initially established as stage III a (prior to neo-adjuvant therapy, if any) with no evidence of disease progression, recurrence, or metastases (for use in a Medicare-approved demonstration project)

● **G9066** Oncology; disease status; limited to non-small cell lung cancer; stage III B- IV at diagnosis, metastatic, locally recurrent, or progressive (for use in a Medicare-approved demonstration project)

● **G9067** Oncology; disease status; limited to non-small cell lung cancer; extent of disease unknown, under evaluation, not yet determined, or not listed (for use in a Medicare-approved demonstration project)

● **G9068** Oncology; disease status; limited to small cell and combined small cell/non-small cell; extent of disease initially established as limited with no evidence of disease progression, recurrence, or metastases (for use in a Medicare-approved demonstration project)

● **G9069** Oncology; disease status; small cell lung cancer, limited to small cell and combined small cell/non-small cell; extensive stage at diagnosis, metastatic, locally recurrent, or progressive (for use in a Medicare-approved demonstration project)

● **G9070** Oncology; disease status; small cell lung cancer, limited to small cell and combined small cell/non-small; extent of disease unknown, under evaluation, pre-surgical, or not listed (for use in a Medicare-approved demonstration project)

● **G9071** Oncology; disease status; invasive female breast cancer (does not include ductal carcinoma in situ); adenocarcinoma as predominant cell type; stage I or stage IIA-IB; OR T3, N1, M0; and ER and/or PR positive; with no evidence of disease progression, recurrence, or metastases (for use in a Medicare-approved demonstration project)

● **G9072** Oncology; disease status; invasive female breast cancer (does not include ductal carcinoma in situ); adenocarcinoma as predominant cell type; stage I, or stage IIA-IIB; or T3, N1, M0; and ER and PR negative; with no evidence of disease progression, recurrence, or metastases (for use in a Medicare-approved demonstration project)

● **G9073** Oncology; disease status; invasive female breast cancer (does not include ductal carcinoma in situ); adenocarcinoma as predominant cell type; stage IIIA-IIIB; and not T3, N1, M0; and ER and/or PR positive; with no evidence of disease progression, recurrence, or metastases (for use in a Medicare-approved demonstration project)

● **G9074** Oncology; disease status; invasive female breast cancer (does not include ductal carcinoma in situ); adenocarcinoma as predominant cell type; stage IIIA-IIIB; and not T3, N1, M0; and ER and PR negative; with no evidence of disease progression, recurrence, or metastases (for use in a Medicare-approved demonstration project)

● **G9075** Oncology; disease status; invasive female breast cancer (does not include ductal carcinoma in situ); adenocarcinoma as predominant cell type; M1 at diagnosis, metastatic, locally recurrent, or progressive (for use in a Medicare-approved demonstration project)

● **G9076** Oncology; disease status; invasive female breast cancer (does not include ductal carcinoma in situ); adenocarcinoma as predominant cell type; extent of disease unknown, under evaluation, pre-surgical or not listed (for use in a Medicare-approved demonstration project)

● **G9077** Oncology; disease status; prostate cancer, limited to adenocarcinoma as predominant cell type; T1-T2C and Gleason 2-7 and PSA < or equal to 20 at diagnosis with no evidence of disease progression, recurrence, or metastases (for use in a Medicare-approved demonstration project)

Special Coverage Instructions   Noncovered by Medicare   Carrier Discretion   ☑ Quantity Alert   ● New Code   ○ Reinstated Code   ▲ Revised Code

2006 HCPCS   **1**-**9** ASC Groups   MED: Pub 100/NCD Reference   ⅃ DMEPOS Paid   ⊘ SNF Excluded   **G Codes — 69**

●   **G9078**   Oncology; disease status; prostate cancer, limited to adenocarcinoma as predominant cell type; T2 or Gleason 8-10 or PSA < 20 at diagnosis with no evidence of disease progression, recurrence, or metastases (for use in a Medicare-approved demonstration project)

●   **G9079**   Oncology; disease status; prostate cancer, limited to adenocarcinoma as predominant cell type; T3B-T4, any N; any T, N1 at diagnosis with no evidence of disease progression, recurrence, or metastases (for use in a Medicare-approved demonstration project)

●   **G9080**   Oncology; disease status; prostate cancer, limited to adenocarcinoma; after initial treatment with rising PSA or failure of PSA decline (for use in a Medicare-approved demonstration project)

●   **G9081**   Oncology; disease status; prostate cancer, limited to adenocarcinoma; non-castrate, incompletely castrate; clinical metastases or M1 at diagnosis (for use in a Medicare-approved demonstration project)

●   **G9082**   Oncology; disease status; prostate cancer, limited to adenocarcinoma; castrate; clinical metastases or M1 at diagnosis (for use in a Medicare-approved demonstration project)

●   **G9083**   Oncology; disease status; prostate cancer, limited to adenocarcinoma; extent of disease unknown, under evaluation or not listed (for use in a Medicare-approved demonstration project)

●   **G9084**   Oncology; disease status; colon cancer, limited to invasive cancer, adenocarcinoma as predominant cell type; extent of disease initially established as T1-3, N0, M0 with no evidence of disease progression, recurrence, or metastases (for use in a Medicare-approved demonstration project)

●   **G9085**   Oncology; disease status; colon cancer, limited to invasive cancer, adenocarcinoma as predominant cell type; extent of disease initially established as T4, N0, M0 with no evidence of disease progression, recurrence, or metastases (for use in a Medicare-approved demonstration project)

●   **G9086**   Oncology; disease status; colon cancer, limited to invasive cancer, adenocarcinoma as predominant cell type; extent of disease initially established as T1-4, N1-2, M0 with no evidence of disease progression, recurrence, or metastases (for use in a Medicare-approved demonstration project)

●   **G9087**   Oncology; disease status; colon cancer, limited to invasive cancer, adenocarcinoma as predominant cell type; M1 at diagnosis, metastatic, locally recurrent, or progressive with current clinical, radiologic, or biochemical evidence of disease (for use in a Medicare-approved demonstration project)

●   **G9088**   Oncology; disease status; colon cancer, limited to invasive cancer, adenocarcinoma as predominant cell type; M1 at diagnosis, metastatic, locally recurrent, or progressive without current clinical, radiologic, or biochemical evidence of disease (for use in a Medicare-approved demonstration project)

●   **G9089**   Oncology; disease status; colon cancer, limited to invasive cancer, adenocarcinoma as predominant cell type; extent of disease unknown, not yet determined, under evaluation, pre-surgical, or not listed (for use in a Medicare-approved demonstration project)

●   **G9090**   Oncology; disease status; rectal cancer, limited to invasive cancer, adenocarcinoma as predominant cell type; extent of disease initially established as T1-2, N0, M0 (prior to neo-adjuvant therapy, if any) with no evidence of disease progression, recurrence, or metastases (for use in a Medicare-approved demonstration project)

●   **G9091**   Oncology; disease status; rectal cancer, limited to invasive cancer, adenocarcinoma as predominant cell type; extent of disease initially established as T3, N0, M0 (prior to neo-adjuvant therapy, if any) with no evidence of disease progression, recurrence, or metastases (for use in a Medicare-approved demonstration project)

●   **G9092**   Oncology; disease status; rectal cancer, limited to invasive cancer, adenocarcinoma as predominant cell type; extent of disease initially established as T1-3, N1-2, M0 (prior to neo-adjuvant therapy, if any) with no evidence of disease progression, recurrence or metastases (for use in a Medicare-approved demonstration project)

●   **G9093**   Oncology; disease status; rectal cancer, limited to invasive cancer, adenocarcinoma as predominant cell type; extent of disease initially established as T4, any N, M0 (prior to neo-adjuvant therapy, if any) with no evidence of disease progression, recurrence, or metastases (for use in a Medicare-approved demonstration project)

●   **G9094**   Oncology; disease status; rectal cancer, limited to invasive cancer, adenocarcinoma as predominant cell type; M1 at diagnosis, metastatic, locally recurrent, or progressive (for use in a Medicare-approved demonstration project)

●   **G9095**   Oncology; disease status; rectal cancer, limited to invasive cancer, adenocarcinoma as predominant cell type; extent of disease unknown, not yet determined, under evaluation, pre-surgical, or not listed (for use in a Medicare-approved demonstration project)

●   **G9096**   Oncology; disease status; esophageal cancer, limited to adenocarcinoma or squamous cell carcinoma as predominant cell type; extent of disease initially established as T1-T3, N0-N1 or NX (prior to neo-adjuvant therapy, if any) with no evidence of disease progression, recurrence, or metastases (for use in a Medicare-approved demonstration project)

●   **G9097**   Oncology; disease status; esophageal cancer, limited to adenocarcinoma or squamous cell carcinoma as predominant cell type; extent of disease initially established as T4, any N, M0 (prior to neo-adjuvant therapy, if any) with no evidence of disease progression, recurrence, or metastases (for use in a Medicare-approved demonstration project)

●   **G9098**   Oncology; disease status; esophageal cancer, limited to adenocarcinoma or squamous cell carcinoma as predominant cell type; M1 at diagnosis, metastatic, locally recurrent, or progressive (for use in a Medicare-approved demonstration project)

●   **G9099**   Oncology; disease status; esophageal cancer, limited to adenocarcinoma or squamous cell carcinoma as predominant cell type; extent of disease unknown, not yet determined, under evaluation, pre-surgical, or not listed (for use in a Medicare-approved demonstration project)

Special Coverage Instructions   Noncovered by Medicare   Carrier Discretion   ☑ Quantity Alert   ● New Code   ○ Reinstated Code   ▲ Revised Code

70 — G Codes   Ⓐ Age   Ⓜ Maternity   ♀ Female Only   ♂ Male Only   Ⓐ-Ⓨ APC Status Indicator   *2006 HCPCS*

● **G9100** Oncology; disease status; gastric cancer, limited to adenocarcinoma as predominant cell type; post R0 resection (with or without neoadjuvant therapy) with no evidence of disease recurrence, progression, or metastases (for use in a Medicare-approved demonstration project)

● **G9101** Oncology; disease status; gastric cancer, limited to adenocarcinoma as predominant cell type; post R1 or R2 resection (with or without neoadjuvant therapy) with no evidence of disease progression, or metastases (for use in a Medicare-approved demonstration project)

● **G9102** Oncology; disease status; gastric cancer, limited to adenocarcinoma as predominant cell type; clinical or pathologic M0, unresectable with no evidence of disease progression, or metastases (for use in a Medicare-approved demonstration project)

● **G9103** Oncology; disease status; gastric cancer, limited to adenocarcinoma as predominant cell type; clinical or pathologic M1 at diagnosis, metastatic, locally recurrent, or progressive (for use in a Medicare-approved demonstration project)

● **G9104** Oncology; disease status; gastric cancer, limited to adenocarcinoma as predominant cell type; extent of disease unknown, under evaluation, not yet determined, pre-surgical, or not listed (for use in a Medicare-approved demonstration project)

● **G9105** Oncology; disease status; pancreatic cancer, limited to adenocarcinoma as predominant cell type; post R0 resection without evidence of disease progression, recurrence, or metastases (for use in a Medicare-approved demonstration project)

● **G9106** Oncology; disease status; pancreatic cancer, limited to adenocarcinoma; post R1 or R2 resection with no evidence of disease progression, or metastases (for use in a Medicare-approved demonstration project)

● **G9107** Oncology; disease status; pancreatic cancer, limited to adenocarcinoma; unresectable at diagnosis, M1 at diagnosis, metastatic, locally recurrent, or progressive (for use in a Medicare-approved demonstration project)

● **G9108** Oncology; disease status; pancreatic cancer, limited to adenocarcinoma; extent of disease unknown, under evaluation, not yet determined, pre-surgical, or not listed (for use in a Medicare-approved demonstration project)

● **G9109** Oncology; disease status; head and neck cancer, limited to cancers of oral cavity, pharynx and larynx with squamous cell as predominant cell type; extent of disease initially established as T1-T2 and N0, M0 (prior to neo-adjuvant therapy, if any) with no evidence of disease progression, recurrence, or metastases (for use in a Medicare-approved demonstration project)

● **G9110** Oncology; disease status; head and neck cancer, limited to cancers of oral cavity, pharynx and larynx with squamous cell as predominant cell type; extent of disease initially established as T3-4 and/or N1-3, M0 (prior to neo-adjuvant therapy, if any) with no evidence of disease progression, recurrence, or metastases (for use in a Medicare-approved demonstration project)

● **G9111** Oncology; disease status; head and neck cancer, limited to cancers of oral cavity, pharynx and larynx with squamous cell as predominant cell type; M1 at diagnosis, metastatic, locally recurrent, or progressive (for use in a Medicare-approved demonstration project)

● **G9112** Oncology; disease status; head and neck cancer, limited to cancers of oral cavity, pharynx and larynx with squamous cell as predominant cell type; extent of disease unknown, not yet determined, pre-surgical, or not listed (for use in a Medicare-approved demonstration project)

● **G9113** Oncology; disease status; ovarian cancer, limited to epithelial cancer; pathologic stage IA-B (grade 1) without evidence of disease progression, recurrence, or metastases (for use in a Medicare-approved demonstration project)

● **G9114** Oncology; disease status; ovarian cancer, limited to epithelial cancer; pathologic stage IA-B (grade 2-3); or stage IC (all grades); or stage II; without evidence of disease progression, recurrence, or metastases (for use in a Medicare-approved demonstration project)

● **G9115** Oncology; disease status; ovarian cancer, limited to epithelial cancer; pathologic stage III-IV; without evidence of progression, recurrence, or metastases (for use in a Medicare-approved demonstration project)

● **G9116** Oncology; disease status; ovarian cancer, limited to epithelial cancer; evidence of disease progression, or recurrence, and/or platinum resistance (for use in a Medicare-approved demonstration project)

● **G9117** Oncology; disease status; ovarian cancer, limited to epithelial cancer; extent of disease unknown, under evaluation, incomplete surgical staging, pre-surgical staging, or not listed (for use in a Medicare-approved demonstration project)

● **G9118** Oncology; disease status; non-Hodgkin's lymphoma, limited to follicular lymphoma, mantle cell lymphoma, diffuse large B-cell lymphoma, peripheral T cell lymphoma; small lymphocytic lymphoma; stage I, II at diagnosis, not relapsed, not refractory (for use in a Medicare-approved demonstration project)

● **G9119** Oncology; disease status; non-Hodgkin's lymphoma, limited to follicular lymphoma, mantle cell lymphoma, diffuse large B-cell lymphoma, peripheral T cell lymphoma, small lymphocytic lymphoma; stage III, IV not relapsed, not refractory (for use in a Medicare-approved demonstration project)

● **G9120** Oncology; disease status; non-Hodgkin's lymphoma; limited to follicular lymphoma, diffuse large B-cell lymphoma; histologically transformed from follicular lymphoma to diffuse large B-cell lymphoma (for use in a Medicare-approved demonstration project)

● **G9121** Oncology; disease status; non-Hodgkin's lymphoma, limited to follicular lymphoma, mantle cell lymphoma, diffuse large B-cell lymphoma, peripheral T cell lymphoma or small lymphocytic lymphoma; stage I, II at diagnosis, not relapsed and not refractory, (for use in a Medicare-approved demonstration project)

Special Coverage Instructions   Noncovered by Medicare   Carrier Discretion   ☑ Quantity Alert   ● New Code   ○ Reinstated Code   ▲ Revised Code

2006 HCPCS   **1**-**9** ASC Groups   MED: Pub 100/NCD Reference   ⅃ DMEPOS Paid   ⊘ SNF Excluded   **G Codes — 71**

Procedures/Professional Services (Temporary)

G9122 — G9130

●   **G9122** Oncology; disease status; non-Hodgkin's lymphoma, limited to follicular lymphoma, mantle cell lymphoma, diffuse large B-cell lymphoma, peripheral T cell lymphoma or small lymphocytic lymphoma; stage III, IV at diagnosis, not relapsed and not refractory (for use in a Medicare-approved demonstration project)

●   **G9123** Oncology; disease status; non-Hodgkin's lymphoma, limited to follicular lymphoma, mantle cell lymphoma, diffuse large B-cell lymphoma, or histologically transformed from follicular lymphoma to diffuse large B-cell lymphoma; relapsed or refractory (for use in a Medicare-approved demonstration project)

●   **G9124** Oncology; disease status; non-Hodgkin's lymphoma, limited to follicular lymphoma, mantle cell lymphoma, diffuse large B-cell lymphoma, peripheral T cell lymphoma or small lympocytic lymphoma; relapsed and refractory (for use in a Medicare-approved demonstration project)

●   **G9125** Oncology; disease status; non-Hodgkin's lymphoma, limited to follicular lymphoma, mantle cell lymphoma, diffuse large B-cell lymphoma, peripheral T cell lymphoma or small lymphocytic lymphoma; diagnostic evaluation, stage not determined, evaluation of possible relapse or non-response to therapy, or not listed (for use in a Medicare-approved demonstration project)

●   **G9126** Oncology; disease status; ovarian cancer, limited to pathologically stage patients with epithelial cancer; stage 1A/1B (for use in a Medicare-approved demonstration project)

●   **G9127** Oncology; disease status; limited to multiple myeloma, systemic disease; smoldering, stage I (for use in a Medicare-approved demonstration project)

●   **G9128** Oncology; disease status; limited to multiple myeloma, systemic disease; stage II or higher (for use in a Medicare-approved demonstration project)

●   **G9129** Oncology; disease status; chronic myelogenous leukemia, limited to Philadelphia chromosome positive and/or Bcr-Abl positive; extent of disease unknown, under evaluation, not listed, or treatment options being considered (for use in a Medicare-approved demonstration project)

●   **G9130** Oncology; disease status; limited to multiple myeloma, systemic disease; extent of disease unknown, under evaluation, or not listed (for use in a Medicare-approved demonstration project)

Special Coverage Instructions   Noncovered by Medicare   Carrier Discretion   ☑ Quantity Alert   ● New Code   ○ Reinstated Code   ▲ Revised Code

72 — G Codes   Ⓐ Age   Ⓜ Maternity   ♀ Female Only   ♂ Male Only   Ⓐ-Ⓨ APC Status Indicator   *2006 HCPCS*

ALCOHOL AND DRUG ABUSE TREATMENT SERVICES
H0001–H2037

The H codes are used by those state Medicaid agencies that are mandated by state law to establish separate codes for identifying mental health services that include alcohol and drug treatment services.

E   **H0001** Alcohol and/or drug assessment

E   **H0002** Behavioral health screening to determine eligibility for admission to treatment program

E   **H0003** Alcohol and/or drug screening; laboratory analysis of specimens for presence of alcohol and/or drugs

E   **H0004** Behavioral health counseling and therapy, per 15 minutes

E   **H0005** Alcohol and/or drug services; group counseling by a clinician

E   **H0006** Alcohol and/or drug services; case management

E   **H0007** Alcohol and/or drug services; crisis intervention (outpatient)

E   **H0008** Alcohol and/or drug services; sub-acute detoxification (hospital inpatient)

E   **H0009** Alcohol and/or drug services; acute detoxification (hospital inpatient)

E   **H0010** Alcohol and/or drug services; sub-acute detoxification (residential addiction program inpatient)

E   **H0011** Alcohol and/or drug services; acute detoxification (residential addiction program inpatient)

E   **H0012** Alcohol and/or drug services; sub-acute detoxification (residential addiction program outpatient)

E   **H0013** Alcohol and/or drug services; acute detoxification (residential addiction program outpatient)

E   **H0014** Alcohol and/or drug services; ambulatory detoxification

E   **H0015** Alcohol and/or drug services; intensive outpatient (treatment program that operates at least 3 hours/day and at least 3 days/week and is based on an individualized treatment plan), including assessment, counseling; crisis intervention, and activity therapies or education

E   **H0016** Alcohol and/or drug services; medical/somatic (medical intervention in ambulatory setting)

E   **H0017** Behavioral health; residential (hospital residential treatment program), without room and board, per diem

E   **H0018** Behavioral health; short-term residential (non-hospital residential treatment program), without room and board, per diem

E   **H0019** Behavioral health; long-term residential (non-medial, non-acute care in a residential treatment program where stay is typically longer than 30 days), without room and board, per diem

E   **H0020** Alcohol and/or drug services; methadone administration and/or service (provision of the drug by a licensed program)

E   **H0021** Alcohol and/or drug training service (for staff and personnel not employed by providers)

E   **H0022** Alcohol and/or drug intervention service (planned facilitation)

E   **H0023** Behavioral health outreach service (planned approach to reach a targeted population)

E   **H0024** Behavioral health prevention information dissemination service (one-way direct or non-direct contact with service audiences to affect knowledge and attitude)

E   **H0025** Behavioral health prevention education service (delivery of services with target population to affect knowledge, attitude and/or behavior)

E   **H0026** Alcohol and/or drug prevention process service, community-based (delivery of services to develop skills of impactors)

E   **H0027** Alcohol and/or drug prevention environmental service (broad range of external activities geared toward modifying systems in order to mainstream prevention through policy and law)

E   **H0028** Alcohol and/or drug prevention problem identification and referral service (e.g., student assistance and employee assistance programs), does not include assessment

E   **H0029** Alcohol and/or drug prevention alternatives service (services for populations that exclude alcohol and other drug use e.g., alcohol free social events)

E   **H0030** Behavioral health hotline service

E   **H0031** Mental health assessment, by nonphysician

E   **H0032** Mental health service plan development by nonphysician

E   **H0033** Oral medication administration, direct observation

E   **H0034** Medication training and support, per 15 minutes

E   **H0035** Mental health partial hospitalization, treatment, less than 24 hours

E   **H0036** Community psychiatric supportive treatment, face-to-face, per 15 minutes

E   **H0037** Community psychiatric supportive treatment program, per diem

E   **H0038** Self-help/peer services, per 15 minutes

E   **H0039** Assertive community treatment, face-to-face, per 15 minutes

E   **H0040** Assertive community treatment program, per diem

E   **H0041** Foster care, child, non-therapeutic, per diem   A

E   **H0042** Foster care, child, non-therapeutic, per month   A

E   **H0043** Supported housing, per diem

E   **H0044** Supported housing, per month

E   **H0045** Respite care services, not in the home, per diem

E   **H0046** Mental health services, not otherwise specified

E   **H0047** Alcohol and/or other drug abuse services, not otherwise specified

E   **H0048** Alcohol and/or other drug testing: collection and handling only, specimens other than blood

E   **H1000** Prenatal care, at-risk assessment   M ♀

E   **H1001** Prenatal care, at-risk enhanced service; antepartum management   M ♀

E   **H1002** Prenatal care, at risk enhanced service; care coordination   M ♀

E   **H1003** Prenatal care, at-risk enhanced service; education   M ♀

E   **H1004** Prenatal care, at-risk enhanced service; follow-up home visit   M ♀

E   **H1005** Prenatal care, at-risk enhanced service package (includes H1001-H1004)   M ♀

E   **H1010** Non-medical family planning education, per session

Special Coverage Instructions   Noncovered by Medicare   Carrier Discretion   ☑ Quantity Alert   ● New Code   ○ Reinstated Code   ▲ Revised Code

2006 HCPCS   1-9 ASC Groups   **MED:** Pub 100/NCD Reference   ఋ DMEPOS Paid   ⊘ SNF Excluded   **H Codes — 73**

Alcohol and Drug Abuse Treatment Services   H0001 — H1010

Alcohol and Drug Abuse Treatment Services

H1011 — H2037

- E   **H1011** Family assessment by licensed behavioral health professional for state defined purposes
- E   **H2000** Comprehensive multidisciplinary evaluation
- E   **H2001** Rehabilitation program, per 1/2 day
- E   **H2010** Comprehensive medication services, per 15 minutes
- E   **H2011** Crisis intervention service, per 15 minutes
- E   **H2012** Behavioral health day treatment, per hour
- E   **H2013** Psychiatric health facility service, per diem
- E   **H2014** Skills training and development, per 15 minutes
- E   **H2015** Comprehensive community support services, per 15 minutes
- E   **H2016** Comprehensive community support services, per diem
- E   **H2017** Psychosocial rehabilitation services, per 15 minutes
- E   **H2018** Psychosocial rehabilitation services, per diem
-    **H2019** Therapeutic behavioral services, per 15 minutes
- E   **H2020** Therapeutic behavioral services, per diem
- E   **H2021** Community-based wrap-around services, per 15 minutes
- E   **H2022** Community-based wrap-around services, per diem

- E   **H2023** Supported employment, per 15 minutes
- E   **H2024** Supported employment, per diem
- E   **H2025** Ongoing support to maintain employment, per 15 minutes
- E   **H2026** Ongoing support to maintain employment, per diem
- E   **H2027** Psychoeducational service, per 15 minutes
- E   **H2028** Sexual offender treatment service, per 15 minutes
- E   **H2029** Sexual offender treatment service, per diem
- E   **H2030** Mental health clubhouse services, per 15 minutes
- E   **H2031** Mental health clubhouse services, per diem
- E   **H2032** Activity therapy, per 15 minutes
- E   **H2033** Multisystemic therapy for juveniles, per 15 minutes
- E   **H2034** Alcohol and/or drug abuse halfway house services, per diem
- E   **H2035** Alcohol and/or other drug treatment program, per hour
- E   **H2036** Alcohol and/or other drug treatment program, per diem
- E   **H2037** Developmental delay prevention activities, dependent child of client, per 15 minutes   A

Special Coverage Instructions   Noncovered by Medicare   Carrier Discretion   ☑ Quantity Alert   ● New Code   ○ Reinstated Code   ▲ Revised Code

74 — H Codes   A Age   M Maternity   ♀ Female Only   ♂ Male Only   A-Y APC Status Indicator   *2006 HCPCS*

DRUGS ADMINISTERED OTHER THAN ORAL METHOD
J0000-J9999

J codes include drugs that ordinarily cannot be self-administered, chemotherapy drugs, immunosuppressive drugs, inhalation solutions, and other miscellaneous drugs and solutions.

EXCEPTION: ORAL IMMUNOSUPPRESSIVE DRUGS

J codes fall under the jurisdiction of the DME Regional office for Medicare, unless incidental or otherwise noted.

Ⓝ ☑ **J0120** Injection, tetracycline, up to 250 mg ⊘
MED: 100-2, 15, 50

Ⓖ ☑ **J0128** Injection, abarelix, 10 mg
Use this code for Plenaxis.

Ⓚ ☑ **J0130** Injection abciximab, 10 mg ⊘
Use this code for ReoPro.
MED: 100-2, 15, 50

● Ⓚ **J0132** Injection, acetylcysteine, 100 mg
Use this code for Acetadote.

● Ⓝ **J0133** Injection, acyclovir, 5 mg
Use this code for Zovirax.

Ⓚ ☑ **J0135** Injection, adalimumab, 20 mg
Use this code for Humira.

Ⓚ ☑ **J0150** Injection, adenosine for therapeutic use, 6 mg (not to be used to report any adenosine phosphate compounds, instead use A9270)
Use this code for Adenocard, Adenoscan.
MED: 100-2, 15, 50
AHA: 2Q, '02, 10

Ⓝ ☑ **J0152** Injection, adenosine for diagnostic use, 30 mg (not to be used to report any adenosine phosphate compounds; instead use A9270) ⊘

Ⓝ ☑ **J0170** Injection, adrenalin, epinephrine, up to 1 ml ampule ⊘
Use this code for Adrenalin Chloride, Epipen, Sus-Phrine.
MED: 100-2, 15, 50

Ⓚ ☑ **J0180** Injection, agalsidase beta, 1 mg
Use this code for Fabrazyme.

Ⓝ ☑ **J0190** Injection, biperiden lactate, per 5 mg ⊘
MED: 100-2, 15, 50

Ⓝ **J0200** Injection, alatrofloxacin mesylate, 100 mg ⊘
Use this code for Trovan IV.
MED: 100-2, 15, 50.5

Ⓚ ☑ **J0205** Injection, alglucerase, per 10 units ⊘
Use this code for Ceredase.
MED: 100-2, 15, 50

Ⓚ ☑ **J0207** Injection, amifostine, 500 mg ⊘
Use this code for Ethyol.
MED: 100-2, 15, 50

Ⓝ ☑ **J0210** Injection, methyldopate HCl, up to 250 mg ⊘
Use this code for Aldomet.
MED: 100-2, 15, 50

Ⓑ ☑ **J0215** Injection, alefacept, 0.5 mg ⊘
Use this for Amevive.

Ⓚ ☑ **J0256** Injection, alpha 1-proteinase inhibitor — human, 10 mg ⊘
Use this code for Prolastin, Zemira.
MED: 100-2, 15, 50

Ⓑ ☑ **J0270** Injection, alprostadil, 1.25 mcg (code may be used for Medicare when drug administered under direct supervision of a physician, not for use when drug is self-administered) ⊘
Use this code for Alprostadil, Caverject, Edex, Prostin VR Pediatric.
MED: 100-2, 15, 50

Ⓑ **J0275** Alprostadil urethral suppository (code may be used for Medicare when drug administered under direct supervision of a physician, not for use when drug is self-administered) ⊘
Use this code for Muse.
MED: 100-2, 15, 50

● Ⓚ **J0278** Injection, amikacin sulfate, 100 mg
Use this code for Amikin.

Ⓝ ☑ **J0280** Injection, aminophyllin, up to 250 mg ⊘
MED: 100-2, 15, 50

Ⓝ ☑ **J0282** Injection, amiodarone HCl, 30 mg ⊘
Use this code for Cordarone IV.
MED: 100-2, 15, 50

Ⓝ ☑ **J0285** Injection, amphotericin B, 50 mg ⊘
Use this for Abelcent, Amphocin, Fungizonef.
MED: 100-2, 15, 50

Ⓚ **J0287** Injection, amphotericin B lipid complex, 10 mg
MED: 100-2, 15, 50

Ⓚ **J0288** Injection, amphotericin B cholesteryl sulfate complex, 10 mg
Use this code for Amphotec.
MED: 100-2, 15, 50

Ⓚ **J0289** Injection, amphotericin B liposome, 10 mg
Use this code for Ambisome.
MED: 100-2, 15, 50

Ⓝ ☑ **J0290** Injection, ampicillin sodium, 500 mg ⊘
MED: 100-2, 15, 50

Ⓝ ☑ **J0295** Injection, ampicillin sodium/sulbactam sodium, per 1.5 g ⊘
Use this code for Unasyn.
MED: 100-2, 15, 50

Ⓝ ☑ **J0300** Injection, amobarbital, up to 125 mg ⊘
Use this code for Amytal.
MED: 100-2, 15, 50

Ⓝ ☑ **J0330** Injection, succinylcholine chloride, up to 20 mg ⊘
Use this code for Anectine, Quelicin.
MED: 100-2, 15, 50

Ⓚ ☑ **J0350** Injection, anistreplase, per 30 units ⊘
Use this code for Eminase.
MED: 100-2, 15, 50

Ⓝ ☑ **J0360** Injection, hydralazine HCl, up to 20 mg ⊘
MED: 100-2, 15, 50

● Ⓚ **J0365** Injection, aprotonin, 10,000 kiu
Use this code for Trasylol.
MED: 100-2, 15, 50

Ⓝ ☑ **J0380** Injection, metaraminol bitartrate, per 10 mg ⊘
Use this code for Aramine.
MED: 100-2, 15, 50

Ⓝ ☑ **J0390** Injection, chloroquine HCl, up to 250 mg ⊘
Use this code for Aralen.
MED: 100-2, 15, 50

N ☑ **J0395** Injection, arbutamine HCl, 1 mg ⊘
MED: 100-2, 15, 50

N ☑ **J0456** Injection, azithromycin, 500 mg ⊘
Use this code for Zithromax.
MED: 100-2, 15, 50.5

N ☑ **J0460** Injection, atropine sulfate, up to 0.3 mg ⊘
Use this code for Atropen.
MED: 100-2, 15, 50

N ☑ **J0470** Injection, dimercaprol, per 100 mg ⊘
Use this code for BAL in oil.
MED: 100-2, 15, 50

N ☑ **J0475** Injection, baclofen, 10 mg ⊘
Use this code for Lioresal.
MED: 100-2, 15, 50

B ☑ **J0476** Injection, baclofen, 50 mcg for intrathecal trial ⊘
Use this code for Lioresal for intrathecal trial.
MED: 100-2, 15, 50

● K **J0480** Injection, basiliximab, 20 mg
Use this code for Simulect.

N ☑ **J0500** Injection, dicyclomine HCl, up to 20 mg ⊘
Use this code for Bentyl.
MED: 100-2, 15, 50

N ☑ **J0515** Injection, benztropine mesylate, per 1 mg ⊘
Use this code for Cogentin.
MED: 100-2, 15, 50

N ☑ **J0520** Injection, bethanechol chloride, Mytonachol or Urecholine, up to 5 mg ⊘
MED: 100-2, 15, 50

N ☑ **J0530** Injection, penicillin G benzathine and penicillin G procaine, up to 600,000 units ⊘
Use this code for Bicillin C-R.
MED: 100-2, 15, 50

N ☑ **J0540** Injection, penicillin G benzathine and penicillin G procaine, up to 1,200,000 units ⊘
Use this code for Bicillin C-R, Bicillin C-R 900/300.
MED: 100-2, 15, 50

N ☑ **J0550** Injection, penicillin G benzathine and penicillin G procaine, up to 2,400,000 units ⊘
Use this code for Bicillin C-R.
MED: 100-2, 15, 50

N ☑ **J0560** Injection, penicillin G benzathine, up to 600,000 units ⊘
Use this code for Bicillin L-A, Permapen.
MED: 100-2, 15, 50

N ☑ **J0570** Injection, penicillin G benzathine, up to 1,200,000 units ⊘
Use this code for Bicillin L-A, Permapen.
MED: 100-2, 15, 50

N ☑ **J0580** Injection, penicillin G benzathine, up to 2,400,000 units ⊘
Use this code for Bicillin L-A, Permapen.
MED: 100-2, 15, 50

G ☑ **J0583** Injection, bivalirudin, 1 mg ⊘
Use this code for Angiomax.

K ☑ **J0585** Botulinum toxin type A, per unit ⊘
Use this code for Botox.
MED: 100-2, 15, 50

K ☑ **J0587** Botulinum toxin type B, per 100 units ⊘
Use this code for Myobloc.
MED: 100-2, 15, 50
AHA: 2Q, '02, 8

N **J0592** Injection, buprenorphine hydrochloride, 0.1 mg
Use this code for Buprenix.
MED: 100-2, 15, 50

N ☑ **J0595** Injection, butorphanol tartrate, 1 mg ⊘
Use this code for Stadol.

N ☑ **J0600** Injection, edetate calcium disodium, up to 1000 mg ⊘
Use this code for Calcium Disodium Versenate, Calcium EDTA.
MED: 100-2, 15, 50

N ☑ **J0610** Injection, calcium gluconate, per 10 ml ⊘
MED: 100-2, 15, 50

N ☑ **J0620** Injection, calcium glycerophosphate and calcium lactate, per 10 ml ⊘
MED: 100-2, 15, 50

N ☑ **J0630** Injection, calcitonin-salmon, up to 400 units ⊘
Use this code for Calcimar, Miacalcin.
MED: 100-2, 15, 50

N **J0636** Injection, calcitriol, 0.1 mcg
Use this code for Calcijex.
MED: 100-2, 15, 50

K **J0637** Injection, caspofungin acetate, 5 mg
Use this code for Cancidas.

N ☑ **J0640** Injection, leucovorin calcium, per 50 mg ⊘
MED: 100-2, 15, 50

N ☑ **J0670** Injection, mepivacaine HCl, per 10 ml ⊘
Use this code for Carbocaine, Polocaine, Isocaine HCl.
MED: 100-2, 15, 50

N ☑ **J0690** Injection, cefazolin sodium, 500 mg ⊘
Use this code for Ancef, Kefzol.
MED: 100-2, 15, 50

N **J0692** Injection, cefepime HCl, 500 mg ⊘
Use this code for Maxipime.

N ☑ **J0694** Injection, cefoxitin sodium, 1 g ⊘
Use this code for Mefoxin.
MED: 100-2, 15, 50
See code(s): Q0090

N ☑ **J0696** Injection, ceftriaxone sodium, per 250 mg ⊘
Use this code for Rocephin.
MED: 100-2, 15, 50

N ☑ **J0697** Injection, sterile cefuroxime sodium, per 750 mg ⊘
MED: 100-2, 15, 50

N ☑ **J0698** Cefotaxime sodium, per g ⊘
Use this code for Claforan.
MED: 100-2, 15, 50

N ☑ **J0702** Injection, betamethasone acetate and betamethasone sodium phosphate, per 3 mg ⊘
Use this code for Celestone Soluspan.
MED: 100-2, 15, 50

N ☑ **J0704** Injection, betamethasone sodium phosphate, per 4 mg ⊘
Use this code for Adbeon.
MED: 100-2, 15, 50

─── Special Coverage Instructions   ─── Noncovered by Medicare   ─── Carrier Discretion   ☑ Quantity Alert   ● New Code   ○ Reinstated Code   ▲ Revised Code

76 — J Codes   A Age   M Maternity   ♀ Female Only   ♂ Male Only   A-Y APC Status Indicator   *2006 HCPCS*

N | | **J0706** | Injection, caffeine citrate, 5 mg ⊘
Use this code for Cafcit.

AHA: 2Q, '02, 8

N ☑ | **J0710** | Injection, cephapirin sodium, up to 1 g ⊘
MED: 100-2, 15, 50

N ☑ | **J0713** | Injection, ceftazidime, per 500 mg ⊘
Use this code for Ceptaz, Fortaz, Tazicef.
MED: 100-2, 15, 50

N ☑ | **J0715** | Injection, ceftizoxime sodium, per 500 mg ⊘
Use this code for Cefizox.
MED: 100-2, 15, 50

N ☑ | **J0720** | Injection, chloramphenicol sodium succinate, up to 1 g ⊘
Use this code for Chloromycetin.
MED: 100-2, 15, 50

N ☑ | **J0725** | Injection, chorionic gonadotropin, per 1,000 USP units ⊘
Use this code for Corgonject-5, Novarel, Pregnyl.
MED: 100-2, 15, 50

N ☑ | **J0735** | Injection, clonidine HCl, 1 mg ⊘
Use this code for Catapres, Duraclon.
MED: 100-2, 15, 50

N ☑ | **J0740** | Injection, cidofovir, 375 mg ⊘
Use this code for Vistide.
MED: 100-2, 15, 50

N ☑ | **J0743** | Injection, cilastatin sodium imipenem, per 250 mg ⊘
Use this code for Primaxin I.M., Primaxin I.V.
MED: 100-2, 15, 50

N | **J0744** | Injection, ciprofloxacin for intravenous infusion, 200 mg ⊘
Use this code for Cipro.

N ☑ | **J0745** | Injection, codeine phosphate, per 30 mg ⊘
MED: 100-2, 15, 50

N ☑ | **J0760** | Injection, colchicine, per 1 mg ⊘
MED: 100-2, 15, 50

N ☑ | **J0770** | Injection, colistimethate sodium, up to 150 mg ⊘
Use this code for Coly-Mycin M.
MED: 100-2, 15, 50

N ☑ | **J0780** | Injection, prochlorperazine, up to 10 mg ⊘
Use this code for Compazine, Cotranzine, Compa-Z, Ultrazine-10.
MED: 100-2, 15, 50

● **K** | **J0795** | Injection, corticorelin ovine triflutate, 1 mcg
MED: 100-2, 15, 50

N ☑ | **J0800** | Injection, corticotropin, up to 40 units ⊘
Use this code for H.P. Acthar.
MED: 100-2, 15, 50

N ☑ | **J0835** | Injection, cosyntropin, per 0.25 mg ⊘
Use this code for Cortrosyn.
MED: 100-2, 15, 50

K ☑ | **J0850** | Injection, cytomegalovirus immune globulin intravenous (human), per vial ⊘
Use this code for Cytogam.
MED: 100-2, 15, 50

G ☑ | **J0878** | Injection, daptomycin, 1 mg
Use this code for Cubicin.

~~J0880 Injection, darbepoetin alfa, 5 mcg~~
See code(s) J0881, J0882.

● **K** | **J0881** | Injection, darbepoetin alfa, 1 mcg (non-ESRD use)
Use this code for Aranesp.
MED: 100-4, 8, 60.4.2

● **B** | **J0882** | Injection, darbepoetin alfa, 1 mcg (for ESRD on dialysis)
Use this code for Aranesp.
MED: 100-4, 8, 60.4.2

● **K** | **J0885** | Injection, epoetin alfa, (for non-ESRD use), 1000 units
Use this code for Epogen, Procrit.
MED: 100-2, 15, 50

● **B** | **J0886** | Injection, epoetin alfa, 1000 units (for ESRD on dialysis)
Use this code for Epogen, Procrit.
MED: 100-4, 8, 60.4.2

N ☑ | **J0895** | Injection, deferoxamine mesylate, 500 mg ⊘
Use this code for Desferal.
MED: 100-2, 15, 50
See code(s): Q0087

N ☑ | **J0900** | Injection, testosterone enanthate and estradiol valerate, up to 1 cc ⊘
Use this code for Deladumone, Andrest 90-4, Andro-Estro 90-4, Androgyn L.A., Delatestadiol, Dua-Gen L.A., Duoval P.A., Estra-Testrin, TEEV, Testadiate, Testradiol 90/4, Valertest No. 1, Valertest No. 2, Deladumone OB, Ditate-DS.
MED: 100-2, 15, 50

N ☑ | **J0945** | Injection, brompheniramine maleate, per 10 mg ⊘
Use this code for Histaject, Cophene-B, Dehist, Nasahist B, ND Stat, Oraminic II, Sinusol-B.
MED: 100-2, 15, 50

N ☑ | **J0970** | Injection, estradiol valerate, up to 40 mg ⊘
Use this code for Clinagen LA, Delestrogen, Gynogen L.A. 10, Gynogen L.A. 20, Gynogen L.A. 40.
MED: 100-2, 15, 50

N ☑ | **J1000** | Injection, depo-estradiol cypionate, up to 5 mg ⊘
Use this code for Estradiol Cypionate, depGynogen, Depogen.
MED: 100-2, 15, 50

N ☑ | **J1020** | Injection, methylprednisolone acetate, 20 mg ⊘
Use this code for Depo-Medrol.
MED: 100-2, 15, 50

N ☑ | **J1030** | Injection, methylprednisolone acetate, 40 mg ⊘
Use this code for Depo-Medrol, depMedalone 40, Sano-Drol.
MED: 100-2, 15, 50

N ☑ | **J1040** | Injection, methylprednisolone acetate, 80 mg ⊘
Use this code for Cortimed, Depmedalone, Depo-Medrol, depMedalone 80, Duro Cort, Methylcotolone, Pri-Methylate, Sano-Drol.
MED: 100-2, 15, 50

N | **J1051** | Injection, medroxyprogesterone acetate, 50 mg
Use this code for Depo-Provera.
MED: 100-2, 15, 50

E ☑ | **J1055** | Injection, medroxyprogesterone acetate for contraceptive use, 150 mg ♀ ⊘
Use this code for Depo-Provera.

E | **J1056** | Injection, medroxyprogesterone acetate/estradiol cypionate, 5 mg/25 mg ♀ ⊘
Use this code for Lunelle monthly contraceptive.

Drugs Administered Other Than Oral Method

J1060 — J1430

N ☑ **J1060** Injection, testosterone cypionate and estradiol cypionate, up to 1 ml ⊘
Use this code for Depo-Testadiol, Duo-Span, Duo-Span II.
MED: 100-2, 15, 50

N ☑ **J1070** Injection, testosterone cypionate, up to 100 mg ⊘
Use this code for depAndro 100, Depo Testosterone Cypionate, Deptestrogen.
MED: 100-2, 15, 50

N ☑ **J1080** Injection, testosterone cypionate, 1 cc, 200 mg ⊘
Use this code for Depandrante, Depo-Testosterone, Virilon.
MED: 100-2, 15, 50

N **J1094** Injection, dexamethasone acetate, 1 mg
Use this code for Cortastat LA, Dalalone L.A., Decadron LA, Dexamethasone Acetate Anhydrous, Dexone LA.
MED: 100-2, 15, 50

N **J1100** Injection, dexamethasone sodium phosphate, 1 mg ⊘
Use this code for Cortastat, Dalalone, Decadron Phosphate.
MED: 100-2, 15, 50

N ☑ **J1110** Injection, dihydroergotamine mesylate, per 1 mg ⊘
Use this code for D.H.E. 45.
MED: 100-2, 15, 50

N ☑ **J1120** Injection, acetazolamide sodium, up to 500 mg ⊘
Use this code for Diamox.
MED: 100-2, 15, 50

N ☑ **J1160** Injection, digoxin, up to 0.5 mg ⊘
Use this code for Lanoxin.
MED: 100-2, 15, 50

● K **J1162** Injection, digoxin immune fab (ovine), per vial
Use this code for Digibind, Digifab.
MED: 100-2, 15, 50

N ☑ **J1165** Injection, phenytoin sodium, per 50 mg ⊘
Use this code for Dilantin.
MED: 100-2, 15, 50

N ☑ **J1170** Injection, hydromorphone, up to 4 mg ⊘
Use this code for Dilaudid, Dilaudid-HP.
MED: 100-2, 15, 50

N ☑ **J1180** Injection, dyphylline, up to 500 mg ⊘
Use this code for Lufyllin, Dilor.
MED: 100-2, 15, 50

K ☑ **J1190** Injection, dexrazoxane HCl, per 250 mg ⊘
Use this code for Zinecard.
MED: 100-2, 15, 50

N ☑ **J1200** Injection, diphenhydramine HCl, up to 50 mg ⊘
Use this code for Benadryl, Benahist 10, Benahist 50, Benoject-10, Benoject-50, Bena-D 10, Bena-D 50, Nordryl, Dihydrex, Dimine, Diphenacen-50, Hyrexin-50, Truxadryl, Wehdryl.
MED: 100-2, 15, 50
AHA: 1Q, '02, 2

N ☑ **J1205** Injection, chlorothiazide sodium, per 500 mg ⊘
Use this code for Diuril Sodium.
MED: 100-2, 15, 50

N ☑ **J1212** Injection, DMSO, dimethyl sulfoxide, 50%, 50 ml ⊘
Use this code for Rimso. DMSO is covered only as a treatment of interstitial cystitis.
MED: 100-2, 15, 50; 100-3, 230.12

N ☑ **J1230** Injection, methadone HCl, up to 10 mg ⊘
Use this code for Dolophine HCl.
MED: 100-2, 15, 50

N ☑ **J1240** Injection, dimenhydrinate, up to 50 mg ⊘
Use this code for Dramamine, Dinate, Dommanate, Dramanate, Dramilin, Dramocen, Dramoject, Dymenate, Hydrate, Marmine, Wehamine.

K ☑ **J1245** Injection, dipyridamole, per 10 mg ⊘
Use this code for Persantine IV.
MED: 100-2, 15, 50

N ☑ **J1250** Injection, dobutamine HCl, per 250 mg ⊘
Use this code for Dobutrex.
MED: 100-2, 15, 50

N ☑ **J1260** Injection, dolasetron mesylate, 10 mg ⊘
Use this code for Anzemet.
MED: 100-2, 15, 50

● N **J1265** Injection, dopamine HCl, 40 mg
Use this code for Intropin.

N **J1270** Injection, doxercalciferol, 1 mcg ⊘
Use this code for Hectorol.

N ☑ **J1320** Injection, amitriptyline HCl, up to 20 mg ⊘
Use this code for Elavil, Enovil, Tryptanol.
MED: 100-2, 15, 50

N ☑ **J1325** Injection, epoprostenol, 0.5 mg ⊘
Use this code for Flolan. See K0455 for infusion pump for epoprosterol.
MED: 100-2, 15, 50

K ☑ **J1327** Injection, eptifibatide, 5 mg ⊘
Use this code for Integrilin.
MED: 100-2, 15, 50

N ☑ **J1330** Injection, ergonovine maleate, up to 0.2 mg ⊘
Medicare jurisdiction: local contractor. Use this code for Ergotrate Maleate.
MED: 100-2, 15, 50

G ☑ **J1335** Injection, ertapenem sodium, 500 mg ⊘
Use this code for Invanz.

N ☑ **J1364** Injection, erythromycin lactobionate, per 500 mg ⊘
MED: 100-2, 15, 50

N ☑ **J1380** Injection, estradiol valerate, up to 10 mg ⊘
Use this code for Delestrogen, Dioval, Dioval XX, Dioval 40, Duragen-10, Duragen-20, Duragen-40, Estradiol L.A., Estradiol L.A. 20, Estradiol L.A. 40, Gynogen L.A. 10, Gynogen L.A. 20, Gynogen L.A. 40, Valergen 10, Valergen 20, Valergen 40, Estra-L 20, Estra-L 40, L.A.E. 20.
MED: 100-2, 15, 50

N ☑ **J1390** Injection, estradiol valerate, up to 20 mg ⊘
Use this code for Delestrogen, Dioval, Dioval XX, Dioval 40, Duragen-10, Duragen-20, Duragen-40, Estradiol L.A., Estradiol L.A. 20, Estradiol L.A. 40, Gynogen L.A. 10, Gynogen L.A. 20, Gynogen L.A. 40, Valergen 10, Valergen 20, Valergen 40, Estra-L 20, Estra-L 40, L.A.E. 20.
MED: 100-2, 15, 50

N ☑ **J1410** Injection, estrogen conjugated, per 25 mg ⊘
Use this code for Natural Estrogenic Substance, Premarin Intravenous, Primestrin Aqueous.
MED: 100-2, 15, 50

● K **J1430** Injection, ethanolamine oleate, 100 mg
Use this code for Ethamolin.

Special Coverage Instructions Noncovered by Medicare Carrier Discretion ☑ Quantity Alert ● New Code ○ Reinstated Code ▲ Revised Code
Ａ Age Ｍ Maternity ♀ Female Only ♂ Male Only Ａ-Ｙ APC Status Indicator

N ☑ **J1435** Injection, estrone, per 1 mg ⊘
Use this code for Estone Aqueous, Estragyn, Estro-A, Estrone, Estronol, Theelin Aqueous, Estone 5, Kestrone 5.
MED: 100-2, 15, 50

N ☑ **J1436** Injection, etidronate disodium, per 300 mg ⊘
Use this code for Didronel.
MED: 100-2, 15, 50

K ☑ **J1438** Injection, etanercept, 25 mg (code may be used for Medicare when drug administered under the direct supervision of a physician, not for use when drug is self-administered) ⊘
Use this code for Enbrel.
MED: 100-2, 15, 50

K ☑ **J1440** Injection, filgrastim (G-CSF), 300 mcg ⊘
Use this code for Neupogen.
MED: 100-2, 15, 50

K ☑ **J1441** Injection, filgrastim (G-CSF), 480 mcg ⊘
Use this code for Neupogen.
MED: 100-2, 15, 50

N ☑ **J1450** Injection, fluconazole, 200 mg ⊘
Use this code for Diflucan.
MED: 100-2, 15, 50.5

● K **J1451** Injection, fomepizole, 15 mg ⊘
Use this code for Antizol.
MED: 100-2, 15, 50

N ☑ **J1452** Injection, fomivirsen sodium, intraocular, 1.65 mg ⊘
Use this code for Vitavene.
MED: 100-2, 15, 50.4; 100-2, 15, 50.4.2

N ☑ **J1455** Injection, foscarnet sodium, per 1,000 mg ⊘
Use this code for Foscavir.
MED: 100-2, 15, 50

☑ **J1457** Injection, gallium nitrate, 1 mg
Use this code for Ganite.

B ☑ **J1460** Injection, gamma globulin, intramuscular, 1 cc ⊘
Use this code for Baygam, Gammar, Gamastan, Flebogamma.
MED: 100-2, 15, 50

B ☑ **J1470** Injection, gamma globulin, intramuscular, 2 cc ⊘
Use this code for Gammar, Gamastan.
MED: 100-2, 15, 50

B ☑ **J1480** Injection, gamma globulin, intramuscular, 3 cc ⊘
Use this code for Gammar, Gamastan.
MED: 100-2, 15, 50

B ☑ **J1490** Injection, gamma globulin, intramuscular, 4 cc ⊘
Use this code for Gammar, Gamastan.
MED: 100-2, 15, 50

B ☑ **J1500** Injection, gamma globulin, intramuscular, 5 cc ⊘
Use this code for Gammar, Gamastan.
MED: 100-2, 15, 50

B ☑ **J1510** Injection, gamma globulin, intramuscular, 6 cc ⊘
Use this code for Gammar, Gamastan.
MED: 100-2, 15, 50

B ☑ **J1520** Injection, gamma globulin, intramuscular, 7 cc ⊘
Use this code for Gammar, Gamastan.
MED: 100-2, 15, 50

B ☑ **J1530** Injection, gamma globulin, intramuscular, 8 cc ⊘
Use this code for Gammar, Gamastan.
MED: 100-2, 15, 50

B ☑ **J1540** Injection, gamma globulin, intramuscular, 9 cc ⊘
Use this code for Gammar, Gamastan.
MED: 100-2, 15, 50

B ☑ **J1550** Injection, gamma globulin, intramuscular, 10 cc ⊘
Use this code for Gammar, Gamastan.
MED: 100-2, 15, 50

B ☑ **J1560** Injection, gamma globulin, intramuscular, over 10 cc ⊘
Use this code for Gammar, Gamastan.
MED: 100-2, 15, 50

~~J1563~~ ~~Injection, immune globulin, intravenous, 1 g~~
See code(s) J1566, J1567.

~~J1564~~ ~~Injection, immune globulin, Intravenous, 10 mg~~
See code(s) J1566, J1567.

K ☑ **J1565** Injection, respiratory syncytial virus immune globulin, intravenous, 50 mg ⊘
Use this code for Respigam.
MED: 100-2, 15, 50

● K **J1566** Injection, immune globulin, intravenous, lyophilized (e.g., powder), 500 mg
MED: 100-2, 15, 50

● K **J1567** Injection, immune globulin, intravenous, non-lyophilized (e.g., liquid), 500 mg
MED: 100-2, 15, 50

K ☑ **J1570** Injection, ganciclovir sodium, 500 mg ⊘
Use this code for Cytovene.
MED: 100-2, 15, 50

N ☑ **J1580** Injection, garamycin, gentamicin, up to 80 mg ⊘
Use this code for Gentamicin Sulfate, Jenamicin.
MED: 100-2, 15, 50

N ☑ **J1590** Injection, gatifloxacin, 10 mg ⊘
Use this code for Tequin.

N ☑ **J1595** Injection, glatiramer acetate, 20 mg ⊘
Use this code for Copaxone.
MED: 100-2, 15, 50

N ☑ **J1600** Injection, gold sodium thiomalate, up to 50 mg ⊘
Use this code for Myochrysine.
MED: 100-2, 15, 50

N ☑ **J1610** Injection, glucagon HCl, per 1 mg ⊘
Use this code for Glucagen.
MED: 100-2, 15, 50

N ☑ **J1620** Injection, gonadorelin HCl, per 100 mcg ⊘
Use this code for Factrel, Lutrepulse.
MED: 100-2, 15, 50

K ☑ **J1626** Injection, granisetron HCl, 100 mcg ⊘
Use this code for Kytril.
MED: 100-2, 15, 50

N ☑ **J1630** Injection, haloperidol, up to 5 mg ⊘
Use this code for Haldol.
MED: 100-2, 15, 50

N ☑ **J1631** Injection, haloperidol decanoate, per 50 mg ⊘
Use this code for Haldol Decanoate-50.
MED: 100-2, 15, 50

● K **J1640** Injection, hemin, 1 mg
Use this code for Panhematin.

Special Coverage Instructions   Noncovered by Medicare   Carrier Discretion   ☑ Quantity Alert   ● New Code   ○ Reinstated Code   ▲ Revised Code

2006 HCPCS   1-9 ASC Groups   MED: Pub 100/NCD Reference   � DMEPOS Paid   ⊘ SNF Excluded   **J Codes — 79**

N ☑ **J1642** Injection, heparin sodium, (heparin lock flush), per 10 units ⊘
Use this code for Hep-Lock, Hep-Lock U/P.
MED: 100-2, 15, 50

N ☑ **J1644** Injection, heparin sodium, per 1,000 units ⊘
Use this code for Heparin Sodium, Liquaemin Sodium.
MED: 100-2, 15, 50

N ☑ **J1645** Injection, dalteparin sodium, per 2500 IU ⊘
Use this code for Fragmin.
MED: 100-2, 15, 50

N ☑ **J1650** Injection, enoxaparin sodium, 10 mg ⊘
Use this code for Lovenox.

N **J1652** Injection, fondaparinux sodium, 0.5 mg ⊘
Use this code for Atrixtra.
MED: 100-2, 15, 50

N ☑ **J1655** Injection, tinzaparin sodium, 1000 IU ⊘
Use this code for Innohep.

N ☑ **J1670** Injection, tetanus immune globulin, human, up to 250 units ⊘
Use this code for Baytet.
MED: 100-2, 15, 50

● B **J1675** Injection, histrelin acetate, 10 mcg
MED: 100-2, 15, 50

N ☑ **J1700** Injection, hydrocortisone acetate, up to 25 mg ⊘
Use this code for Hydrocortone Acetate.
MED: 100-2, 15, 50

N ☑ **J1710** Injection, hydrocortisone sodium phosphate, up to 50 mg ⊘
Use this code for Hydrocortone Phosphate.
MED: 100-2, 15, 50

N ☑ **J1720** Injection, hydrocortisone sodium succinate, up to 100 mg ⊘
Use this code for Solu-Cortef, A-Hydrocort.
MED: 100-2, 15, 50

N ☑ **J1730** Injection, diazoxide, up to 300 mg ⊘
Use this code for Hyperstat IV.
MED: 100-2, 15, 50

N ☑ **J1742** Injection, ibutilide fumarate, 1 mg ⊘
Use this code for Corvert.
MED: 100-2, 15, 50

K ☑ **J1745** Injection, infliximab, 10 mg ⊘
Use this code for Remicade.
MED: 100-2, 15, 50

~~J1750 Injection, iron dextran, 50 mg~~
See code(s) J1751, J1752.

● K **J1751** Injection, iron dextran 165, 50 mg
● K **J1752** Injection, iron dextran 267, 50 mg
N **J1756** Injection, iron sucrose, 1 mg
Use this code for Venofer.

K ☑ **J1785** Injection, imiglucerase, per unit ⊘
Use this code for Cerezyme.
MED: 100-2, 15, 50

N ☑ **J1790** Injection, droperidol, up to 5 mg ⊘
Use this code for Inapsine.
MED: 100-2, 15, 50

N ☑ **J1800** Injection, propranolol HCl, up to 1 mg ⊘
Use this code for Inderal.
MED: 100-2, 15, 50

E ☑ **J1810** Injection, droperidol and fentanyl citrate, up to 2 ml ampule ⊘
Use this code for Innovar.
MED: 100-2, 15, 50
AHA: 2Q, '02, 8

N **J1815** Injection, insulin, per 5 units
Use this code for Humalog, Humulin, Iletin, Insulin Lispo, Novo Nordisk, NPH, Pork insulin, Regular insulin, Ultralente, Velosulin, Humulin R, Iletin II Regular Port, Insulin Purified Pork, Relion, Lente Iletin I, Novolin R, Humulin R U-500.
MED: 100-2, 15, 50; 100-3, 280.14

N **J1817** Insulin for administration through DME (i.e., insulin pump) per 50 units
Use this code for Humalog, Humulin, Vesolin BR, Iletin II NPH Pork, Lantus, Lispro-PFC, Novolin, Novolog, Novolog Flexpen, Novolog Mix, Relion Novolin.

E ☑ **J1825** Injection, interferon beta-1a, 33 mcg ⊘
Use this code for Avonex, Rebif.

K ☑ **J1830** Injection interferon beta-1b, 0.25 mg (code may be used for Medicare when drug administered under direct supervision of a physician, not for use when drug is self-administered) ⊘
Use this code for Actimmune and Betaseron.
MED: 100-2, 15, 50

N ☑ **J1835** Injection, itraconazole, 50 mg ⊘
Use this code for Sporonox IV.

N ☑ **J1840** Injection, kanamycin sulfate, up to 500 mg ⊘
Use this code for Kantrex, Klebcil.
MED: 100-2, 15, 50

N ☑ **J1850** Injection, kanamycin sulfate, up to 75 mg ⊘
Use this code for Kantrex, Klebcil.
MED: 100-2, 15, 50

N ☑ **J1885** Injection, ketorolac tromethamine, per 15 mg ⊘
Use this code for Toradol.
MED: 100-2, 15, 50

N ☑ **J1890** Injection, cephalothin sodium, up to 1 g ⊘
Use this code for Cephalothin Sodium, Keflin.
MED: 100-2, 15, 50

☑ **J1931** Injection, laronidase, 0.1 mg
Use this code for Aldurazyme.

N ☑ **J1940** Injection, furosemide, up to 20 mg ⊘
Use this code for Lasix, Furomide M.D., Furocot.
MED: 100-2, 15, 50

● K **J1945** Injection, lepirudin, 50 mg
Use this code for Refludan.
MED: 100-2, 15, 50

K ☑ **J1950** Injection, leuprolide acetate (for depot suspension), per 3.75 mg ⊘
Use this code for Lupron Depot.
MED: 100-2, 15, 50

B ☑ **J1955** Injection, levocarnitine, per 1 g ⊘
Use this code for Carnitor, L-Carnitine.
MED: 100-2, 15, 50

N ☑ **J1956** Injection, levofloxacin, 250 mg ⊘
Use this code for Levaquin.
MED: 100-2, 15, 50

Special Coverage Instructions　　Noncovered by Medicare　　Carrier Discretion　　☑ Quantity Alert　● New Code　○ Reinstated Code　▲ Revised Code

80 — J Codes　　A Age　　M Maternity　　♀ Female Only　　♂ Male Only　　A-Y APC Status Indicator　　*2006 HCPCS*

N ☑ **J1960** Injection, levorphanol tartrate, up to 2 mg ⊘
Use this code for Levo-Dromoran.
MED: 100-2, 15, 50

N **J1980** Injection, hyoscyamine sulfate, up to 0.25 mg ⊘
Use this code for Levsin.
MED: 100-2, 15, 50

N ☑ **J1990** Injection, chlordiazepoxide HCl, up to 100 mg ⊘
Use this code for Librium.
MED: 100-2, 15, 50

N ☑ **J2001** Injection, lidocaine HCl for intravenous infusion, 10 mg ⊘
Use this code for Xylocaine.
MED: 100-2, 15, 50

N ☑ **J2010** Injection, lincomycin HCl, up to 300 mg ⊘
Use this code for Lincocin, Bactramycin.
MED: 100-2, 15, 50

K ☑ **J2020** Injection, linezolid, 200 mg ⊘
Use this code for Zyvok.
AHA: 2Q, '02, 8

N ☑ **J2060** Injection, lorazepam, 2 mg ⊘
Use this code for Ativan.
MED: 100-2, 15, 50

N ☑ **J2150** Injection, mannitol, 25% in 50 ml ⊘
Use this code for Osmitrol.
MED: 100-2, 15, 50

N ☑ **J2175** Injection, meperidine HCl, per 100 mg ⊘
Use this code for Demerol.
MED: 100-2, 15, 50

N ☑ **J2180** Injection, meperidine and promethazine HCl, up to 50 mg ⊘
Use this code for Mepergan Injection.
MED: 100-2, 15, 50

N ☑ **J2185** Injection, meropenem, 100 mg ⊘

N ☑ **J2210** Injection, methylergonovine maleate, up to 0.2 mg ⊘
Use this code for Methergine.
MED: 100-2, 15, 50

N ☑ **J2250** Injection, midazolam HCl, per 1 mg ⊘
Use this code for Versed.
MED: 100-2, 15, 50

K ☑ **J2260** Injection, milrinone lactate, 5 mg ⊘
Use this code for Primacor.
MED: 100-2, 15, 50

N ☑ **J2270** Injection, morphine sulfate, up to 10 mg ⊘
Use this code for Infumorph.
MED: 100-2, 15, 50

N ☑ **J2271** Injection, morphine sulfate, 100 mg ⊘
Use this code for Infumorph.
MED: 100-2, 15, 50; 100-3, 280.14

N ☑ **J2275** Injection, morphine sulfate (preservative-free sterile solution), per 10 mg ⊘
Use this code for Astramorph PF, Duramorph, Infumorph.
MED: 100-2, 15, 50; 100-3, 280.14

● G **J2278** Injection, ziconotide, 1 mcg

N ☑ **J2280** Injection, moxifloxacin, 100 mg ⊘
Use this code for Avelox.

N ☑ **J2300** Injection, nalbuphine HCl, per 10 mg ⊘
Use this code for Nubain.
MED: 100-2, 15, 50

N ☑ **J2310** Injection, naloxone HCl, per 1 mg ⊘
Use this code for Narcan.
MED: 100-2, 15, 50

N ☑ **J2320** Injection, nandrolone decanoate, up to 50 mg ⊘
Use this code for Deca-Durabolin, Hybolin Decanoate, Decolone-50, Neo-Durabolic, Pri-Andriol LA.
MED: 100-2, 15, 50

N ☑ **J2321** Injection, nandrolone decanoate, up to 100 mg ⊘
Use this code for Deca-Durabolin, Hybolin Decanoate, Decolone-100, Neo-Durabolic, Anabolin LA 100, Androlone-D 100, Nandrobolic L.A.
MED: 100-2, 15, 50

N ☑ **J2322** Injection, nandrolone decanoate, up to 200 mg ⊘
Use this code for Deca-Durabolin, Neo-Durabolic.
MED: 100-2, 15, 50

~~**J2324** Injection, nesiritide, 0.25 mg~~
See code(s) J2325.

● K **J2325** Injection, nesiritide, 0.1 mg
Use this code for Natrecor.
MED: 100-2, 15, 50

K ☑ **J2353** Injection, octreotide, depot form for intramuscular injection, 1 mg ⊘
Use this code for Sandostatin LAR.

K ☑ **J2354** Injection, octreotide, non-depot form for subcutaneous or intravenous injection, 25 mcg ⊘
Use this code for Sandostatin.

K ☑ **J2355** Injection, oprelvekin, 5 mg ⊘
Use this code for Neumega.
MED: 100-2, 15, 50

☑ **J2357** Injection, omalizumab, 5 mg
Use this code for Xolair.

N ☑ **J2360** Injection, orphenadrine citrate, up to 60 mg ⊘
Use this code for Antiflex, Mio Rel, Myophen, Norflex, Banflex, Flexoject, Flexon, K-Flex, Myolin, Neocyten, O-Flex, Orphenate.
MED: 100-2, 15, 50

N ☑ **J2370** Injection, phenylephrine HCl, up to 1 ml ⊘
Use this code for Neo-Synephrine.
MED: 100-2, 15, 50

N ☑ **J2400** Injection, chloroprocaine HCl, per 30 ml ⊘
Use this code for Nesacaine, Nesacaine-MPF.
MED: 100-2, 15, 50

N ☑ **J2405** Injection, ondansetron HCl, per 1 mg ⊘
Use this code for Zofran.
MED: 100-2, 15, 50

N ☑ **J2410** Injection, oxymorphone HCl, up to 1 mg ⊘
Use this code for Numorphan, Numorphan H.P., Oxymorphone HCl.
MED: 100-2, 15, 50

● K **J2425** Injection, palifermin, 50 mcg

K ☑ **J2430** Injection, pamidronate disodium, per 30 mg ⊘
Use this code for Aredia, Argatroban.
MED: 100-2, 15, 50

N ☑ **J2440** Injection, papaverine HCl, up to 60 mg ⊘
MED: 100-2, 15, 50

Special Coverage Instructions   Noncovered by Medicare   Carrier Discretion   ☑ Quantity Alert   ● New Code   ○ Reinstated Code   ▲ Revised Code

2006 HCPCS   1-9 ASC Groups   MED: Pub 100/NCD Reference   ⅚ DMEPOS Paid   ⊘ SNF Excluded   **J Codes — 81**

Drugs Administered Other Than Oral Method

J2460 — J2794

N ☑ **J2460** Injection, oxytetracycline HCl, up to 50 mg ⊘
Use this code for Terramycin IM.
MED: 100-2, 15, 50

☑ **J2469** Injection, palonosetron HCl, 25 mcg
Use this code for Aloxi.

N **J2501** Injection, paricalcitol, 1 mcg
Use this code For Zemplar.
MED: 100-2, 15, 50

● G **J2503** Injection, pegaptanib sodium, 0.3 mg
Use this code for Mucagen.

● K **J2504** Injection, pegademase bovine, 25 IU
Use this code for Adagen.
MED: 100-2, 15, 50

G ☑ **J2505** Injection, pegfilgrastim, 6 mg ⊘
Use this code for Neulasta.

N ☑ **J2510** Injection, penicillin G procaine, aqueous, up to
600,000 units ⊘
Use this code for Wycillin, Duracillin A.S., Pfizerpen A.S.,
Crysticillin 300 A.S., Crysticillin 600 A.S.
MED: 100-2, 15, 50

● K **J2513** Injection, pentastarch, 10% solution, 100 ml
MED: 100-2, 15, 50

N ☑ **J2515** Injection, pentobarbital sodium, per 50 mg ⊘
Use this code for Nembutal Sodium Solution.
MED: 100-2, 15, 50

N ☑ **J2540** Injection, penicillin G potassium, up to 600,000
units ⊘
Use this code for Pfizerpen.
MED: 100-2, 15, 50

N ☑ **J2543** Injection, piperacillin sodium/tazobactam
sodium, 1 g/0.125 g (1.125 g) ⊘
Use this code for Zosyn.
MED: 100-2, 15, 50

Y ☑ **J2545** Pentamidine isethionate, inhalation solution, per
300 mg, administered through a DME ⊘
Use this code for Nebupent, PentacaRinat, Pentam 300.
MED: 100-2, 15, 50
See code(s): Q0077

N ☑ **J2550** Injection, promethazine HCl, up to 50 mg ⊘
Use this code for Anergan 25, Anergan 50, Antinaus,
Phenazine 25, Phenazine 50, Phenergan, Prorex-25, Prorex-50,
Prothazine, V-Gan 25, V-Gan 50.
MED: 100-2, 15, 50

N ☑ **J2560** Injection, phenobarbital sodium, up to 120 mg ⊘
Use this code for Luminal Sodium, Nembutal Sodium.
MED: 100-2, 15, 50

N ☑ **J2590** Injection, oxytocin, up to 10 units ⊘
Use this code for Pitocin, Syntocinon.
MED: 100-2, 15, 50

N ☑ **J2597** Injection, desmopressin acetate, per 1 mcg ⊘
Use this code for DDAVP.
MED: 100-2, 15, 50

N ☑ **J2650** Injection, prednisolone acetate, up to 1 ml ⊘
Use this code for Colotone, Key-Pred 25, Key-Pred 50,
Predacort, Predcor-25, Predcor-50, Predoject-50, Predalone-
50, Predicort-50.
MED: 100-2, 15, 50

N ☑ **J2670** Injection, tolazoline HCl, up to 25 mg ⊘
Use this code for Priscoline HCl.
MED: 100-2, 15, 50

N **J2675** Injection, progesterone, per 50 mg ⊘
Use this code for Gesterone, Gestrin.
MED: 100-2, 15, 50

N ☑ **J2680** Injection, fluphenazine decanoate, up to 25 mg ⊘
Use this code for Prolixin Decanoate.
MED: 100-2, 15, 50

N ☑ **J2690** Injection, procainamide HCl, up to 1 g ⊘
Use this code for Pronestyl.
MED: 100-2, 15, 50

N ☑ **J2700** Injection, oxacillin sodium, up to 250 mg ⊘
Use this code for Bactocill, Prostaphlin.
MED: 100-2, 15, 50

N ☑ **J2710** Injection, neostigmine methylsulfate, up to
0.5 mg ⊘
Use this code for Prostigmin.
MED: 100-2, 15, 50

N ☑ **J2720** Injection, protamine sulfate, per 10 mg ⊘
MED: 100-2, 15, 50

N ☑ **J2725** Injection, protirelin, per 250 mcg ⊘
Use this code for Relefact TRH, Thypinone, Thyrel TRH.
MED: 100-2, 15, 50

N ☑ **J2730** Injection, pralidoxime chloride, up to 1 g ⊘
Use this code for Protopam Chloride.

N ☑ **J2760** Injection, phentolamine mesylate, up to 5 mg ⊘
Use this code for Regitine.
MED: 100-2, 15, 50

N ☑ **J2765** Injection, metoclopramide HCl, up to 10 mg ⊘
Use this code for Ocatmide PFS, Reglan.
MED: 100-2, 15, 50

N ☑ **J2770** Injection, quinupristin/dalfopristin, 500 mg
(150/350) ⊘
Use this code for Synercid.
MED: 100-2, 15, 50

N ☑ **J2780** Injection, ranitidine HCl, 25 mg ⊘
Use this code for Zantac.
MED: 100-2, 15, 50

G ☑ **J2783** Injection, rasburicase, 0.5 mg ⊘
Use this code for Elitek.

K **J2788** Injection, Rho D immune globulin, human,
minidose, 50 mcg
Use this code for RhoGam, BAYRho-D, HYPRho-D,
MICRhoGAM Ultra-Filtered.
MED: 100-2, 15, 50

K ☑ **J2790** Injection, Rho D immune globulin, human, full dose,
300 mcg ⊘
Use this code for Gamulin RH, HypRho-D, BayRho-D, RhoGam,
Rhophylac.
MED: 100-2, 15, 50

K ☑ **J2792** Injection, Rho D immune globulin, intravenous,
human, solvent detergent, 100 IU ⊘
Use this code for BAYRho-D, Rhophylac, WINRho SDF.
MED: 100-2, 15, 50

☑ **J2794** Injection, risperidone, long acting, 0.5 mg
Use this code for Risperidal Costa Long Acting.

N ☑ **J2795** Injection, ropivacaine HCl, 1 mg ⊘
Use this code for Naropin.

N ☑ **J2800** Injection, methocarbamol, up to 10 ml ⊘
Use this code for Robaxin, Carbacot, Methocarbamol, Relaxin.
MED: 100-2, 15, 50

● K **J2805** Injection, sincalide, 5 mcg

N ☑ **J2810** Injection, theophylline, per 40 mg ⊘
MED: 100-2, 15, 50

K ☑ **J2820** Injection, sargramostim (GM-CSF), 50 mcg ⊘
Use this code for Leukine, Prokine.
MED: 100-2, 15, 50

● K **J2850** Injection, secretin, synthetic, human, 1 mcg

N ☑ **J2910** Injection, aurothioglucose, up to 50 mg ⊘
Use this code for Solganal.
MED: 100-2, 15, 50

N ☑ **J2912** Injection, sodium chloride, 0.9%, per 2 ml ⊘
Use this code for normal saline, Syrex.
MED: 100-2, 15, 50

N **J2916** Injection, sodium ferric gluconate complex in
sucrose injection, 12.5 mg
Use this code for Ferrlecit, Sodium Ferric Gluconate Complex.
MED: 100-2, 15, 50.2; 100-2, 15, 50.2

N ☑ **J2920** Injection, methylprednisolone sodium succinate, up
to 40 mg ⊘
Use this code for Solu-Medrol, A-methaPred.
MED: 100-2, 15, 50

N ☑ **J2930** Injection, methylprednisolone sodium succinate, up
to 125 mg ⊘
Use this code for Solu-Medrol, A-methaPred.
MED: 100-2, 15, 50

N ☑ **J2940** Injection, somatrem, 1 mg ⊘
Use this code for Protropin.
MED: 100-2, 15, 50
AHA: 2Q, '02, 8

K ☑ **J2941** Injection, somatropin, 1 mg ⊘
Use this code for Humatrope, Genotropin Nutropin, Biotropin,
Genotropin, Genotropin Miniquick, Norditropin, Nutropin,
Nutropin AQ, Saizen, Saizen Somatropin RDNA Origin,
Serostim, Serostim RDNA Origin, Zorbtive.
MED: 100-2, 15, 50
AHA: 2Q, '02, 8

N ☑ **J2950** Injection, promazine HCl, up to 25 mg ⊘
Use this code for Sparine, Prozine-50.
MED: 100-2, 15, 50

K ☑ **J2993** Injection, reteplase, 18.1 mg ⊘
Use this code for Retavase
MED: 100-2, 15, 50

K ☑ **J2995** Injection, streptokinase, per 250,000 IU ⊘
Use this code for Kabikinase, Streptase.
MED: 100-2, 15, 50

K ☑ **J2997** Injection, alteplase recombinant, 1 mg ⊘
Use this code for Activase, Cathflo.
MED: 100-2, 15, 50

N ☑ **J3000** Injection, streptomycin, up to 1 g ⊘
Use this code for Streptomycin Sulfate.
MED: 100-2, 15, 50

N ☑ **J3010** Injection, fentanyl citrate, 0.1 mg ⊘
Use this code for Sublimaze.
MED: 100-2, 15, 50

N ☑ **J3030** Injection, sumatriptan succinate, 6 mg (code may be
used for Medicare when drug administered under
the direct supervision of a physician, not for use
when drug is self administered) ⊘
Use this code for Imitrex.
MED: 100-2, 15, 50

N ☑ **J3070** Injection, pentazocine, 30 mg ⊘
Use this code for Talwin.
MED: 100-2, 15, 50

K ☑ **J3100** Injection, tenecteplase, 50 mg ⊘
Use this code for TNKase.
AHA: 2Q, '02, 8

N ☑ **J3105** Injection, terbutaline sulfate, up to 1 mg ⊘
Use this code for Brethine, Bricanyl Subcutaneous. For
terbutaline in inhalation solution, see K0525 and K0526.
MED: 100-2, 15, 50

☑ **J3110** Injection, teriparatide, 10 mcg
Use this code for Forteo.

N ☑ **J3120** Injection, testosterone enanthate, up to 100 mg ⊘
Use this code for Everone, Delatest, Delatestryl, Andropository
100, Testone LA 100.
MED: 100-2, 15, 50

N ☑ **J3130** Injection, testosterone enanthate, up to 200 mg ⊘
Use this code for Everone, Delatestryl, Andro L.A. 200, Andryl
200, Durathate-200, Testone LA 200, Testrin PA.
MED: 100-2, 15, 50

N ☑ **J3140** Injection, testosterone suspension, up to 50 mg ⊘
Use this code for Andronaq 50, Testosterone Aqueous,
Testaqua, Testoject-50, Histerone 50, Histerone 100.
MED: 100-2, 15, 50

N ☑ **J3150** Injection, testosterone propionate, up to 100 mg ⊘
Use this code for Testex.
MED: 100-2, 15, 50

N ☑ **J3230** Injection, chlorpromazine HCl, up to 50 mg ⊘
Use this code for Thorazine.
MED: 100-2, 15, 50

K ☑ **J3240** Injection, thyrotropin alpha, 0.9 mg, provided in 1.1
mg vial ⊘
Use this code for Thyrogen, Thytropar.
MED: 100-2, 15, 50

☑ **J3246** Injection, tirofiban HCl, 0.25mg
Use this code for Aggrastat.

N ☑ **J3250** Injection, trimethobenzamide HCl, up to 200 mg ⊘
Use this code for Tigan, Ticon, Tiject-20, Arrestin.
MED: 100-2, 15, 50

N ☑ **J3260** Injection, tobramycin sulfate, up to 80 mg ⊘
Use this code for Nebcin.
MED: 100-2, 15, 50

N ☑ **J3265** Injection, torsemide, 10 mg/ml ⊘
Use this code for Demadex, Torsemide.
MED: 100-2, 15, 50

N ☑ **J3280** Injection, thiethylperazine maleate, up to 10 mg ⊘
Use this code for Norzine, Torecan.
MED: 100-2, 15, 50

● K **J3285** Injection, treprostinil, 1 mg
Use this code for Remodulin.

Special Coverage Instructions   Noncovered by Medicare   Carrier Discretion   ☑ Quantity Alert   ● New Code   ○ Reinstated Code   ▲ Revised Code

2006 HCPCS   **1-9** ASC Groups   MED: Pub 100/NCD Reference   ᵬ DMEPOS Paid   ⊘ SNF Excluded   **J Codes — 83**

Drugs Administered Other Than Oral Method

J3301 — J7050

N ☑ **J3301** Injection, triamcinolone acetonide, per 10 mg ⃠
Use this code for Kenalog-10, Kenalog-40, Tri-Kort, Kenaject-40, Cenacort A-40, Triam-A, Trilog. For triamcinolone in inhalation solution, see K0527 and K0528.
MED: 100-2, 15, 50

N ☑ **J3302** Injection, triamcinolone diacetate, per 5 mg ⃠
Use this code for Aristocort, Aristocort Intralesional, Aristocort Forte, Amcort, Trilone, Cenacort Forte.
MED: 100-2, 15, 50

N ☑ **J3303** Injection, triamcinolone hexacetonide, per 5 mg ⃠
Use this code for Aristospan Intralesional, Aristospan Intra-articular.
MED: 100-2, 15, 50

K ☑ **J3305** Injection, trimetrexate glucoronate, per 25 mg ⃠
Use this code for Neutrexin.
MED: 100-2, 15, 50

N ☑ **J3310** Injection, perphenazine, up to 5 mg ⃠
Use this code for Trilafon.
MED: 100-2, 15, 50

G **J3315** Injection, triptorelin pamoate, 3.75 mg
Use this code for Trelstar Depot, Trelstar Depot Plus Debioclip Kit, Trelstar LA.
MED: 100-2, 15, 50

N ☑ **J3320** Injection, spectinomycin dihydrochloride, up to 2 g ⃠
Use this code for Trobicin.
MED: 100-2, 15, 50

N ☑ **J3350** Injection, urea, up to 40 g ⃠
Use this code for Ureaphil.
MED: 100-2, 15, 50

● K **J3355** Injection, urofollitropin, 75 IU
Use this code for Metrodin, Bravelle.

N ☑ **J3360** Injection, diazepam, up to 5 mg ⃠
Use this code for Diastat, Dizac, Valium, Zetran.
MED: 100-2, 15, 50

N ☑ **J3364** Injection, urokinase, 5,000 IU vial ⃠
Use this code for Abbokinase Open-Cath.
MED: 100-2, 15, 50

K ☑ **J3365** Injection, IV, urokinase, 250,000 IU vial ⃠
Use this code for Abbokinase.
MED: 100-2, 15, 50
See code(s): Q0089

N ☑ **J3370** Injection, vancomycin HCl, 500 mg ⃠
Use this code for Varocin, Vancoled.
MED: 100-2, 15, 50; 100-3, 280.14

☑ **J3396** Injection, verteporfin, 0.1 mg
MED: 100-3, 80.2; 100-3, 80.2; 100-3, 80.3; 100-3, 80.3; 100-3, 80.3; 100-3, 80.3; 100-3, 80.3; 100-3, 80.3; 100-3, 80.3; 100-3, 80.3

N ☑ **J3400** Injection, triflupromazine HCl, up to 20 mg ⃠
MED: 100-2, 15, 50

N ☑ **J3410** Injection, hydroxyzine HCl, up to 25 mg ⃠
Use this code for Vistaril, Vistaject-25, Hyzine, Hyzine-50.
MED: 100-2, 15, 50

N ☑ **J3411** Injection, thiamine HCl, 100 mg ⃠

N ☑ **J3415** Injection, pyridoxine HCl, 100 mg ⃠

N ☑ **J3420** Injection, vitamin B-12 cyanocobalamin, up to 1,000 mcg ⃠
Use this code for Sytobex, Redisol, Rubramin PC, Betalin 12, Berubigen, Cobex, Cobal, Crystal B12, Cyano, Cyanocobalamin, Hydroxocobalamin, Hydroxycobal, Nutri-Twelve.
MED: 100-2, 15, 50; 100-3, 150.6

N ☑ **J3430** Injection, phytonadione (vitamin K), per 1 mg ⃠
Use this code for AquaMephyton, Konakion, Menadione, Phytonadione.
MED: 100-2, 15, 50

N ☑ **J3465** Injection, voriconazole, 10 mg ⃠
MED: 100-2, 15, 50

N ☑ **J3470** Injection, hyaluronidase, up to 150 units ⃠
Use this code for Wydase.
MED: 100-2, 15, 50

● K **J3471** Injection, hyaluronidase, ovine, preservative free, per 1 USP unit (up to 999 USP units)

● K **J3472** Injection, hyaluronidase, ovine, preservative free, per 1000 USP units

N ☑ **J3475** Injection, magnesium sulphate, per 500 mg ⃠
Use this code for Mag Sul, Sulfa Mag.
MED: 100-2, 15, 50

N ☑ **J3480** Injection, potassium chloride, per 2 meq ⃠
MED: 100-2, 15, 50

N ☑ **J3485** Injection, zidovudine, 10 mg ⃠
Use this code for Retrovir, Zidovudine.
MED: 100-2, 15, 50

G ☑ **J3486** Injection, ziprasidone mesylate, 10 mg ⃠
Use this code for Geodon.

G **J3487** Injection, zoledronic acid, 1 mg
Use this code for Zometa.

N **J3490** Unclassified drugs ⃠
MED: 100-2, 15, 50

E ☑ **J3520** Edetate disodium, per 150 mg ⃠
Use this code for Endrate, Disotate, Meritate. This drug is used in chelation therapy, a treatment for atherosclerosis that is not covered by Medicare.
MED: 100-3, 20.21; 100-3, 20.22

E **J3530** Nasal vaccine inhalation ⃠
MED: 100-2, 15, 50

E **J3535** Drug administered through a metered dose inhaler ⃠

E **J3570** Laetrile, amygdalin, vitamin B-17 ⃠
The FDA has found Laetrile to have no safe or effective therapeutic purpose.
MED: 100-3, 30.7

N **J3590** Unclassified biologics

MISCELLANEOUS DRUGS AND SOLUTIONS

N ☑ **J7030** Infusion, normal saline solution, 1,000 cc ⃠
MED: 100-2, 15, 50

N ☑ **J7040** Infusion, normal saline solution, sterile (500 ml = 1 unit) ⃠
MED: 100-2, 15, 50

☑ **J7042** 5% dextrose/normal saline (500 ml = 1 unit) ⃠
MED: 100-2, 15, 50

N ☑ **J7050** Infusion, normal saline solution, 250 cc ⃠
MED: 100-2, 15, 50

▨ Special Coverage Instructions ▨ Noncovered by Medicare ▨ Carrier Discretion ☑ Quantity Alert ● New Code ○ Reinstated Code ▲ Revised Code

84 — J Codes A Age M Maternity ♀ Female Only ♂ Male Only A-Y APC Status Indicator *2006 HCPCS*

~~J7051 Sterile saline or water, up to 5 cc~~

N ☑ **J7060 5% dextrose/water (500 ml = 1 unit)** ⊘
MED: 100-2, 15, 50

N ☑ **J7070 Infusion, D-5-W, 1,000 cc** ⊘
MED: 100-2, 15, 50

N ☑ **J7100 Infusion, dextran 40, 500 ml** ⊘
Use this code for Gentran, 10% LMD, Rheomacrodex.
MED: 100-2, 15, 50

N ☑ **J7110 Infusion, dextran 75, 500 ml** ⊘
Use this code for Gentran 75.
MED: 100-2, 15, 50

N ☑ **J7120 Ringer's lactate infusion, up to 1,000 cc** ⊘
MED: 100-2, 15, 50

N ☑ **J7130 Hypertonic saline solution, 50 or 100 meq, 20 cc vial** ⊘
MED: 100-2, 15, 50

● K **J7188 Injection, Von Willebrand factor complex, human, IU**
MED: 100-2, 15, 50.5.5; 100-3, 110.8

● K **J7189 Factor VIIa (antihemophilic Factor, recombinant), per 1 mcg**
MED: 100-2, 15, 50

K ☑ **J7190 Factor VIII (antihemophilic factor, human) per IU**
Use this code for Monarc-M, Koate-HP, Alphanate, Hemofil-M, Koate-DVI, Kogenate, Monoclate-P.
Medicare jurisdiction: local contractor.
MED: 100-2, 15, 50

K ☑ **J7191 Factor VIII (antihemophilic factor (porcine), per IU**
Use this code for Hyate:C. Medicare jurisdiction: local contractor.
MED: 100-2, 15, 50

K ☑ **J7192 Factor VIII (antihemophilic factor, recombinant) per IU**
Use this code for Recombinate, Kogenate, Bioclate, Helixate, Advate rAHF-PFM, Antihemophilic Factor Human Method M Monoclonal Purified, Genarc, Refacto. Medicare jurisdiction: local contractor.
MED: 100-2, 15, 50

K ☑ **J7193 Factor IX (antihemophilic factor, purified, non-recombinant) per IU**
Use this code for AlphaNine SD, Mononine.
MED: 100-2, 15, 50
AHA: 2Q, '02, 8

K ☑ **J7194 Factor IX complex, per IU**
Use this code for Konyne-80, Profilnine Heat-Treated, Proplex T, Proplex SX-T, Alphanine SD, Bebulin VH, factor IX+ complex, Profilnine SD. Medicare jurisdiction: local contractor.
MED: 100-2, 15, 50

K ☑ **J7195 Factor IX (antihemophilic factor, recombinant) per IU**
Use this code for Benefix, Konyne 80, Proplex T.
MED: 100-2, 15, 50
AHA: 2Q, '02, 8

N ☑ **J7197 Antithrombin III (human), per IU**
Medicare jurisdiction: local contractor. Use this code for Throbate III, ATnativ.
MED: 100-2, 15, 50

K ☑ **J7198 Anti-inhibitor, per IU**
Medicare jurisdiction: local contractor. Use this code for Autoplex T, Feiba VH AICC.
MED: 100-2, 15, 50; 100-3, 110.3; 100-3, 110.3; 100-3, 110.3; 100-3, 110.3; 100-3, 110.3; 100-3, 110.3; 100-3, 110.3; 100-3, 110.3

B **J7199 Hemophilia clotting factor, not otherwise classified**
Medicare jurisdiction: local contractor.
MED: 100-2, 15, 50; 100-3, 110.3; 100-3, 110.3; 100-3, 110.3; 100-3, 110.3; 100-3, 110.3; 100-3, 110.3; 100-3, 110.3; 100-3, 110.3

E **J7300 Intrauterine copper contraceptive** ⊘
Use this code for Paragard T380A.

E ☑ **J7302 Levonorgestrel-releasing intrauterine contraceptive system, 52 mg** ♀ ⊘
Use this code for Mirena.

E ☑ **J7303 Contraceptive supply, hormone containing vaginal ring, each** ♀ ⊘
Use this code for Nuvaring Vaginal Ring.

☑ **J7304 Contraceptive supply, hormone containing patch, each**

● E **J7306 Levonorgestrel (contraceptive) implant system, including implants and supplies**

N ☑ **J7308 Aminolevulinic acid HCl for topical administration, 20%, single unit dosage form (354 mg)** ⊘

K ☑ **J7310 Ganciclovir, 4.5 mg, long-acting implant** ⊘
Use this code for Vitrasert.
MED: 100-2, 15, 50

K **J7317 Sodium hyaluronate, per 20 to 25 mg dose for intra-articular injection**

K ☑ **J7320 Hylan G-F 20, 16 mg, for intra-articular injection**

B ☑ **J7330 Autologous cultured chondrocytes, implant** ⊘
Medicare jurisdiction: local contractor. Use this code for Carticel.

▲ K ☑ **J7340 Dermal and epidermal, (substitute) tissue of human origin, with or without bioengineered or processed elements, with metabolically active elements, per square centimeter**
Use this code for Apligraf, Orcel, TransCyte.

● K **J7341 Dermal (substitute) tissue of nonhuman origin, with or without other bioengineered or processed elements, with metabolically active elements, per square centimeter**

▲ K ☑ **J7342 Dermal (substitute) tissue of human origin, with or without other bioengineered or processed elements, with metabolically active elements, per square centimeter**
Use this code for Dermagraft , Dermagraft TC.

▲ K **J7343 Dermal and epidermal, (substitute) tissue of non-human origin, with or without other bioengineered or processed elements, without metabolically active elements, per square centimeter**
Use this code for Integra.

▲ K **J7344 Dermal (substitute) tissue of human origin, with or without other bioengineered or processed elements, without metabolically active elements, per square centimeter**

▲ K ☑ **J7350 Dermal (substitute) tissue of human origin, injectable, with or without other bioengineered or processed elements, but without metabolized active elements, per 10 mg**

N ☑ **J7500 Azathioprine, oral, 50 mg**
Use this code for Azasan, Imuran.
MED: 100-2, 15, 50.5

Drugs Administered Other Than Oral Method

J7501 — J7635

N ☑ **J7501** Azathioprine, parenteral, 100 mg
Use this code for Imuran.
MED: 100-2, 15, 50

K ☑ **J7502** Cyclosporine, oral, 100 mg
Use this code for Neoral, Sandimmune, Gengraf, Sangcya.
See also code: C9438
MED: 100-2, 15, 50.5

K ☑ **J7504** Lymphocyte immune globulin, antithymocyte globulin, equine, parenteral, 250 mg
Use this code for Atgam.
MED: 100-2, 15, 50; 100-3, 260.7

K ☑ **J7505** Muromonab-CD3, parenteral, 5 mg
Use this code for Orthoclone OKT3.
MED: 100-2, 15, 50

N ☑ **J7506** Prednisone, oral, per 5 mg
Use this code for Deltasone, Liquid Pred Syrup, Levoxyl, Predone, Prednicot, Sterapred.
MED: 100-2, 15, 50.5

K ☑ **J7507** Tacrolimus, oral, per 1 mg
Use this code for Prograf.
MED: 100-2, 15, 50.5

N ☑ **J7509** Methylprednisolone, oral, per 4 mg
Use this code for Medrol, Methylpred.
MED: 100-2, 15, 50.5

N ☑ **J7510** Prednisolone, oral, per 5 mg
Use this code for Delta-Cortef, Cotolone, Pediapred, Prednoral, Prelone.
MED: 100-2, 15, 50.5

K ☑ **J7511** Lymphocyte immune globulin, antithymocyte globulin, rabbit, parenteral, 25 mg
Use this code for Thymoglobulin.
AHA: 2Q, '02, 8

K ☑ **J7513** Daclizumab, parenteral, 25 mg
Use this code for Zenapax.
MED: 100-2, 15, 50.5

N ☑ **J7515** Cyclosporine, oral, 25 mg   ⊘
Use this code for Gengraf, Neoral, Sandimmune.

N ☑ **J7516** Cyclosporine, parenteral, 250 mg   ⊘
Use this code for Neoral, Sandimmune.

G ☑ **J7517** Mycophenolate mofetil, oral, 250 mg
Use this code for CellCept.

☑ **J7518** Mycophenolic acid, oral, 180 mg
Use this code for Myfortic Delayed Release.
MED: 100-4, 17, 80.3.1; 100-4, 8, 120.1

K ☑ **J7520** Sirolimus, oral, 1 mg   ⊘
Use this code for Rapamune.
MED: 100-2, 15, 50.5

K ☑ **J7525** Tacrolimus, parenteral, 5 mg
Use this code for Prograf.
MED: 100-2, 15, 50.5

N **J7599** Immunosuppressive drug, NOC   ⊘
Determine if an alternative HCPCS Level II or a CPT code better describes the service being reported. This code should be used only if a more specific code is unavailable.
MED: 100-2, 15, 50.5

INHALATION SOLUTIONS

Y ☑ **J7608** Acetylcysteine, inhalation solution administered through DME, unit dose form, per g   ⊘
Use this code for Acetadote, Mucomyst, Mucosil.
MED: 100-2, 15, 110.3

☑ **J7611** Albuterol, inhalation solution, administered through DME, concentrated form, 1 mg
Use this code for Accuneb, Proventil, Respirol, Ventolin.
MED: 100-2, 15, 110.3

☑ **J7612** Levalbuterol, inhalation solution, administered through DME, concentrated form, 0.5 mg
Use this code for Xopenex.
MED: 100-2, 15, 110.3

☑ **J7613** Albuterol, inhalation solution, administered through DME, unit dose, 1 mg
Use this code for Accuneb, Proventil, Respirol, Ventolin.
MED: 100-2, 15, 110.3

☑ **J7614** Levalbuterol, inhalation solution, administered through DME, unit dose, 0.5 mg
Use this code for Xopenex.
MED: 100-2, 15, 110.3

~~**J7616** Albuterol, up to 5 mg and ipratropium bromide, up to 1 mg, compounded inhalation solution, administered through DME~~

~~**J7617** Levalbuterol, up to 2.5 mg and ipratropium bromide, up to 1 mg, compounded inhalation solution, administered through DME~~

○ B **J7620** Albuterol, up to 2.5 mg and ipratropium bromide, up to 0.5 mg, non-compounded

A **J7622** Beclomethasone, inhalation solution administered through DME, unit dose form, per mg   ⊘
Use this code for Beclovent, Beconase.

A ☑ **J7624** Betamethasone, inhalation solution administered through DME, unit dose form, per mg   ⊘

▲ B ☑ **J7626** Budesonide inhalation solution, non-compounded, administered through DME, unit dose form, up to 0.5 mg
Use this code for Pulmicort Respules.

○ B **J7627** Budesonide, powder, compounded for inhalation solution, administered through

Y ☑ **J7628** Bitolterol mesylate, inhalation solution administered through DME, concentrated form, per mg   ⊘
Use this code for Tornalate.
MED: 100-2, 15, 110.3

Y ☑ **J7629** Bitolterol mesylate, inhalation solution administered through DME, unit dose form, per mg   ⊘
Use this code for Tornalate.
MED: 100-2, 15, 110.3

Y ☑ **J7631** Cromolyn sodium, inhalation solution administered through DME, unit dose form, per 10 mg   ⊘
Use this code for Intal, Nasalcrom, Gastrocrom.
MED: 100-2, 15, 110.3

N **J7633** Budesonide, inhalation solution administered through DME, concentrated form, per 0.25 milligram
Use this code for Pumocort.

Y ☑ **J7635** Atropine, inhalation solution administered through DME, concentrated form, per mg   ⊘
MED: 100-2, 15, 110.3

Special Coverage Instructions   Noncovered by Medicare   Carrier Discretion   ☑ Quantity Alert   ● New Code   ○ Reinstated Code   ▲ Revised Code

86 — J Codes   A Age   M Maternity   ♀ Female Only   ♂ Male Only   A-Y APC Status Indicator   *2006 HCPCS*

☑ ☑ **J7636** Atropine, inhalation solution administered through DME, unit dose form, per mg ⊘
MED: 100-2, 15, 110.3

☑ ☑ **J7637** Dexamethasone, inhalation solution administered through DME, concentrated form, per mg ⊘
MED: 100-2, 15, 110.3

☑ ☑ **J7638** Dexamethasone, inhalation solution administered through DME, unit dose form, per mg ⊘
MED: 100-2, 15, 110.3

☑ ☑ **J7639** Dornase alpha, inhalation solution administered through DME, unit dose form, per mg
Use this code for Pulmozyme.
MED: 100-2, 15, 110.3

○ Ⓔ **J7640** Formoterol, inhalation solution, administered through DME, unit dose form, 12 micrograms

Ⓐ **J7641** Flunisolide, inhalation solution administered through DME, unit dose, per mg ⊘
Use this code for Aerobid, Flunisolide.

☑ ☑ **J7642** Glycopyrrolate, inhalation solution administered through DME, concentrated form, per mg ⊘
MED: 100-2, 15, 110.3

☑ ☑ **J7643** Glycopyrrolate, inhalation solution administered through DME, unit dose form, per mg ⊘
Use this code for Robinul.
MED: 100-2, 15, 110.3

☑ ☑ **J7644** Ipratropium bromide, inhalation solution administered through DME, unit dose form, per mg ⊘
Use this code for Atrovent.
MED: 100-2, 15, 110.3

☑ ☑ **J7648** Isoetharine HCl, inhalation solution administered through DME, concentrated form, per mg ⊘
Use this code for Beta-2.
MED: 100-2, 15, 110.3

☑ ☑ **J7649** Isoetharine HCl, inhalation solution administered through DME, unit dose form, per mg ⊘
MED: 100-2, 15, 110.3

☑ ☑ **J7658** Isoproterenol HCl, inhalation solution administered through DME, concentrated form, per mg ⊘
Use this code for Isuprel HCl, Medihaler-ISO.
MED: 100-2, 15, 110.3

☑ ☑ **J7659** Isoproterenol HCl, inhalation solution administered through DME, unit dose form, per mg ⊘
Use this code for Isuprel HCl, Medihaler-ISO.
MED: 100-2, 15, 110.3

☑ ☑ **J7668** Metaproterenol sulfate, inhalation solution administered through DME, concentrated form, per 10 mg ⊘
Use this code for Alupent, Metaprel.
MED: 100-2, 15, 110.3

☑ ☑ **J7669** Metaproterenol sulfate, inhalation solution administered through DME, unit dose form, per 10 mg ⊘
Use this code for Alupent.
MED: 100-2, 15, 110.3

☑ **J7674** Methacholine chloride administered as inhalation solution through a nebulizer, per 1 mg
Use this code for Provocholine Powder.

☑ ☑ **J7680** Terbutaline sulfate, inhalation solution administered through DME, concentrated form, per mg ⊘
Use this code for Brethine, Bricanyl.
MED: 100-2, 15, 110.3

☑ ☑ **J7681** Terbutaline sulfate, inhalation solution administered through DME, unit dose form, per mg ⊘
Use this code for Brethine, Bricanyl.
MED: 100-2, 15, 110.3

☑ ☑ **J7682** Tobramycin, unit dose form, 300 mg, inhalation solution, administered through DME ⊘
Use this code for Tobi.
MED: 100-2, 15, 110.3

☑ ☑ **J7683** Triamcinolone, inhalation solution administered through DME, concentrated form, per mg ⊘
Use this code for Azmacort.
MED: 100-2, 15, 110.3

☑ ☑ **J7684** Triamcinolone, inhalation solution administered through DME, unit dose form, per mg ⊘
Use this code for Azmacort.
MED: 100-2, 15, 110.3

☑ **J7699** NOC drugs, inhalation solution administered through DME ⊘
MED: 100-2, 15, 110.3

☑ **J7799** NOC drugs, other than inhalation drugs, administered through DME ⊘
MED: 100-2, 15, 110.3

● Ⓑ **J8498** Antiemetic drug, rectal/suppository, not otherwise specified

Ⓔ **J8499** Prescription drug, oral, nonchemotherapeutic, NOS ⊘
MED: 100-2, 15, 50

☑ **J8501** Aprepitant, oral, 5 mg
Use this code for Emend.

Ⓚ ☑ **J8510** Bulsulfan, oral, 2 mg
Use this code for Busulfex, Myleran.
MED: 100-2, 15, 50.5

● Ⓔ **J8515** Cabergoline, oral, 0.25 mg
Use this code for Dostinex.
MED: 100-2, 15, 50.5

Ⓚ ☑ **J8520** Capecitabine, oral, 150 mg
Use this code for Xeloda.
MED: 100-2, 15, 50.5

Ⓔ ☑ **J8521** Capecitabine, oral, 500 mg
Use this code for Xeloda.
MED: 100-2, 15, 50.5

Ⓝ ☑ **J8530** Cyclophosphamide, oral, 25 mg
Use this code for Cytoxan.
MED: 100-2, 15, 50.5

● Ⓚ **J8540** Dexamethasone, oral, 0.25 mg
Use this code for Decadron.

Ⓚ ☑ **J8560** Etoposide, oral, 50 mg
Use this code for VePesid.
MED: 100-2, 15, 50.5

☑ **J8565** Gefitinib, oral, 250 mg
Use this code for Iressa.

● Ⓝ **J8597** Antiemetic drug, oral, not otherwise specified

Chemotherapy Drugs

J8600 — J9140

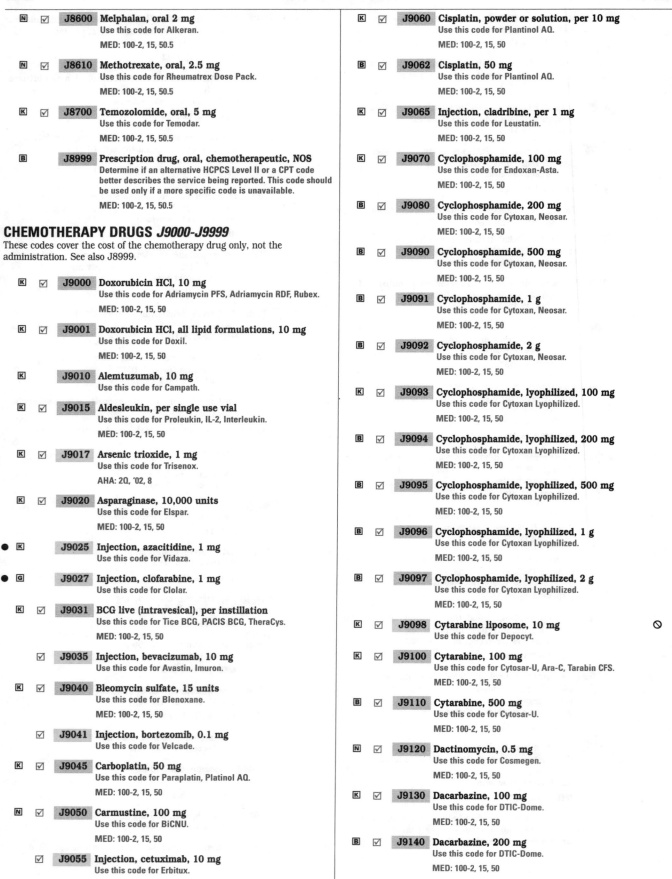

N ☑ **J8600** Melphalan, oral 2 mg
Use this code for Alkeran.
MED: 100-2, 15, 50.5

N ☑ **J8610** Methotrexate, oral, 2.5 mg
Use this code for Rheumatrex Dose Pack.
MED: 100-2, 15, 50.5

K ☑ **J8700** Temozolomide, oral, 5 mg
Use this code for Temodar.
MED: 100-2, 15, 50.5

B **J8999** Prescription drug, oral, chemotherapeutic, NOS
Determine if an alternative HCPCS Level II or a CPT code better describes the service being reported. This code should be used only if a more specific code is unavailable.
MED: 100-2, 15, 50.5

CHEMOTHERAPY DRUGS *J9000-J9999*

These codes cover the cost of the chemotherapy drug only, not the administration. See also J8999.

K ☑ **J9000** Doxorubicin HCl, 10 mg
Use this code for Adriamycin PFS, Adriamycin RDF, Rubex.
MED: 100-2, 15, 50

K ☑ **J9001** Doxorubicin HCl, all lipid formulations, 10 mg
Use this code for Doxil.
MED: 100-2, 15, 50

K **J9010** Alemtuzumab, 10 mg
Use this code for Campath.

K ☑ **J9015** Aldesleukin, per single use vial
Use this code for Proleukin, IL-2, Interleukin.
MED: 100-2, 15, 50

K ☑ **J9017** Arsenic trioxide, 1 mg
Use this code for Trisenox.
AHA: 2Q, '02, 8

K ☑ **J9020** Asparaginase, 10,000 units
Use this code for Elspar.
MED: 100-2, 15, 50

● **K** **J9025** Injection, azacitidine, 1 mg
Use this code for Vidaza.

● **G** **J9027** Injection, clofarabine, 1 mg
Use this code for Clolar.

K ☑ **J9031** BCG live (intravesical), per instillation
Use this code for Tice BCG, PACIS BCG, TheraCys.
MED: 100-2, 15, 50

☑ **J9035** Injection, bevacizumab, 10 mg
Use this code for Avastin, Imuron.

K ☑ **J9040** Bleomycin sulfate, 15 units
Use this code for Blenoxane.
MED: 100-2, 15, 50

☑ **J9041** Injection, bortezomib, 0.1 mg
Use this code for Velcade.

K ☑ **J9045** Carboplatin, 50 mg
Use this code for Paraplatin, Platinol AQ.
MED: 100-2, 15, 50

N ☑ **J9050** Carmustine, 100 mg
Use this code for BiCNU.
MED: 100-2, 15, 50

☑ **J9055** Injection, cetuximab, 10 mg
Use this code for Erbitux.

K ☑ **J9060** Cisplatin, powder or solution, per 10 mg
Use this code for Plantinol AQ.
MED: 100-2, 15, 50

B ☑ **J9062** Cisplatin, 50 mg
Use this code for Plantinol AQ.
MED: 100-2, 15, 50

K ☑ **J9065** Injection, cladribine, per 1 mg
Use this code for Leustatin.
MED: 100-2, 15, 50

K ☑ **J9070** Cyclophosphamide, 100 mg
Use this code for Endoxan-Asta.
MED: 100-2, 15, 50

B ☑ **J9080** Cyclophosphamide, 200 mg
Use this code for Cytoxan, Neosar.
MED: 100-2, 15, 50

B ☑ **J9090** Cyclophosphamide, 500 mg
Use this code for Cytoxan, Neosar.
MED: 100-2, 15, 50

B ☑ **J9091** Cyclophosphamide, 1 g
Use this code for Cytoxan, Neosar.
MED: 100-2, 15, 50

B ☑ **J9092** Cyclophosphamide, 2 g
Use this code for Cytoxan, Neosar.
MED: 100-2, 15, 50

K ☑ **J9093** Cyclophosphamide, lyophilized, 100 mg
Use this code for Cytoxan Lyophilized.
MED: 100-2, 15, 50

B ☑ **J9094** Cyclophosphamide, lyophilized, 200 mg
Use this code for Cytoxan Lyophilized.
MED: 100-2, 15, 50

B ☑ **J9095** Cyclophosphamide, lyophilized, 500 mg
Use this code for Cytoxan Lyophilized.
MED: 100-2, 15, 50

B ☑ **J9096** Cyclophosphamide, lyophilized, 1 g
Use this code for Cytoxan Lyophilized.
MED: 100-2, 15, 50

B ☑ **J9097** Cyclophosphamide, lyophilized, 2 g
Use this code for Cytoxan Lyophilized.
MED: 100-2, 15, 50

K ☑ **J9098** Cytarabine liposome, 10 mg   ⊘
Use this code for Depocyt.

K ☑ **J9100** Cytarabine, 100 mg
Use this code for Cytosar-U, Ara-C, Tarabin CFS.
MED: 100-2, 15, 50

B ☑ **J9110** Cytarabine, 500 mg
Use this code for Cytosar-U.
MED: 100-2, 15, 50

N ☑ **J9120** Dactinomycin, 0.5 mg
Use this code for Cosmegen.
MED: 100-2, 15, 50

K ☑ **J9130** Dacarbazine, 100 mg
Use this code for DTIC-Dome.
MED: 100-2, 15, 50

B ☑ **J9140** Dacarbazine, 200 mg
Use this code for DTIC-Dome.
MED: 100-2, 15, 50

Special Coverage Instructions   Noncovered by Medicare   Carrier Discretion   ☑ Quantity Alert   ● New Code   ○ Reinstated Code   ▲ Revised Code

88 — J Codes   **A** Age   **M** Maternity   ♀ Female Only   ♂ Male Only   **A**-**Y** APC Status Indicator   *2006 HCPCS*

K ☑ **J9150** Daunorubicin HCl, 10 mg
Use this code for Cerubidine.
MED: 100-2, 15, 50

K ☑ **J9151** Daunorubicin citrate, liposomal formulation, 10 mg
Use this code for Daunoxome.
MED: 100-2, 15, 50

K ☑ **J9160** Denileukin diftitox, 300 mcg
Use this code for Ontak.

N ☑ **J9165** Diethylstilbestrol diphosphate, 250 mg
Use this code for Stilphostrol.
MED: 100-2, 15, 50

K ☑ **J9170** Docetaxel, 20 mg
Use this code for Taxotere.
MED: 100-2, 15, 50

● N **J9175** Injection, Eliotts' B solution, 1 ml
Use this code for dextrose/electsol, IV
MED: 100-2, 15, 50

K ☑ **J9178** Injection, epirubicin HCl, 2 mg
Use this code for Ellence.

K ☑ **J9181** Etoposide, 10 mg
Use this code for VePesid, Toposar.
MED: 100-2, 15, 50

B ☑ **J9182** Etoposide, 100 mg
Use this code for VePesid, Toposar.
MED: 100-2, 15, 50

K ☑ **J9185** Fludarabine phosphate, 50 mg
Use this code for Fludara.
MED: 100-2, 15, 50

N ☑ **J9190** Fluorouracil, 500 mg
Use this code for Adrucil.
MED: 100-2, 15, 50

K ☑ **J9200** Floxuridine, 500 mg
Use this code for FUDR.
MED: 100-2, 15, 50

K ☑ **J9201** Gemcitabine HCl, 200 mg
Use this code for Gemzar.
MED: 100-2, 15, 50

K ☑ **J9202** Goserelin acetate implant, per 3.6 mg
Use this code for Zoladex.
MED: 100-2, 15, 50

K ☑ **J9206** Irinotecan, 20 mg
Use this code for Camptosar.
MED: 100-2, 15, 50

K ☑ **J9208** Ifosfamide, per 1 g
Use this code for IFEX, Mitoxana.
MED: 100-2, 15, 50

K ☑ **J9209** Mesna, 200 mg
Use this code for Mesnex.
MED: 100-2, 15, 50

K ☑ **J9211** Idarubicin HCl, 5 mg
Use this code for Idamycin.
MED: 100-2, 15, 50

N ☑ **J9212** Injection, interferon alfacon-1, recombinant, 1 mcg
Use this code for Infergen.
MED: 100-2, 15, 50

K ☑ **J9213** Interferon alfa-2A, recombinant, 3 million units
Use this code for Roferon-A.
MED: 100-2, 15, 50

K ☑ **J9214** Interferon alfa-2B, recombinant, 1 million units
Use this code for Intron A, Rebetron Kit.
MED: 100-2, 15, 50

K ☑ **J9215** Interferon alfa-N3, (human leukocyte derived), 250,000 IU
Use this code for Alferon N.
MED: 100-2, 15, 50

K ☑ **J9216** Interferon gamma-1B, 3 million units
Use this code for Actimmune.
MED: 100-2, 15, 50

K ☑ **J9217** Leuprolide acetate (for depot suspension), 7.5 mg
Use this code for Lupron Depot, Eligard.
MED: 100-2, 15, 50

K ☑ **J9218** Leuprolide acetate, per 1 mg
Use this code for Lupron, Eligard.
MED: 100-2, 15, 50

K ☑ **J9219** Leuprolide acetate implant, 65 mg
Use this code for Lupron Implant.
MED: 100-2, 15, 50
AHA: 4Q, '01, 5

● K **J9225** Histrelin implant, 50 mg
Use this code for Vantas.
MED: 100-2, 15, 50

N ☑ **J9230** Mechlorethamine HCl, (nitrogen mustard), 10 mg
Use this code for Mustargen.
MED: 100-2, 15, 50

K ☑ **J9245** Injection, melphalan HCl, 50 mg
Use this code for Alkeran, L-phenylalanine mustard.
MED: 100-2, 15, 50

N ☑ **J9250** Methotrexate sodium, 5 mg
Use this code for Folex, Folex PFS, Methotrexate LPF.
MED: 100-2, 15, 50

B ☑ **J9260** Methotrexate sodium, 50 mg
Use this code for Folex, Folex PFS, Methotrexate LPF.
MED: 100-2, 15, 50

B ☑ **J9263** Injection, oxaliplatin, 0.5 mg
Use this code for Eloxatin.

● G **J9264** Injection, paclitaxel protein-bound particles, 1 mg
Use this code for Abraxane.

K ☑ **J9265** Paclitaxel, 30 mg
Use this code for Taxol, Nov-Onxol.
MED: 100-2, 15, 50

N ☑ **J9266** Pegaspargase, per single dose vial
Use this code for Oncaspar.
MED: 100-2, 15, 50
AHA: 2Q, '02, 8

K ☑ **J9268** Pentostatin, per 10 mg
Use this code for Nipent.
MED: 100-2, 15, 50

K ☑ **J9270** Plicamycin, 2.5 mg
Use this code for Mithacin.
MED: 100-2, 15, 50

K ☑ **J9280** **Mitomycin, 5 mg**
Use this code for Mutamycin.

MED: 100-2, 15, 50

B ☑ **J9290** **Mitomycin, 20 mg**
Use this code for Mutamycin.

MED: 100-2, 15, 50

B ☑ **J9291** **Mitomycin, 40 mg**
Use this code for Mutamycin.

MED: 100-2, 15, 50

K ☑ **J9293** **Injection, mitoxantrone HCl, per 5 mg**
Use this code for Navantrone.

MED: 100-2, 15, 50

K **J9300** **Gemtuzumab ozogamicin, 5 mg**
Use this code for Mylotarg.

AHA: 2Q, '02, 8

☑ **J9305** **Injection, pemetrexed, 10 mg**
Use this code for Alimta.

K ☑ **J9310** **Rituximab, 100 mg**
Use this code for RituXan.

MED: 100-2, 15, 50

K ☑ **J9320** **Streptozocin, 1 g**
Use this code for Zanosar.

MED: 100-2, 15, 50

K ☑ **J9340** **Thiotepa, 15 mg**
Use this code for Thioplex.

MED: 100-2, 15, 50

K ☑ **J9350** **Topotecan, 4 mg**
Use this code for Hycamtin.

MED: 100-2, 15, 50

K ☑ **J9355** **Trastuzumab, 10 mg**
Use this code for Herceptin.

K ☑ **J9357** **Valrubicin, intravesical, 200 mg**
Use this code for Valstar.

MED: 100-2, 15, 50

N ☑ **J9360** **Vinblastine sulfate, 1 mg**
Use this code for Velban.

MED: 100-2, 15, 50

N ☑ **J9370** **Vincristine sulfate, 1 mg**
Use this code for Oncovin, Vincasar PFS.

MED: 100-2, 15, 50

B ☑ **J9375** **Vincristine sulfate, 2 mg**
Use this code for Oncovin, Vincasar PFS.

MED: 100-2, 15, 50

B ☑ **J9380** **Vincristine sulfate, 5 mg**
Use this code for Oncovin.

MED: 100-2, 15, 50

K ☑ **J9390** **Vinorelbine tartrate, per 10 mg**
Use this code for Navelbine.

MED: 100-2, 15, 50

G ☑ **J9395** **Injection, fulvestrant, 25 mg**
Use this code for Fastodex.

K ☑ **J9600** **Porfimer sodium, 75 mg**
Use this code for Photofrin.

MED: 100-2, 15, 50

N **J9999** **NOC, antineoplastic drug**
Determine if an alternative HCPCS Level II or a CPT code better describes the service being reported. This code should be used only if a more specific code is unavailable.

MED: 100-2, 15, 50; 100-3, 110.2

| Special Coverage Instructions | Noncovered by Medicare | Carrier Discretion | ☑ Quantity Alert | ● New Code | ○ Reinstated Code | ▲ Revised Code |

90 — J Codes   A Age   M Maternity   ♀ Female Only   ♂ Male Only   A-Y APC Status Indicator   *2006 HCPCS*

TEMPORARY CODES *K0000-K9999*

The K codes were established for use by the durable medical equipment regional carriers (DMERCs). The K codes are developed when the currently existing permanent national codes for supplies and certain product categories do not include the codes needed to implement a DMERC medical review policy.

K CODES ASSIGNED TO DURABLE MEDICAL EQUIPMENT REGIONAL CARRIERS (DMERC)

WHEELCHAIR AND WHEELCHAIR ACCESSORIES

- K0001 Standard wheelchair
- K0002 Standard hemi (low seat) wheelchair
- K0003 Lightweight wheelchair
- K0004 High strength, lightweight wheelchair
- K0005 Ultralightweight wheelchair
- K0006 Heavy-duty wheelchair
- K0007 Extra heavy-duty wheelchair
- K0009 Other manual wheelchair/base
- K0010 Standard-weight frame motorized/power wheelchair
- K0011 Standard-weight frame motorized/power wheelchair with programmable control parameters for speed adjustment, tremor dampening, acceleration control and braking
- K0012 Lightweight portable motorized/power wheelchair
- K0014 Other motorized/power wheelchair base
- K0015 Detachable, nonadjustable height armrest, each
- K0017 Detachable, adjustable height armrest, base, each
- K0018 Detachable, adjustable height armrest, upper portion, each
- K0019 Arm pad, each
- K0020 Fixed, adjustable height armrest, pair
- K0037 High mount flip-up footrest, each
- K0038 Leg strap, each
- K0039 Leg strap, H style, each
- K0040 Adjustable angle footplate, each
- K0041 Large size footplate, each
- K0042 Standard size footplate, each
- K0043 Footrest, lower extension tube, each
- K0044 Footrest, upper hanger bracket, each
- K0045 Footrest, complete assembly
- K0046 Elevating legrest, lower extension tube, each
- K0047 Elevating legrest, upper hanger bracket, each
- K0050 Ratchet assembly
- K0051 Cam release assembly, footrest or legrest, each
- K0052 Swingaway, detachable footrests, each
- K0053 Elevating footrests, articulating (telescoping), each
- K0056 Seat height less than 17 in. or equal to or greater than 21 in. for a high strength, lightweight, or ultralightweight wheelchair
- ~~K0064~~ ~~Zero-pressure tube (flat free insert), any size, each~~
  See code(s) E2213.
- K0065 Spoke protectors, each

- ~~K0066~~ ~~Solid tire, any size, each~~
  See code(s) E2220.
- ~~K0067~~ ~~Pneumatic tire, any size, each~~
  See code(s) E2211.
- ~~K0068~~ ~~Pneumatic tire tube, each~~
  See code(s) E2212.
- K0069 Rear wheel assembly, complete, with solid tire, spokes or molded, each
- K0070 Rear wheel assembly, complete with pneumatic tire, spokes or molded, each
- K0071 Front caster assembly, complete, with pneumatic tire, each
- K0072 Front caster assembly, complete, with semipneumatic tire, each
- K0073 Caster pin lock, each
- ~~K0074~~ ~~Pneumatic caster tire, any size, each~~
  See code(s) E2214.
- ~~K0075~~ ~~Semipneumatic caster tire, any size, each~~
  See code(s) E2219.
- ~~K0076~~ ~~Solid caster tire, any size, each~~
  See code(s) E2221.
- K0077 Front caster assembly, complete, with solid tire, each
- ~~K0078~~ ~~Pneumatic caster tire tube, each~~
  See code(s) E2215.
- K0090 Rear wheel tire for power wheelchair, any size, each
- K0091 Rear wheel tire tube other than zero pressure for power wheelchair, any size, each
- K0092 Rear wheel assembly for power wheelchair, complete, each
- K0093 Rear wheel zero pressure tire tube (flat free insert) for power wheelchair, any size, each
- K0094 Wheel tire for power base, any size, each
- K0095 Wheel tire tube other than zero pressure for each base, any size, each
- K0096 Wheel assembly for power base, complete, each
- K0097 Wheel zero-pressure tire tube (flat free insert) for power base, any size, each
- K0098 Drive belt for power wheelchair
- K0099 Front caster for power wheelchair
- ~~K0102~~ ~~Crutch and cane holder, each~~
  See code(s) E2207.
- ~~K0104~~ ~~Cylinder tank carrier, each~~
  See code(s) E2208.
- K0105 IV hanger, each
- ~~K0106~~ ~~Arm trough, each~~
  See code(s) E2209.
- K0108 Other accessories
- K0195 Elevating legrest, pair (for use with capped rental wheelchair base)
  MED: 100-3, 230.10
- ~~K0415~~ ~~Prescription antiemetic drug, oral, per 1 mg, for use in conjunction with oral anti-cancer drug, NOS~~
- ~~K0416~~ ~~Prescription antiemetic drug, rectal, per 1 mg, for use in conjunction with oral anti-cancer drug, NOS~~
- ~~K0452~~ ~~Wheelchair bearings, any type~~
  See code(s) E2210.

Special Coverage Instructions   Noncovered by Medicare   Carrier Discretion   ☑ Quantity Alert   ● New Code   ○ Reinstated Code   ▲ Revised Code

2006 HCPCS   1-9 ASC Groups   MED: Pub 100/NCD Reference   ⅄ DMEPOS Paid   ⊘ SNF Excluded   **K Codes — 91**

Temporary Codes

K0455 — K0635

☑   **K0455** Infusion pump used for uninterrupted parenteral administration of medication, (e.g., epoprostenol or treprostinol)   ♿○
MED: 100-3, 280.14

☑   **K0462** Temporary replacement for patient owned equipment being repaired, any type   ○
MED: 100-4, 20, 40.2

☑ ☑ **K0552** Supplies for external drug infusion pump, syringe type cartridge, sterile, each   ♿○
MED: 100-3, 280.14

~~**K0600** Functional neuromuscular stimulator, transcutaneous stimulation of muscles of ambulation with computer control, used for walking by spinal cord injured, entire system, after completion of training program~~
See code(s) E0762.

☑ ☑ **K0601** Replacement battery for external infusion pump owned by patient, silver oxide, 1.5 volt, each   ♿○
AHA: 2Q, '03, 7

☑ ☑ **K0602** Replacement battery for external infusion pump owned by patient, silver oxide, 3 volt, each   ♿○
AHA: 2Q, '03, 7

☑ ☑ **K0603** Replacement battery for external infusion pump owned by patient, alkaline, 1.5 volt, each   ♿○
AHA: 2Q, '03, 7

☑ ☑ **K0604** Replacement battery for external infusion pump owned by patient, lithium, 3.6 volt, each   ♿○
AHA: 2Q, '03, 7

☑ ☑ **K0605** Replacement battery for external infusion pump owned by patient, lithium, 4.5 volt, each   ♿○
AHA: 2Q, '03, 7

☑   **K0606** Automatic external defibrillator, with integrated electrocardiogram analysis, garment type   ♿○
AHA: 4Q, '03, 4

☑ ☑ **K0607** Replacement battery for automated external defibrillator, garment type only, each   ♿○
AHA: 4Q, '03, 4

☑ ☑ **K0608** Replacement garment for use with automated external defibrillator, each   ♿○
AHA: 4Q, '03, 4

☑ ☑ **K0609** Replacement electrodes for use with automated external defibrillator, garment type only, each ♿○
AHA: 4Q, '03, 4

~~**K0618** TLSO, sagittal coronal control, modular segmented spinal system, two rigid plastic shells, posterior extends from the sacrococcygeal junction and terminates just inferior to the scapular spine, anterior extends from the symphysis pubis to the xiphoid, soft liner, restricts gross trunk motion in the sagittal and coronal planes, lateral strength is provided by overlapping plastic and stabilizing closures, includes straps and closures, prefabricated, includes fitting and adjustment~~
See code(s) L0491.

~~**K0610** TLSO, sagittal coronal control, modular segmented spinal system, three rigid plastic shells, posterior extends from the sacrococcygeal junction and terminates just inferior to the scapular spine, anterior extends from the symphysis pubis to the xiphoid, soft liner, restricts gross trunk motion in the sagittal and coronal planes, lateral strength is provided by overlapping plastic and stabilizing closures, includes straps and closures, prefabricated, includes fitting and adjustment~~
See code(s) L0492.

~~**K0620** Tubular elastic dressing, any width, per linear yard~~
See code(s) A6457.

~~**K0628** For diabetics only, multiple density insert, direct formed, molded to foot after external heat source of 230 degrees fahrenheit or higher, total contact with patient's foot, including arch, base layer minimum of 1/4 in. material of Shore A 35 durometer or 3/16 in. material of Shore A 40 (or higher), prefabricated, each~~
See code(s) A5512.

~~**K0629** For diabetics only, multiple density insert, custom molded from model of patient's foot, total contact with patient's foot, including arch, base layer minimum of 3/16 in. material of Shore A 35 durometer or higher, includes arch filler and other shaping material, custom fabricated, each~~
See code(s) A5513.

~~**K0630** SO, flexible, provides pelvic sacral support, reduces motion about the sacroiliac joint, includes straps, closures, may include pendulous abdomen design, prefabricated, includes fitting and adjustment~~
See code(s) L0621.

~~**K0631** SO, flexible, provides pelvic sacral support, reduces motion about the sacroiliac joint, includes straps, closures, may include pendulous abdomen design, custom fabricated~~
See code(s) L0622.

~~**K0632** SO, provides pelvic sacral support, with rigid or semi rigid panels over the sacrum and abdomen, reduces motion about the sacroiliac joint, includes straps, closures, may include pendulous abdomen design, prefabricated, includes fitting and adjustment~~
See code(s) L0623.

~~**K0633** SO, provides pelvic sacral support, with rigid or semi rigid panels placed over the sacrum and abdomen, reduces motion about the sacroiliac joint, includes straps, closures, may include pendulous abdomen design, custom fabricated~~
See code(s) L0624.

~~**K0634** LO, flexible, provides lumbar support, posterior extends from L 1 to below L 5 vertebra, produces intracavitary pressure to reduce load on the intervertebral discs, includes straps, closures, may include pendulous abdomen design, shoulder straps, stays, prefabricated, includes fitting and adjustment~~
See code(s) L0625.

~~**K0635** LO, sagittal control, with rigid posterior panel(s), posterior extends from L 1 to below L 5 vertebrae, produces intracavitary pressure to reduce load on the intervertebral discs, includes straps, closures, may include padding, stays, shoulder straps, pendulous abdomen design, prefabricated, includes fitting and adjustment~~
See code(s) L0626.

K0636 ~~LO, sagittal control, with rigid anterior and posterior panels, posterior extends from L 1 to below L 5 vertebra, produces intracavitary pressure to reduce load on the intervertebral discs, includes straps, closures, may include padding, shoulder straps, pendulous abdomen design, prefabricated, includes fitting and adjustment~~
See code(s) L0627.

K0637 ~~LSO, flexible, provides lumbo sacral support, posterior extends from sacrococcygeal junction to T 9 vertebra, produces intracavitary pressure to reduce load on the intervertebral discs, includes straps, closures, may include stays, shoulder straps, pendulous abdomen design, prefabricated, includes fitting and adjustment~~
See code(s) L0628.

K0638 ~~LSO, flexible, provides lumbo sacral support, posterior extends from sacrococcygeal junction to T 9 vertebra, produces intracavitary pressure to reduce load on the intervertebral discs, includes straps, closures, may include stays, shoulder straps, pendulous abdomen design, custom fabricated~~
See code(s) L0629.

K0639 ~~LSO, sagittal control, with rigid posterior panel(s), posterior extends from sacrococcygeal junction to T 9 vertebra, produces intracavitary pressure to reduce load on the intervertebral discs, includes straps, closures, may include padding, stays, shoulder straps, pendulous abdomen design, prefabricated, includes fitting and adjustment~~
See code(s) L0630.

K0640 ~~LSO, sagittal control, with rigid anterior and posterior panels, posterior extends from sacrococcygeal junction to T 9 vertebra, produces intracavitary pressure to reduce load on the intervertebral disks, includes straps, closures, may include padding, shoulder straps, pendulous abdomen design, prefabricated, includes fitting and adjustment~~
See code(s) L0631.

K0641 ~~LSO, sagittal control, with rigid anterior and posterior panels, posterior extends from sacrococcygeal junction to T 9 vertebra, produces intracavitary pressure to reduce load on the intervertebral discs, includes straps, closures, may include padding, shoulder straps, pendulous abdomen design, custom fabricated~~
See code(s) L0632.

K0642 ~~LSO, sagittal coronal control, with rigid posterior frame/panel(s), posterior extends from sacrococcygeal junction to T 9 vertebra, lateral strength provided by rigid lateral frame/panels, produces intracavitary pressure to reduce load on intervertebral discs, includes straps, closures, may include padding, stays, shoulder straps, pendulous abdomen design, prefabricated, includes fitting and adjustment~~
See code(s) L0633.

K0643 ~~LSO, sagittal coronal control, with rigid posterior frame/panel(s), posterior extends from sacrococcygeal junction to T 9 vertebra, lateral strength provided by rigid lateral frame/panels, produces intracavitary pressure to reduce load on intervertebral discs, includes straps, closures, may include padding, stays, shoulder straps, pendulous abdomen design, custom fabricated~~
See code(s) L0634.

K0644 ~~LSO, sagittal coronal control, lumbar flexion, rigid posterior frame/panels, lateral articulating design to flex the lumbar spine, posterior extends from sacrococcygeal junction to T 9 vertebra, lateral strength provided by rigid lateral frame/panels, produces intracavitary pressure to reduce load on intervertebral discs, includes straps, closures, may include padding, anterior panel, pendulous abdomen design, prefabricated, includes fitting and adjustment~~
See code(s) L0635.

K0645 ~~LSO, sagittal coronal control, lumbar flexion, rigid posterior frame/panels, lateral articulating design to flex the lumbar spine, posterior extends from sacrococcygeal junction to T 9 vertebra, lateral strength provided by rigid lateral frame/panels, produces intracavitary pressure to reduce load on intervertebral discs, includes straps, closures, may include padding, anterior panel, pendulous abdomen design, custom fabricated~~
See code(s) L0636.

K0646 ~~LSO, sagittal coronal control, with rigid anterior and posterior frame/panels, posterior extends from sacrococcygeal junction to T 9 vertebra, lateral strength provided by rigid lateral frame/panels, produces intracavitary pressure to reduce load on intervertebral discs, includes straps, closures, may include padding, shoulder straps, pendulous abdomen design, prefabricated, includes fitting and adjustment~~
See code(s) L0637.

K0647 ~~LSO, sagittal coronal control, with rigid anterior and posterior frame/panels, posterior extends from sacrococcygeal junction to T 9 vertebra, lateral strength provided by rigid lateral frame/panels, produces intracavitary pressure to reduce load on intervertebral discs, includes straps, closures, may include padding, shoulder straps, pendulous abdomen design, custom fabricated~~
See code(s) L0638.

K0648 ~~LSO, sagittal coronal control, rigid shell(s)/panel(s), posterior extends from sacrococcygeal junction to T 9 vertebra, anterior extends from symphysis pubis to xiphoid, produces intracavitary pressure to reduce load on the intervertebral discs, overall strength is provided by overlapping rigid plastic and stabilizing closures, includes straps, closures, may include soft interface, pendulous abdomen design, prefabricated, includes fitting and adjustment~~
See code(s) L0639.

K0649 ~~LSO, sagittal coronal control, rigid shell(s)/panel(s), posterior extends from sacrococcygeal junction to T 9 vertebra, anterior extends from symphysis pubis to xiphoid, produces intracavitary pressure to reduce load on the intervertebral discs, overall strength is provided by overlapping rigid plastic and stabilizing closures, includes straps, closures, may include soft interface, pendulous abdomen design, custom fabricated~~
See code(s) L0640.

▲ ☑ K0669 Wheelchair accessory, wheelchair seat or back cushion, does not meet specific code criteria or no written coding verification from SADMERC

K0670 ~~Addition to lower extremity prosthesis, endoskeletal knee shin system, microprocessor control feature, stance phase only, includes electronic sensor(s), any type~~
See code(s) L5858.

Special Coverage Instructions | Noncovered by Medicare | Carrier Discretion | ☑ Quantity Alert | ● New Code | ○ Reinstated Code | ▲ Revised Code

2006 HCPCS | **1**-**9** ASC Groups | **MED:** Pub 100/NCD Reference | ♿ DMEPOS Paid | Ⓢ SNF Excluded | **K Codes — 93**

Temporary Codes

K0671 — K0732

~~K0671~~ ~~Portable oxygen concentrator, rental~~
See code(s) E1392.

● ☑   **K0730** Controlled dose inhalation drug delivery system

~~K0731~~ ~~Lithium ion battery for use with cochlear implant device speech processor, other than ear level, replacement, each~~
See code(s) L8623.

~~K0732~~ ~~Lithium ion battery for use with cochlear implant device speech processor, ear level, replacement, each~~
See code(s) L8624.

| Special Coverage Instructions | Noncovered by Medicare | Carrier Discretion | ☑ Quantity Alert | ● New Code | ○ Reinstated Code | ▲ Revised Code |

94 — K Codes   Ⓐ Age   Ⓜ Maternity   ♀ Female Only   ♂ Male Only   Ⓐ-☑ APC Status Indicator   *2006 HCPCS*

Orthotic Procedures and Devices

ORTHOTIC PROCEDURES AND DEVICES *L0000-L4999*

L codes include orthotic and prosthetic procedures and devices, as well as scoliosis equipment, orthopedic shoes, and prosthetic implants.

ORTHOTIC DEVICES — SPINAL

CERVICAL

Medicare claims for L codes fall under the jurisdiction of the DME regional contractor, unless otherwise noted.

A ☑ **L0100** Cranial orthosis (helmet), with or without soft interface, molded to patient model &

A ☑ **L0110** Cranial orthosis (helmet), with or without soft-interface, non-molded &

A **L0112** Cranial cervical orthosis, congenital torticollis type, with or without soft interface material, adjustable range of motion joint, custom fabricated &

A **L0120** Cervical, flexible, nonadjustable (foam collar) &

A **L0130** Cervical, flexible, thermoplastic collar, molded to patient &

A **L0140** Cervical, semi-rigid, adjustable (plastic collar) &

A **L0150** Cervical, semi-rigid, adjustable molded chin cup (plastic collar with mandibular/occipital piece) &

A **L0160** Cervical, semi-rigid, wire frame occipital/mandibular support &

A **L0170** Cervical, collar, molded to patient model &

A ☑ **L0172** Cervical, collar, semi-rigid thermoplastic foam, two piece &

A ☑ **L0174** Cervical, collar, semi-rigid, thermoplastic foam, two piece with thoracic extension &

MULTIPLE POST COLLAR

A **L0180** Cervical, multiple post collar, occipital/mandibular supports, adjustable &

A **L0190** Cervical, multiple post collar, occipital/mandibular supports, adjustable cervical bars (SOMI, Guilford, Taylor types) &

A **L0200** Cervical, multiple post collar, occipital/mandibular supports, adjustable cervical bars, and thoracic extension &

THORACIC

A **L0210** Thoracic, rib belt &

A **L0220** Thoracic, rib belt, custom fabricated &

L0430 Spinal orthosis, anterior-posterior-lateral control, with interface material, custom fitted (dewall posture protector only)

A **L0450** TLSO, flexible, provides trunk support, upper thoracic region, produces intracavitary pressure to reduce load on the intervertebral disks with rigid stays or panel(s), includes shoulder straps and closures, prefabricated, includes fitting and adjustment &

A **L0452** TLSO, flexible, provides trunk support, upper thoracic region, produces intracavitary pressure to reduce load on the intervertebral disks with rigid stays or panel(s), includes shoulder straps and closures, custom fabricated &

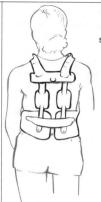

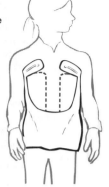

TLSO brace with adjustable straps and pads (L0450). The model at right and similar devices such as the Boston brace are molded polymer over foam and may be bivalve (front and back components)

Thoracic lumbar sacral orthosis (TLSO)

A **L0454** TLSO flexible, provides trunk support, extends from sacrococcygeal junction to above T-9 vertebra, restricts gross trunk motion in the sagittal plane, produces intracavitary pressure to reduce load on the intervertebral disks with rigid stays or panel(s), includes shoulder straps and closures, prefabricated, includes fitting and adjustment &

A **L0456** TLSO, flexible, provides trunk support, thoracic region, rigid posterior panel and soft anterior apron, extends from the sacrococcygeal junction and terminates just inferior to the scapular spine, restricts gross trunk motion in the sagittal plane, produces intracavitary pressure to reduce load on the intervertebral disks, includes straps and closures, prefabricated, includes fitting and adjustment &

A **L0458** TLSO, triplanar control, modular segmented spinal system, two rigid plastic shells, posterior extends from the sacrococcygeal junction and terminates just inferior to the scapular spine, anterior extends from the symphysis pubis to the xiphoid, soft liner, restricts gross trunk motion in the sagittal, coronal, and transverse planes, lateral strength is provided by overlapping plastic and stabilizing closures, includes straps and closures, prefabricated, includes fitting and adjustment &

A **L0460** TLSO, triplanar control, modular segmented spinal system, two rigid plastic shells, posterior extends from the sacrococcygeal junction and terminates just inferior to the scapular spine, anterior extends from the symphysis pubis to the sternal notch, soft liner, restricts gross trunk motion in the sagittal, coronal, and transverse planes, lateral strength is provided by overlapping plastic and stabilizing closures, includes straps and closures, prefabricated, includes fitting and adjustment &

A **L0462** TLSO, triplanar control, modular segmented spinal system, three rigid plastic shells, posterior extends from the sacrococcygeal junction and terminates just inferior to the scapular spine, anterior extends from the symphysis pubis to the sternal notch, soft liner, restricts gross trunk motion in the sagittal, coronal, and transverse planes, lateral strength is provided by overlapping plastic and stabilizing closures, includes straps and closures, prefabricated, includes fitting and adjustment &

L0100 — L0462

| Special Coverage Instructions | | Noncovered by Medicare | | Carrier Discretion | | ☑ Quantity Alert | ● New Code | ○ Reinstated Code | ▲ Revised Code |

2006 HCPCS | **1-9** ASC Groups | **MED:** Pub 100/NCD Reference | & DMEPOS Paid | ⃠ SNF Excluded | **L Codes — 95**

Orthotic Procedures and Devices

L0464 — L0622

Ⓐ **L0464** TLSO, triplanar control, modular segmented spinal system, four rigid plastic shells, posterior extends from sacrococcygeal junction and terminates just inferior to scapular spine, anterior extends from symphysis pubis to the sternal notch, soft liner, restricts gross trunk motion in sagittal, coronal, and transverse planes, lateral strength is provided by overlapping plastic and stabilizing closures, includes straps and closures, prefabricated, includes fitting and adjustment   ♿

Ⓐ **L0466** TLSO, sagittal control, rigid posterior frame and flexible soft anterior apron with straps, closures and padding, restricts gross trunk motion in sagittal plane, produces intracavitary pressure to reduce load on intervertebral disks, includes fitting and shaping the frame, prefabricated, includes fitting and adjustment   ♿

Ⓐ **L0468** TLSO, sagittal-coronal control, rigid posterior frame and flexible soft anterior apron with straps, closures and padding, extends from sacrococcygeal junction over scapulae, lateral strength provided by pelvic, thoracic, and lateral frame pieces, restricts gross trunk motion in sagittal, and coronal planes, produces intracavitary pressure to reduce load on intervertebral disks, includes fitting and shaping the frame, prefabricated, includes fitting and adjustment   ♿

Ⓐ **L0470** TLSO, triplanar control, rigid posterior frame and flexible soft anterior apron with straps, closures and padding, extends from sacrococcygeal junction to scapula, lateral strength provided by pelvic, thoracic, and lateral frame pieces, rotational strength provided by subclavicular extensions, restricts gross trunk motion in sagittal, coronal, and transverse planes, produces intracavitary pressure to reduce load on the intervertebral disks, includes fitting and shaping the frame, prefabricated, includes fitting and adjustment   ♿

Ⓐ **L0472** TLSO, triplanar control, hyperextension, rigid anterior and lateral frame extends from symphysis pubis to sternal notch with two anterior components (one pubic and one sternal), posterior and lateral pads with straps and closures, limits spinal flexion, restricts gross trunk motion in sagittal, coronal, and transverse planes, includes fitting and shaping the frame, prefabricated, includes fitting and adjustment   ♿

Ⓐ **L0480** TLSO, triplanar control, one piece rigid plastic shell without interface liner, with multiple straps and closures, posterior extends from sacrococcygeal junction and terminates just inferior to scapular spine, anterior extends from symphysis pubis to sternal notch, anterior or posterior opening, restricts gross trunk motion in sagittal, coronal, and transverse planes, includes a carved plaster or CAD-CAM model, custom fabricated

Ⓐ **L0482** TLSO, triplanar control, one piece rigid plastic shell with interface liner, multiple straps and closures, posterior extends from sacrococcygeal junction and terminates just inferior to scapular spine, anterior extends from symphysis pubis to sternal notch, anterior or posterior opening, restricts gross trunk motion in sagittal, coronal, and transverse planes, includes a carved plaster or CAD-CAM model, custom fabricated   ♿

Ⓐ **L0484** TLSO, triplanar control, two piece rigid plastic shell without interface liner, with multiple straps and closures, posterior extends from sacrococcygeal junction and terminates just inferior to scapular spine, anterior extends from symphysis pubis to sternal notch, lateral strength is enhanced by overlapping plastic, restricts gross trunk motion in the sagittal, coronal, and transverse planes, includes a carved plaster or CAD-CAM model, custom fabricated   ♿

Ⓐ **L0486** TLSO, triplanar control, two piece rigid plastic shell with interface liner, multiple straps and closures, posterior extends from sacrococcygeal junction and terminates just inferior to scapular spine, anterior extends from symphysis pubis to sternal notch, lateral strength is enhanced by overlapping plastic, restricts gross trunk motion in the sagittal, coronal, and transverse planes, includes a carved plaster or CAD-CAM model, custom fabricated   ♿

Ⓐ **L0488** TLSO, triplanar control, one piece rigid plastic shell with interface liner, multiple straps and closures, posterior extends from sacrococcygeal junction and terminates just inferior to scapular spine, anterior extends from symphysis pubis to sternal notch, anterior or posterior opening, restricts gross trunk motion in sagittal, coronal, and transverse planes, prefabricated, includes fitting and adjustment   ♿

Ⓐ **L0490** TLSO, sagittal-coronal control, one piece rigid plastic shell, with overlapping reinforced anterior, with multiple straps and closures, posterior extends from sacrococcygeal junction and terminates at or before the T-9 vertebra, anterior extends from symphysis pubis to xiphoid, anterior opening, restricts gross trunk motion in sagittal and coronal planes, prefabricated, includes fitting and adjustment   ♿

● Ⓐ **L0491** TLSO, sagittal-coronal control, modular segmented spinal sytem, two rigid plastic shells, posterior extends from the sacrococcygeal junction and terminates just inferior to the scapular spine, anterior extends from the symphysis pubis to the xiphoid, soft liner, restricts gross trunk motion in the sagittal and coronal planes, lateral strength is provided by overlapping plastic and stabilizing closures, includes straps and closures, prefabricated, includes fitting and adjustment

● Ⓐ **L0492** TLSO, sagittal-coronal control, modular segmented spinal system, three rigid plastic shells, posterior extends from the sacrococcygeal junction and terminates just inferior to the scapular spine, anterior extends from the symphysis pubis to the xiphoid, soft liner, restricts gross trunk motion in the sagittal and coronal planes, lateral strength is provided by overlapping plastic and stabilizing closures, includes straps and closures, prefabricated, includes fitting and adjustment

CERVICAL-THORACIC-LUMBAR-SACRAL ORTHOSIS (CTLSO)

● Ⓐ **L0621** Sacroiliac orthosis, flexible, provides pelvic-sacral support, reduces motion about the sacroiliac joint, includes straps, closures, may include pendulous abdomen design, prefabricated, includes fitting and adjustment

● Ⓐ **L0622** Sacroiliac orthosis, flexible, provides pelvic-sacral support, reduces motion about the sacroiliac joint, includes straps, closures, may include pendulous abdomen design, custom fabricated

Special Coverage Instructions   Noncovered by Medicare   Carrier Discretion   ☑ Quantity Alert   ● New Code   ○ Reinstated Code   ▲ Revised Code

96 — L Codes   Ⓐ Age   Ⓜ Maternity   ♀ Female Only   ♂ Male Only   Ⓐ-Ⓨ APC Status Indicator   **2006 HCPCS**

● Ⓐ **L0623** Sacroiliac orthosis, provides pelvic-sacral support, with rigid or semi-rigid panels over the sacrum and abdomen, reduces motion about the sacroiliac joint, includes straps, closures, may include pendulous abdomen design, prefabricated, includes fitting and adjustment

● Ⓐ **L0624** Sacroiliac orthosis, provides pelvic-sacral support, with rigid or semi-rigid panels placed over the sacrum and abdomen, reduces motion about the sacroiliac joint, includes straps, closures, may include pendulous abdomen design, custom fabricated

● Ⓐ **L0625** Lumbar orthosis, flexible, provides lumbar support, posterior extends from L-1 to below L-5 vertebra, produces intracavitary pressure to reduce load on the intervertebral discs, includes straps, closures, may include pendulous abdomen design, shoulder straps, stays, prefabricated, includes fitting and adjustment

● Ⓐ **L0626** Lumbar orthosis, sagittal control, with rigid posterior panel(s), posterior extends from L-1 to below L-5 vertebra, produces intracavitary pressure to reduce load on the intervertebral discs, includes straps, closures, may include padding, stays, shoulder straps, pendulous abdomen design, prefabricated, includes fitting and adjustment

● Ⓐ **L0627** Lumbar orthosis, sagittal control, with rigid anterior and posterior panels, posterior extends from L-1 to below L-5 vertebra, produces intracavitary pressure to reduce load on the intervertebral discs, includes straps, closures, may include padding, shoulder straps, pendulous abdomen design, prefabricated, includes fitting and adjustment

● Ⓐ **L0628** LSO, flexible, provides lumbo-sacral support, posterior extends from sacrococcygeal junction to T-9 vertebra, produces intracavitary pressure to reduce load on the intervertebral discs, includes straps, closures, may include stays, shoulder straps, pendulous abdomen design, prefabricated, includes fitting and adjustment

● Ⓐ **L0629** LSO, flexible, provides lumbo-sacral support, posterior extends from sacrococcygeal junction to T-9 vertebra, produces intracavitary pressure to reduce load on the intervertebral discs, includes straps, closures, may include stays, shoulder straps, pendulous abdomen design, custom fabricated

● Ⓐ **L0630** LSO, sagittal control, with rigid posterior panel(s), posterior extends from sacrococcygeal junction to T-9 vertebra, produces intracavitary pressure to reduce load on the intervertebral discs, includes straps, closures, may include padding, stays, shoulder straps, pendulous abdomen design, prefabricated, includes fitting and adjustment

● Ⓐ **L0631** LSO, sagittal control, with rigid anterior and posterior panels, posterior extends from sacrococcygeal junction to T-9 vertebra, produces intracavitary pressure to reduce load on the intervertebral discs, includes straps, pendulous abdomen design, prefabricated, includes fitting and adjustment

● Ⓐ **L0632** LSO, sagittal control, with rigid anterior and posterior panels, posterior extends from sacrococcygeal junction to T-9 vertebra, produces intracavitary pressure to reduce load on the intervertebral discs, includes straps, closures, may include padding, shoulder straps, pendulous abdomen design, custom fabricated

● Ⓐ **L0633** LSO, sagittal-coronal control, with rigid posterior frame/panel(s), posterior extends from sacrococcygeal junction to T-9 vertebra, lateral strength provided by rigid lateral frame/panels, produces intracavitary pressure to reduce load on intervertebral discs, includes straps, closures, may include padding, stays, shoulder straps, pendulous abdomen design, prefabricated, includes fitting and adjustment

● Ⓐ **L0634** LSO, sagittal-coronal control, with rigid posterior frame/panel(s), posterior extends from sacrococcygeal junction to T-9 vertebra, lateral strength provided by rigid lateral frame/panel(s), produces intracavitary pressure to reduce load on intervertebral discs, includes straps, closures, may include padding, stays, shoulder straps, pendulous abdomen design, custom fabricated

● Ⓐ **L0635** LSO, sagittal-coronal control, lumbar flexion, rigid posterior frame/panel(s), lateral articulating design to flex the lumbar spine, posterior extends from sacrococcygeal junction to T-9 vertebra, lateral strength provided by rigid lateral frame/panel(s), produces intracavitary pressure to reduce load on intervertebral discs, includes straps, closures, may include padding, anterior panel, pendulous abdomen design, prefabricated, includes fitting and adjustment

● Ⓐ **L0636** LSO, sagittal-coronal control, lumbar flexion, rigid posterior frame/panels, lateral articulating design to flex the lumbar spine, posterior extends from sacrococcygeal junction to T-9 vertebra, lateral strength provided by rigid lateral frame/panels, produces intracavitary pressure to reduce load on intervertebral discs, includes straps, closures, may include padding, anterior panel, pendulous abdomen design, custom fabricated

● Ⓐ **L0637** LSO, sagittal-coronal control, with rigid anterior and posterior frame/panels, posterior extends from sacrococcygeal junction to T-9 vertebra, lateral strength provided by rigid lateral frame/panels, produces intracavitary pressure to reduce load on intervertebral discs, includes straps, closures, may include padding, shoulder straps, pendulous abdomen design, prefabricated, includes fitting and adjustment

● Ⓐ **L0638** LSO, sagittal-coronal control, with rigid anterior and posterior frame/panels, posterior extends from sacrococcygeal junction to T-9 vertebra, lateral strength provided by rigid lateral frame/panels, produces intracavitary pressure to reduce load on intervertebral discs, includes straps, closures, may include padding, shoulder straps, pendulous abdomen design, custom fabricated

● Ⓐ **L0639** LSO, sagittal-coronal control, rigid shell(s)/panel(s), posterior extends from sacrococcygeal junction to T-9 vertebra, anterior extends from symphysis pubis to xyphoid, produces intracavitary pressure to reduce load on the intervertebral discs, overall strength is provided by overlapping rigid material and stabilizing closures, includes straps, closures, may include soft interface, pendulous abdomen design, prefabricated, includes fitting and adjustment

---

Special Coverage Instructions　　　Noncovered by Medicare　　　Carrier Discretion　　　☑ Quantity Alert　　● New Code　　○ Reinstated Code　　▲ Revised Code

2006 HCPCS　　　**1**-**9** ASC Groups　　**MED:** Pub 100/NCD Reference　　🗄 DMEPOS Paid　　⊘ SNF Excluded　　**L Codes — 97**

● Ⓐ **L0640** LSO, sagittal-coronal control, rigid shell(s)/panel(s), posterior extends from sacrococcygeal junction to T-9 vertebra, anterior extends from symphysis pubis to xyphoid, produces intracavitary pressure to reduce load on the intervertebral discs, overall strength is provided by overlapping rigid material and stabilizing closures, includes straps, closures, may include soft interface, pendulous abdomen design, custom fabricated

ANTERIOR-POSTERIOR-LATERAL CONTROL

Ⓐ **L0700** CTLSO, anterior-posterior-lateral control, molded to patient model (Minerva type) ♿

Ⓐ **L0710** CTLSO, anterior-posterior-lateral control, molded to patient model, with interface material (Minerva type) ♿

HALO PROCEDURE

Ⓐ **L0810** Halo procedure, cervical halo incorporated into jacket vest ♿

Ⓐ **L0820** Halo procedure, cervical halo incorporated into plaster body jacket ♿

Ⓐ **L0830** Halo procedure, cervical halo incorporated into Milwaukee type orthosis ♿

● Ⓐ **L0859** Addition to halo procedure, magnetic resonance image compatible systems, rings and pins, any material

~~**L0860** Addition to halo procedure, magnetic resonance image compatible system~~
See code(s) L0859.

Ⓐ **L0861** Addition to halo procedure, replacement liner/interface material ♿

Ⓔ **L0960** Torso support, postsurgical support, pads for postsurgical support ♿

ADDITIONS TO SPINAL ORTHOSIS

Ⓐ **L0970** TLSO, corset front ♿

Ⓐ **L0972** LSO, corset front ♿

Ⓐ **L0974** TLSO, full corset ♿

Ⓐ **L0976** LSO, full corset ♿

Ⓐ **L0978** Axillary crutch extension ♿

Ⓐ ☑ **L0980** Peroneal straps, pair ♿

Ⓐ ☑ **L0982** Stocking supporter grips, set of four (4) ♿

Ⓐ ☑ **L0984** Protective body sock, each ♿

Ⓐ **L0999** Addition to spinal orthosis, NOS
Determine if an alternative HCPCS Level II or a CPT code better describes the service being reported. This code should be used only if a more specific code is unavailable.

ORTHOTIC DEVICES — SCOLIOSIS PROCEDURES

The orthotic care of scoliosis differs from other orthotic care in that the treatment is more dynamic in nature and uses continual modification of the orthosis to the patient's changing condition. This coding structure uses the proper names — or eponyms — of the procedures because they have historic and universal acceptance in the profession. It should be recognized that variations to the basic procedures described by the founders/developers are accepted in various medical and orthotic practices throughout the country. All procedures include model of patient when indicated.

CERVICAL-THORACIC-LUMBAR-SACRAL ORTHOSIS (CTLSO)

Ⓐ **L1000** CTLSO (Milwaukee), inclusive of furnishing initial orthosis, including model ♿

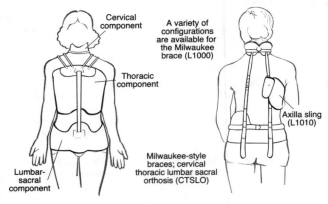

Cervical component

A variety of configurations are available for the Milwaukee brace (L1000)

Thoracic component

Axilla sling (L1010)

Milwaukee-style braces; cervical thoracic lumbar sacral orthosis (CTSLO)

Lumbar-sacral component

Ⓐ **L1005** Tension based scoliosis orthosis and accessory pads, includes fitting and adjustment ♿

Ⓐ **L1010** Addition to CTLSO or scoliosis orthosis, axilla sling ♿

Ⓐ **L1020** Addition to CTLSO or scoliosis orthosis, kyphosis pad ♿

Ⓐ **L1025** Addition to CTLSO or scoliosis orthosis, kyphosis pad, floating ♿

Ⓐ **L1030** Addition to CTLSO or scoliosis orthosis, lumbar bolster pad ♿

Ⓐ **L1040** Addition to CTLSO or scoliosis orthosis, lumbar or lumbar rib pad ♿

Ⓐ **L1050** Addition to CTLSO or scoliosis orthosis, sternal pad ♿

Ⓐ **L1060** Addition to CTLSO or scoliosis orthosis, thoracic pad ♿

Ⓐ **L1070** Addition to CTLSO or scoliosis orthosis, trapezius sling ♿

Ⓐ **L1080** Addition to CTLSO or scoliosis orthosis, outrigger ♿

Ⓐ **L1085** Addition to CTLSO or scoliosis orthosis, outrigger, bilateral with vertical extensions ♿

Ⓐ **L1090** Addition to CTLSO or scoliosis orthosis, lumbar sling ♿

Ⓐ **L1100** Addition to CTLSO or scoliosis orthosis, ring flange, plastic or leather ♿

Ⓐ **L1110** Addition to CTLSO or scoliosis orthosis, ring flange, plastic or leather, molded to patient model ♿

Ⓐ ☑ **L1120** Addition to CTLSO, scoliosis orthosis, cover for upright, each ♿

THORACIC-LUMBAR-SACRAL ORTHOSIS (TLSO) (LOW PROFILE)

Ⓐ **L1200** TLSO, inclusive of furnishing initial orthosis only ♿

Ⓐ **L1210** Addition to TLSO, (low profile), lateral thoracic extension ♿

Ⓐ **L1220** Addition to TLSO, (low profile), anterior thoracic extension ♿

Ⓐ **L1230** Addition to TLSO, (low profile), Milwaukee type superstructure ♿

Ⓐ **L1240** Addition to TLSO, (low profile), lumbar derotation pad ♿

Ⓐ **L1250** Addition to TLSO, (low profile), anterior ASIS pad ♿

Ⓐ **L1260** Addition to TLSO, (low profile), anterior thoracic derotation pad ♿

Ⓐ **L1270** Addition to TLSO, (low profile), abdominal pad ♿

Special Coverage Instructions | Noncovered by Medicare | Carrier Discretion | ☑ Quantity Alert ● New Code ○ Reinstated Code ▲ Revised Code

98 — L Codes | Ⓐ Age | Ⓜ Maternity | ♀ Female Only | ♂ Male Only | Ⓐ-Ⓨ APC Status Indicator | *2006 HCPCS*

Ⓐ ☑ **L1280** Addition to TLSO, (low profile), rib gusset (elastic), each ♿

Ⓐ **L1290** Addition to TLSO, (low profile), lateral trochanteric pad ♿

OTHER SCOLIOSIS PROCEDURES

Ⓐ **L1300** Other scoliosis procedure, body jacket molded to patient model ♿

Ⓐ **L1310** Other scoliosis procedure, postoperative body jacket ♿

Ⓐ **L1499** Spinal orthosis, not otherwise specified
Determine if an alternative HCPCS Level II or a CPT code better describes the service being reported. This code should be used only if a more specific code is unavailable.

THORACIC-HIP-KNEE-ANKLE ORTHOSIS (THKAO)

Ⓐ **L1500** THKAO, mobility frame (Newington, Parapodium types) ♿

Ⓐ **L1510** THKAO, standing frame, with or without tray and accessories ♿

Ⓐ **L1520** THKAO, swivel walker ♿

ORTHOTIC DEVICES — LOWER LIMB

The procedures in L1600-L2999 are considered as "base" or "basic procedures" and may be modified by listing procedure from the "additions" sections and adding them to the base procedures.

HIP ORTHOSIS (HO) — FLEXIBLE

Ⓐ **L1600** HO, abduction control of hip joints, flexible, Frejka type with cover, prefabricated, includes fitting and adjustment ♿

Ⓐ **L1610** HO, abduction control of hip joints, flexible, (Frejka cover only), prefabricated, includes fitting and adjustment ♿

Ⓐ **L1620** HO, abduction control of hip joints, flexible, (Pavlik harness), prefabricated, includes fitting and adjustment ♿

Ⓐ **L1630** HO, abduction control of hip joints, semi-flexible (Von Rosen type), custom fabricated ♿

Ⓐ **L1640** HO, abduction control of hip joints, static, pelvic band or spreader bar, thigh cuffs, custom fabricated ♿

Ⓐ **L1650** HO, abduction control of hip joints, static, adjustable (Ilfled type), prefabricated, includes fitting and adjustment ♿

Ⓐ **L1652** HO, bilateral thigh cuffs with adjustable abductor spreader bar, adult size, prefabricated, includes fitting and adjustment, any type ♿

Ⓐ **L1660** HO, abduction control of hip joints, static, plastic, prefabricated, includes fitting and adjustment ♿

Ⓐ **L1680** HO, abduction control of hip joints, dynamic, pelvic control, adjustable hip motion control, thigh cuffs (Rancho hip action type), custom fabricated ♿

Ⓐ **L1685** HO, abduction control of hip joint, postoperative hip abduction type, custom fabricated ♿

Ⓐ **L1686** HO, abduction control of hip joint, postoperative hip abduction type, prefabricated, includes fitting and adjustments ♿

Ⓐ **L1690** Combination, bilateral, lumbo-sacral, hip, femur orthosis providing adduction and internal rotation control, prefabricated, includes fitting and adjustment ♿

LEGG PERTHES

Ⓐ **L1700** Legg Perthes orthosis, (Toronto type), custom fabricated ♿

Ⓐ **L1710** Legg Perthes orthosis, (Newington type), custom fabricated ♿

Ⓐ **L1720** Legg Perthes orthosis, trilateral, (Tachdijan type), custom fabricated ♿

Ⓐ **L1730** Legg Perthes orthosis, (Scottish Rite type), custom fabricated ♿

~~**L1750** Legg Perthes orthosis, Legg Perthes sling (Sam Brown type), prefabricated, includes fitting and adjustment~~
See code(s) A4565.

Ⓐ **L1755** Legg Perthes orthosis, (Patten bottom type), custom fabricated ♿

KNEE ORTHOSIS (KO)

Ⓐ **L1800** KO, elastic with stays, prefabricated, includes fitting and adjustment ♿

Ⓐ **L1810** KO, elastic with joints, prefabricated, includes fitting and adjustment ♿

Ⓐ **L1815** KO, elastic or other elastic type material with condylar pad(s), prefabricated, includes fitting and adjustment ♿

Ⓐ **L1820** KO, elastic with condylar pads and joints, with or without patellar control, prefabricated, includes fitting and adjustment ♿

Ⓐ **L1825** KO, elastic knee cap, prefabricated, includes fitting and adjustment ♿

Ⓐ **L1830** KO, immobilizer, canvas longitudinal, prefabricated, includes fitting and adjustment ♿

Ⓐ **L1831** KO, locking knee joint(s), positional orthosis, prefabricated, includes fitting and adjustment ♿

▲ Ⓐ **L1832** Knee orthosis, adjustable knee joints (unicentric or polycentric), positional orthosis, rigid support, prefabricated, includes fitting and adjustment ♿

Ⓐ **L1834** KO, without knee joint, rigid, custom fabricated ♿

Ⓐ **L1836** KO, rigid, without joint(s), includes soft interface material, prefabricated, includes fitting and adjustment ♿

Ⓐ **L1840** KO, derotation, medial-lateral, anterior cruciate ligament, custom fabricated ♿

▲ Ⓐ **L1843** Knee orthosis, single upright, thigh and calf, with adjustable flexion and extension joint (unicentric or polycentric), medial-lateral and rotation control, with or without varus/valgus adjustment, prefabricated, includes fitting and adjustment ♿

▲ Ⓐ **L1844** Knee orthosis, single upright, thigh and calf, with adjustable flexion and extension joint (unicentric or polycentric), medial-lateral and rotation control, with or without varus/valgus adjustment, custom fabricated ♿

▲ Ⓐ **L1845** Knee orthosis, double upright, thigh and calf, with adjustable flexion and extension joint (unicentric or polycentric), medial-lateral and rotation control, with or without varus/valgus adjustment, prefabricated, includes fitting and adjustment ♿

▲ Ⓐ **L1846** Knee orthosis, double upright, thigh and calf, with adjustable flexion and extension joint (unicentric or polycentric), medial-lateral and rotation control, with or without varus/valgus adjustment, custom fabricated ♿

| Special Coverage Instructions | Noncovered by Medicare | Carrier Discretion | ☑ Quantity Alert | ● New Code | ○ Reinstated Code | ▲ Revised Code |

2006 HCPCS   **1**-**9** ASC Groups   MED: Pub 100/NCD Reference   ♿ DMEPOS Paid   ⊘ SNF Excluded   **L Codes — 99**

Ⓐ **L1847** KO, double upright with adjustable joint, with inflatable air support chamber(s), prefabricated, includes fitting and adjustment ৬

Ⓐ **L1850** KO, Swedish type, prefabricated, includes fitting and adjustment ৬

Ⓐ **L1855** KO, molded plastic, thigh and calf sections, with double upright knee joints, custom fabricated ৬

Ⓐ **L1858** KO, molded plastic, polycentric knee joints, pneumatic knee pads (CTI), custom fabricated ৬

Ⓐ **L1860** KO, modification of supracondylar prosthetic socket, custom fabricated (SK) ৬

Ⓐ **L1870** KO, double upright, thigh and calf lacers, with knee joints, custom fabricated ৬

Ⓐ **L1880** KO, double upright, nonmolded thigh and calf cuffs/lacers with knee joints, custom fabricated ৬

ANKLE-FOOT ORTHOSIS (AFO)

Ⓐ **L1900** AFO, spring wire, dorsiflexion assist calf band, custom fabricated ৬

Ⓐ **L1901** Ankle orthosis, elastic, prefabricated, includes fitting and adjustment (e.g., neoprene, Lycra) ৬

Ⓐ **L1902** AFO, ankle gauntlet, prefabricated, includes fitting and adjustment ৬

Ⓐ **L1904** AFO, molded ankle gauntlet, custom fabricated ৬

Ⓐ **L1906** AFO, multiligamentous ankle support, prefabricated, includes fitting and adjustment ৬

Ⓐ **L1907** AFO, supramalleolar with straps, with or without interface/pads, custom fabricated ৬

Ⓐ **L1910** AFO, posterior, single bar, clasp attachment to shoe counter, prefabricated, includes fitting and adjustment ৬

Ⓐ **L1920** AFO, single upright with static or adjustable stop (Phelps or Perlstein type), custom fabricated ৬

Ⓐ **L1930** AFO, plastic or other material, prefabricated, includes fitting and adjustment ৬

L1932 AFO, rigid anterior tibial section, total carbon fiber or equal material, prefabricated, includes fitting and adjustment

Ⓐ **L1940** AFO, plastic or other material, custom-fabricated ৬

Ⓐ **L1945** AFO, molded to patient model, plastic, rigid anterior tibial section (floor reaction), custom fabricated ৬

Ⓐ **L1950** AFO, spiral, (Institute of Rehabilitative Medicine type), plastic, custom-fabricated ৬

Ⓐ **L1951** AFO, spiral, (Institute of Rehabilitative Medicine type), plastic or other material, prefabricated, includes fitting and adjustment ৬

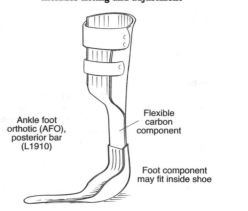

Ankle foot orthotic (AFO), posterior bar (L1910)

Flexible carbon component

Foot component may fit inside shoe

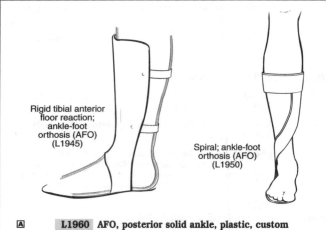

Rigid tibial anterior floor reaction; ankle-foot orthosis (AFO) (L1945)

Spiral; ankle-foot orthosis (AFO) (L1950)

Ⓐ **L1960** AFO, posterior solid ankle, plastic, custom fabricated ৬

Ⓐ **L1970** AFO, plastic, with ankle joint, custom fabricated ৬

Ⓐ **L1971** AFO, plastic or other material with ankle joint, prefabricated, includes fitting and adjustment ৬

Ⓐ **L1980** AFO, single upright free plantar dorsiflexion, solid stirrup, calf band/cuff (single bar BK orthosis), custom fabricated ৬

Ⓐ **L1990** AFO, double upright free plantar dorsiflexion, solid stirrup, calf band/cuff (double bar BK orthosis), custom fabricated ৬

KNEE-ANKLE-FOOT ORTHOSIS (KAFO) — OR ANY COMBINATION

Ⓐ **L2000** KAFO, single upright, free knee, free ankle, solid stirrup, thigh and calf bands/cuffs (single bar AK orthosis), custom fabricated ৬

L2005 KAFO, any material, single or double upright, stance control, automatic lock and swing phase release, mechanical activation, includes ankle joint, any type, custom fabricated

Ⓐ **L2010** KAFO, single upright, free ankle, solid stirrup, thigh and calf bands/cuffs (single bar AK orthosis), without knee joint, custom fabricated ৬

Ⓐ **L2020** KAFO, double upright, free knee, free ankle, solid stirrup, thigh and calf bands/cuffs (double bar AK orthosis), custom fabricated ৬

Ⓐ **L2030** KAFO, double upright, free ankle, solid stirrup, thigh and calf bands/cuffs, (double bar AK orthosis), without knee joint, custom fabricated ৬

● **L2034** KAFO, full plastic, single upright, with or without free motion knee, medial lateral rotation control, with or without free motion ankle, custom fabricated

Ⓐ **L2035** KAFO, full plastic, static (pediatric size), without free motion ankle, prefabricated, includes fitting and adjustment ৬

▲ Ⓐ **L2036** KAFO, full plastic, double upright, with or without free motion knee, with or without free motion ankle, custom fabricated ৬

▲ Ⓐ **L2037** Knee ankle foot orthosis, full plastic, single upright, with or without free motion knee, with or without free motion ankle, custom fabricated ৬

▲ Ⓐ **L2038** Knee ankle foot orthosis, full plastic, with or without free motion knee, multi-axis ankle, custom fabKnee ankle foot orthosis, full plastic, with or without free motion knee, multi-axis ankle, custom fabricated ৬

Special Coverage Instructions　　　Noncovered by Medicare　　　Carrier Discretion　　☑ Quantity Alert　● New Code　○ Reinstated Code　▲ Revised Code

100 — L Codes　　Ⓐ Age　　Ⓜ Maternity　　♀ Female Only　　♂ Male Only　　Ⓐ-Y APC Status Indicator　　***2006 HCPCS***

L2039 KAFO, full plastic, single-upright, poly-axial hinge, medial-lateral rotation control, with or without free motion ankle, custom fabricated

TORSION CONTROL: HIP-KNEE-ANKLE-FOOT ORTHOSIS (HKAFO)

Ⓐ **L2040** HKAFO, torsion control, bilateral rotation straps, pelvic band/belt, custom fabricated ⴟ

Ⓐ **L2050** HKAFO, torsion control, bilateral torsion cables, hip joint, pelvic band/belt, custom fabricated ⴟ

Ⓐ **L2060** HKAFO, torsion control, bilateral torsion cables, ball bearing hip joint, pelvic band/ belt, custom fabricated ⴟ

Ⓐ **L2070** HKAFO, torsion control, unilateral rotation straps, pelvic band/belt, custom fabricated ⴟ

Ⓐ **L2080** HKAFO, torsion control, unilateral torsion cable, hip joint, pelvic band/belt, custom fabricated ⴟ

Ⓐ **L2090** HKAFO, torsion control, unilateral torsion cable, ball bearing hip joint, pelvic band/belt, custom fabricated ⴟ

Ⓐ **L2106** AFO, fracture orthosis, tibial fracture cast orthosis, thermoplastic type casting material, custom fabricated ⴟ

Ⓐ **L2108** AFO, fracture orthosis, tibial fracture cast orthosis, custom fabricated ⴟ

Ⓐ **L2112** AFO, fracture orthosis, tibial fracture orthosis, soft, prefabricated, includes fitting and adjustment ⴟ

Ⓐ **L2114** AFO, fracture orthosis, tibial fracture orthosis, semi-rigid, prefabricated, includes fitting and adjustment ⴟ

Ⓐ **L2116** AFO, fracture orthosis, tibial fracture orthosis, rigid, prefabricated, includes fitting and adjustment ⴟ

Ⓐ **L2126** KAFO, fracture orthosis, femoral fracture cast orthosis, thermoplastic type casting material, custom fabricated ⴟ

Ⓐ **L2128** KAFO, fracture orthosis, femoral fracture cast orthosis, custom fabricated ⴟ

Ⓐ **L2132** KAFO, fracture orthosis, femoral fracture cast orthosis, soft, prefabricated, includes fitting and adjustment ⴟ

Ⓐ **L2134** KAFO, fracture orthosis, femoral fracture cast orthosis, semi-rigid, prefabricated, includes fitting and adjustment ⴟ

Ⓐ **L2136** KAFO, fracture orthosis, femoral fracture cast orthosis, rigid, prefabricated, includes fitting and adjustment ⴟ

ADDITIONS TO FRACTURE ORTHOSIS

Ⓐ **L2180** Addition to lower extremity fracture orthosis, plastic shoe insert with ankle joints ⴟ

Ⓐ **L2182** Addition to lower extremity fracture orthosis, drop lock knee joint ⴟ

Ⓐ **L2184** Addition to lower extremity fracture orthosis, limited motion knee joint ⴟ

Ⓐ **L2186** Addition to lower extremity fracture orthosis, adjustable motion knee joint, Lerman type ⴟ

Ⓐ **L2188** Addition to lower extremity fracture orthosis, quadrilateral brim ⴟ

Ⓐ **L2190** Addition to lower extremity fracture orthosis, waist belt ⴟ

Ⓐ **L2192** Addition to lower extremity fracture orthosis, hip joint, pelvic band, thigh flange, and pelvic belt ⴟ

ADDITIONS TO LOWER EXTREMITY ORTHOSIS: SHOE-ANKLE-SHIN-KNEE

Ⓐ ☑ **L2200** Addition to lower extremity, limited ankle motion, each joint ⴟ

Ⓐ ☑ **L2210** Addition to lower extremity, dorsiflexion assist (plantar flexion resist), each joint ⴟ

Ⓐ ☑ **L2220** Addition to lower extremity, dorsiflexion and plantar flexion assist/resist, each joint ⴟ

Ⓐ **L2230** Addition to lower extremity, split flat caliper stirrups and plate attachment ⴟ

L2232 Addition to lower extremity orthosis, rocker bottom for total contact ankle foot orthosis, for custom fabricated orthosis only

Ⓐ **L2240** Addition to lower extremity, round caliper and plate attachment ⴟ

Ⓐ **L2250** Addition to lower extremity, foot plate, molded to patient model, stirrup attachment ⴟ

Ⓐ **L2260** Addition to lower extremity, reinforced solid stirrup (Scott-Craig type) ⴟ

Ⓐ **L2265** Addition to lower extremity, long tongue stirrup ⴟ

Ⓐ **L2270** Addition to lower extremity, varus/valgus correction (T) strap, padded/lined or malleolus pad ⴟ

Ⓐ **L2275** Addition to lower extremity, varus/valgus correction, plastic modification, padded/lined ⴟ

Ⓐ **L2280** Addition to lower extremity, molded inner boot ⴟ

Ⓐ **L2300** Addition to lower extremity, abduction bar (bilateral hip involvement), jointed, adjustable ⴟ

Ⓐ **L2310** Addition to lower extremity, abduction bar, straight ⴟ

Ⓐ **L2320** Addition to lower extremity, non-molded lacer, for custom fabricated orthosis only ⴟ

Ⓐ **L2330** Addition to lower extremity, lacer molded to patient model, for custom fabricated orthosis only ⴟ

Ⓐ **L2335** Addition to lower extremity, anterior swing band ⴟ

Ⓐ **L2340** Addition to lower extremity, pretibial shell, molded to patient model ⴟ

Ⓐ **L2350** Addition to lower extremity, prosthetic type, (BK) socket, molded to patient model, (used for PTB, AFO orthoses) ⴟ

Ⓐ **L2360** Addition to lower extremity, extended steel shank ⴟ

Ⓐ **L2370** Addition to lower extremity, Patten bottom ⴟ

Ⓐ **L2375** Addition to lower extremity, torsion control, ankle joint and half solid stirrup ⴟ

Ⓐ ☑ **L2380** Addition to lower extremity, torsion control, straight knee joint, each joint ⴟ

Ⓐ ☑ **L2385** Addition to lower extremity, straight knee joint, heavy duty, each joint ⴟ

● **L2387** Addition to lower extremity, polycentric knee joint, for custom fabricated knee ankle foot orthosis, each joint

Ⓐ ☑ **L2390** Addition to lower extremity, offset knee joint, each joint ⴟ

Ⓐ ☑ **L2395** Addition to lower extremity, offset knee joint, heavy duty, each joint ⴟ

Ⓐ **L2397** Addition to lower extremity orthosis, suspension sleeve ⴟ

ADDITIONS TO STRAIGHT KNEE OR OFFSET KNEE JOINTS

▲ Ⓐ ☑ **L2405** Addition to knee joint, drop lock, each ⴟ

| Special Coverage Instructions | Noncovered by Medicare | Carrier Discretion | ☑ Quantity Alert | ● New Code | ○ Reinstated Code | ▲ Revised Code |

2006 HCPCS   **1**-**9** ASC Groups   MED: Pub 100/NCD Reference   ⴟ DMEPOS Paid   ⊘ SNF Excluded   **L Codes — 101**

Orthotic Procedures and Devices

L2415 — L3010

Ⓐ ☑ **L2415** Addition to knee lock with integrated release mechanism (bail, cable, or equal), any material, each joint

Ⓐ ☑ **L2425** Addition to knee joint, disc or dial lock for adjustable knee flexion, each joint

Ⓐ ☑ **L2430** Addition to knee joint, ratchet lock for active and progressive knee extension, each joint

Ⓐ **L2492** Addition to knee joint, lift loop for drop lock ring

ADDITIONS: THIGH/WEIGHT BEARING — GLUTEAL/ISCHIAL WEIGHT BEARING

Ⓐ **L2500** Addition to lower extremity, thigh/weight bearing, gluteal/ischial weight bearing, ring

Ⓐ **L2510** Addition to lower extremity, thigh/weight bearing, quadri-lateral brim, molded to patient model

Ⓐ **L2520** Addition to lower extremity, thigh/weight bearing, quadri-lateral brim, custom fitted

Ⓐ **L2525** Addition to lower extremity, thigh/weight bearing, ischial containment/narrow M-L brim molded to patient model

Ⓐ **L2526** Addition to lower extremity, thigh/weight bearing, ischial containment/narrow M-L brim, custom fitted

Ⓐ **L2530** Addition to lower extremity, thigh/weight bearing, lacer, nonmolded

Ⓐ **L2540** Addition to lower extremity, thigh/weight bearing, lacer, molded to patient model

Ⓐ **L2550** Addition to lower extremity, thigh/weight bearing, high roll cuff

ADDITIONS: PELVIC AND THORACIC CONTROL

Ⓐ ☑ **L2570** Addition to lower extremity, pelvic control, hip joint, Clevis type, two position joint, each

Ⓐ **L2580** Addition to lower extremity, pelvic control, pelvic sling

Ⓐ ☑ **L2600** Addition to lower extremity, pelvic control, hip joint, Clevis type, or thrust bearing, free, each

Ⓐ ☑ **L2610** Addition to lower extremity, pelvic control, hip joint, Clevis or thrust bearing, lock, each

Ⓐ ☑ **L2620** Addition to lower extremity, pelvic control, hip joint, heavy-duty, each

Ⓐ ☑ **L2622** Addition to lower extremity, pelvic control, hip joint, adjustable flexion, each

Ⓐ ☑ **L2624** Addition to lower extremity, pelvic control, hip joint, adjustable flexion, extension, abduction control, each

Ⓐ **L2627** Addition to lower extremity, pelvic control, plastic, molded to patient model, reciprocating hip joint and cables

Ⓐ **L2628** Addition to lower extremity, pelvic control, metal frame, reciprocating hip joint and cables

Ⓐ **L2630** Addition to lower extremity, pelvic control, band and belt, unilateral

Ⓐ **L2640** Addition to lower extremity, pelvic control, band and belt, bilateral

Ⓐ ☑ **L2650** Addition to lower extremity, pelvic and thoracic control, gluteal pad, each

Ⓐ **L2660** Addition to lower extremity, thoracic control, thoracic band

Ⓐ **L2670** Addition to lower extremity, thoracic control, paraspinal uprights

Ⓐ **L2680** Addition to lower extremity, thoracic control, lateral support uprights

ADDITIONS: GENERAL

Ⓐ ☑ **L2750** Addition to lower extremity orthosis, plating chrome or nickel, per bar

Ⓐ **L2755** Addition to lower extremity orthosis, high strength, lightweight material, all hybrid lamination/prepreg composite, per segment, for custom fabricated orthosis only

Ⓐ ☑ **L2760** Addition to lower extremity orthosis, extension, per extension, per bar (for lineal adjustment for growth)

Ⓐ ☑ **L2768** Orthotic side bar disconnect device, per bar

Ⓐ ☑ **L2770** Addition to lower extremity orthosis, any material, per bar or joint

Ⓐ ☑ **L2780** Addition to lower extremity orthosis, noncorrosive finish, per bar

Ⓐ ☑ **L2785** Addition to lower extremity orthosis, drop lock retainer, each

Ⓐ **L2795** Addition to lower extremity orthosis, knee control, full kneecap

Ⓐ **L2800** Addition to lower extremity orthosis, knee control, knee cap, medial or lateral pull, for use with custom fabricated orthosis only

Ⓐ **L2810** Addition to lower extremity orthosis, knee control, condylar pad

Ⓐ **L2820** Addition to lower extremity orthosis, soft interface for molded plastic, below knee section

Ⓐ **L2830** Addition to lower extremity orthosis, soft interface for molded plastic, above knee section

Ⓐ ☑ **L2840** Addition to lower extremity orthosis, tibial length sock, fracture or equal, each

Ⓐ ☑ **L2850** Addition to lower extremity orthosis, femoral length sock, fracture or equal, each

Ⓐ ☑ **L2860** Addition to lower extremity joint, knee or ankle, concentric adjustable torsion style mechanism, each

Ⓐ **L2999** Lower extremity orthoses, NOS
Determine if an alternative HCPCS Level II or a CPT code better describes the service being reported. This code should be used only if a more specific code is unavailable.

ORTHOPEDIC SHOES

INSERTS

Ⓑ ☑ **L3000** Foot insert, removable, molded to patient model, UCB type, Berkeley shell, each
MED: 100-2, 15, 290

Ⓑ ☑ **L3001** Foot insert, removable, molded to patient model, Spenco, each
MED: 100-2, 15, 290

Ⓑ ☑ **L3002** Foot insert, removable, molded to patient model, Plastazote or equal, each
MED: 100-2, 15, 290

Ⓑ ☑ **L3003** Foot insert, removable, molded to patient model, silicone gel, each
MED: 100-2, 15, 290

Ⓑ ☑ **L3010** Foot insert, removable, molded to patient model, longitudinal arch support, each
MED: 100-2, 15, 290

Orthotic Procedures and Devices

L3020 — L3251

| B | ☑ | **L3020** | Foot insert, removable, molded to patient model, longitudinal/metatarsal support, each
MED: 100-2, 15, 290 | ⊘ |

| B | ☑ | **L3030** | Foot insert, removable, formed to patient foot, each
MED: 100-2, 15, 290 | ⊘ |

| E | ☑ | **L3031** | Foot, insert/plate, removable, addition to lower extremity orthosis, high strength, lightweight material, all hybrid lamination/prepreg composite, each | ⊘ |

ARCH SUPPORT, REMOVABLE, PREMOLDED

| B | ☑ | **L3040** | Foot, arch support, removable, premolded, longitudinal, each
MED: 100-2, 15, 290 | ⊘ |

| B | ☑ | **L3050** | Foot, arch support, removable, premolded, metatarsal, each
MED: 100-2, 15, 290 | ⊘ |

| B | ☑ | **L3060** | Foot, arch support, removable, premolded, longitudinal/metatarsal, each
MED: 100-2, 15, 290 | ⊘ |

ARCH SUPPORT, NONREMOVABLE, ATTACHED TO SHOE

| B | ☑ | **L3070** | Foot, arch support, nonremovable, attached to shoe, longitudinal, each
MED: 100-2, 15, 290 | ⊘ |

| B | ☑ | **L3080** | Foot, arch support, nonremovable, attached to shoe, metatarsal, each
MED: 100-2, 15, 290 | ⊘ |

| B | ☑ | **L3090** | Foot, arch support, nonremovable, attached to shoe, longitudinal/metatarsal, each
MED: 100-2, 15, 290 | ⊘ |

| B | | **L3100** | Hallus-valgus night dynamic splint
MED: 100-2, 15, 290 | ⊘ |

ABDUCTION AND ROTATION BARS

| B | | **L3140** | Foot, abduction rotation bar, including shoes
MED: 100-2, 15, 290 | ⊘ |

| B | | **L3150** | Foot, abduction rotation bar, without shoes
MED: 100-2, 15, 290 | ⊘ |

| B | | **L3160** | Foot, adjustable shoe-styled positioning device | ⊘ |

| ▲ A | | **L3170** | Foot, plastic, silicone or equal, heel stabilizer, each
MED: 100-2, 15, 290 | ᵭ⊘ |

A Denis-Browne style splint is a bar that can be applied by strapping or mounted on a shoe. This type of splint generally corrects congenital conditions such as genu varus

Denis-Browne splint

The angle may be adjusted on a plate on the sole of the shoe

ORTHOPEDIC FOOTWEAR

| B | | **L3201** | Orthopedic shoe, Oxford with supinator or pronator, infant
MED: 100-2, 15, 290 | A ⊘ |

| B | | **L3202** | Orthopedic shoe, Oxford with supinator or pronator, child
MED: 100-2, 15, 290 | A ⊘ |

| B | | **L3203** | Orthopedic shoe, Oxford with supinator or pronator, junior
MED: 100-2, 15, 290 | A ⊘ |

| B | | **L3204** | Orthopedic shoe, hightop with supinator or pronator, infant
MED: 100-2, 15, 290 | A ⊘ |

| B | | **L3206** | Orthopedic shoe, hightop with supinator or pronator, child
MED: 100-2, 15, 290 | A ⊘ |

| B | | **L3207** | Orthopedic shoe, hightop with supinator or pronator, junior
MED: 100-2, 15, 290 | A ⊘ |

| B | ☑ | **L3208** | Surgical boot, each, infant
MED: 100-2, 15, 100 | A ⊘ |

| B | ☑ | **L3209** | Surgical boot, each, child
MED: 100-2, 15, 100 | A ⊘ |

| B | ☑ | **L3211** | Surgical boot, each, junior
MED: 100-2, 15, 100 | A ⊘ |

| B | ☑ | **L3212** | Benesch boot, pair, infant
MED: 100-2, 15, 100 | A ⊘ |

| B | ☑ | **L3213** | Benesch boot, pair, child
MED: 100-2, 15, 100 | A ⊘ |

| B | ☑ | **L3214** | Benesch boot, pair, junior
MED: 100-2, 15, 100 | A ⊘ |

| ▲ A | | **L3215** | Orthopedic footwear, ladies shoe, oxford, each | A ♀ ⊘ |

| ▲ A | | **L3216** | Orthopedic footwear, ladies shoe, depth inlay, each | A ♀ ⊘ |

| ▲ A | | **L3217** | Orthopedic footwear, ladies shoe, hightop, depth inlay, each | A ♀ ⊘ |

| ▲ A | | **L3219** | Orthopedic footwear, mens shoe, oxford, each | A ♂ ⊘ |

| ▲ A | | **L3221** | Orthopedic footwear, mens shoe, depth inlay, each | A ♂ ⊘ |

| ▲ A | | **L3222** | Orthopedic footwear, mens shoe, hightop, depth inlay, each | A ♂ ⊘ |

| A | | **L3224** | Orthopedic footwear, woman's shoe, Oxford, used as an integral part of a brace (orthosis)
MED: 100-2, 15, 290 | ♀ ᵭ |

| A | | **L3225** | Orthopedic footwear, man's shoe, Oxford, used as an integral part of a brace (orthosis)
MED: 100-2, 15, 290 | ♂ ᵭ |

| ▲ A | | **L3230** | Orthopedic footwear, custom shoe, depth inlay, each
MED: 100-2, 15, 290 | ⊘ |

| B | ☑ | **L3250** | Orthopedic footwear, custom molded shoe, removable inner mold, prosthetic shoe, each
MED: 100-2, 15, 290 | ⊘ |

| B | ☑ | **L3251** | Foot, shoe molded to patient model, silicone shoe, each
MED: 100-2, 15, 290 | ⊘ |

| Special Coverage Instructions | Noncovered by Medicare | Carrier Discretion | ☑ Quantity Alert | ● New Code | ○ Reinstated Code | ▲ Revised Code |

2006 HCPCS   **1**-**9** ASC Groups   **MED:** Pub 100/NCD Reference   ᵭ DMEPOS Paid   ⊘ SNF Excluded   **L Codes — 103**

Orthotic Procedures and Devices

L3252 — L3630

B ☑ **L3252** Foot, shoe molded to patient model, Plastazote (or similar), custom fabricated, each ⊘
MED: 100-2, 15, 290

B ☑ **L3253** Foot, molded shoe Plastazote (or similar), custom fitted, each ⊘
MED: 100-2, 15, 290

B **L3254** Nonstandard size or width ⊘
MED: 100-2, 15, 290

B **L3255** Nonstandard size or length ⊘
MED: 100-2, 15, 290

B **L3257** Orthopedic footwear, additional charge for split size ⊘
MED: 100-2, 15, 290

B ☑ **L3260** Surgical boot/shoe, each ⊘
MED: 100-2, 15, 100

B ☑ **L3265** Plastazote sandal, each ⊘

SHOE MODIFICATION — LIFTS

B ☑ **L3300** Lift, elevation, heel, tapered to metatarsals, per inch ⊘
MED: 100-2, 15, 290

B ☑ **L3310** Lift, elevation, heel and sole, neoprene, per inch ⊘
MED: 100-2, 15, 290

B ☑ **L3320** Lift, elevation, heel and sole, cork, per inch ⊘
MED: 100-2, 15, 290

B **L3330** Lift, elevation, metal extension (skate) ⊘

B ☑ **L3332** Lift, elevation, inside shoe, tapered, up to one-half inch ⊘
MED: 100-2, 15, 290

B ☑ **L3334** Lift, elevation, heel, per inch ⊘
MED: 100-2, 15, 290

SHOE MODIFICATION — WEDGES

B **L3340** Heel wedge, SACH ⊘
MED: 100-2, 15, 290

B **L3350** Heel wedge ⊘
MED: 100-2, 15, 290

B **L3360** Sole wedge, outside sole ⊘
MED: 100-2, 15, 290

B **L3370** Sole wedge, between sole ⊘
MED: 100-2, 15, 290

B **L3380** Clubfoot wedge ⊘
MED: 100-2, 15, 290

B **L3390** Outflare wedge ⊘
MED: 100-2, 15, 290

B **L3400** Metatarsal bar wedge, rocker ⊘
MED: 100-2, 15, 290

B **L3410** Metatarsal bar wedge, between sole ⊘
MED: 100-2, 15, 290

B **L3420** Full sole and heel wedge, between sole ⊘
MED: 100-2, 15, 290

SHOE MODIFICATIONS — HEELS

B **L3430** Heel, counter, plastic reinforced ⊘
MED: 100-2, 15, 290

B **L3440** Heel, counter, leather reinforced ⊘
MED: 100-2, 15, 290

B **L3450** Heel, SACH cushion type ⊘
MED: 100-2, 15, 290

B **L3455** Heel, new leather, standard ⊘
MED: 100-2, 15, 290

B **L3460** Heel, new rubber, standard ⊘
MED: 100-2, 15, 290

B **L3465** Heel, Thomas with wedge ⊘
MED: 100-2, 15, 290

B **L3470** Heel, Thomas extended to ball ⊘
MED: 100-2, 15, 290

B **L3480** Heel, pad and depression for spur ⊘
MED: 100-2, 15, 290

B **L3485** Heel, pad, removable for spur ⊘
MED: 100-2, 15, 290

MISCELLANEOUS SHOE ADDITIONS

B **L3500** Orthopedic shoe addition, insole, leather ⊘
MED: 100-2, 15, 290

B **L3510** Orthopedic shoe addition, insole, rubber ⊘
MED: 100-2, 15, 290

B **L3520** Orthopedic shoe addition, insole, felt covered with leather ⊘
MED: 100-2, 15, 290

B **L3530** Orthopedic shoe addition, sole, half ⊘
MED: 100-2, 15, 290

B **L3540** Orthopedic shoe addition, sole, full ⊘
MED: 100-2, 15, 290

B **L3550** Orthopedic shoe addition, toe tap, standard
MED: 100-2, 15, 290

B **L3560** Orthopedic shoe addition, toe tap, horseshoe
MED: 100-2, 15, 290

B **L3570** Orthopedic shoe addition, special extension to instep (leather with eyelets)
MED: 100-2, 15, 290

B **L3580** Orthopedic shoe addition, convert instep to Velcro closure
MED: 100-2, 15, 290

B **L3590** Orthopedic shoe addition, convert firm shoe counter to soft counter
MED: 100-2, 15, 290

B **L3595** Orthopedic shoe addition, March bar
MED: 100-2, 15, 290

TRANSFER OR REPLACEMENT

B **L3600** Transfer of an orthosis from one shoe to another, caliper plate, existing
MED: 100-2, 15, 290

B **L3610** Transfer of an orthosis from one shoe to another, caliper plate, new
MED: 100-2, 15, 290

B **L3620** Transfer of an orthosis from one shoe to another, solid stirrup, existing
MED: 100-2, 15, 290

B **L3630** Transfer of an orthosis from one shoe to another, solid stirrup, new
MED: 100-2, 15, 290

Special Coverage Instructions   Noncovered by Medicare   Carrier Discretion   ☑ Quantity Alert   ● New Code   ○ Reinstated Code   ▲ Revised Code

104 — L Codes   A Age   M Maternity   ♀ Female Only   ♂ Male Only   A-Y APC Status Indicator   *2006 HCPCS*

| B | L3640 | Transfer of an orthosis from one shoe to another, Dennis Browne splint (Riveton), both shoes
MED: 100-2, 15, 290 |

| B | L3649 | Orthopedic shoe, modification, addition or transfer, NOS
Determine if an alternative HCPCS Level II or a CPT code better describes the service being reported. This code should be used only if a more specific code is unavailable.
MED: 100-2, 15, 290 |

ORTHOTIC DEVICES — UPPER LIMB

The procedures in this section are considered as "base" or "basic procedures" and may be modified by listing procedures from the "additions" sections and adding them to the base procedure.

SHOULDER ORTHOSIS (SO)

A	L3650	SO, figure of eight design abduction restrainer, prefabricated, includes fitting and adjustment 🦽
A	L3651	SO, single shoulder, elastic, prefabricated, includes fitting and adjustment (e.g., neoprene, Lycra) 🦽
A	L3652	SO, double shoulder, elastic, prefabricated, includes fitting and adjustment (e.g., neoprene, Lycra) 🦽
A	L3660	SO, figure of eight design abduction restrainer, canvas and webbing, prefabricated, includes fitting and adjustment 🦽
A	L3670	SO, acromio/clavicular (canvas and webbing type), prefabricated, includes fitting and adjustment 🦽
● A	L3671	SO, shoulder cap design, without joints, may include soft interface, straps, custom fabricated, includes fitting and adjustment
● A	L3672	SO, abduction positioning (airplane design), thoracic component and support bar, without joints, may inlcude soft interface, straps, custom fabricated, includes fitting and adjustment
● A	L3673	Shoulder orthosis, abduction positioning (airplane design), thoracic component and support bar, includes nontorsion joint/turnbuckle, may include soft interface, straps, custom fabricated, includes fitting and adjustment
A	L3675	SO, vest type abduction restrainer, canvas webbing type, or equal, prefabricated, includes fitting and adjustment 🦽
E	L3677	SO, hard plastic, shoulder stabilizer, prefabricated, includes fitting and adjustment MED: 100-2, 15, 120

ELBOW ORTHOSIS (EO)

A	L3700	EO, elastic with stays, prefabricated, includes fitting and adjustment 🦽
A	L3701	EO, elastic, prefabricated, includes fitting and adjustment (e.g., neoprene, Lycra) 🦽
● A	L3702	Elbow orthosis, without joints, may include soft interface, straps, custom fabricated, includes fitting and adjustment
A	L3710	EO, elastic with metal joints, prefabricated, includes fitting and adjustment 🦽
A	L3720	EO, double upright with forearm/arm cuffs, free motion, custom fabricated 🦽
A	L3730	EO, double upright with forearm/arm cuffs, extension/flexion assist, custom fabricated 🦽
A	L3740	EO, double upright with forearm/arm cuffs, adjustable position lock with active control, custom fabricated 🦽

A	L3760	EO, with adjustable position locking joint(s), prefabricated, includes fitting and adjustments, any type 🦽
A	L3762	EO, rigid, without joints, includes soft interface material, prefabricated, includes fitting and adjustment 🦽
● A	L3763	EWHO, rigid, without joints, may include soft interface, straps, custom fabricated, includes fitting and adjustment
● A	L3764	EWHO, includes one or more nontorsion joints, elastic bands, turnbuckles, may include soft interface, straps, custom fabricated, includes fitting and adjustment
● A	L3765	EWHFO, rigid, without joints, may include soft interface, straps, custom fabricated, includes fitting and adjustment
● A	L3766	EWHFO, includes one or more nontorsion joints, elastic bands, turnbuckles, may include soft interface, straps, custom fabricated, includes fitting and adjustment

WRIST-HAND-FINGER ORTHOSIS (WHFO)

A	L3800	WHFO, short opponens, no attachments, custom fabricated 🦽
A	L3805	WHFO, long opponens, no attachment, custom fabricated 🦽
A	L3807	WHFO, without joint(s), prefabricated, includes fitting and adjustments, any type 🦽

ADDITIONS

A	L3810	WHFO, addition to short and long opponens, thumb abduction (C) bar 🦽
A	L3815	WHFO, addition to short and long opponens, second M.P. abduction assist 🦽
A	L3820	WHFO, addition to short and long opponens, I.P. extension assist, with M.P. extension stop 🦽
A	L3825	WHFO, addition to short and long opponens, M.P. extension stop 🦽
A	L3830	WHFO, addition to short and long opponens, M.P. extension assist 🦽
A	L3835	WHFO, addition to short and long opponens, M.P. spring extension assist 🦽
A	L3840	WHFO, addition to short and long opponens, spring swivel thumb 🦽
A	L3845	WHFO, addition to short and long opponens, thumb I.P. extension assist, with M.P. stop 🦽
A	L3850	WHFO, addition to short and long opponens, action wrist, with dorsiflexion assist 🦽
A	L3855	WHFO, addition to short and long opponens, adjustable M.P. flexion control 🦽
A	L3860	WHFO, addition to short and long opponens, adjustable M.P. flexion control and I.P. 🦽
B	L3890	Addition to upper extremity joint, wrist or elbow, concentric adjustable torsion style mechanism, each

DYNAMIC FLEXOR HINGE, RECIPROCAL WRIST EXTENSION/FLEXION, FINGER FLEXION/EXTENSION

| A | L3900 | WHFO, dynamic flexor hinge, reciprocal wrist extension/flexion, finger flexion/extension, wrist or finger driven, custom fabricated 🦽 |

Special Coverage Instructions　　　Noncovered by Medicare　　　Carrier Discretion　　　☑ Quantity Alert　　● New Code　　○ Reinstated Code　　▲ Revised Code

2006 HCPCS　　　1-9 ASC Groups　　　MED: Pub 100/NCD Reference　　🦽 DMEPOS Paid　　⊘ SNF Excluded　　**L Codes — 105**

A L3901 WHFO, dynamic flexor hinge, reciprocal wrist extension/flexion, finger flexion/extension, cable driven, custom fabricated

EXTERNAL POWER

E L3902 WHFO, external powered, compressed gas, custom fabricated

A L3904 WHFO, external powered, electric, custom fabricated

OTHER WHFOS — CUSTOM FITTED

● A L3905 WHO, includes one or more nontorsion joints, elastic bands, turnbuckles, may include soft interface, straps, custom fabricated, includes fitting and adjustment

▲ A L3906 WHO, without joints, may include soft interface, straps, custom fabricated, includes fitting and adjustment

A L3907 WHFO, wrist gauntlet with thumb spica, molded to patient model, custom fabricated

A L3908 WHO, wrist extension control cock-up, nonmolded, prefabricated, includes fitting and adjustment

A L3909 WO, elastic, prefabricated, includes fitting and adjustment (e.g., neoprene, Lycra)

A L3910 WHFO, Swanson design, prefabricated, includes fitting and adjustment

A L3911 WHFO, elastic, prefabricated, includes fitting and adjustment (e.g., neoprene, Lycra)

A L3912 HFO, flexion glove with elastic finger control, prefabricated, includes fitting and adjustment

● A L3913 HFO, without joints, may include soft interface, straps, custom fabricated, includes fitting and adjustment

A L3914 WHO, wrist extension cock-up, prefabricated, includes fitting and adjustment

A L3916 WHFO, wrist extension cock-up, with outrigger, prefabricated, includes fitting and adjustment

A L3917 HO, metacarpal fracture orthosis, prefabricated, includes fitting and adjustment

A L3918 HFO, knuckle bender, prefabricated, includes fitting and adjustment

● A L3919 Hand orthosis, without joints, may include soft interface, straps, custom fabricated, includes fitting and adjustment

A L3920 HFO, knuckle bender, with outrigger, prefabricated, includes fitting and adjustment

● A L3921 HFO, includes one or more nontorsion joints, elastic bands, turnbuckles, may include soft interface, straps, custom fabricated, includes fitting and adjustment

A L3922 HFO, knuckle bender, two segment to flex joints, prefabricated, includes fitting and adjustment

▲ A L3923 HFO, without joints, may include soft interface, straps, prefabricated, includes fitting and adjustment

A L3924 WHFO, Oppenheimer, prefabricated, includes fitting and adjustment

A L3926 WHFO, Thomas suspension, prefabricated, includes fitting and adjustment

A L3928 HFO, finger extension, with clock spring, prefabricated, includes fitting and adjustment

A L3930 WHFO, finger extension, with wrist support, prefabricated, includes fitting and adjustment

A L3932 FO, safety pin, spring wire, prefabricated, includes fitting and adjustment

● A L3933 Finger orthosis, without joints, may include soft interface, custom fabricated, includes fitting and adjustment

A L3934 FO, safety pin, modified, prefabricated, includes fitting and adjustment

● A L3935 Finger orthosis, nontorsion joint, may include soft interface, custom fabricated, includes fitting and adjustment

A L3936 WHFO, Palmer, prefabricated, includes fitting and adjustment

A L3938 WHFO, dorsal wrist, prefabricated, includes fitting and adjustment

A L3940 WHFO, dorsal wrist, with outrigger attachment, prefabricated, includes fitting and adjustment

A L3942 HFO, reverse knuckle bender, prefabricated, includes fitting and adjustment

A L3944 HFO, reverse knuckle bender, with outrigger, prefabricated, includes fitting and adjustment

A L3946 HFO, composite elastic, prefabricated, includes fitting and adjustment

A L3948 FO, finger knuckle bender, prefabricated, includes fitting and adjustment

A L3950 WHFO, combination Oppenheimer, with knuckle bender and two attachments, prefabricated, includes fitting and adjustment

A L3952 WHFO, combination Oppenheimer, with reverse knuckle and two attachments, prefabricated, includes fitting and adjustment

A L3954 HFO, spreading hand, prefabricated, includes fitting and adjustment

A ☑ L3956 Addition of joint to upper extremity orthosis, any material; per joint

SHOULDER-ELBOW-WRIST-HAND ORTHOSIS (SEWHO)

ABDUCTION POSITION, CUSTOM FITTED

A L3960 SEWHO, abduction positioning, airplane design, prefabricated, includes fitting and adjustment

● A L3961 SEWHO, shoulder cap design, without joints, may include soft interface, straps, custom fabricated, includes fitting and adjustment

A L3962 SEWHO, abduction positioning, Erb's palsy design, prefabricated, includes fitting and adjustment

~~L3963~~ ~~SEWHO, molded shoulder, arm, forearm, and wrist, with articulating elbow joint, custom fabricated~~
See code(s) L3963.

Y L3964 SEO, mobile arm support attached to wheelchair, balanced, adjustable, prefabricated, includes fitting and adjustment

Y L3965 SEO, mobile arm support attached to wheelchair, balanced, adjustable Rancho type, prefabricated, includes fitting and adjustment

Y L3966 SEO, mobile arm support attached to wheelchair, balanced, reclining, prefabricated, includes fitting and adjustment

Special Coverage Instructions | Noncovered by Medicare | Carrier Discretion | ☑ Quantity Alert | ● New Code | ○ Reinstated Code | ▲ Revised Code

106 — L Codes | A Age | M Maternity | ♀ Female Only | ♂ Male Only | A-Y APC Status Indicator | 2006 HCPCS

● Ⓐ   **L3967**   SEWHO, abduction positioning (airplane design), thoracic component and support bar, without joints, may include soft interface, straps, custom fabricated, includes fitting and adjustment

Ⓨ   **L3968**   SEO, mobile arm support attached to wheelchair, balanced, friction arm support (friction dampening to proximal and distal joints), prefabricated, includes fitting and adjustment   ઠ

Ⓨ   **L3969**   SEO, mobile arm support, monosuspension arm and hand support, overhead elbow forearm hand sling support, yoke type arm suspension support, prefabricated, includes fitting and adjustment   ઠ

ADDITIONS TO MOBILE ARM SUPPORTS

Ⓨ   **L3970**   SEO, addition to mobile arm support, elevating proximal arm   ઠ

● Ⓐ   **L3971**   SEWHO, shoulder cap design, includes one or more nontorsion joints, elastic bands, turnbuckles, may include soft interface, straps, custom fabricated, includes fitting and adjustment

Ⓨ   **L3972**   SEO, addition to mobile arm support, offset or lateral rocker arm with elastic balance control   ઠ

● Ⓐ   **L3973**   SEWHO, abduction positioning (airplane design), thoracic component and support bar, includes one or more nontorsion joints, elastic bands, turnbuckles, may include soft interface, straps, custom fabricated, includes fitting and adjustment

Ⓨ   **L3974**   SEO, addition to mobile arm support, supinator   ઠ

● Ⓐ   **L3975**   SEWHFO, shoulder cap design, without joints, may include soft interface, straps, custom fabricated, includes fitting and adjustment

● Ⓐ   **L3976**   SEWHFO, abduction positioning (airplane design), thoracic component and support bar, without joints, may include soft interface, straps, custom fabricated, includes fitting and adjustment

● Ⓐ   **L3977**   SEWHFO, shoulder cap design, includes one or more nontorsion joints, elastic bands, turnbuckles, may include soft interface, straps, custom fabricated, includes fitting and adjustment

● Ⓐ   **L3978**   SEWHFO, abduction positioning (airplane design), thoracic component and support bar, includes one or more nontorsion joints, elastic bands, turnbuckles, may include soft interface, straps, custom fabricated, includes fitting and adjustment

FRACTURE ORTHOSIS

Ⓐ   **L3980**   Upper extremity fracture orthosis, humeral, prefabricated, includes fitting and adjustment   ઠ

Ⓐ   **L3982**   Upper extremity fracture orthosis, radius/ulnar, prefabricated, includes fitting and adjustment   ઠ

Ⓐ   **L3984**   Upper extremity fracture orthosis, wrist, prefabricated, includes fitting and adjustment   ઠ

Ⓐ   **L3985**   Upper extremity fracture orthosis, forearm, hand with wrist hinge, custom fabricated

Ⓐ   **L3986**   Upper extremity fracture orthosis, combination of humeral, radius/ulnar, wrist (example: Colles' fracture), custom fabricated   ઠ

Ⓐ   **L3995**   Addition to upper extremity orthosis, sock, fracture or equal, each   ઠ

Ⓐ   **L3999**   Upper limb orthosis, NOS

SPECIFIC REPAIR

Ⓐ   **L4000**   Replace girdle for spinal orthosis (CTLSO or SO)   ઠ

Ⓐ   **L4002**   Replacement strap, any orthosis, includes all components, any length, any type

Ⓐ   **L4010**   Replace trilateral socket brim   ઠ

Ⓐ   **L4020**   Replace quadrilateral socket brim, molded to patient model   ઠ

Ⓐ   **L4030**   Replace quadrilateral socket brim, custom fitted ઠ

Ⓐ   **L4040**   Replace molded thigh lacer, for custom fabricated orthosis only   ઠ

Ⓐ   **L4045**   Replace non-molded thigh lacer, for custom fabricated orthosis only   ઠ

Ⓐ   **L4050**   Replace molded calf lacer, for custom fabricated orthosis only   ઠ

Ⓐ   **L4055**   Replace non-molded calf lacer, for custom fabricated orthosis only   ઠ

Ⓐ   **L4060**   Replace high roll cuff   ઠ

Ⓐ   **L4070**   Replace proximal and distal upright for KAFO   ઠ

Ⓐ   **L4080**   Replace metal bands KAFO, proximal thigh   ઠ

Ⓐ   **L4090**   Replace metal bands KAFO-AFO, calf or distal thigh   ઠ

Ⓐ   **L4100**   Replace leather cuff KAFO, proximal thigh   ઠ

Ⓐ   **L4110**   Replace leather cuff KAFO-AFO, calf or distal thigh   ઠ

Ⓐ   **L4130**   Replace pretibial shell   ઠ

REPAIRS

Ⓐ   ☑   **L4205**   Repair of orthotic device, labor component, per 15 minutes
MED: 100-2, 15, 110.2

Ⓐ   **L4210**   Repair of orthotic device, repair or replace minor parts
MED: 100-2, 15, 110.2; 100-2, 15, 120; 100-2, 15, 120

Ⓐ   **L4350**   Ankle control orthosis, stirrup style, rigid, includes any type interface (e.g., pneumatic, gel), prefabricated, includes fitting and adjustment   ઠ

Ⓐ   **L4360**   Walking boot, pneumatic, with or without joints, with or without interface material, prefabricated, includes fitting and adjustment   ઠ

Ⓐ   **L4370**   Pneumatic full leg splint, prefabricated, includes fitting and adjustment   ઠ

Ⓐ   **L4380**   Pneumatic knee splint, prefabricated, includes fitting and adjustment   ઠ

Ⓐ   **L4386**   Walking boot, non-pneumatic, with or without joints, with or without interface material, prefabricated, includes fitting and adjustment   ઠ

Ⓐ   **L4392**   Replacement soft interface material, static AFO ઠ

Ⓐ   **L4394**   Replace soft interface material, foot drop splint ઠ

Ⓐ   **L4396**   Static ankle foot orthosis, including soft interface material, adjustable for fit, for positioning, pressure reduction, may be used for minimal ambulation, prefabricated, includes fitting and adjustment   ઠ

Ⓐ   **L4398**   Foot drop splint, recumbent positioning device, prefabricated, includes fitting and adjustment   ઠ

| Special Coverage Instructions | Noncovered by Medicare | Carrier Discretion | ☑ Quantity Alert | ● New Code | ○ Reinstated Code | ▲ Revised Code |

2006 HCPCS   1-9 ASC Groups   MED: Pub 100/NCD Reference   ઠ DMEPOS Paid   ⊘ SNF Excluded   **L Codes — 107**

Prosthetic Procedures

L5000 — L5520

PROSTHETIC PROCEDURES *L5000-L9999*

LOWER LIMB

The procedures in this section are considered as "base" or "basic procedures" and may be modified by listing items/procedures or special materials from the "additions" sections and adding them to the base procedure.

PARTIAL FOOT

Ⓐ   **L5000** Partial foot, shoe insert with longitudinal arch, toe filler
       MED: 100-2, 15, 290

Ⓐ   **L5010** Partial foot, molded socket, ankle height, with toe filler
       MED: 100-2, 15, 290

Ⓐ   **L5020** Partial foot, molded socket, tibial tubercle height, with toe filler
       MED: 100-2, 15, 290

ANKLE

Ⓐ   **L5050** Ankle, Symes, molded socket, SACH foot

Ⓐ   **L5060** Ankle, Symes, metal frame, molded leather socket, articulated ankle/foot

BELOW KNEE

Ⓐ   **L5100** Below knee, molded socket, shin, SACH foot

Ⓐ   **L5105** Below knee, plastic socket, joints and thigh lacer, SACH foot

KNEE DISARTICULATION

Ⓐ   **L5150** Knee disarticulation (or through knee), molded socket, external knee joints, shin, SACH foot

Ⓐ   **L5160** Knee disarticulation (or through knee), molded socket, bent knee configuration, external knee joints, shin, SACH foot

ABOVE KNEE

Ⓐ   **L5200** Above knee, molded socket, single axis constant friction knee, shin, SACH foot

Ⓐ ☑ **L5210** Above knee, short prosthesis, no knee joint (stubbies), with foot blocks, no ankle joints, each

Ⓐ ☑ **L5220** Above knee, short prosthesis, no knee joint (stubbies), with articulated ankle/foot, dynamically aligned, each

Ⓐ   **L5230** Above knee, for proximal femoral focal deficiency, constant friction knee, shin, SACH foot

HIP DISARTICULATION

Ⓐ   **L5250** Hip disarticulation, Canadian type; molded socket, hip joint, single axis constant friction knee, shin, SACH foot

Ⓐ   **L5270** Hip disarticulation, tilt table type; molded socket, locking hip joint, single axis constant friction knee, shin, SACH foot

HEMIPELVECTOMY

Ⓐ   **L5280** Hemipelvectomy, Canadian type; molded socket, hip joint, single axis constant friction knee, shin, SACH foot

Ⓐ   **L5301** Below knee, molded socket, shin, SACH foot, endoskeletal system

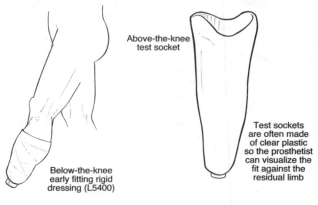

Above-the-knee test socket

Test sockets are often made of clear plastic so the prosthetist can visualize the fit against the residual limb

Below-the-knee early fitting rigid dressing (L5400)

Ⓐ   **L5311** Knee disarticulation (or through knee), molded socket, external knee joints, shin, SACH foot, endoskeletal system

Ⓐ   **L5321** Above knee, molded socket, open end, SACH foot, endoskeletal system, single axis knee

Ⓐ   **L5331** Hip disarticulation, Canadian type, molded socket, endoskeletal system, hip joint, single axis knee, SACH foot

Ⓐ   **L5341** Hemipelvectomy, Canadian type, molded socket, endoskeletal system, hip joint, single axis knee, SACH foot

IMMEDIATE POSTSURGICAL OR EARLY FITTING PROCEDURES

Ⓐ ☑ **L5400** Immediate postsurgical or early fitting, application of initial rigid dressing, including fitting, alignment, suspension, and one cast change, below knee

Ⓐ ☑ **L5410** Immediate postsurgical or early fitting, application of initial rigid dressing, including fitting, alignment and suspension, below knee, each additional cast change and realignment

Ⓐ ☑ **L5420** Immediate postsurgical or early fitting, application of initial rigid dressing, including fitting, alignment and suspension and one cast change AK or knee disarticulation

Ⓐ ☑ **L5430** Immediate postsurgical or early fitting, application of initial rigid dressing, including fitting, alignment and suspension, AK or knee disarticulation, each additional cast change and realignment

Ⓐ   **L5450** Immediate postsurgical or early fitting, application of nonweight bearing rigid dressing, below knee

Ⓐ   **L5460** Immediate postsurgical or early fitting, application of nonweight bearing rigid dressing, above knee

INITIAL PROSTHESIS

Ⓐ   **L5500** Initial, below knee PTB type socket, non-alignable system, pylon, no cover, SACH foot, plaster socket, direct formed

Ⓐ   **L5505** Initial, above knee — knee disarticulation, ischial level socket, non-alignable system, pylon, no cover, SACH foot plaster socket, direct formed

PREPARATORY PROSTHESIS

Ⓐ   **L5510** Preparatory, below knee PTB type socket, non-alignable system, pylon, no cover, SACH foot, plaster socket, molded to model

Ⓐ   **L5520** Preparatory, below knee PTB type socket, non-alignable system, pylon, no cover, SACH foot, thermoplastic or equal, direct formed

Special Coverage Instructions   Noncovered by Medicare   Carrier Discretion   ☑ Quantity Alert   ● New Code   ○ Reinstated Code   ▲ Revised Code

108 — L Codes   Ⓐ Age   Ⓜ Maternity   ♀ Female Only   ♂ Male Only   Ⓐ-Ⓨ APC Status Indicator   *2006 HCPCS*

Ⓐ   **L5530**   Preparatory, below knee PTB type socket, non-alignable system, pylon, no cover, SACH foot, thermoplastic or equal, molded to model   ႕

Ⓐ   **L5535**   Preparatory, below knee PTB type socket, non-alignable system, pylon, no cover, SACH foot, prefabricated, adjustable open end socket   ႕

Ⓐ   **L5540**   Preparatory, below knee PTB type socket, non-alignable system, pylon, no cover, SACH foot, laminated socket, molded to model   ႕

Ⓐ   **L5560**   Preparatory, above knee — knee disarticulation, ischial level socket, non-alignable system, pylon, no cover, SACH foot, plaster socket, molded to model ႕

Ⓐ   **L5570**   Preparatory, above knee — knee disarticulation, ischial level socket, non-alignable system, pylon, no cover, SACH foot, thermoplastic or equal, direct formed   ႕

Ⓐ   **L5580**   Preparatory, above knee — knee disarticulation, ischial level socket, non-alignable system, pylon, no cover, SACH foot, thermoplastic or equal, molded to model   ႕

Ⓐ   **L5585**   Preparatory, above knee — knee disarticulation, ischial level socket, non-alignable system, pylon, no cover, SACH foot, prefabricated adjustable open end socket   ႕

Ⓐ   **L5590**   Preparatory, above knee — knee disarticulation, ischial level socket, non-alignable system, pylon, no cover, SACH foot, laminated socket, molded to model   ႕

Ⓐ   **L5595**   Preparatory, hip disarticulation — hemipelvectomy, pylon, no cover, SACH foot, thermoplastic or equal, molded to patient model   ႕

Ⓐ   **L5600**   Preparatory, hip disarticulation — hemipelvectomy, pylon, no cover, SACH foot, laminated socket, molded to patient model   ႕

ADDITIONS: LOWER EXTREMITY

Ⓐ   **L5610**   Addition to lower extremity, endoskeletal system, above knee, hydracadence system   ႕

Ⓐ   **L5611**   Addition to lower extremity, endoskeletal system, above knee — knee disarticulation, 4-bar linkage, with friction swing phase control   ႕

Ⓐ   **L5613**   Addition to lower extremity, endoskeletal system, above knee — knee disarticulation, 4-bar linkage, with hydraulic swing phase control   ႕

Ⓐ   **L5614**   Addition to lower extremity, endoskeletal system, above knee — knee disarticulation, 4-bar linkage, with pneumatic swing phase control   ႕

Ⓐ   **L5616**   Addition to lower extremity, endoskeletal system, above knee, universal multiplex system, friction swing phase control   ႕

Ⓐ ☑   **L5617**   Addition to lower extremity, quick change self-aligning unit, above or below knee, each   ႕

ADDITIONS: TEST SOCKETS

Ⓐ   **L5618**   Addition to lower extremity, test socket, Symes ႕

Ⓐ   **L5620**   Addition to lower extremity, test socket, below knee   ႕

Ⓐ   **L5622**   Addition to lower extremity, test socket, knee disarticulation   ႕

Ⓐ   **L5624**   Addition to lower extremity, test socket, above knee   ႕

Ⓐ   **L5626**   Addition to lower extremity, test socket, hip disarticulation   ႕

Ⓐ   **L5628**   Addition to lower extremity, test socket, hemipelvectomy   ႕

Ⓐ   **L5629**   Addition to lower extremity, below knee, acrylic socket   ႕

ADDITIONS: SOCKET VARIATIONS

Ⓐ   **L5630**   Addition to lower extremity, Symes type, expandable wall socket   ႕

Ⓐ   **L5631**   Addition to lower extremity, above knee or knee disarticulation, acrylic socket   ႕

Ⓐ   **L5632**   Addition to lower extremity, Symes type, PTB brim design socket   ႕

Ⓐ   **L5634**   Addition to lower extremity, Symes type, posterior opening (Canadian) socket   ႕

Ⓐ   **L5636**   Addition to lower extremity, Symes type, medial opening socket   ႕

Ⓐ   **L5637**   Addition to lower extremity, below knee, total contact   ႕

Ⓐ   **L5638**   Addition to lower extremity, below knee, leather socket   ႕

Ⓐ   **L5639**   Addition to lower extremity, below knee, wood socket   ႕

Ⓐ   **L5640**   Addition to lower extremity, knee disarticulation, leather socket   ႕

Ⓐ   **L5642**   Addition to lower extremity, above knee, leather socket   ႕

Ⓐ   **L5643**   Addition to lower extremity, hip disarticulation, flexible inner socket, external frame   ႕

Ⓐ   **L5644**   Addition to lower extremity, above knee, wood socket   ႕

Ⓐ   **L5645**   Addition to lower extremity, below knee, flexible inner socket, external frame   ႕

Ⓐ   **L5646**   Addition to lower extremity, below knee, air, fluid, gel or equal, cushion socket   ႕

Ⓐ   **L5647**   Addition to lower extremity, below knee, suction socket   ႕

Ⓐ   **L5648**   Addition to lower extremity, above knee, air, fluid, gel or equal, cushion socket   ႕

Ⓐ   **L5649**   Addition to lower extremity, ischial containment/narrow M-L socket   ႕

Ⓐ   **L5650**   Addition to lower extremity, total contact, above knee or knee disarticulation socket   ႕

Ⓐ   **L5651**   Addition to lower extremity, above knee, flexible inner socket, external frame   ႕

Ⓐ   **L5652**   Addition to lower extremity, suction suspension, above knee or knee disarticulation socket   ႕

Ⓐ   **L5653**   Addition to lower extremity, knee disarticulation, expandable wall socket   ႕

ADDITIONS: SOCKET INSERT AND SUSPENSION

Ⓐ   **L5654**   Addition to lower extremity, socket insert, Symes (Kemblo, Pelite, Aliplast, Plastazote or equal)   ႕

Ⓐ   **L5655**   Addition to lower extremity, socket insert, below knee (Kemblo, Pelite, Aliplast, Plastazote or equal) ႕

Ⓐ   **L5656**   Addition to lower extremity, socket insert, knee disarticulation (Kemblo, Pelite, Aliplast, Plastazote or equal)   ႕

Ⓐ   **L5658**   Addition to lower extremity, socket insert, above knee (Kemblo, Pelite, Aliplast, Plastazote or equal) ႕

Ⓐ   **L5661**   Addition to lower extremity, socket insert, multidurometer, Symes   ႕

Special Coverage Instructions	Noncovered by Medicare	Carrier Discretion	☑ Quantity Alert	● New Code	○ Reinstated Code	▲ Revised Code

Prosthetic Procedures

L5665 — L5726

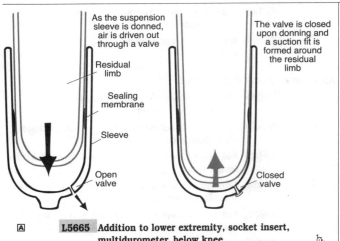

As the suspension sleeve is donned, air is driven out through a valve

Residual limb

Sealing membrane

Sleeve

Open valve

The valve is closed upon donning and a suction fit is formed around the residual limb

Closed valve

[A] **L5665** Addition to lower extremity, socket insert, multidurometer, below knee ♿

[A] **L5666** Addition to lower extremity, below knee, cuff suspension ♿

[A] **L5668** Addition to lower extremity, below knee, molded distal cushion ♿

[A] **L5670** Addition to lower extremity, below knee, molded supracondylar suspension (PTS or similar) ♿

[A] **L5671** Addition to lower extremity, below knee/above knee suspension locking mechanism (shuttle, lanyard or equal), excludes socket insert ♿

[A] **L5672** Addition to lower extremity, below knee, removable medial brim suspension ♿

[A] **L5673** Addition to lower extremity, below knee/above knee, custom fabricated from existing mold or prefabricated, socket insert, silicone gel, elastomeric or equal, for use with locking mechanism ♿

[A] ☑ **L5676** Addition to lower extremity, below knee, knee joints, single axis, pair ♿

[A] ☑ **L5677** Addition to lower extremity, below knee, knee joints, polycentric, pair ♿

[A] ☑ **L5678** Addition to lower extremity, below knee joint covers, pair ♿

[A] **L5679** Addition to lower extremity, below knee/above knee, custom fabricated from existing mold or prefabricated, socket insert, silicone gel, elastomeric or equal, not for use with locking mechanism ♿

[A] **L5680** Addition to lower extremity, below knee, thigh lacer, nonmolded ♿

[A] **L5681** Addition to lower extremity, below knee/above knee, custom fabricated socket insert for congenital or atypical traumatic amputee, silicone gel, elastomeric or equal, for use with or without locking mechanism, initial only (for other than initial, use code L5673 or L5679) ♿

[A] **L5682** Addition to lower extremity, below knee, thigh lacer, gluteal/ischial, molded ♿

[A] **L5683** Addition to lower extremity, below knee/above knee, custom fabricated socket insert for other than congenital or atypical traumatic amputee, silicone gel, elastomeric or equal, for use with or without locking mechanism, initial only (for other than initial, use code L5673 or L5679) ♿

[A] **L5684** Addition to lower extremity, below knee, fork strap ♿

L5685 Addition to lower extremity prosthesis, below knee, suspension/sealing sleeve, with or without valve, any material, each

[A] **L5686** Addition to lower extremity, below knee, back check (extension control) ♿

[A] **L5688** Addition to lower extremity, below knee, waist belt, webbing ♿

[A] **L5690** Addition to lower extremity, below knee, waist belt, padded and lined ♿

[E] **L5692** Addition to lower extremity, above knee, pelvic control belt, light ♿

[A] **L5694** Addition to lower extremity, above knee, pelvic control belt, padded and lined ♿

[A] ☑ **L5695** Addition to lower extremity, above knee, pelvic control, sleeve suspension, neoprene or equal, each ♿

[A] **L5696** Addition to lower extremity, above knee or knee disarticulation, pelvic joint ♿

[A] **L5697** Addition to lower extremity, above knee or knee disarticulation, pelvic band ♿

[A] **L5698** Addition to lower extremity, above knee or knee disarticulation, Silesian bandage ♿

[A] **L5699** All lower extremity prostheses, shoulder harness ♿

REPLACEMENTS

[A] **L5700** Replacement, socket, below knee, molded to patient model ♿

[A] **L5701** Replacement, socket, above knee/knee disarticulation, including attachment plate, molded to patient model ♿

[A] **L5702** Replacement, socket, hip disarticulation, including hip joint, molded to patient model ♿

● [A] **L5703** Ankle, symes, molded to patient model, socket without solid ankle cushion heel ♿

[A] **L5704** Custom shaped protective cover, below knee ♿

[A] **L5705** Custom shaped protective cover, above knee ♿

[A] **L5706** Custom shaped protective cover, knee disarticulation ♿

[A] **L5707** Custom shaped protective cover, hip disarticulation ♿

ADDITIONS: EXOSKELETAL KNEE-SHIN SYSTEM

[A] **L5710** Addition, exoskeletal knee-shin system, single axis, manual lock ♿

[A] **L5711** Addition, exoskeletal knee-shin system, single axis, manual lock, ultra-light material ♿

[A] **L5712** Addition, exoskeletal knee-shin system, single axis, friction swing and stance phase control (safety knee) ♿

[A] **L5714** Addition, exoskeletal knee-shin system, single axis, variable friction swing phase control ♿

[A] **L5716** Addition, exoskeletal knee-shin system, polycentric, mechanical stance phase lock ♿

[A] **L5718** Addition, exoskeletal knee-shin system, polycentric, friction swing and stance phase control ♿

[A] **L5722** Addition, exoskeletal knee-shin system, single axis, pneumatic swing, friction stance phase control ♿

[A] **L5724** Addition, exoskeletal knee-shin system, single axis, fluid swing phase control ♿

[A] **L5726** Addition, exoskeletal knee-shin system, single axis, external joints, fluid swing phase control ♿

| ▨ Special Coverage Instructions | | ▨ Noncovered by Medicare | | ▨ Carrier Discretion | ☑ Quantity Alert | ● New Code | ○ Reinstated Code | ▲ Revised Code |

110 — L Codes   [A] Age   [M] Maternity   ♀ Female Only   ♂ Male Only   [A]-[Y] APC Status Indicator   *2006 HCPCS*

Ⓐ **L5728** Addition, exoskeletal knee-shin system, single axis, fluid swing and stance phase control ♿

Ⓐ **L5780** Addition, exoskeletal knee-shin system, single axis, pneumatic/hydra pneumatic swing phase control ♿

Ⓐ **L5781** Addition to lower limb prosthesis, vacuum pump, residual limb volume management and moisture evacuation system ♿

Ⓐ **L5782** Addition to lower limb prosthesis, vacuum pump, residual limb volume management and moisture evacuation system, heavy duty ♿

COMPONENT MODIFICATION

Ⓐ **L5785** Addition, exoskeletal system, below knee, ultra-light material (titanium, carbon fiber or equal) ♿

Ⓐ **L5790** Addition, exoskeletal system, above knee, ultra-light material (titanium, carbon fiber or equal) ♿

Ⓐ **L5795** Addition, exoskeletal system, hip disarticulation, ultra-light material (titanium, carbon fiber or equal) ♿

ADDITIONS: ENDOSKELETAL KNEE-SHIN SYSTEM

Ⓐ **L5810** Addition, endoskeletal knee-shin system, single axis, manual lock ♿

Ⓐ **L5811** Addition, endoskeletal knee-shin system, single axis, manual lock, ultra-light material ♿

Ⓐ **L5812** Addition, endoskeletal knee-shin system, single axis, friction swing and stance phase control (safety knee) ♿

Ⓐ **L5814** Addition, endoskeletal knee-shin system, polycentric, hydraulic swing phase control, mechanical stance phase lock ♿

Ⓐ **L5816** Addition, endoskeletal knee-shin system, polycentric, mechanical stance phase lock ♿

Ⓐ **L5818** Addition, endoskeletal knee-shin system, polycentric, friction swing and stance phase control ♿

Ⓐ **L5822** Addition, endoskeletal knee-shin system, single axis, pneumatic swing, friction stance phase control ♿

Ⓐ **L5824** Addition, endoskeletal knee-shin system, single axis, fluid swing phase control ♿

Ⓐ **L5826** Addition, endoskeletal knee-shin system, single axis, hydraulic swing phase control, with miniature high activity frame ♿

Ⓐ **L5828** Addition, endoskeletal knee-shin system, single axis, fluid swing and stance phase control ♿

Ⓐ **L5830** Addition, endoskeletal knee-shin system, single axis, pneumatic/swing phase control ♿

Ⓐ **L5840** Addition, endoskeletal knee-shin system, 4-bar linkage or multiaxial, pneumatic swing phase control ♿

Ⓐ **L5845** Addition, endoskeletal knee-shin system, stance flexion feature, adjustable ♿

Ⓐ **L5848** Addition to endoskeletal, knee-shin system, hydraulic stance extension, dampening feature, with or without adjustability ♿

Ⓐ **L5850** Addition, endoskeletal system, above knee or hip disarticulation, knee extension assist ♿

Ⓐ **L5855** Addition, endoskeletal system, hip disarticulation, mechanical hip extension assist ♿

Ⓐ **L5856** Addition to lower extremity prosthesis, endoskeletal knee-shin system, microprocessor control feature, swing and stance phase, includes electronic sensor(s), any type

Ⓐ **L5857** Addition to lower extremity prosthesis, endoskeletal knee-shin system, microprocessor control feature, swing phase only, includes electronic sensor(s), any type

● Ⓐ **L5858** Addition to lower extremity prosthesis, endoskeletal knee shin system, microprocessor control feature, stance phase only, includes electronic sensor(s), any type

Ⓐ **L5910** Addition, endoskeletal system, below knee, alignable system ♿

Ⓐ **L5920** Addition, endoskeletal system, above knee or hip disarticulation, alignable system ♿

Ⓐ **L5925** Addition, endoskeletal system, above knee, knee disarticulation or hip disarticulation, manual lock ♿

Ⓐ **L5930** Addition, endoskeletal system, high activity knee control frame ♿

Ⓐ **L5940** Addition, endoskeletal system, below knee, ultra-light material (titanium, carbon fiber or equal) ♿

Ⓐ **L5950** Addition, endoskeletal system, above knee, ultra-light material (titanium, carbon fiber or equal) ♿

Ⓐ **L5960** Addition, endoskeletal system, hip disarticulation, ultra-light material (titanium, carbon fiber or equal) ♿

Ⓐ **L5962** Addition, endoskeletal system, below knee, flexible protective outer surface covering system ♿

Ⓐ **L5964** Addition, endoskeletal system, above knee, flexible protective outer surface covering system ♿

Ⓐ **L5966** Addition, endoskeletal system, hip disarticulation, flexible protective outer surface covering system ♿

Ⓐ **L5968** Addition to lower limb prosthesis, multiaxial ankle with swing phase active dorsiflexion feature ♿

Ⓐ **L5970** All lower extremity prostheses, foot, external keel, SACH foot ♿

● Ⓐ **L5971** All lower extremity prosthesis, solid ankle cushion heel (SACH) foot, replacement only

Ⓐ **L5972** All lower extremity prostheses, flexible keel foot (safe, sten, bock dynamic or equal) ♿

Ⓐ **L5974** All lower extremity prostheses, foot, single axis ankle/foot ♿

Ⓐ **L5975** All lower extremity prosthesis, combination single axis ankle and flexible keel foot ♿

Ⓐ **L5976** All lower extremity prostheses, energy storing foot (Seattle carbon copy II or equal) ♿

Foot prosthesis
(L5974)

Energy storing foot
(L5976)

Carbon

| Special Coverage Instructions | Noncovered by Medicare | Carrier Discretion | ☑ Quantity Alert | ● New Code | ○ Reinstated Code | ▲ Revised Code |

2006 HCPCS   **1-9** ASC Groups   **MED:** Pub 100/NCD Reference   ♿ DMEPOS Paid   Ⓢ SNF Excluded   **L Codes — 111**

Prosthetic Procedures

L5978 — L6386

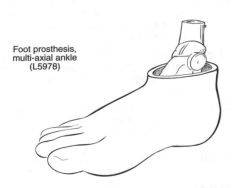

Foot prosthesis,
multi-axial ankle
(L5978)

Ⓐ   **L5978** All lower extremity prostheses, foot, multi-axial ankle/foot   ♿

Ⓐ   **L5979** All lower extremity prostheses, multi-axial ankle, dynamic response foot, one piece system   ♿

Ⓐ   **L5980** All lower extremity prostheses, flex-foot system ♿

Ⓐ   **L5981** All lower extremity prostheses, flex-walk system or equal   ♿

Ⓐ   **L5982** All exoskeletal lower extremity prostheses, axial rotation unit   ♿

Ⓐ   **L5984** All endoskeletal lower extremity prosthesis, axial rotation unit, with or without adjustability   ♿

Ⓐ   **L5985** All endoskeletal lower extremity prostheses, dynamic prosthetic pylon   ♿

Ⓐ   **L5986** All lower extremity prostheses, multi-axial rotation unit (MCP or equal)   ♿

Ⓐ   **L5987** All lower extremity prosthesis, shank foot system with vertical loading pylon   ♿

Ⓐ   **L5988** Addition to lower limb prosthesis, vertical shock reducing pylon feature   ♿

Ⓐ   **L5990** Addition to lower extremity prosthesis, user adjustable heel height   ♿

Ⓐ   **L5995** Addition to lower extremity prosthesis, heavy duty feature (for patient weight > 300 lbs.)   ♿

Ⓐ   **L5999** Lower extremity prosthesis, not otherwise specified
Determine if an alternative HCPCS Level II or a CPT code better describes the service being reported. This code should be used only if a more specific code is unavailable.

UPPER LIMB

The procedures in L6000-L6590 are considered as "base" or "basic procedures" and may be modified by listing procedures from the "addition" sections. The base procedures include only standard friction wrist and control cable system unless otherwise specified.

PARTIAL HAND

Ⓐ   **L6000** Partial hand, Robin-Aids, thumb remaining (or equal)   ♿

Ⓐ   **L6010** Partial hand, Robin-Aids, little and/or ring finger remaining (or equal)   ♿

Ⓐ   **L6020** Partial hand, Robin-Aids, no finger remaining (or equal)   ♿

Ⓐ   **L6025** Transcarpal/metacarpal or partial hand disarticulation prosthesis, external power, self-suspended, inner socket with removable forearm section, electrodes and cables, two batteries, charger, myoelectric control of terminal device   ♿

WRIST DISARTICULATION

Ⓐ   **L6050** Wrist disarticulation, molded socket, flexible elbow hinges, triceps pad   ♿

Ⓐ   **L6055** Wrist disarticulation, molded socket with expandable interface, flexible elbow hinges, triceps pad   ♿

BELOW ELBOW

Ⓐ   **L6100** Below elbow, molded socket, flexible elbow hinge, triceps pad   ♿

Ⓐ   **L6110** Below elbow, molded socket (Muenster or Northwestern suspension types)   ♿

Ⓐ   **L6120** Below elbow, molded double wall split socket, step-up hinges, half cuff   ♿

Ⓐ   **L6130** Below elbow, molded double wall split socket, stump activated locking hinge, half cuff   ♿

ELBOW DISARTICULATION

Ⓐ   **L6200** Elbow disarticulation, molded socket, outside locking hinge, forearm   ♿

Ⓐ   **L6205** Elbow disarticulation, molded socket with expandable interface, outside locking hinges, forearm   ♿

ABOVE ELBOW

Ⓐ   **L6250** Above elbow, molded double wall socket, internal locking elbow, forearm   ♿

SHOULDER DISARTICULATION

Ⓐ   **L6300** Shoulder disarticulation, molded socket, shoulder bulkhead, humeral section, internal locking elbow, forearm   ♿

Ⓐ   **L6310** Shoulder disarticulation, passive restoration (complete prosthesis)   ♿

Ⓐ   **L6320** Shoulder disarticulation, passive restoration (shoulder cap only)   ♿

INTERSCAPULAR THORACIC

Ⓐ   **L6350** Interscapular thoracic, molded socket, shoulder bulkhead, humeral section, internal locking elbow, forearm   ♿

Ⓐ   **L6360** Interscapular thoracic, passive restoration (complete prosthesis)   ♿

Ⓐ   **L6370** Interscapular thoracic, passive restoration (shoulder cap only)   ♿

IMMEDIATE AND EARLY POSTSURGICAL PROCEDURES

Ⓐ   **L6380** Immediate postsurgical or early fitting, application of initial rigid dressing, including fitting alignment and suspension of components, and one cast change, wrist disarticulation or below elbow   ♿

Ⓐ ☑   **L6382** Immediate postsurgical or early fitting, application of initial rigid dressing including fitting alignment and suspension of components, and one cast change, elbow disarticulation or above elbow   ♿

Ⓐ ☑   **L6384** Immediate postsurgical or early fitting, application of initial rigid dressing including fitting alignment and suspension of components, and one cast change, shoulder disarticulation or interscapular thoracic   ♿

Ⓐ ☑   **L6386** Immediate postsurgical or early fitting, each additional cast change and realignment   ♿

Special Coverage Instructions	Noncovered by Medicare	Carrier Discretion	☑ Quantity Alert ● New Code ○ Reinstated Code ▲ Revised Code

112 — L Codes   Ⓐ Age   Ⓜ Maternity   ♀ Female Only   ♂ Male Only   Ⓐ-Ⓨ APC Status Indicator   *2006 HCPCS*

Ⓐ L6388 Immediate postsurgical or early fitting, application of rigid dressing only ⅃

ENDOSKELETAL: BELOW ELBOW

Ⓐ L6400 Below elbow, molded socket, endoskeletal system, including soft prosthetic tissue shaping ⅃

ENDOSKELETAL: ELBOW DISARTICULATION

Ⓐ L6450 Elbow disarticulation, molded socket, endoskeletal system, including soft prosthetic tissue shaping ⅃

ENDOSKELETAL: ABOVE ELBOW

Ⓐ L6500 Above elbow, molded socket, endoskeletal system, including soft prosthetic tissue shaping ⅃

ENDOSKELETAL: SHOULDER DISARTICULATION

Ⓐ L6550 Shoulder disarticulation, molded socket, endoskeletal system, including soft prosthetic tissue shaping ⅃

ENDOSKELETAL: INTERSCAPULAR THORACIC

Ⓐ L6570 Interscapular thoracic, molded socket, endoskeletal system, including soft prosthetic tissue shaping ⅃

Ⓐ L6580 Preparatory, wrist disarticulation or below elbow, single wall plastic socket, friction wrist, flexible elbow hinges, figure of eight harness, humeral cuff, Bowden cable control, USMC or equal pylon, no cover, molded to patient model

Ⓐ L6582 Preparatory, wrist disarticulation or below elbow, single wall socket, friction wrist, flexible elbow hinges, figure of eight harness, humeral cuff, Bowden cable control, USMC or equal pylon, no cover, direct formed ⅃

Ⓐ L6584 Preparatory, elbow disarticulation or above elbow, single wall plastic socket, friction wrist, locking elbow, figure of eight harness, fair lead cable control, USMC or equal pylon, no cover, molded to patient model ⅃

Ⓐ L6586 Preparatory, elbow disarticulation or above elbow, single wall socket, friction wrist, locking elbow, figure of eight harness, fair lead cable control, USMC or equal pylon, no cover, direct formed ⅃

Ⓐ L6588 Preparatory, shoulder disarticulation or interscapular thoracic, single wall plastic socket, shoulder joint, locking elbow, friction wrist, chest strap, fair lead cable control, USMC or equal pylon, no cover, molded to patient model ⅃

Ⓐ L6590 Preparatory, shoulder disarticulation or interscapular thoracic, single wall socket, shoulder joint, locking elbow, friction wrist, chest strap, fair lead cable control, USMC or equal pylon, no cover, direct formed ⅃

ADDITIONS: UPPER LIMB

The following procedures/modifications/components may be added to other base procedures. The items in this section should reflect the additional complexity of each modification procedure, in addition to the base procedure, at the time of the original order.

Ⓐ ☑ L6600 Upper extremity additions, polycentric hinge, pair ⅃

Ⓐ ☑ L6605 Upper extremity additions, single pivot hinge, pair ⅃

Ⓐ ☑ L6610 Upper extremity additions, flexible metal hinge, pair ⅃

Ⓐ L6615 Upper extremity addition, disconnect locking wrist unit ⅃

Ⓐ ☑ L6616 Upper extremity addition, additional disconnect insert for locking wrist unit, each ⅃

Ⓐ L6620 Upper extremity addition, flexion/extension wrist unit, with or without friction ⅃

● Ⓐ L6621 Upper extremity prosthesis addition, flexion/extension wrist with or without friction, for use with external powered terminal device

Ⓐ L6623 Upper extremity addition, spring assisted rotational wrist unit with latch release ⅃

Ⓐ L6625 Upper extremity addition, rotation wrist unit with cable lock ⅃

Ⓐ L6628 Upper extremity addition, quick disconnect hook adapter, Otto Bock or equal ⅃

Ⓐ L6629 Upper extremity addition, quick disconnect lamination collar with coupling piece, Otto Bock or equal ⅃

Ⓐ L6630 Upper extremity addition, stainless steel, any wrist ⅃

Ⓐ ☑ L6632 Upper extremity addition, latex suspension sleeve, each ⅃

Ⓐ L6635 Upper extremity addition, lift assist for elbow ⅃

Ⓐ L6637 Upper extremity addition, nudge control elbow lock ⅃

Ⓐ L6638 Upper extremity addition to prosthesis, electric locking feature, only for use with manually powered elbow ⅃

Ⓐ ☑ L6640 Upper extremity additions, shoulder abduction joint, pair ⅃

Ⓐ L6641 Upper extremity addition, excursion amplifier, pulley type ⅃

Ⓐ L6642 Upper extremity addition, excursion amplifier, lever type ⅃

Ⓐ ☑ L6645 Upper extremity addition, shoulder flexion-abduction joint, each ⅃

Ⓐ L6646 Upper extremity addition, shoulder joint, multipositional locking, flexion, adjustable abduction friction control, for use with body powered or external powered system ⅃

Ⓐ L6647 Upper extremity addition, shoulder lock mechanism, body powered actuator ⅃

Ⓐ L6648 Upper extremity addition, shoulder lock mechanism, external powered actuator ⅃

Ⓐ ☑ L6650 Upper extremity addition, shoulder universal joint, each ⅃

Ⓐ L6655 Upper extremity addition, standard control cable, extra ⅃

Ⓐ L6660 Upper extremity addition, heavy duty control cable ⅃

Ⓐ L6665 Upper extremity addition, Teflon, or equal, cable lining ⅃

Ⓐ L6670 Upper extremity addition, hook to hand, cable adapter ⅃

Ⓐ L6672 Upper extremity addition, harness, chest or shoulder, saddle type ⅃

Ⓐ L6675 Upper extremity addition, harness, (e.g., figure of eight type), single cable design ⅃

Ⓐ L6676 Upper extremity addition, harness, (e.g., figure of eight type), dual cable design ⅃

Special Coverage Instructions Noncovered by Medicare Carrier Discretion ☑ Quantity Alert ● New Code ○ Reinstated Code ▲ Revised Code

2006 HCPCS ❶-❾ ASC Groups MED: Pub 100/NCD Reference ⅃ DMEPOS Paid Ⓢ SNF Excluded **L Codes — 113**

Prosthetic Procedures

L6677 — L6809

● Ⓐ **L6677** Upper extremity addition, harness, triple control, simultaneous operation of terminal device and elbow

Ⓐ **L6680** Upper extremity addition, test socket, wrist disarticulation or below elbow ♿

Ⓐ **L6682** Upper extremity addition, test socket, elbow disarticulation or above elbow ♿

Ⓐ **L6684** Upper extremity addition, test socket, shoulder disarticulation or interscapular thoracic ♿

Ⓐ **L6686** Upper extremity addition, suction socket ♿

Ⓐ **L6687** Upper extremity addition, frame type socket, below elbow or wrist disarticulation ♿

Ⓐ **L6688** Upper extremity addition, frame type socket, above elbow or elbow disarticulation ♿

Ⓐ **L6689** Upper extremity addition, frame type socket, shoulder disarticulation ♿

Ⓐ **L6690** Upper extremity addition, frame type socket, interscapular-thoracic ♿

Ⓐ ☑ **L6691** Upper extremity addition, removable insert, each ♿

Ⓐ ☑ **L6692** Upper extremity addition, silicone gel insert or equal, each ♿

Ⓐ **L6693** Upper extremity addition, locking elbow, forearm counterbalance ♿

L6694 Addition to upper extremity prosthesis, below elbow/above elbow, custom fabricated from existing mold or prefabricated, socket insert, silicone gel, elastomeric or equal, for use with locking mechanism

L6695 Addition to upper extremity prosthesis, below elbow/above elbow, custom fabricated from existing mold or prefabricated, socket insert, silicone gel, elastomeric or equal, not for use with locking mechanism

L6696 Addition to upper extremity prosthesis, below elbow/above elbow, custom fabricated socket insert for congenital or atypical traumatic amputee, silicone gel, elastomeric or equal, for use with or without locking mechanism, initial only (for other than initial, use code L6694 or L6695)

L6697 Addition to upper extremity prosthesis, below elbow/above elbow, custom fabricated socket insert for other than congenital or atypical traumatic amputee, silicone gel, elastomeric or equal, for use with or without locking mechanism, initial only (for other than initial, use code L6694 or L6695)

L6698 Addition to upper extremity prosthesis, below elbow/above elbow, lock mechanism, excludes socket insert

TERMINAL DEVICES

HOOKS

Ⓐ **L6700** Terminal device, hook, Dorrance or equal, model #3 ♿
MED: 100-2, 15, 120

Ⓐ **L6705** Terminal device, hook, Dorrance or equal, model #5 ♿
MED: 100-2, 15, 120

Ⓐ **L6710** Terminal device, hook, Dorrance or equal, model #5X ♿
MED: 100-2, 15, 120

Ⓐ **L6715** Terminal device, hook, Dorrance or equal, model #5XA ♿
MED: 100-2, 15, 120

Ⓐ **L6720** Terminal device, hook, Dorrance or equal, model #6 ♿
MED: 100-2, 15, 120

Ⓐ **L6725** Terminal device, hook, Dorrance or equal, model #7 ♿
MED: 100-2, 15, 120

Ⓐ **L6730** Terminal device, hook, Dorrance or equal, model #7LO ♿
MED: 100-2, 15, 120

Ⓐ **L6735** Terminal device, hook, Dorrance or equal, model #8 ♿
MED: 100-2, 15, 120

Ⓐ **L6740** Terminal device, hook, Dorrance or equal, model #8X ♿
MED: 100-2, 15, 120

Ⓐ **L6745** Terminal device, hook, Dorrance or equal, model #88X ♿
MED: 100-2, 15, 120

Ⓐ **L6750** Terminal device, hook, Dorrance or equal, model #10P ♿
MED: 100-2, 15, 120

Ⓐ **L6755** Terminal device, hook, Dorrance or equal, model #10X ♿
MED: 100-2, 15, 120

Ⓐ **L6765** Terminal device, hook, Dorrance or equal, model #12P ♿
MED: 100-2, 15, 120

Ⓐ **L6770** Terminal device, hook, Dorrance or equal, model #99X ♿
MED: 100-2, 15, 120

Ⓐ **L6775** Terminal device, hook, Dorrance or equal, model #555 ♿
MED: 100-2, 15, 120

Ⓐ **L6780** Terminal device, hook, Dorrance or equal, model #SS555 ♿
MED: 100-2, 15, 120

Ⓐ **L6790** Terminal device, hook, Accu hook or equal ♿
MED: 100-2, 15, 120

Ⓐ **L6795** Terminal device, hook, 2 load or equal ♿
MED: 100-2, 15, 120

Ⓐ **L6800** Terminal device, hook, APRL VC or equal ♿
MED: 100-2, 15, 120

Ⓐ **L6805** Terminal device, modifier wrist flexion unit ♿
MED: 100-2, 15, 120

Ⓐ **L6806** Terminal device, hook, TRS Grip, Grip III, VC, or equal ♿
MED: 100-2, 15, 120

Ⓐ **L6807** Terminal device, hook, Grip I, Grip II, VC, or equal ♿
MED: 100-2, 15, 120

Ⓐ **L6808** Terminal device, hook, TRS Adept, infant or child, VC, or equal ♿
MED: 100-2, 15, 120

Ⓐ **L6809** Terminal device, hook, TRS Super Sport, passive ♿
MED: 100-2, 15, 120

Special Coverage Instructions   Noncovered by Medicare   Carrier Discretion   ☑ Quantity Alert   ● New Code   ○ Reinstated Code   ▲ Revised Code

114 — L Codes   Ⓐ Age   Ⓜ Maternity   ♀ Female Only   ♂ Male Only   Ⓐ-Ⓨ APC Status Indicator   *2006 HCPCS*

A   L6810   Terminal device, Pincher tool, Otto Bock or equal   ら
MED: 100-2, 15, 120

HANDS

A   L6825   Terminal device, hand, Dorrance, VO   ら
MED: 100-2, 15, 120

A   L6830   Terminal device, hand, APRL, VC   ら
MED: 100-2, 15, 120

A   L6835   Terminal device, hand, Sierra, VO   ら
MED: 100-2, 15, 120

A   L6840   Terminal device, hand, Becker Imperial   ら
MED: 100-2, 15, 120

A   L6845   Terminal device, hand, Becker Lock Grip   ら
MED: 100-2, 15, 120

A   L6850   Terminal device, hand, Becker Plylite   ら
MED: 100-2, 15, 120

A   L6855   Terminal device, hand, Robin-Aids, VO   ら
MED: 100-2, 15, 120

A   L6860   Terminal device, hand, Robin-Aids, VO soft   ら
MED: 100-2, 15, 120

A   L6865   Terminal device, hand, passive hand   ら
MED: 100-2, 15, 120

A   L6867   Terminal device, hand, Detroit infant hand (mechanical)   A ら
MED: 100-2, 15, 120

A   L6868   Terminal device, hand, passive infant hand, Steeper, Hosmer or equal   A ら
MED: 100-2, 15, 120

A   L6870   Terminal device, hand, child mitt   ら
MED: 100-2, 15, 120

A   L6872   Terminal device, hand, NYU child hand   ら
MED: 100-2, 15, 120

A   L6873   Terminal device, hand, mechanical infant hand, steeper or equal   ら
MED: 100-2, 15, 120

A   L6875   Terminal device, hand, Bock, VC   ら
MED: 100-2, 15, 120

A   L6880   Terminal device, hand, Bock, VO   ら
MED: 100-2, 15, 120

A   L6881   Automatic grasp feature, addition to upper limb prosthetic terminal device   ら

A   L6882   Microprocessor control feature, addition to upper limb prosthetic terminal device   ら
MED: 100-2, 15, 120

● A   L6883   Replacement socket, below elbow/wrist disarticulation, molded to patient model, for use with or without external power

● A   L6884   Replacement socket, above elbow disarticulation, molded to patient model, for use with or without external power

● A   L6885   Replacement socket, shoulder disarticulation/interscapular thoracic, molded to patient model, for use with or without external power

GLOVES FOR ABOVE HANDS

A   L6890   Addition to upper extremity prosthesis, glove for terminal device, any material, prefabricated, includes fitting and adjustment   ら

A   L6895   Addition to upper extremity prosthesis, glove for terminal device, any material, custom fabricated ら

HAND RESTORATION

A   L6900   Hand restoration (casts, shading and measurements included), partial hand, with glove, thumb or one finger remaining   ら

A   L6905   Hand restoration (casts, shading and measurements included), partial hand, with glove, multiple fingers remaining   ら

A   L6910   Hand restoration (casts, shading and measurements included), partial hand, with glove, no fingers remaining   ら

A   L6915   Hand restoration (shading and measurements included), replacement glove for above   ら

EXTERNAL POWER

BASE DEVICES

A   L6920   Wrist disarticulation, external power, self-suspended inner socket, removable forearm shell, Otto Bock or equal switch, cables, two batteries and one charger, switch control of terminal device   ら

A   L6925   Wrist disarticulation, external power, self-suspended inner socket, removable forearm shell, Otto Bock or equal electrodes, cables, two batteries and one charger, myoelectronic control of terminal device ら

A   L6930   Below elbow, external power, self-suspended inner socket, removable forearm shell, Otto Bock or equal switch, cables, two batteries and one charger, switch control of terminal device   ら

A   L6935   Below elbow, external power, self-suspended inner socket, removable forearm shell, Otto Bock or equal electrodes, cables, two batteries and one charger, myoelectronic control of terminal device   ら

A   L6940   Elbow disarticulation, external power, molded inner socket, removable humeral shell, outside locking hinges, forearm, Otto Bock or equal switch, cables, two batteries and one charger, switch control of terminal device   ら

A   L6945   Elbow disarticulation, external power, molded inner socket, removable humeral shell, outside locking hinges, forearm, Otto Bock or equal electrodes, cables, two batteries and one charger, myoelectronic control of terminal device   ら

A   L6950   Above elbow, external power, molded inner socket, removable humeral shell, internal locking elbow, forearm, Otto Bock or equal switch, cables, two batteries and one charger, switch control of terminal device   ら

A   L6955   Above elbow, external power, molded inner socket, removable humeral shell, internal locking elbow, forearm, Otto Bock or equal electrodes, cables, two batteries and one charger, myoelectronic control of terminal device

A   L6960   Shoulder disarticulation, external power, molded inner socket, removable shoulder shell, shoulder bulkhead, humeral section, mechanical elbow, forearm, Otto Bock or equal switch, cables, two batteries and one charger, switch control of terminal device   ら

Special Coverage Instructions   Noncovered by Medicare   Carrier Discretion   ☑ Quantity Alert   ● New Code   ○ Reinstated Code   ▲ Revised Code

2006 HCPCS   1-9 ASC Groups   MED: Pub 100/NCD Reference   ら DMEPOS Paid   ⊘ SNF Excluded   **L Codes — 115**

Prosthetic Procedures

L6965 — L8030

[A] **L6965** Shoulder disarticulation, external power, molded inner socket, removable shoulder shell, shoulder bulkhead, humeral section, mechanical elbow, forearm, Otto Bock or equal electrodes, cables, two batteries and one charger, myoelectronic control of terminal device   🦽

[A] **L6970** Interscapular-thoracic, external power, molded inner socket, removable shoulder shell, shoulder bulkhead, humeral section, mechanical elbow, forearm, Otto Bock or equal switch, cables, two batteries and one charger, switch control of terminal device   🦽

[A] **L6975** Interscapular-thoracic, external power, molded inner socket, removable shoulder shell, shoulder bulkhead, humeral section, mechanical elbow, forearm, Otto Bock or equal electrodes, cables, two batteries and one charger, myoelectronic control of terminal device   🦽

[A] **L7010** Electronic hand, Otto Bock, Steeper or equal, switch controlled   🦽

[A] **L7015** Electronic hand, System Teknik, Variety Village or equal, switch controlled   🦽

[A] **L7020** Electronic Greifer, Otto Bock or equal, switch controlled   🦽

[A] **L7025** Electronic hand, Otto Bock or equal, myoelectronically controlled   🦽

[A] **L7030** Electronic hand, System Teknik, Variety Village or equal, myoelectronically controlled   🦽

[A] **L7035** Electronic Greifer, Otto Bock or equal, myoelectronically controlled   🦽

[A] **L7040** Prehensile actuator, Hosmer or equal, switch controlled   🦽

[A] **L7045** Electronic hook, child, Michigan or equal, switch controlled   🦽

ELBOW

[A] **L7170** Electronic elbow, Hosmer or equal, switch controlled   🦽

[A] **L7180** Electronic elbow, microprocessor sequential control of elbow and terminal device   🦽

L7181 Electronic elbow, microprocessor simultaneous control of elbow and terminal device

[A] **L7185** Electronic elbow, adolescent, Variety Village or equal, switch controlled   🦽

[A] **L7186** Electronic elbow, child, Variety Village or equal, switch controlled   🦽

[A] **L7190** Electronic elbow, adolescent, Variety Village or equal, myoelectronically controlled   🦽

[A] **L7191** Electronic elbow, child, Variety Village or equal, myoelectronically controlled   🦽

[A] **L7260** Electronic wrist rotator, Otto Bock or equal   🦽

[A] **L7261** Electronic wrist rotator, for Utah Arm   🦽

[A] **L7266** Servo control, Steeper or equal   🦽

[A] **L7272** Analogue control, UNB or equal   🦽

[A] **L7274** Proportional control, 6-12 volt, Liberty, Utah or equal   🦽

BATTERY COMPONENTS

[A] **L7360** Six volt battery, Otto Bock or equal, each   🦽

[A] **L7362** Battery charger, six volt, Otto Bock or equal   🦽

[A] **L7364** Twelve volt battery, Utah or equal, each   🦽

[A] **L7366** Battery charger, twelve volt, Utah or equal   🦽

[A] **L7367** Lithium ion battery, replacement   🦽

[A] **L7368** Lithium ion battery charger   🦽

● [A] **L7400** Addition to upper extremity prosthesis, below elbow/wrist disarticulation, ultralight material (titanium, carbon fiber or equal)

● [A] **L7401** Addition to upper extremity prosthesis, above elbow disarticulation, ultralight material (titanium, carbon fiber or equal)

● [A] **L7402** Addition to upper extremity prosthesis, shoulder disarticulation/interscapular thoracic, ultralight material (titanium, carbon fiber or equal)

● [A] **L7403** Addition to upper extremity prosthesis, below elbow/wrist disarticulation, acrylic material

● [A] **L7404** Addition to upper extremity prosthesis, above elbow disarticulation, acrylic material

● [A] **L7405** Addition to upper extremity prosthesis, shoulder disarticulation/interscapular thoracic, acrylic material

[A] **L7499** Upper extremity prosthesis, NOS   ⊘

REPAIRS

[A] **L7500** Repair of prosthetic device, hourly rate
Medicare jurisdiction: local contractor if repair or implanted prosthetic device.

MED: 100-2, 15, 110.2; 100-2, 15, 120; 100-2, 15, 120

[A] **L7510** Repair of prosthetic device, repair or replace minor parts
Medicare jurisdiction: local contractor if repair of implanted prosthetic device.

MED: 100-2, 15, 110.2; 100-2, 15, 120; 100-2, 15, 120

[A] ☑ **L7520** Repair prosthetic device, labor component, per 15 minutes
Medicare jurisdiction: local contractor if repair of implanted prosthetic device.

● [S] **L7600** Prosthetic donning sleeve, any material, each

GENERAL

[A] **L7900** Male vacuum erection system   [A] ♂ 🦽

PROSTHESIS

[A] **L8000** Breast prosthesis, mastectomy bra   [A] ♀ 🦽
MED: 100-2, 15, 120

[A] **L8001** Breast prosthesis, mastectomy bra, with integrated breast prosthesis form, unilateral   [A] ♀ 🦽
MED: 100-2, 15, 120

[A] **L8002** Breast prosthesis, mastectomy bra, with integrated breast prosthesis form, bilateral   [A] ♀ 🦽
MED: 100-2, 15, 120

[A] **L8010** Breast prosthesis, mastectomy sleeve   [A] ♀
MED: 100-2, 15, 120

[A] **L8015** External breast prosthesis garment, with mastectomy form, postmastectomy   [A] ♀ 🦽
MED: 100-2, 15, 120

[A] **L8020** Breast prosthesis, mastectomy form   [A] ♀ 🦽
MED: 100-2, 15, 120

[A] **L8030** Breast prosthesis, silicone or equal   [A] ♀ 🦽
MED: 100-2, 15, 120

Special Coverage Instructions   Noncovered by Medicare   Carrier Discretion   ☑ Quantity Alert   ● New Code   ○ Reinstated Code   ▲ Revised Code

116 — L Codes   [A] Age   [M] Maternity   ♀ Female Only   ♂ Male Only   [A]-[Y] APC Status Indicator   **2006 HCPCS**

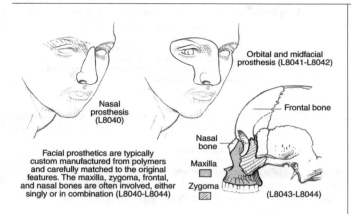

Facial prosthetics are typically custom manufactured from polymers and carefully matched to the original features. The maxilla, zygoma, frontal, and nasal bones are often involved, either singly or in combination (L8040-L8044)

Nasal prosthesis (L8040)

Orbital and midfacial prosthesis (L8041-L8042)

Frontal bone

Nasal bone

Maxilla

Zygoma

(L8043-L8044)

Ⓐ	**L8035**	Custom breast prosthesis, postmastectomy, molded to patient model MED: 100-2, 15, 120	Ⓐ ♀ ⅙
Ⓐ	**L8039**	Breast prosthesis, NOS	Ⓐ ♀
Ⓐ	**L8040**	Nasal prosthesis, provided by a nonphysician	⅙
Ⓐ	**L8041**	Midfacial prosthesis, provided by a nonphysician	⅙
Ⓐ	**L8042**	Orbital prosthesis, provided by a nonphysician	⅙
Ⓐ	**L8043**	Upper facial prosthesis, provided by a nonphysician	⅙
Ⓐ	**L8044**	Hemi-facial prosthesis, provided by a nonphysician	⅙
Ⓐ	**L8045**	Auricular prosthesis, provided by a nonphysician	⅙
Ⓐ	**L8046**	Partial facial prosthesis, provided by a nonphysician	⅙
Ⓐ	**L8047**	Nasal septal prosthesis, provided by a nonphysician	⅙
Ⓐ	**L8048**	Unspecified maxillofacial prosthesis, by report, provided by a nonphysician	
Ⓐ	**L8049**	Repair or modification of maxillofacial prosthesis, labor component, 15 minute increments, provided by a nonphysician	

ELASTIC SUPPORTS

L8100 ~~Gradient compression stocking, below knee, 18-30 mmHg, each~~
See code(s) A6530.

L8110 ~~Gradient compression stocking, below knee, 30-40 mmHg, each~~
See code(s) A6531.

L8120 ~~Gradient compression stocking, below knee, 40-50 mmHg, each~~
See code(s) A6532.

L8130 ~~Gradient compression stocking, thigh length, 18-30 mmHg, each~~
See code(s) A6533.

L8140 ~~Gradient compression stocking, thigh length, 30-40 mmHg, each~~
See code(s) A6534.

L8150 ~~Gradient compression stocking, thigh length, 40-50 mmHg, each~~
See code(s) A6535.

L8160 ~~Gradient compression stocking, full length/chap style, 18-30 mmHg, each~~
See code(s) A6536.

L8170 ~~Gradient compression stocking, full length/chap style, 30-40 mmHg, each~~
See code(s) A6537.

L8180 ~~Gradient compression stocking, full length/chap style, 40-50 mmHg, each~~
See code(s) A6538.

L8190 ~~Gradient compression stocking, waist length, 18-30 mmHg, each~~
See code(s) A6539.

L8195 ~~Gradient compression stocking, waist length, 30-40 mmHg, each~~
See code(s) A6540.

L8200 ~~Gradient compression stocking, waist length, 40-50 mmHg, each~~
See code(s) A6541.

L8210 ~~Gradient compression stocking, custom-made~~
See code(s) A6542.

L8220 ~~Gradient compression stocking, lymphedema~~
See code(s) A6543.

L8230 ~~Gradient compression stocking, garter belt~~
See code(s) A6544.

L8239 ~~Gradient compression stocking, NOS~~
See code(s) A6549.

TRUSSES

Ⓐ	**L8300**	Truss, single with standard pad MED: 100-2, 15, 120; 100-3, 280.11; 100-3, 280.12	⅙
Ⓐ	**L8310**	Truss, double with standard pads MED: 100-2, 15, 120; 100-3, 280.11; 100-3, 280.12	⅙
Ⓐ	**L8320**	Truss, addition to standard pad, water pad MED: 100-2, 15, 120; 100-3, 280.11; 100-3, 280.12	⅙
Ⓐ	**L8330**	Truss, addition to standard pad, scrotal pad MED: 100-2, 15, 120; 100-3, 280.11; 100-3, 280.12	♂ ⅙

PROSTHETIC SOCKS

Ⓐ	☑	**L8400**	Prosthetic sheath, below knee, each MED: 100-2, 15, 120	⅙
Ⓐ	☑	**L8410**	Prosthetic sheath, above knee, each MED: 100-2, 15, 120	⅙
Ⓐ	☑	**L8415**	Prosthetic sheath, upper limb, each MED: 100-2, 15, 120	⅙
Ⓐ	☑	**L8417**	Prosthetic sheath/sock, including a gel cushion layer, below knee or above knee, each	⅙
Ⓐ	☑	**L8420**	Prosthetic sock, multiple ply, below knee, each MED: 100-2, 15, 120	⅙
Ⓐ	☑	**L8430**	Prosthetic sock, multiple ply, above knee, each MED: 100-2, 15, 120	⅙
Ⓐ	☑	**L8435**	Prosthetic sock, multiple ply, upper limb, each MED: 100-2, 15, 120	⅙
Ⓐ	☑	**L8440**	Prosthetic shrinker, below knee, each MED: 100-2, 15, 120	⅙
Ⓐ	☑	**L8460**	Prosthetic shrinker, above knee, each MED: 100-2, 15, 120	⅙
Ⓐ	☑	**L8465**	Prosthetic shrinker, upper limb, each MED: 100-2, 15, 120	⅙
Ⓐ	☑	**L8470**	Prosthetic sock, single ply, fitting, below knee, each MED: 100-2, 15, 120	⅙

Special Coverage Instructions | Noncovered by Medicare | Carrier Discretion | ☑ Quantity Alert | ● New Code | ○ Reinstated Code | ▲ Revised Code

2006 HCPCS | **1-9** ASC Groups | MED: Pub 100/NCD Reference | ⅙ DMEPOS Paid | ⊘ SNF Excluded | **L Codes — 117**

Prosthetic Procedures

L8480 — L8624

Ⓐ ☑ **L8480** Prosthetic sock, single ply, fitting, above knee, each ♿
MED: 100-2, 15, 120

Ⓐ ☑ **L8485** Prosthetic sock, single ply, fitting, upper limb, each ♿
MED: 100-2, 15, 120

Ⓐ **L8499** Unlisted procedure for miscellaneous prosthetic services
Determine if an alternative HCPCS Level II or a CPT code better describes the service being reported. This code should be used only if a more specific code is unavailable.

PROSTHETIC IMPLANTS

INTEGUMENTARY SYSTEM

Ⓐ **L8500** Artificial larynx, any type ♿
MED: 100-2, 15, 120; 100-3, 50.2

Ⓐ **L8501** Tracheostomy speaking valve ♿
MED: 100-3, 50.4

Ⓐ **L8505** Artificial larynx replacement battery/accessory, any type

Ⓐ **L8507** Tracheo-esophageal voice prosthesis, patient inserted, any type, each ♿

Ⓐ **L8509** Tracheo-esophageal voice prosthesis, inserted by a licensed health care provider, any type ♿

Ⓐ **L8510** Voice amplifier ♿
MED: 100-3, 50.2

Ⓐ ☑ **L8511** Insert for indwelling tracheoesophageal prosthesis, with or without valve, replacement only, each ♿

Ⓐ ☑ **L8512** Gelatin capsules or equivalent, for use with tracheoesophageal voice prosthesis, replacement only, per 10 ♿

Ⓐ ☑ **L8513** Cleaning device used with tracheoesophageal voice prosthesis, pipet, brush, or equal, replacement only, each ♿

Ⓐ ☑ **L8514** Tracheoesophageal puncture dilator, replacement only, each ♿

☑ **L8515** Gelatin capsule, application device for use with tracheoesophageal voice prosthesis, each

Ⓝ **L8600** Implantable breast prosthesis, silicone or equal Ⓐ ♀ ♿
Medicare covers implants inserted in post-mastectomy reconstruction in a breast cancer patient. Always report concurrent to the implant procedure. Medicare jurisdiction: local contractor.
MED: 100-2, 15, 120; 100-3, 140.2

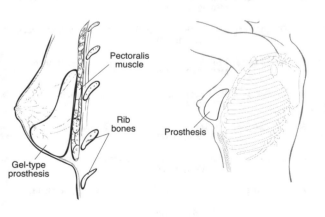

Pectoralis muscle

Rib bones

Prosthesis

Gel-type prosthesis

Ⓝ ☑ **L8603** Injectable bulking agent, collagen implant, urinary tract, 2.5 ml syringe, includes shipping and necessary supplies ♿
Medicare covers up to five separate collagen implant treatments in patients with intrinsic sphincter deficiency. Who have passed a collagen sensitivity test. Medicare jurisdiction: local contractor.
MED: 100-3, 230.10

Ⓝ ☑ **L8606** Injectable bulking agent, synthetic implant, urinary tract, 1 ml syringe, includes shipping and necessary supplies ♿
MED: 100-3, 230.10

● Ⓝ **L8609** Artificial cornea

HEAD: SKULL, FACIAL BONES, AND TEMPOROMANDIBULAR JOINT

Ⓝ **L8610** Ocular implant ♿
Medicare jurisdiction: local contractor.
MED: 100-2, 15, 120

Ⓝ **L8612** Aqueous shunt ♿
Medicare jurisdiction: local contractor.
MED: 100-2, 15, 120
See code(s): Q0074

Ⓝ **L8613** Ossicular implant ♿
Medicare jurisdiction: local contractor.
MED: 100-2, 15, 120

Ⓝ **L8614** Cochlear device/system ♿
A cochlear implant is covered by Medicare when the patient has bilateral sensorineural deafness. Medicare jurisdiction: local contractor.
MED: 100-2, 15, 120; 100-3, 50.3
AHA: 3Q, '02, 5; 4Q, '03, 8

L8615 Headset/headpiece for use with cochlear implant device, replacement
MED: 100-3, 50.3

L8616 Microphone for use with cochlear implant device, replacement
MED: 100-3, 50.3

L8617 Transmitting coil for use with cochlear implant device, replacement
MED: 100-3, 50.3

L8618 Transmitter cable for use with cochlear implant device, replacement
MED: 100-3, 50.3

Ⓐ **L8619** Cochlear implant external speech processor, replacement ♿
Medicare jurisdiction: local contractor.
MED: 100-3, 50.3

~~**L8620** Lithium ion battery for use with cochlear implant device, replacement, each~~
See code(s) L8623, L8624.

L8621 Zinc air battery for use with cochlear implant device, replacement, each

☑ **L8622** Alkaline battery for use with cochlear implant device, any size, replacement, each

● Ⓐ **L8623** Lithium ion battery for use with cochlear implant device speech processor ♿

● Ⓐ **L8624** Lithium ion battery for use with cochlear implant device speech processor, ear ♿

Special Coverage Instructions   Noncovered by Medicare   Carrier Discretion   ☑ Quantity Alert   ● New Code   ○ Reinstated Code   ▲ Revised Code

118 — L Codes   Ⓐ Age   Ⓜ Maternity   ♀ Female Only   ♂ Male Only   Ⓐ-Ⓨ APC Status Indicator   *2006 HCPCS*

Bone is cut at the MP joint (arthroplasty)

Bone may be hollowed out in both metacarpal and phalangeal sides in preparation for a prosthesis

Prosthetic joint implant

Prosthesis in place

Metacarpophalangeal prosthetic implant

UPPER EXTREMITY

N   **L8630**   Metacarpophalangeal joint implant   &b;
Medicare jurisdiction: local contractor.
MED: 100-2, 15, 120

A   **L8631**   Metacarpal phalangeal joint replacement, two or more pieces, metal (e.g., stainless steel or cobalt chrome), ceramic-like material (e.g., pyrocarbon), for surgical implantation (all sizes, includes entire system)   &b;
MED: 100-2, 15, 120

LOWER EXTREMITY — JOINT: KNEE, ANKLE, TOE

N   **L8641**   Metatarsal joint implant   &b;
Medicare jurisdiction: local contractor.
MED: 100-2, 15, 120

N   **L8642**   Hallux implant   &b;
Medicare jurisdiction: local contractor.
MED: 100-2, 15, 120
See code(s): Q0073

MISCELLANEOUS MUSCULAR-SKELETAL

N   **L8658**   Interphalangeal joint spacer, silicone or equal, each   &b;
Medicare jurisdiction: local contractor.
MED: 100-2, 15, 120

A   **L8659**   Interphalangeal finger joint replacement, two or more pieces, metal (e.g., stainless steel or cobalt chrome), ceramic-like material (e.g., pyrocarbon) for surgical implantation, any size   &b;
MED: 100-2, 15, 120

CARDIOVASCULAR SYSTEM

N   **L8670**   Vascular graft material, synthetic, implant   &b;
Medicare jurisdiction: local contractor.
MED: 100-2, 15, 120

GENERAL

● **B**   **L8680**   Implantable neurostimulator electrode, each

● **A**   **L8681**   Patient programmer (external) for use with implantable programmable neurostimulator pulse generator
MED: 100-3, 160.7

● **N**   **L8682**   Implantable neurostimulator radiofrequency receiver
MED: 100-3, 160.7

● **A**   **L8683**   Radiofrequency transmitter (external) for use with implantable neurostimulator radiofrequency receiver
MED: 100-3, 160.7

● **A**   **L8684**   Radiofrequency transmitter (external) for use with implantable sacral root neurostimulator receiver for bowel and bladder management, replacement
MED: 100-3, 160.7

● **B**   **L8685**   Implantable neurostimulator pulse generator, single array, rechargeable, includes extension
MED: 100-3, 160.7

● **B**   **L8686**   Implantable neurostimulator pulse generator, single array, non-rechargeable, includes extension
MED: 100-3, 160.7

● **B**   **L8687**   Implantable neurostimulator pulse generator, dual array, rechargeable, includes extension
MED: 100-3, 160.7

● **B**   **L8688**   Implantable neurostimulator pulse generator, dual array, non-rechargeable, includes extension
MED: 100-3, 160.7

● **A**   **L8689**   External recharging system for implanted neurostimulator, replacement only
MED: 100-3, 160.7

N   **L8699**   Prosthetic implant, not otherwise specified
Determine if an alternative HCPCS Level II or a CPT code better describes the service being reported. This code should be used only if a more specific code is unavailable. Medicare jurisdiction: local contractor.

A   **L9900**   Orthotic and prosthetic supply, accessory, and/or service component of another HCPCS L code

MEDICAL SERVICES *M0000-M0301*

OTHER MEDICAL SERVICES

M codes include office services, cellular therapy, prolotherapy, intragastric hypothermia, IV chelation therapy, and fabric wrapping of an abdominal aneurysm (MNP).

M codes fall under the jurisdiction of the local contractor

☒   `M0064` **Brief office visit for the sole purpose of monitoring or changing drug prescriptions used in the treatment of mental psychoneurotic and personality disorders** ⊘
MED: 100-4, 12, 210.1

Ⓔ   `M0075` **Cellular therapy** ⊘
The therapeutic efficacy of injecting foreign proteins has not been established.

MED: 100-3, 30.8

Ⓔ   `M0076` **Prolotherapy** ⊘
The therapeutic efficacy of prolotherapy and joint sclerotherapy has not been established.

MED: 100-3, 150.7

Ⓔ   `M0100` **Intragastric hypothermia using gastric freezing** ⊘
Code with caution: This procedure is considered obsolete.

MED: 100-3, 100.6

CARDIOVASCULAR SERVICES

Ⓔ   `M0300` **IV chelation therapy (chemical endarterectomy)** ⊘
Chelation therapy is considered experimental in the United States.

MED: 100-3, 20.21

Ⓔ   `M0301` **Fabric wrapping of abdominal aneurysm** ⊘
Code with caution: This procedure has largely been replaced with more effective treatment modalities. Submit documentation.

MED: 100-3, 20.23

Special Coverage Instructions   **Noncovered by Medicare**   **Carrier Discretion**   ☑ Quantity Alert   ● New Code   ○ Reinstated Code   ▲ Revised Code

2006 HCPCS   **1**-**9** ASC Groups   **MED:** Pub 100/NCD Reference   ♿ DMEPOS Paid   ⊘ SNF Excluded   **M Codes — 121**

PATHOLOGY AND LABORATORY SERVICES *P0000-P9999*
P codes include chemistry, toxicology, and microbiology tests, screening Papanicolaou procedures, and various blood products.

CHEMISTRY AND TOXICOLOGY TESTS
P codes fall under the jurisdiction of the local contractor.

Ⓐ **P2028** Cephalin flocculation, blood ⊘
Code with caution: This test is considered obsolete. Submit documentation.
MED: 100-3, 300.1

Ⓐ **P2029** Congo red, blood ⊘
Code with caution: This test is considered obsolete. Submit documentation.
MED: 100-3, 300.1

Ⓔ **P2031** Hair analysis (excluding arsenic) ⊘
For hair analysis for arsenic, see CPT codes 83015, 82175.
MED: 100-3, 190.6

Ⓐ **P2033** Thymol turbidity, blood ⊘
Code with caution: This test is considered obsolete. Submit documentation.
MED: 100-3, 300.1

Ⓐ **P2038** Mucoprotein, blood (seromucoid) (medical necessity procedure) ⊘
Code with caution: This test is considered obsolete. Submit documentation.
MED: 100-3, 300.1

PATHOLOGY SCREENING TESTS

Ⓐ **P3000** Screening Papanicolaou smear, cervical or vaginal, up to three smears, by technician under physician supervision Ⓐ ♀
One Pap test is covered by Medicare every two years, unless the physician suspects cervical abnormalities and shortens the interval. See also G0123-G0124.
MED: 100-3, 190.2

Ⓑ **P3001** Screening Papanicolaou smear, cervical or vaginal, up to three smears, requiring interpretation by physician Ⓐ ♀ ⊘
One Pap test is covered by Medicare every two years, unless the physician suspects cervical abnormalities and shortens the interval. See also G0123-G0124.
MED: 100-3, 190.2

MICROBIOLOGY TESTS

Ⓔ **P7001** Culture, bacterial, urine; quantitative, sensitivity study ⊘

MISCELLANEOUS

Ⓚ ☑ **P9010** Blood (whole), for transfusion, per unit
MED: 100-1, 3, 20.5

Ⓚ ☑ **P9011** Blood (split unit), specify amount
MED: 100-1, 3, 20.5

Ⓚ ☑ **P9012** Cryoprecipitate, each unit
MED: 100-1, 3, 20.5

Ⓚ ☑ **P9016** Red blood cells, leukocytes reduced, each unit
MED: 100-1, 3, 20.5

Ⓚ ☑ **P9017** Fresh frozen plasma (single donor), frozen within 8 hours of collection, each unit
MED: 100-1, 3, 20.5

Ⓚ ☑ **P9019** Platelets, each unit
MED: 100-1, 3, 20.5

Ⓚ ☑ **P9020** Platelet rich plasma, each unit
MED: 100-1, 3, 20.5

Ⓚ ☑ **P9021** Red blood cells, each unit
MED: 100-1, 3, 20.5

Ⓚ ☑ **P9022** Red blood cells, washed, each unit
MED: 100-1, 3, 20.5

Ⓚ ☑ **P9023** Plasma, pooled multiple donor, solvent/detergent treated, frozen, each unit
MED: 100-1, 3, 20.5

Ⓚ ☑ **P9031** Platelets, leukocytes reduced, each unit
MED: 100-1, 3, 20.5; 100-1, 3, 20.5.2; 100-1, 3, 20.5.3

Ⓚ ☑ **P9032** Platelets, irradiated, each unit
MED: 100-1, 3, 20.5; 100-1, 3, 20.5.2; 100-1, 3, 20.5.3

Ⓚ ☑ **P9033** Platelets, leukocytes reduced, irradiated, each unit
MED: 100-1, 3, 20.5; 100-1, 3, 20.5.2; 100-1, 3, 20.5.3

Ⓚ ☑ **P9034** Platelets, pheresis, each unit
MED: 100-1, 3, 20.5; 100-1, 3, 20.5.2; 100-1, 3, 20.5.3

Ⓚ ☑ **P9035** Platelets, pheresis, leukocytes reduced, each unit
MED: 100-1, 3, 20.5; 100-1, 3, 20.5.2; 100-1, 3, 20.5.3

Ⓚ ☑ **P9036** Platelets, pheresis, irradiated, each unit
MED: 100-1, 3, 20.5; 100-1, 3, 20.5.2; 100-1, 3, 20.5.3

Ⓚ ☑ **P9037** Platelets, pheresis, leukocytes reduced, irradiated, each unit
MED: 100-1, 3, 20.5; 100-1, 3, 20.5.2; 100-1, 3, 20.5.3

Ⓚ ☑ **P9038** Red blood cells, irradiated, each unit
MED: 100-1, 3, 20.5; 100-1, 3, 20.5.2; 100-1, 3, 20.5.3

Ⓚ ☑ **P9039** Red blood cells, deglycerolized, each unit
MED: 100-1, 3, 20.5; 100-1, 3, 20.5.2; 100-1, 3, 20.5.3

Ⓚ ☑ **P9040** Red blood cells, leukocytes reduced, irradiated, each unit
MED: 100-1, 3, 20.5; 100-1, 3, 20.5.2; 100-1, 3, 20.5.3

Ⓚ ☑ **P9041** Infusion, albumin (human), 5%, 50 ml
Not considered a blood product for OPPS effective July 1, 2005.

Ⓚ ☑ **P9043** Infusion, plasma protein fraction (human), 5%, 50 ml
MED: 100-1, 3, 20.5

Ⓚ ☑ **P9044** Plasma, cryoprecipitate reduced, each unit
MED: 100-1, 3, 20.5

Ⓚ ☑ **P9045** Infusion, albumin (human), 5%, 250 ml
Not considered a blood product for OPPS effective July 1, 2005.

Ⓚ ☑ **P9046** Infusion, albumin (human), 25%, 20 ml
Not considered a blood product for OPPS effective July 1, 2005.

Ⓚ ☑ **P9047** Infusion, albumin (human), 25%, 50 ml
Not considered a blood product for OPPS effective July 1, 2005.

Ⓚ ☑ **P9048** Infusion, plasma protein fraction (human), 5%, 250 ml

Ⓚ ☑ **P9050** Granulocytes, pheresis, each unit

Ⓚ ☑ **P9051** Whole blood or red blood cells, leukocytes reduced, CMV-negative, each unit

Ⓚ ☑ **P9052** Platelets, HLA-matched leukocytes reduced, apheresis/pheresis, each unit

Ⓚ ☑ **P9053** Platelets, pheresis, leukocytes reduced, CMV-negative, irradiated, each unit

Pathology and Laboratory Services

P9054 — P9615

K	☑	**P9054**	Whole blood or red blood cells, leukocytes reduced, frozen, deglycerol, washed, each unit
K	☑	**P9055**	Platelets, leukocytes reduced, CMV-negative, apheresis/pheresis, each unit
K	☑	**P9056**	Whole blood, leukocytes reduced, irradiated, each unit
K	☑	**P9057**	Red blood cells, frozen/deglycerolized/washed, leukocytes reduced, irradiated, each unit
K	☑	**P9058**	Red blood cells, leukocytes reduced, CMV-negative, irradiated, each unit
K	☑	**P9059**	Fresh frozen plasma between 8-24 hours of collection, each unit
K	☑	**P9060**	Fresh frozen plasma, donor retested, each unit

A	☑	**P9603**	Travel allowance one way in connection with medically necessary laboratory specimen collection drawn from homebound or nursing home bound patient; prorated miles actually traveled MED: 100-4, 16, 60
A	☑	**P9604**	Travel allowance one way in connection with medically necessary laboratory specimen collection drawn from homebound or nursing home bound patient; prorated trip charge MED: 100-4, 16, 60
N		**P9612**	Catheterization for collection of specimen, single patient, all places of service ⊘ See also new CPT catheterization codes 51701-51703 MED: 100-4, 16, 60
N		**P9615**	Catheterization for collection of specimen(s) (multiple patients) See also new CPT catheterization codes 51701-51703 MED: 100-4, 16, 60

Special Coverage Instructions   Noncovered by Medicare   Carrier Discretion   ☑ Quantity Alert   ● New Code   ○ Reinstated Code   ▲ Revised Code

124 — P Codes   A Age   M Maternity   ♀ Female Only   ♂ Male Only   A-Y APC Status Indicator   *2006 HCPCS*

Q CODES (TEMPORARY) *Q0000-Q9999*

New temporary Q codes to pay health care providers for the supplies used in creating casts were established to replace the removal of the practice expense for all HCPCS codes, including the CPT codes for fracture management and for casts and splints. Coders should continue to use the appropriate CPT code to report the work and practice expenses involved with creating the cast or splint; the temporary Q codes replace less specific coding for the casting and splinting supplies.

Q codes fall under the jurisdiction of the local contractor unless they represent an incidental service or are otherwise specified.

⊠ **Q0035** Cardiokymography
Covered only in conjunction with electrocardiographic stress testing in male patients with atypical angina or nonischemic chest pain, or female patients with angina.
MED: 100-3, 20.24

Ⓣ **Q0081** Infusion therapy, using other than chemotherapeutic drugs, per visit ⊘
MED: 100-3, 280.14
AHA: 1Q, '02, 7; 2Q, '02, 9, 10; 4Q, '02, 7

Ⓢ **Q0083** Chemotherapy administration by other than infusion technique only (e.g., subcutaneous, intramuscular, push), per visit
AHA: 1Q, '02, 1, 7

Ⓢ ☑ **Q0084** Chemotherapy administration by infusion technique only, per visit
MED: 100-3, 280.14
AHA: 1Q, '02, 1, 7

Ⓔ ☑ **Q0085** Chemotherapy administration by both infusion technique and other technique(s) (e.g., subcutaneous, intramuscular, push), per visit
AHA: 1Q, '02, 1, 7

Ⓣ **Q0091** Screening Papanicolaou smear; obtaining, preparing and conveyance of cervical or vaginal smear to laboratory Ⓐ ♀
One pap test is covered by Medicare every two years for low risk patients and every one year for high risk patients. Q0091 can be reported with an E/M code when a separately identifiable E/M service is provided.
MED: 100-3, 190.2
AHA: 4Q, '02, 8

Ⓝ **Q0092** Set-up portable x-ray equipment
MED: 100-2, 15, 80.4; 100-4, 13, 90

Ⓐ **Q0111** Wet mounts, including preparations of vaginal, cervical or skin specimens

Ⓐ **Q0112** All potassium hydroxide (KOH) preparations

Ⓐ **Q0113** Pinworm examination

Ⓐ **Q0114** Fern test ♀

Ⓐ **Q0115** Post-coital direct, qualitative examinations of vaginal or cervical mucous Ⓐ ♀

~~**Q0136** Injection, epoetin alpha, (for non ESRD use), per 1,000 units~~
See code(s) J0885.

~~**Q0137** Injection, darbepoetin alfa, 1 mcg (non ESRD use)~~
See code(s) J0881.

Ⓔ **Q0144** Azithromycin dihydrate, oral, capsules/powder, 1 gram ⊘
Use this code for Zithromax, Zithromax Z-PAK.

Ⓝ **Q0163** Diphenhydramine HCl, 50 mg, oral, FDA approved prescription anti-emetic, for use as a complete therapeutic substitute for an IV anti-emetic at time of chemotherapy treatment not to exceed a 48-hour dosage regimen
See also J1200. Medicare covers at the time of chemotherapy if regimen doesn't exceed 48 hours. Submit on the same claim as the chemotherapy. Use this code for Truxadryl.
MED: 100-4, 17, 80.2
AHA: 1Q, '02, 2

Ⓝ **Q0164** Prochlorperazine maleate, 5 mg, oral, FDA approved prescription anti-emetic, for use as a complete therapeutic substitute for an IV anti-emetic at the time of chemotherapy treatment, not to exceed a 48-hour dosage regimen
Medicare covers at the time of chemotherapy if regimen doesn't exceed 48 hours. Submit on the same claim as the chemotherapy. Medicare jurisdiction: DME regional contractor. Use this code for Compazine.
MED: 100-4, 17, 80.2

Ⓑ **Q0165** Prochlorperazine maleate, 10 mg, oral, FDA approved prescription anti-emetic, for use as a complete therapeutic substitute for an IV anti-emetic at the time of chemotherapy treatment, not to exceed a 48-hour dosage regimen
Medicare covers at the time of chemotherapy if regimen doesn't exceed 48 hours. Submit on the same claim as the chemotherapy. Medicare jurisdiction: DME regional contractor. Use this code for Compazine.
MED: 100-4, 17, 80.2

Ⓚ **Q0166** Granisetron HCl, 1 mg, oral, FDA approved prescription anti-emetic, for use as a complete therapeutic substitute for an IV anti-emetic at the time of chemotherapy treatment, not to exceed a 24-hour dosage regimen
Medicare covers at the time of chemotherapy if regimen doesn't exceed 48 hours. Submit on the same claim as the chemotherapy. Medicare jurisdiction: DME regional contractor. Use this code for Kytril.
MED: 100-4, 17, 80.2

Ⓝ **Q0167** Dronabinol, 2.5 mg, oral, FDA approved prescription anti-emetic, for use as a complete therapeutic substitute for an IV anti-emetic at the time of chemotherapy treatment, not to exceed a 48-hour dosage regimen
Medicare covers at the time of chemotherapy if regimen doesn't exceed 48 hours. Submit on the same claim as the chemotherapy. Medicare jurisdiction: DME regional contractor. Use this code for Marinol.
MED: 100-4, 17, 80.2

Ⓑ **Q0168** Dronabinol, 5 mg, oral, FDA approved prescription anti-emetic, for use as a complete therapeutic substitute for an IV anti-emetic at the time of chemotherapy treatment, not to exceed a 48-hour dosage regimen
Medicare jurisdiction: DME regional contractor. Use this code for Marinol.
MED: 100-4, 17, 80.2

Ⓝ **Q0169** Promethazine HCl, 12.5 mg, oral, FDA approved prescription anti-emetic, for use as a complete therapeutic substitute for an IV anti-emetic at the time of chemotherapy treatment, not to exceed a 48-hour dosage regimen
Medicare covers at the time of chemotherapy if regimen doesn't exceed 48 hours. Submit on the same claim as the chemotherapy. Medicare jurisdiction: DME regional contractor. Use this code for Phenergan, Amergan.
MED: 100-4, 17, 80.2

Special Coverage Instructions · Noncovered by Medicare · Carrier Discretion · ☑ Quantity Alert · ● New Code · ○ Reinstated Code · ▲ Revised Code

2006 HCPCS · ❶-❾ ASC Groups · MED: Pub 100/NCD Reference · ㄥ DMEPOS Paid · ⊘ SNF Excluded · Q Codes — 125

B **Q0170** Promethazine HCl, 25 mg, oral, FDA approved prescription anti-emetic, for use as a complete therapeutic substitute for an IV anti-emetic at the time of chemotherapy treatment, not to exceed a 48-hour dosage regimen
Medicare covers at the time of chemotherapy if regimen doesn't exceed 48 hours. Submit on the same claim as the chemotherapy. Medicare jurisdiction: DME regional contractor. Use this code for Phenergan, Amergan.
MED: 100-4, 17, 80.2

N **Q0171** Chlorpromazine HCl, 10 mg, oral, FDA approved prescription anti-emetic, for use as a complete therapeutic substitute for an IV anti-emetic at the time of chemotherapy treatment, not to exceed a 48-hour dosage regimen
Medicare covers at the time of chemotherapy if regimen doesn't exceed 48 hours. Submit on the same claim as the chemotherapy. Medicare jurisdiction: DME regional contractor. Use this code for Thorazine.
MED: 100-4, 17, 80.2

B **Q0172** Chlorpromazine HCl, 25 mg, oral, FDA approved prescription anti-emetic, for use as a complete therapeutic substitute for an IV anti-emetic at the time of chemotherapy treatment, not to exceed a 48-hour dosage regimen
Medicare covers at the time of chemotherapy if regimen doesn't exceed 48 hours. Submit on the same claim as the chemotherapy. Medicare jurisdiction: DME regional contractor. Use this code for Thorazine.
MED: 100-4, 17, 80.2

N **Q0173** Trimethobenzamide HCl, 250 mg, oral, FDA approved prescription anti-emetic, for use as a complete therapeutic substitute for an IV anti-emetic at the time of chemotherapy treatment, not to exceed a 48-hour dosage regimen
Medicare covers at the time of chemotherapy if regimen doesn't exceed 48 hours. Submit on the same claim as the chemotherapy. Medicare jurisdiction: DME regional contractor. Use this code for Tebamide, T-Gen, Ticon, Tigan, Triban, Thimazide.
MED: 100-4, 17, 80.2

N **Q0174** Thiethylperazine maleate, 10 mg, oral, FDA approved prescription anti-emetic, for use as a complete therapeutic substitute for an IV anti-emetic at the time of chemotherapy treatment, not to exceed a 48-hour dosage regimen
Medicare covers at the time of chemotherapy if regimen doesn't exceed 48 hours. Submit on the same claim as the chemotherapy. Medicare jurisdiction: DME regional contractor. Use this code for Torecan.
MED: 100-4, 17, 80.2

N **Q0175** Perphenazine, 4 mg, oral, FDA approved prescription anti-emetic, for use as a complete therapeutic substitute for an IV anti-emetic at the time of chemotherapy treatment, not to exceed a 48-hour dosage regimen
Medicare covers at the time of chemotherapy if regimen doesn't exceed 48 hours. Submit on the same claim as the chemotherapy. Medicare jurisdiction: DME regional contractor. Use this code for Trilifon.
MED: 100-4, 17, 80.2

B **Q0176** Perphenazine, 8 mg, oral, FDA approved prescription anti-emetic, for use as a complete therapeutic substitute for an IV anti-emetic at the time of chemotherapy treatment, not to exceed a 48-hour dosage regimen
Medicare covers at the time of chemotherapy if regimen doesn't exceed 48 hours. Submit on the same claim as the chemotherapy. Medicare jurisdiction: DME regional contractor. Use this code for Trilifon.
MED: 100-4, 17, 80.2

N **Q0177** Hydroxyzine pamoate, 25 mg, oral, FDA approved prescription anti-emetic, for use as a complete therapeutic substitute for an IV anti-emetic at the time of chemotherapy treatment, not to exceed a 48-hour dosage regimen
Medicare covers at the time of chemotherapy if regimen doesn't exceed 48 hours. Submit on the same claim as the chemotherapy. Medicare jurisdiction: DME regional contractor. Use this code for Vistaril.
MED: 100-4, 17, 80.2

B **Q0178** Hydroxyzine pamoate, 50 mg, oral, FDA approved prescription anti-emetic, for use as a complete therapeutic substitute for an IV anti-emetic at the time of chemotherapy treatment, not to exceed a 48-hour dosage regimen
Medicare covers at the time of chemotherapy if regimen doesn't exceed 48 hours. Submit on the same claim as the chemotherapy.
MED: 100-4, 17, 80.2

N **Q0179** Ondansetron HCl 8 mg, oral, FDA approved prescription anti-emetic, for use as a complete therapeutic substitute for an IV anti-emetic at the time of chemotherapy treatment, not to exceed a 48-hour dosage regimen
Medicare covers at the time of chemotherapy if regimen doesn't exceed 48 hours. Submit on the same claim as the chemotherapy. Medicare jurisdiction: DME regional contractor. Use this code for Zofran.
MED: 100-4, 17, 80.2

K **Q0180** Dolasetron mesylate, 100 mg, oral, FDA approved prescription anti-emetic, for use as a complete therapeutic substitute for an IV anti-emetic at the time of chemotherapy treatment, not to exceed a 24-hour dosage regimen
Medicare covers at the time of chemotherapy if regimen doesn't exceed 24 hours. Submit on the same claim as the chemotherapy. Medicare jurisdiction: DME regional contractor. Use this code for Anzemet.
MED: 100-4, 17, 80.2

E **Q0181** Unspecified oral dosage form, FDA approved prescription anti-emetic, for use as a complete therapeutic substitute for an IV anti-emetic at the time of chemotherapy treatment, not to exceed a 48-hour dosage regimen
Medicare covers at the time of chemotherapy if regimen doesn't exceed 48-hours. Submit on the same claim as the chemotherapy. Medicare jurisdiction: DME regional contractor.
MED: 100-4, 17, 80.2

~~**Q0187** Factor VIIa (coagulation factor, recombinant) per 1.2 mg~~
See code(s) J7189.

● A **Q0480** Driver for use with pneumatic ventricular assist device, replacement only
AHA: 3Q, '05, 2

● A **Q0481** Microprocessor control unit for use with electric ventricular assist device, replacement only
AHA: 3Q, '05, 2

Special Coverage Instructions   Noncovered by Medicare   Carrier Discretion   ☑ Quantity Alert   ● New Code   ○ Reinstated Code   ▲ Revised Code

126 — Q Codes   A Age   M Maternity   ♀ Female Only   ♂ Male Only   A-Y APC Status Indicator   *2006 HCPCS*

● Ⓐ **Q0482** Microprocessor control unit for use with electric/pneumatic combination ventricular assist device, replacement only ♿
AHA: 3Q, '05, 2

● Ⓐ **Q0483** Monitor/display module for use with electric ventricular assist device, replacement only ♿
AHA: 3Q, '05, 2

● Ⓐ **Q0484** Monitor/display module for use with electric or electric/pneumatic ventricular assist device, replacement only ♿
AHA: 3Q, '05, 2

● Ⓐ **Q0485** Monitor control cable for use with electric ventricular assist device, replacement only ♿
AHA: 3Q, '05, 2

● Ⓐ **Q0486** Monitor control cable for use with electric/pneumatic ventricular assist device, replacement only ♿
AHA: 3Q, '05, 2

● Ⓐ **Q0487** Leads (pneumatic/electrical) for use with any type electric/pneumatic ventricular assist device, replacement only ♿
AHA: 3Q, '05, 2

● Ⓐ **Q0488** Power pack base for use with electric ventricular assist device, replacement only
AHA: 3Q, '05, 2

● Ⓐ **Q0489** Power pack base for use with electric/pneumatic ventricular assist device, replacement only ♿
AHA: 3Q, '05, 2

● Ⓐ **Q0490** Emergency power source for use with electric ventricular assist device, replacement only ♿
AHA: 3Q, '05, 2

● Ⓐ **Q0491** Emergency power source for use with electric/pneumatic ventricular assist device, replacement only ♿
AHA: 3Q, '05, 2

● Ⓐ **Q0492** Emergency power supply cable for use with electric ventricular assist device, replacement only ♿
AHA: 3Q, '05, 2

● Ⓐ **Q0493** Emergency power supply cable for use with electric/pneumatic ventricular assist device, replacement only ♿
AHA: 3Q, '05, 2

● Ⓐ **Q0494** Emergency hand pump for use with electric/pneumatic ventricular assist device, replacement only ♿
AHA: 3Q, '05, 2

● Ⓐ **Q0495** Battery/power pack charger for use with electric or electric/pneumatic ventricular assist device, replacement only ♿
AHA: 3Q, '05, 2

● Ⓐ **Q0496** Battery for use with electric or electric/pneumatic ventricular assist device, replacement only ♿
AHA: 3Q, '05, 2

● Ⓐ **Q0497** Battery clips for use with electric or electric/pneumatic ventricular assist device, replacement only ♿
AHA: 3Q, '05, 2

● Ⓐ **Q0498** Holster for use with electric or electric/pneumatic ventricular assist device, replacement only ♿
AHA: 3Q, '05, 2

● Ⓐ **Q0499** Belt/vest for use with electric or electric/pneumatic ventricular assist device, replacement only ♿
AHA: 3Q, '05, 2

● Ⓐ ☑ **Q0500** Filters for use with electric or electric/pneumatic ventricular assist device, replacement only ♿
The base unit for this code is for each filter.
AHA: 3Q, '05, 2

● Ⓐ **Q0501** Shower cover for use with electric or electric/pneumatic ventricular assist device, replacement only ♿
AHA: 3Q, '05, 2

● Ⓐ **Q0502** Mobility cart for pneumatic ventricular assist device, replacement only ♿
AHA: 3Q, '05, 2

● Ⓐ **Q0503** Battery for pneumatic ventricular assist device, replacement only, each ♿
AHA: 3Q, '05, 2

● Ⓐ **Q0504** Power adapter for pneumatic ventricular assist device, replacement only, vehicle type ♿
AHA: 3Q, '05, 2

● Ⓐ **Q0505** Miscellaneous supply or accessory for use with ventricular assist device
AHA: 3Q, '05, 2

● Ⓑ **Q0510** Pharmacy supply fee for initial immunosuppressive drug(s), first month following transplant

● Ⓑ **Q0511** Pharmacy supply fee for oral anti-cancer, oral anti-emetic or immunosuppressive drug(s); for the first prescription In a 30-day period

● Ⓜ **Q0512** Pharmacy supply fee for oral anti-cancer, oral anti-emetic or immunosuppressive drug(s); for a subsequent prescription in a 30-day period

● Ⓑ **Q0513** Pharmacy dispensing fee for inhalation drug(s); per 30 days

● Ⓑ **Q0514** Pharmacy dispensing fee for inhalation drug(s); per 90 days

● Ⓝ **Q0515** Injection, sermorelin acetate, 1 mcg
MED: 100-2, 15, 50

~~**Q1001** New technology intraocular lens category 1 as defined in Federal Register notice, Vol. 65, date May 3, 2000~~

~~**Q1002** New technology intraocular lens category 2 as defined in Federal Register notice, Vol. 65, dated May 3, 2000~~

Ⓑ **Q1003** New technology intraocular lens category 3 as defined in Federal Register notice ⊘

Ⓑ **Q1004** New technology intraocular lens category 4 as defined in Federal Register notice ⊘

Ⓑ **Q1005** New technology intraocular lens category 5 as defined in Federal Register notice ⊘

~~**Q2001** Oral, cabergoline, 0.5 mg~~
See code(s) J8515.

~~**Q2002** Injection, Elliott's B solution, per ml~~
See code(s) J9175.

~~**Q2003** Injection, aprotinin, 10,000 kiu~~
See code(s) J0365.

Ⓝ ☑ **Q2004** Irrigation solution for treatment of bladder calculi, for example renacidin, per 500 ml

~~**Q2005** Injection, corticorelin ovine triflutate, per dose~~
See code(s) J0795.

| Special Coverage Instructions | Noncovered by Medicare | Carrier Discretion | ☑ Quantity Alert | ● New Code | ○ Reinstated Code | ▲ Revised Code |

2006 HCPCS   **1**-**9** ASC Groups   **MED:** Pub 100/NCD Reference   ♿ DMEPOS Paid   ⊘ SNF Excluded   **Q Codes — 127**

Q Codes (Temporary)

Q2006 — Q4016

~~Q2006 Injection, digoxin immune fab (ovine), per vial~~
See code(s) J1162.

~~Q2007 Injection, ethanolamine oleate, 100 mg~~
See code(s) J1430.

~~Q2008 Injection, fomepizole, 15 mg~~
See code(s) J1451.

☒ ☑ **Q2009** Injection, fosphenytoin, 50 mg ⊘
Use this code for Cerebryx.
MED: 100-2, 15, 50

~~Q2011 Injection, hemin, per 1 mg~~
See code(s) J1640.

~~Q2012 Injection, pegademase bovine, 25 IU~~
See code(s) J2504.

~~Q2013 Injection, pentastarch, 10% solution, per 100 ml~~
See code(s) J2513.

~~Q2014 Injection, sermorelin acetate, 0.5 mg~~
See code(s) Q0515.

☒ ☑ **Q2017** Injection, teniposide, 50 mg ⊘
Use this code for Vumon.
MED: 100-2, 15, 50

~~Q2018 Injection, urofollitropin, 75 IU~~
See code(s) J3355.

~~Q2019 Injection, basiliximab, 20 mg~~
See code(s) J0480.

~~Q2020 Injection, histrelin acetate, 10 mg~~
See code(s) J1675.

~~Q2021 Injection, lepirudin, 50 mg~~
See code(s) J1945.

~~Q2022 Von Willebrand factor complex, human, per IU~~
See code(s) J7188.

~~Q3000 Supply of radiopharmaceutical diagnostic imaging agent, rubidium RB 82, per dose~~
See code(s) A9555.

☒ ☑ **Q3001** Radioelements for brachytherapy, any type, each⊘
MED: 100-4, 12, 70; 100-4, 13, 20; 100-4, 13, 90

~~Q3002 Supply of radiopharmaceutical diagnostic imaging agent, gallium Ga 67, per mCi~~
See code(s) A9556.

~~Q3003 Supply of radiopharmaceutical diagnostic imaging agent, technetium Te 00m bicisate, per unit dose~~
See code(s) A9557.

~~Q3004 Supply of radiopharmaceutical diagnostic imaging agent, xenon Xe 133, per 10 mCi~~
See code(s) A9558.

~~Q3005 Supply of radiopharmaceutical diagnostic imaging agent, technetium Te 00m mertiatide, per mCi~~
See code(s) A9562.

~~Q3006 Supply of radiopharmaceutical diagnostic imaging agent, technetium Te 00m glucepatate, per 5 mCi~~
See code(s) A9550.

~~Q3007 Supply of radiopharmaceutical diagnostic imaging agent, sodium phosphate P32, per mCi~~
See code(s) A9563.

~~Q3008 Supply of radiopharmaceutical diagnostic imaging agent, indium 111 ,Äi in pentetreotide, per 3 mCi~~
See code(s) A9565.

~~Q3000 Supply of radiopharmaceutical diagnostic imaging agent, technetium Te 00m oxidronate, per mCi~~
See code(s) A9561.

~~Q3010 Supply of radiopharmaceutical diagnostic imaging agent, technetium Te 00m ,Äi labeled red blood cells, per mCi~~
See code(s) A9560.

~~Q3011 Supply of radiopharmaceutical diagnostic imaging agent, chromic phosphate P32 suspension, per mCi~~
See code(s) A9564.

~~Q3012 Supply of oral radiopharmaceutical diagnostic imaging agent, cyanocobalamin cobalt Co 57, per 0.5 mCi~~
See code(s) A9559.

Ⓐ **Q3014** Telehealth originating site facility fee ⊘

Ⓐ **Q3019** ALS vehicle used, emergency transport, no ALS level services furnished

Ⓐ **Q3020** ALS vehicle used, non-emergency transport, no ALS level service furnished

☒ **Q3025** Injection, interferon beta-1A, 11 mcg for intramuscular use
Use this code for Avonex, Rebif. See also J1825.
MED: 100-2, 15, 50

Ⓔ **Q3026** Injection, interferon beta-1A, 11 mcg for subcutaneous use
Use this code for Avonex Rebif. See also J1825.

Ⓝ **Q3031** Collagen skin test
MED: 100-3, 230.10

Ⓑ **Q4001** Casting supplies, body cast adult, with or without head, plaster Ⓐ

Ⓑ **Q4002** Cast supplies, body cast adult, with or without head, fiberglass Ⓐ

Ⓑ **Q4003** Cast supplies, shoulder cast, adult (11 years +), plaster Ⓐ

Ⓑ **Q4004** Cast supplies, shoulder cast, adult (11 years +), fiberglass Ⓐ

Ⓑ **Q4005** Cast supplies, long arm cast, adult (11 years +), plaster Ⓐ

Ⓑ **Q4006** Cast supplies, long arm cast, adult (11 years +), fiberglass Ⓐ

Ⓑ **Q4007** Cast supplies, long arm cast, pediatric (0-10 years), plaster Ⓐ

Ⓑ **Q4008** Cast supplies, long arm cast, pediatric (0-10 years), fiberglass Ⓐ

Ⓑ **Q4009** Cast supplies, short arm cast, adult (11 years +), plaster Ⓐ

Ⓑ **Q4010** Cast supplies, short arm cast, adult (11 years +), fiberglass Ⓐ

Ⓑ **Q4011** Cast supplies, short arm cast, pediatric (0-10 years), plaster Ⓐ

Ⓑ **Q4012** Cast supplies, short arm cast, pediatric (0-10 years), fiberglass Ⓐ

Ⓑ **Q4013** Cast supplies, gauntlet cast (includes lower forearm and hand), adult (11 years +), plaster Ⓐ

Ⓑ **Q4014** Cast supplies, gauntlet cast (includes lower forearm and hand), adult (11 years +), fiberglass Ⓐ

Ⓑ **Q4015** Cast supplies, gauntlet cast (includes lower forearm and hand), pediatric (0-10 years), plaster Ⓐ

Ⓑ **Q4016** Cast supplies, gauntlet cast (includes lower forearm and hand), pediatric (0-10 years), fiberglass Ⓐ

Special Coverage Instructions   Noncovered by Medicare   Carrier Discretion   ☑ Quantity Alert ● New Code ○ Reinstated Code ▲ Revised Code

128 — Q Codes   Ⓐ Age   Ⓜ Maternity   ♀ Female Only   ♂ Male Only   Ⓐ-Ⓨ APC Status Indicator   **2006 HCPCS**

Ⓑ   **Q4017** Cast supplies, long arm splint, adult (11 years +), plaster   Ⓐ

Ⓑ   **Q4018** Cast supplies, long arm splint, adult (11 years +), fiberglass   Ⓐ

Ⓑ   **Q4019** Cast supplies, long arm splint, pediatric (0-10 years), plaster   Ⓐ

Ⓑ   **Q4020** Cast supplies, long arm splint, pediatric (0-10 years), fiberglass   Ⓐ

Ⓑ   **Q4021** Cast supplies, short arm splint, adult (11 years +), plaster   Ⓐ

Ⓑ   **Q4022** Cast supplies, short arm splint, adult (11 years +), fiberglass   Ⓐ

Ⓑ   **Q4023** Cast supplies, short arm splint, pediatric (0-10 years), plaster   Ⓐ

Ⓑ   **Q4024** Cast supplies, short arm splint, pediatric (0-10 years), fiberglass   Ⓐ

Ⓑ   **Q4025** Cast supplies, hip spica (one or both legs), adult (11 years +), plaster   Ⓐ

Ⓑ   **Q4026** Cast supplies, hip spica (one or both legs), adult (11 years +), fiberglass   Ⓐ

Ⓑ   **Q4027** Cast supplies, hip spica (one or both legs), pediatric (0-10 years), plaster   Ⓐ

Ⓑ   **Q4028** Cast supplies, hip spica (one or both legs), pediatric (0-10 years), fiberglass   Ⓐ

Ⓑ   **Q4029** Cast supplies, long leg cast, adult (11 years +), plaster   Ⓐ

Ⓑ   **Q4030** Cast supplies, long leg cast, adult (11 years +), fiberglass   Ⓐ

Ⓑ   **Q4031** Cast supplies, long leg cast, pediatric (0-10 years), plaster   Ⓐ

Ⓑ   **Q4032** Cast supplies, long leg cast, pediatric (0-10 years), fiberglass   Ⓐ

Ⓑ   **Q4033** Cast supplies, long leg cylinder cast, adult (11 years +), plaster   Ⓐ

Ⓑ   **Q4034** Cast supplies, long leg cylinder cast, adult (11 years +), fiberglass   Ⓐ

Ⓑ   **Q4035** Cast supplies, long leg cylinder cast, pediatric (0-10 years), plaster   Ⓐ

Ⓑ   **Q4036** Cast supplies, long leg cylinder cast, pediatric (0-10 years), fiberglass   Ⓐ

Ⓑ   **Q4037** Cast supplies, short leg cast, adult (11 years +), plaster   Ⓐ

Ⓑ   **Q4038** Cast supplies, short leg cast, adult (11 years +), fiberglass   Ⓐ

Ⓑ   **Q4039** Cast supplies, short leg cast, pediatric (0-10 years), plaster   Ⓐ

Ⓑ   **Q4040** Cast supplies, short leg cast, pediatric (0-10 years), fiberglass   Ⓐ

Ⓑ   **Q4041** Cast supplies, long leg splint, adult (11 years +), plaster   Ⓐ

Ⓑ   **Q4042** Cast supplies, long leg splint, adult (11 years +), fiberglass   Ⓐ

Ⓑ   **Q4043** Cast supplies, long leg splint, pediatric (0-10 years), plaster   Ⓐ

Ⓑ   **Q4044** Cast supplies, long leg splint, pediatric (0-10 years), fiberglass   Ⓐ

Ⓑ   **Q4045** Cast supplies, short leg splint, adult (11 years +), plaster   Ⓐ

Ⓑ   **Q4046** Cast supplies, short leg splint, adult (11 years +), fiberglass   Ⓐ

Ⓑ   **Q4047** Cast supplies, short leg splint, pediatric (0-10 years), plaster   Ⓐ

Ⓑ   **Q4048** Cast supplies, short leg splint, pediatric (0-10 years), fiberglass   Ⓐ

Ⓑ   **Q4049** Finger splint, static

Ⓑ   **Q4050** Cast supplies, for unlisted types and materials of casts

Ⓑ   **Q4051** Splint supplies, miscellaneous (includes thermoplastics, strapping, fasteners, padding and other supplies)

Q4054 ~~Injection, darbepoetin alfa, 1 mcg (for ESRD on dialysis)~~
See code(s) J0882.

Q4055 ~~Injection, epoetin alfa, 1000 units (for ESRD on dialysis)~~
See code(s) J0886.

Q4075 ~~Injection, acyclovir, 5 mg~~
See code(s) J0133.

Q4076 ~~Injection, dopamine HCl, 40 mg~~
See code(s) J1265.

Q4077 ~~Injection, treprostinil, 1 mg~~
See code(s) J3285.

● Ⓖ   **Q4079** Injection, natalizumab, per 1 mg
AHA: 2Q, '05, 11

● Ⓑ   **Q4080** Iloprost, inhalation solution, administered through DME, 20 mcg
AHA: 3Q, '05, 7

Q0041 ~~Injection, immune globulin, intravenous, lyophilized, 1 g~~
See code(s) J1566.

Q0042 ~~Injection, immune globulin, intravenous, lyophilized, 10 mg~~
See code(s) J1566.

Q0043 ~~Injection, immune globulin, intravenous, nonlyophilized, 1 g~~
See code(s) J1567.

Q0044 ~~Injection, immune globulin, intravenous, nonlyophilized, 10 mg~~
See code(s) J1567.

● Ⓚ   **Q9945** Low osmolar contrast material, up to 149 mg/ml iodine concentration, per ml
MED: 100-4, 13, 20; 100-4, 13, 90

● Ⓚ   **Q9946** Low osmolar contrast material, 150-199 mg/ml iodine concentration, per ml
MED: 100-4, 12, 70; 100-4, 13, 20; 100-4, 13, 90

● Ⓚ   **Q9947** Low osmolar contrast material, 200-249 mg/ml iodine concentration, per ml
MED: 100-4, 12, 70; 100-4, 13, 20; 100-4, 13, 90

● Ⓚ   **Q9948** Low osmolar contrast material, 250-299 mg/ml iodine concentration, per ml
MED: 100-4, 12, 70; 100-4, 13, 20; 100-4, 13, 90

● Ⓚ   **Q9949** Low osmolar contrast material, 300-349 mg/ml iodine concentration, per ml
MED: 100-4, 12, 70; 100-4, 13, 20; 100-4, 13, 90

● Ⓚ   **Q9950** Low osmolar contrast material, 350-399 mg/ml iodine concentration, per ml
MED: 100-4, 12, 70; 100-4, 13, 20; 100-4, 13, 90

● Ⓚ   **Q9951** Low osmolar contrast material, 400 or greater mg/ml iodine concentration, per ml
MED: 100-4, 12, 70; 100-4, 13, 20; 100-4, 13, 90

Special Coverage Instructions		☑ Quantity Alert	● New Code	○ Reinstated Code	▲ Revised Code
Noncovered by Medicare					
2006 HCPCS	**1**-**9** ASC Groups MED: Pub 100/NCD Reference	⅃ DMEPOS Paid	Ⓢ SNF Excluded		**Q Codes — 129**

Carrier Discretion

● K **Q9952** Injection, gadolinium-based magnetic resonance contrast agent, per ml
MED: 100-4, 12, 70; 100-4, 13, 20; 100-4, 13, 90

● K **Q9953** Injection, iron-based magnetic resonance contrast agent, per ml
MED: 100-4, 12, 70; 100-4, 13, 20; 100-4, 13, 90

● K **Q9954** Oral magnetic resonance contrast agent, per ml
MED: 100-4, 12, 70; 100-4, 13, 20; 100-4, 13, 90

● K **Q9955** Injection, perflexane lipid microspheres, per ml

● K **Q9956** Injection, octafluoropropane microspheres, per ml

● K **Q9957** Injection, perflutren lipid microspheres, per ml

● K **Q9958** High osmolar contrast material, up to 149 mg/ml iodine concentration, per ml
MED: 100-4, 12, 70; 100-4, 13, 20; 100-4, 13, 90

AHA: 3Q, '05, 7

● N **Q9959** High osmolar contrast material, 150-199 mg/ml iodine concentration, per ml
MED: 100-4, 12, 70; 100-4, 13, 20; 100-4, 13, 90

AHA: 3Q, '05, 7

● K **Q9960** High osmolar contrast material, 200-249 mg/ml iodine concentration, per ml
MED: 100-4, 12, 70; 100-4, 13, 20; 100-4, 13, 90

AHA: 3Q, '05, 7

● K **Q9961** High osmolar contrast material, 250-299 mg/ml iodine concentration, per ml
MED: 100-4, 12, 70; 100-4, 13, 20; 100-4, 13, 90

AHA: 3Q, '05, 7

● K **Q9962** High osmolar contrast material, 300-349 mg/ml iodine concentration, per ml
MED: 100-4, 12, 70; 100-4, 13, 20; 100-4, 13, 90

AHA: 3Q, '05, 7

● K **Q9963** High osmolar contrast material, 350-399 mg/ml iodine concentration, per ml
MED: 100-4, 12, 70; 100-4, 13, 20; 100-4, 13, 90

AHA: 3Q, '05, 7

● K **Q9964** High osmolar contrast material, 400 or greater mg/ml iodine concentration, per ml
MED: 100-4, 12, 70; 100-4, 13, 20; 100-4, 13, 90

AHA: 3Q, '05, 7

Special Coverage Instructions   Noncovered by Medicare   Carrier Discretion   ☑ Quantity Alert   ● New Code   ○ Reinstated Code   ▲ Revised Code

130 — Q Codes   A Age   M Maternity   ♀ Female Only   ♂ Male Only   A-Y APC Status Indicator   *2006 HCPCS*

DIAGNOSTIC RADIOLOGY SERVICES *R0000-R5999*

R codes are used for the transportation of portable x-ray and/or EKG equipment.

R codes fall under the jurisdiction of the local contractor.

Ⓝ ☑ **R0070 Transportation of portable x-ray equipment and personnel to home or nursing home, per trip to facility or location, one patient seen**
Only a single, reasonable transportation charge is allowed for each trip the portable x-ray supplier makes to a location. When more than one patient is x-rayed at the same location, prorate the single allowable transport charge among all patients.

MED: 100-2, 15, 80.4; 100-4, 13, 90; 100-4, 13, 90

Ⓝ ☑ **R0075 Transportation of portable x-ray equipment and personnel to home or nursing home, per trip to facility or location, more than one patient seen**
Only a single, reasonable transportation charge is allowed for each trip the portable x-ray supplier makes to a location. When more than one patient is x-rayed at the same location, prorate the single allowable transport charge among all patients.

MED: 100-2, 15, 80.4; 100-4, 13, 90; 100-4, 13, 90

Ⓝ ☑ **R0076 Transportation of portable EKG to facility or location, per patient** ⊘
Only a single, reasonable transportation charge is allowed for each trip the portable EKG supplier makes to a location. When more than one patient is tested at the same location, prorate the single allowable transport charge among all patients.

MED: 100-1, 5, 90.2; 100-2, 15, 80.1; 100-2, 15, 80.4; 100-3, 20.15; 100-4, 13, 90; 100-4, 16, 10; 100-4, 16, 10.1; 100-4, 16, 110.4

Special Coverage Instructions   Noncovered by Medicare   Carrier Discretion   ☑ Quantity Alert   ● New Code   ○ Reinstated Code   ▲ Revised Code

2006 HCPCS   ❶-❾ ASC Groups   MED: Pub 100/NCD Reference   ♿ DMEPOS Paid   ⊘ SNF Excluded   **R Codes — 131**

TEMPORARY NATIONAL CODES (NON-MEDICARE)
S0000-S9999

The S codes are used by the Blue Cross/Blue Shield Association (BCBSA) and the Health Insurance Association of America (HIAA) to report drugs, services, and supplies for which there are no national codes but for which codes are needed by the private sector to implement policies, programs, or claims processing. They are for the purpose of meeting the particular needs of the private sector. These codes are also used by the Medicaid program, but they are not payable by Medicare.

☑ **S0012** Butorphanol tartrate, nasal spray, 25 mg
Use this code for Stadol NS.

☑ **S0014** Tacrine HCl, 10 mg
Use this code for Cognex.

~~**S0016** Injection, amikacin sulfate, 500 mg~~

☑ **S0017** Injection, aminocaproic acid, 5 grams
Use this code for Amicar.

☑ **S0020** Injection, bupivacaine HCl, 30 ml
Use this code for Marcaine, Sensorcaine.

☑ **S0021** Injection, cefoperazone sodium, 1 gram
Use this code for Cefobid.

☑ **S0023** Injection, cimetidine HCl, 300 mg
Use this code for Tagamet HCl.

☑ **S0028** Injection, famotidine, 20 mg
Use this code for Pepcid.

☑ **S0030** Injection, metronidazole, 500 mg
Use this code for Flagyl IV RTU.

☑ **S0032** Injection, nafcillin sodium, 2 grams
Use this code for Nallpen, Unipen.

☑ **S0034** Injection, ofloxacin, 400 mg
Use this code for Floxin IV.

☑ **S0039** Injection, sulfamethoxazole and trimethoprim, 10 ml
Use this code for Bactrim IV, Septra IV, SMZ-TMP, Sulfutrim.

☑ **S0040** Injection, ticarcillin disodium and clavulanate potassium, 3.1 grams
Use this code for Timentin.

~~**S0071** Injection, acyclovir sodium, 50 mg~~
See code(s) J0133.

~~**S0072** Injection, amikacin sulfate, 100 mg~~
See code(s) J0278.

☑ **S0073** Injection, aztreonam, 500 mg
Use this code for Azactam.

☑ **S0074** Injection, cefotetan disodium, 500 mg
Use this code for Cefotan.

☑ **S0077** Injection, clindamycin phosphate, 300 mg
Use this code for Cleocin Phosphate.

☑ **S0078** Injection, fosphenytoin sodium, 750 mg
Use this code for Cerebryx.

☑ **S0080** Injection, pentamidine isethionate, 300 mg
Use this code for NebuPent, Pentam 300, Pentacarinat. See also code J2545.

☑ **S0081** Injection, piperacillin sodium, 500 mg
Use this code for Pipracil.

☑ **S0088** Imatinib 100 mg
Use this code for Gleevec.

☑ **S0090** Sildenafil citrate, 25 mg   ▲
Use this code for Viagra.

☑ **S0091** Granisetron hydrochloride, 1 mg (for circumstances falling under the Medicare statute, use Q0166)
Use this code for Kytril.

☑ **S0092** Injection, hydromorphone hydrochloride, 250 mg (loading dose for infusion pump)
Use this code for Dilaudid, Hydromophone. See also J1170.

☑ **S0093** Injection, morphine sulfate, 500 mg (loading dose for infusion pump)
Use this code for Duramorph, MS Contin, Morphine Sulfate. See also J2270, J2271, J2275.

S0104 Zidovudine, oral 100 mg
See also J3485 for Retrovir.

☑ **S0106** Bupropion HCl sustained release tablet, 150 mg, per bottle of 60 tablets
Use this code for Wellbutrin SR tablets.

~~**S0107** Injection, omalizumab, 25 mg~~

S0108 Mercaptopurine, oral, 50 mg
Use this code for Purinethol oral.

☑ **S0109** Methadone, oral, 5mg
Use this code for Dolophine.

~~**S0114** Injection, treprostinil sodium, 0.5 mg~~
See code(s) J3285.

☑ **S0116** Bevacizumab, 100 mg

☑ **S0117** Tretinoin, topical 5 grams

~~**S0118** Injection, ziconotide, for intrathecal infusion, 1 mcg~~

S0122 Injection, menotropins, 75 IU
Use this code for Humegon, Pergonal, Repronex.

S0126 Injection, follitropin alfa, 75 IU
Use this code for Gonal-F.

S0128 Injection, follitropin beta, 75 IU   ♀
Use this code for Follistim.

S0132 Injection, ganirelix acetate, 250 mcg   ♀
Use this code for Antagon.

● **S0133** Histerelin, implant, 50 mg
Use this code for Vantas.

☑ **S0136** Clozapine, 25 mg
Use this code for Clozaril.

☑ **S0137** Didanosine (ddi), 25 mg
Use this code for Videx.

☑ **S0138** Finasteride, 5 mg   ♂
Use this code for Propecia (oral), Proscar (oral).

☑ **S0139** Minoxidil, 10 mg
Use this code for Loniten (oral).

☑ **S0140** Saquinavir, 200 mg
Use this code for Fortovase (oral), Invirase (oral).

☑ **S0141** Zalcitabine (ddC), 0.375 mg
Use this code for Hivid (oral).

● **S0142** Colistimethate sodium, inhalation solution administrated through DME, concentrated form, per mg

● **S0143** Aztreonam, inhalation solution administered through DME, concentrated form, per gram

● **S0145** Injection, pegylated interferon alfa-2a, 180 mcg per ml
Use this code for Pegasys.

● **S0146** Injection, pegylated interferon alfa-2b, 10 mcg per 0.5 ml

☑ **S0155** Sterile dilutant for epoprostenol, 50 ml
Use this code for Flolan.

☑ **S0156** Exemestane, 25 mg
Use this code for Aromasin.

☑ **S0157** Becaplermin gel 0.01%, 0.5 gm
Use this code for Regraex Gel.

~~**S0158** Injection, laronidase, 0.58 mg~~

~~**S0159** Injection, agalsidase beta, 35 mg~~

☑ **S0160** Dextroamphetamine sulfate, 5 mg

☑ **S0161** Calcitrol, 0.25 mcg

☑ **S0162** Injection, efalizumab, 125 mg
Use this code for Raptiva.

☑ **S0164** Injection, pantoprazole sodium, 40 mg
Use this code for Protonix IV.

☑ **S0166** Injection, olanzapine, 2.5 mg
Use this code for Zyprexa.

☑ **S0167** Injection, apomorphine hydrochloride, 1 mg

~~**S0168** Injection, azacitidine, 100 mg~~
See code(s) J9025.

☑ **S0170** Anastrozole, oral, 1mg
Use this code for Arimidex.

☑ **S0171** Injection, bumetanide, 0.5 mg
Use this code for Bumex.

☑ **S0172** Chlorambucil, oral, 2 mg
Use this code for Leukeran.

~~**S0173** Dexamethasone, oral, 4 mg~~
See code(s) J8540.

☑ **S0174** Dolasetron mesylate, oral 50 mg (for circumstances falling under the Medicare statute, use Q0180)
Use this code for Anzemet.

☑ **S0175** Flutamide, oral, 125 mg
Use this code for Eulexin.

☑ **S0176** Hydroxyurea, oral, 500 mg
Use this code for Droxia, Hydrea, Mylocel.

☑ **S0177** Levamisole HCl, oral, 50 mg
Use this code for Ergamisol.

☑ **S0178** Lomustine, oral, 10 mg
Use this code for Ceenu.

☑ **S0179** Megestrol acetate, oral, 20 mg
Use this code for Megace.

☑ **S0181** Ondansetron HCl, oral, 4 mg (for circumstances falling under the Medicare statute, use Q0179)
Use this code for Zofran.

☑ **S0182** Procarbazine HCl, oral, 50 mg
Use this code for Matulane.

☑ **S0183** Prochlorperazine maleate, oral, 5 mg (for circumstances falling under the Medicare statute, use Q0164-Q0165)
Use this code for Compazine.

☑ **S0187** Tamoxifen citrate, oral, 10 mg
Use this code for Nolvadex.

☑ **S0189** Testosterone pellet, 75 mg

☑ **S0190** Mitepristone, oral, 200 mg ♀
Use this code for Mifoprex 200 mg oral.

☑ **S0191** Misoprostol, oral, 200 mcg

☑ **S0194** Dialysis/stress vitamin supplement, oral, 100 capsules

S0195 Pneumococcal conjugate vaccine, polyvalent, intramuscular, for children from five years to nine years of age who have not previously received the vaccine Ⓐ
Use this code for Pneumovax II.

☑ **S0196** Injectable poly-l-lactic acid, restorative implant, 1 ml, face (deep dermis, subcutaneous layers)

● ☑ **S0197** Prenatal vitamins, 30-day supply Ⓜ ♀

● ☑ **S0198** Injection, pegaptanib sodium, 0.3 mg
Use this code for Macugen.

S0199 Medically induced abortion by oral ingestion of medication including all associated services and supplies (e.g., patient counseling, office visits, confirmation of pregnancy by HCG, ultrasound to confirm duration of pregnancy, ultrasound to confirm completion of abortion) except drugs ♀

S0201 Partial hospitalization services, less than 24 hours, per diem

S0207 Paramedic intercept, non-hospital based ALS service (non-voluntary), non-transport

S0208 Paramedic intercept, hospital-based ALS service (non-voluntary), non-transport

S0209 Wheelchair van, mileage, per mile

S0215 Non-emergency transportation; mileage, per mile
See also codes A0021-A0999 for transportation.

S0220 Medical conference by a physician with interdisciplinary team of health professionals or representatives of community agencies to coordinate activities of patient care (patient is present); approximately 30 minutes

S0221 Medical conference by a physician with interdisciplinary team of health professionals or representatives of community agencies to coordinate activities of patient care (patient is present); approximately 60 minutes

S0250 Comprehensive geriatric assessment and treatment planning performed by assessment team Ⓐ

S0255 Hospice referral visit (advising patient and family of care options) performed by nurse, social worker, or other designated staff

S0257 Counseling and discussion regarding advance directives or end of life care planning and decisions, with patient and/or surrogate (list separately in addition to code for appropriate evaluation and management service)

S0260 History and physical (outpatient or office) related to surgical procedure (list separately in addition to code for appropriate evaluation and management service)

● ☑ **S0265** Genetic counseling, under physician supervision, each 15 minutes

S0302 Completed early periodic screening diagnosis and treatment (EPSDT) service (list in addition to code for appropriate evaluation and management service)

S0310 Hospitalist services (list separately in addition to code for appropriate evaluation and management service)

S0315 Disease management program; initial assessment and initiation of the program

S0316 Follow-up/reassessment

Special Coverage Instructions   **Noncovered by Medicare**   **Carrier Discretion**   ☑ Quantity Alert   ● New Code   ○ Reinstated Code   ▲ Revised Code

134 — S Codes   Ⓐ Age   Ⓜ Maternity   ♀ Female Only   ♂ Male Only   Ⓐ-Ⓥ APC Status Indicator   *2006 HCPCS*

☑ **S0317** Disease management program; per diem

S0320 Telephone calls by a registered nurse to a disease management program member for monitoring purposes; per month

S0340 Lifestyle modification program for management of coronary artery disease, including all supportive services; first quarter/stage

S0341 Lifestyle modification program for management of coronary artery disease, including all supportive services; second or third quarter/stage

S0342 Lifestyle modification program for management of coronary artery disease, including all supportive services; fourth quarter/stage

S0390 Routine foot care; removal and/or trimming of corns, calluses and/or nails and preventive maintenance in specific medical conditions (e.g., diabetes), per visit
See also CPT code 11719-11721.

S0395 Impression casting of a foot performed by a practitioner other than the manufacturer of the orthotic

S0400 Global fee for extracorporeal shock wave lithotripsy treatment of kidney stone(s)
See CPT code 50590.

☑ **S0500** Disposable contact lens, per lens

☑ **S0504** Single vision prescription lens (safety, athletic, or sunglass), per lens

☑ **S0506** Bifocal vision prescription lens (safety, athletic, or sunglass), per lens

☑ **S0508** Trifocal vision prescription lens (safety, athletic, or sunglass), per lens

☑ **S0510** Non-prescription lens (safety, athletic, or sunglass), per lens

☑ **S0512** Daily wear specialty contact lens, per lens

☑ **S0514** Color contact lens, per lens

S0515 Scleral lens, liquid bandage device, per lens

S0516 Safety eyeglass frames

S0518 Sunglasses frames

S0580 Polycarbonate lens (list this code in addition to the basic code for the lens)

S0581 Nonstandard lens (list this code in addition to the basic code for the lens)

S0590 Integral lens service, miscellaneous services reported separately

S0592 Comprehensive contact lens evaluation

● **S0595** Dispensing new spectacle lenses for patient supplied frame

S0601 Screening proctoscopy   ♂

S0605 Digital rectal examination, annual

S0610 Annual gynecological examination; new patient   ♀

S0612 Annual gynecological examination; established patient   ♀

● **S0613** Annual gynecological examination, clinical breast examination without pelvic examination   ♀

S0618 Audiometry for hearing aid evaluation to determine the level and degree of hearing loss

S0620 Routine ophthalmological examination including refraction; new patient

S0621 Routine ophthalmological examination including refraction; established patient

S0622 Physical exam for college, new or established patient (list separately in addition to appropriate evaluation and management code)   ▲

● **S0625** Retinal telescreening by digital imaging of multiple different fundus areas to screen for vision threatening conditions, including imaging, interpretation and report

S0630 Removal of sutures by a physician other than the physician who originally closed the wound

S0800 Laser in situ keratomileusis (LASIK)

S0810 Photorefractive keratectomy (PRK)

S0812 Phototherapeutic keratectomy (PTK)

S0820 Computerized corneal topography, unilateral

S1001 Deluxe item, patient aware (list in addition to code for basic item)

S1002 Customized item (list in addition to code for basic item)

S1015 IV tubing extension set

S1016 Non-PVC (polyvinylchloride) intravenous administration set, for use with drugs that are not stable in PVC e.g., Paclitaxel

S1025 Inhaled nitric oxide for the treatment of hypoxic respiratory failure in the neonate; per diem

S1030 Continuous noninvasive glucose monitoring device, purchase (for physician interpretation of data, use CPT code)

S1031 Continuous noninvasive glucose monitoring device, rental, including sensor, sensor replacement, and download to monitor (for physician interpretation of data, use CPT code)

S1040 Cranial remolding orthosis, rigid, with soft interface material, custom fabricated, includes fitting and adjustment(s)

S2053 Transplantation of small intestine, and liver allografts

S2054 Transplantation of multivisceral organs

S2055 Harvesting of donor multivisceral organs, with preparation and maintenance of allografts; from cadaver donor

S2060 Lobar lung transplantation

S2061 Donor lobectomy (lung) for transplantation, living donor

S2065 Simultaneous pancreas kidney transplantation

● **S2068** Breast reconstruction with deep inferior epigastric perforator (deep) flap, including microvascular anastomosis and closure of donor site, unilateral ♀

S2070 Cystourethroscopy, with ureteroscopy and/or pyeloscopy; with endoscopic laser treatment of ureteral calculi (includes ureteral catheterization)

● **S2075** Laparoscopy, surgical; repair incisional or ventral hernia

● **S2076** Laparoscopy, surgical; repair umbilical hernia

● **S2077** Laparoscopy, surgical; implantation of mesh or other prosthesis for incisional or ventral hernia repair (List separately in addition to code for the incisional or ventral hernia repair) ♀

● **S2078** Laparoscopic supracervical hysterectomy (subtotal hysterectomy), with or without removal of tube(s), with or without removal of ovary(s)

| Special Coverage Instructions | | Noncovered by Medicare | Carrier Discretion | ☑ Quantity Alert | ● New Code | ○ Reinstated Code | ▲ Revised Code |

2006 HCPCS   **1**-**9** ASC Groups   MED: Pub 100/NCD Reference   ♿ DMEPOS Paid   ⊘ SNF Excluded   **S Codes — 135**

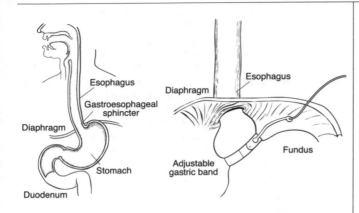

Esophagus

Gastroesophageal sphincter

Diaphragm

Stomach

Duodenum

Diaphragm

Esophagus

Fundus

Adjustable gastric band

● **S2079** Laparoscopic esophagomyotomy (Heller type)

S2080 Laser-assisted uvulopalatoplasty (LAUP)

~~**S2082** Laparoscopy, surgical; gastric restrictive procedure, adjustable gastric band includes placement of subcutaneous port~~
See code(s) 43770.

S2083 Adjustment of gastric band diameter via subcutanous port by injection or aspiration of saline

~~**S2000** Ablation, open, one or more renal tumor(s), cryosurgical~~
See code(s) 50250.

~~**S2001** Ablation, percutaneous, one or more renal tumor(s), cryosurgical~~
See code(s) 0135T.

S2095 Transcatheter occlusion or embolization for tumor destruction, percutaneous, any method, using yttrium 90 microspheres

S2102 Islet cell tissue transplant from pancreas; allogeneic

S2103 Adrenal tissue transplant to brain

S2107 Adoptive immunotherapy, i.e., development of specific anti-tumor reactivity (e.g., tumor-infiltrating lymphocyte therapy) per course of treatment

S2112 Arthroscopy, knee, surgical for harvesting of cartilage (chondrocyte cells)

● **S2114** Arthroscopy, shoulder, surgical; tenodesis of biceps

S2115 Osteotomy, periacetabular, with internal fixation

● **S2117** Arthroereisis, subtalar

S2120 Low density lipoprotein (LDL) apheresis using heparin-induced extracorporeal LDL precipitation

S2135 Neurolysis, by injection, of metatarsal neuroma/interdigital neuritis, any interspace of the foot

S2140 Cord blood harvesting for transplantation, allogeneic

S2142 Cord blood-derived stem-cell transplantation, allogeneic

S2150 Bone marrow or blood-derived stem cells (peripheral or umbilical), allogeneic or autologous, harvesting, transplantation, and related complications; including: pheresis and cell preparation/storage; marrow ablative therapy; drugs, supplies, hospitalization with outpatient follow-up; medical/surgical, diagnostic, emergency, and rehabilitative services; and the number of days of pre-and post-transplant care in the global definition

S2152 Solid organ(s), complete or segmental, single organ or combination of organs; deceased or living donor(s), procurement, transplantation, and related complications including: drugs; supplies; hospitalization with outpatient follow-up; medical/surgical, diagnostic, emergency, and rehabilitative services; and the number of days of pre- and post-transplant care in the global definition

S2202 Echosclerotherapy

S2205 Minimally invasive direct coronary artery bypass surgery involving mini-thoracotomy or mini-sternotomy surgery, performed under direct vision; using arterial graft(s), single coronary arterial graft

S2206 Minimally invasive direct coronary artery bypass surgery involving mini-thoracotomy or mini-sternotomy surgery, performed under direct vision; using arterial graft(s), two coronary arterial grafts

S2207 Minimally invasive direct coronary artery bypass surgery involving mini-thoracotomy or mini-sternotomy surgery, performed under direct vision; using venous graft only, single coronary venous graft

S2208 Minimally invasive direct coronary artery bypass surgery involving mini-thoracotomy or mini-sternotomy surgery, performed under direct vision; using single arterial and venous graft(s), single venous graft

S2209 Minimally invasive direct coronary artery bypass surgery involving mini-thoracotomy or mini-sternotomy surgery, performed under direct vision; using two arterial grafts and single venous graft

S2213 Implantation of gastric electrical stimulation device

~~**S2215** Upper gastrointestinal endoscopy, including esophagus, stomach, and either the duodenum and/or jejunum as appropriate; with injection of implant material into and along the muscle of the lower esophageal sphincter for treatment of gastroesophageal reflux disease~~
See code(s) 0133T.

S2225 Myringotomy, laser-assisted

S2230 Implantation of magnetic component of semi-implantable hearing device on ossicles in middle ear

S2235 Implantation of auditory brain stem implant

S2250 Uterine artery embolization for uterine fibroids A ♀

S2260 Induced abortion, 17 to 24 weeks, any surgical method M ♀

S2262 Abortion for maternal indication, 25 weeks or greater M ♀

S2265 Abortion for fetal indication, 25-28 weeks M ♀

S2266 Abortion for fetal indication, 29-31 weeks M ♀

S2267 Abortion for fetal indication, 32 weeks or greater M ♀

S2300 Arthroscopy, shoulder, surgical; with thermally-induced capsulorrhaphy

S2340 Chemodenervation of abductor muscle(s) of vocal cord

S2341 Chemodenervation of adductor muscle(s) of vocal cord

S2342 Nasal endoscopy for post-operative debridement following functional endoscopic sinus surgery, nasal and/or sinus cavity(s), unilateral or bilateral

Special Coverage Instructions   Noncovered by Medicare   Carrier Discretion   ☑ Quantity Alert   ● New Code   ○ Reinstated Code   ▲ Revised Code

136 — S Codes   A Age   M Maternity   ♀ Female Only   ♂ Male Only   A-Y APC Status Indicator   *2006 HCPCS*

S2348	Decompression procedure, percutaneous, of nucleus pulposus of intervertebral disc, using radiofrequency energy, single or multiple levels, lumbar	
S2350	Diskectomy, anterior, with decompression of spinal cord and/or nerve root(s), including osteophytectomy; lumbar, single interspace	
S2351	Diskectomy, anterior, with decompression of spinal cord and/or nerve root(s), including osteophytectomy; lumbar, each additional interspace (list separately in addition to code for primary procedure)	
S2360	Percutaneous vertebroplasty, one vertebral body, unilateral or bilateral injection; cervical	
S2361	Each additional cervical vertebral body (list separately in addition to code for primary procedure)	
S2362	Kyphoplasty, one vertebral body, unilateral or bilateral injection	
☑ S2363	Kyphoplasty, one vertebral body, unilateral or bilateral injection; each additional vertebral body (list separately in addition to code for primary procedure)	
S2400	Repair, congenital diaphragmatic hernia in the fetus using temporary tracheal occlusion, procedure performed in utero M ♀ Repair, congenital diaphragmatic hernia in the fetus using temporary tracheal occlusion, procedure performed in utero.	
S2401	Repair, urinary tract obstruction in the fetus, procedure performed in utero M ♀	
S2402	Repair, congenital cystic adenomatoid malformation in the fetus, procedure performed in utero M ♀	
S2403	Repair, extralobar pulmonary sequestration in the fetus, procedure performed in utero M ♀	
S2404	Repair, myelomeningocele in the fetus, procedure performed in utero M ♀	
S2405	Repair of sacrococcygeal teratoma in the fetus, procedure performed in utero M ♀	
S2409	Repair, congenital malformation of fetus, procedure performed in utero, not otherwise classified M ♀	
S2411	Fetoscopic laser therapy for treatment of twin-to-twin transfusion syndrome M ♀	
● S2900	Surgical techniques requiring use of robotic surgical system (list separately in addition to code for primary procedure)	
S3000	Diabetic indicator; retinal eye exam, dilated, bilateral	
● S3005	Performance measurement, evaluation of patient self assessment, depression	
S3600	STAT laboratory request (situations other than S3601)	
S3601	Emergency STAT laboratory charge for patient who is homebound or residing in a nursing facility	
☑ S3620	Newborn metabolic screening panel, includes test kit, postage and the laboratory tests specified by the state for inclusion in this panel (e.g., galactose; hemoglobin, electrophoresis; hydroxyprogesterone, 17-d; phenylanine (PKU); and thyroxine, total) A	
S3625	Maternal serum triple marker screen including alpha-fetoprotein (AFP), estriol, and human chorionic gonadotropin (hcG) M ♀	
● S3626	Maternal serum quadruple marker screen including alpha-fetoprotein (AFP), estriol, human chorionic gonadotropin (hcG), and inhibin A	

S3630	Eosinophil count, blood, direct
S3645	HIV-1 antibody testing of oral mucosal transudate
S3650	Saliva test, hormone level; during menopause A ♀
S3652	Saliva test, hormone level; to assess preterm labor risk M ♀
S3655	Antisperm antibodies test (immunobead) A ♀
S3701	Immunoassay for nuclear matrix protein 22 (NMP-22), quantitative
S3708	Gastrointestinal fat absorption study
S3818	Complete gene sequence analysis; BRCA 1 gene
S3819	Complete gene sequence analysis; BRCA 2 gene
S3820	Complete BRCA 1 and BRCA 2 gene sequence analysis for susceptibility to breast and ovarian cancer ♀
S3822	Single mutation analysis (in individual with a known BRCA 1 or BRCA 2 mutation in the family) for susceptibility to breast and ovarian cancer ♀
S3823	Three-mutation BRCA 1 and BRCA 2 analysis for susceptibility to breast and ovarian cancer in Ashkenazi individuals ♀
S3828	Complete gene sequence analysis; MLH 1 gene
S3829	Complete gene sequence analysis; MLH 2 gene
S3830	Complete MLH 1 and MLH 2 gene sequence analysis for hereditary nonpolyposis colorectal cancer (HNPCC) genetic testing
S3831	Single-mutation analysis (in individual with a known MLH 1 and MLH 2 mutation in the family) for hereditary nonpolyposis colorectal cancer (HNPCC) genetic testing
S3833	Complete APC gene sequence analysis for susceptibility to familial adenomatous polyposis (FAP) and attenuated FAP
S3834	Single-mutation analysis (in individual with a known APC mutation in the family) for susceptibility to familial adenomatous polyposis (FAP) and attenuated FAP
S3835	Complete gene sequence analysis for cystic fibrosis genetic testing
S3837	Complete gene sequence analysis for hemochromatosis genetic testing
S3840	DNA analysis for germline mutations of the RET proto-oncogene for susceptibility to multiple endocrine neoplasia type 2
S3841	Genetic testing for retinoblastoma
S3842	Genetic testing for Von Hippel-Lindau disease
S3843	DNA analysis of the F5 gene for susceptibility to factor V Leiden thrombophilia
S3844	DNA analysis of the connexin 26 gene (GJB2) for susceptibility to congenital, profound deafness
S3845	Genetic testing for alpha-thalassemia
S3846	Genetic testing for hemoglobin E beta-thalassemia
S3847	Genetic testing for Tay-Sachs disease
S3848	Genetic testing for Gaucher disease
S3849	Genetic testing for Niemann-Pick disease
S3850	Genetic testing for sickle cell anemia
S3851	Genetic testing for Canavan disease
S3852	DNA analysis for APOE epilson 4 allele for susceptibility to Alzheimer's disease
S3853	Genetic testing for myotonic muscular dystrophy

Special Coverage Instructions   Noncovered by Medicare   Carrier Discretion   ☑ Quantity Alert   ● New Code   ○ Reinstated Code   ▲ Revised Code

2006 HCPCS   🯄-🯆 ASC Groups   MED: Pub 100/NCD Reference   ℞ DMEPOS Paid   ⊘ SNF Excluded   S Codes — 137

●   **S3854** Gene expression profiling panel for use in the management of breast cancer treatment

S3890 DNA analysis, fecal, for colorectal cancer screening

S3900 Surface electromyography (EMG)

S3902 Ballistocardiogram

S3904 Masters two step

S4005 Interim labor facility global (labor occurring but not resulting in delivery)   Ⓜ ♀

S4011 In vitro fertilization; including but not limited to identification and incubation of mature oocytes, fertilization with sperm, incubation of embryo(s), and subsequent visualization for determination of development   Ⓜ ♀

S4013 Complete cycle, gamete intrafallopian transfer (GIFT), case rate   Ⓜ ♀

S4014 Complete cycle, zygote intrafallopian transfer (ZIFT), case rate   Ⓜ ♀

S4015 Complete in vitro fertilization cycle, not otherwise specified, case rate   Ⓜ ♀

S4016 Frozen in vitro fertilization cycle, case rate   ♀

S4017 Incomplete cycle, treatment canceled prior to stimulation, case rate   ♀

S4018 Frozen embryo transfer procedure canceled before transfer, case rate   ♀

S4020 In vitro fertilization procedure canceled before aspiration, case rate   ♀

S4021 In vitro fertilization procedure canceled after aspiration, case rate   ♀

S4022 Assisted oocyte fertilization, case rate   ♀

S4023 Donor egg cycle, incomplete, case rate   ♀

S4025 Donor services for in vitro fertilization (sperm or embryo), case rate   Ⓐ

S4026 Procurement of donor sperm from sperm bank   Ⓐ

S4027 Storage of previously frozen embryos

S4028 Microsurgical epididymal sperm aspiration (MESA)   Ⓐ ♂

S4030 Sperm procurement and cryopreservation services; initial visit   Ⓐ ♂

S4031 Sperm procurement and cryopreservation services; subsequent visit   Ⓐ ♂

S4035 Stimulated intrauterine insemination (IUI), case rate   ♀

S4036 Intravaginal culture (IVC), case rate   ♀

S4037 Cryopreserved embryo transfer, case rate

S4040 Monitoring and storage of cryopreserved embryos, per 30 days

S4042 Management of ovulation induction (interpretation of diagnostic tests and studies, non-face-to-face medical management of the patient), per cycle

S4981 Insertion of levonorgestrel-releasing intrauterine system   ♀

S4989 Contraceptive intrauterine device (e.g., Progestacert IUD), including implants and supplies   ♀

☑   **S4990** Nicotine patches, legend

☑   **S4991** Nicotine patches, non-legend

S4993 Contraceptive pills for birth control   ♀

S4995 Smoking cessation gum

☑   **S5000** Prescription drug, generic

☑   **S5001** Prescription drug, brand name

☑   **S5010** 5% dextrose and 45% normal saline, 1000 ml

☑   **S5011** 5% dextrose in lactated ringer's, 1000 ml

☑   **S5012** 5% dextrose with potassium chloride, 1000 ml

☑   **S5013** 5% dextrose/45% normal saline with potassium chloride and magnesium sulfate, 1000 ml

☑   **S5014** 5% dextrose/0.45% normal saline with potassium chloride and magnesium sulfate, 1500 ml

S5035 Home infusion therapy, routine service of infusion device (e.g., pump maintenance)

S5036 Home infusion therapy, repair of infusion device (e.g., pump repair)

S5100 Day care services, adult; per 15 minutes   Ⓐ

S5101 Day care services, adult; per half day   Ⓐ

S5102 Day care services, adult; per diem   Ⓐ

S5105 Day care services, center-based; services not included in program fee, per diem

☑   **S5108** Home care training to home care client, per 15 minutes

☑   **S5109** Home care training to home care client, per session

S5110 Home care training, family; per 15 minutes

S5111 Home care training, family; per session

S5115 Home care training, non-family; per 15 minutes

S5116 Home care training, non-family; per session

S5120 Chore services; per 15 minutes

S5121 Chore services; per diem

S5125 Attendant care services; per 15 minutes

S5126 Attendant care services; per diem

S5130 Homemaker service, NOS; per 15 minutes

S5131 Homemaker service, NOS; per diem

S5135 Companion care, adult (e.g., IADL/ADL); per 15 minutes   Ⓐ

S5136 Companion care, adult (e.g., IADL/ADL); per diem   Ⓐ

S5140 Foster care, adult; per diem   Ⓐ

S5141 Foster care, adult; per month   Ⓐ

S5145 Foster care, therapeutic, child; per diem   Ⓐ

S5146 Foster care, therapeutic, child; per month   Ⓐ

S5150 Unskilled respite care, not hospice; per 15 minutes

S5151 Unskilled respite care, not hospice; per diem

S5160 Emergency response system; installation and testing

S5161 Emergency response system; service fee, per month (excludes installation and testing)

S5162 Emergency response system; purchase only

S5165 Home modifications; per service

S5170 Home delivered meals, including preparation; per meal

S5175 Laundry service, external, professional; per order

S5180 Home health respiratory therapy, initial evaluation

S5181 Home health respiratory therapy, NOS, per diem

S5185 Medication reminder services, non-face-to-face; per month

S5190 Wellness assessment, performed by nonphysician

S5199 Personal care item, NOS, each

Special Coverage Instructions   Noncovered by Medicare   Carrier Discretion   ☑ Quantity Alert   ● New Code   ○ Reinstated Code   ▲ Revised Code

138 — S Codes   Ⓐ Age   Ⓜ Maternity   ♀ Female Only   ♂ Male Only   Ⓐ-☑ APC Status Indicator   **2006 HCPCS**

S5497 Home infusion therapy, catheter care/maintenance, not otherwise classified; includes administrative services, professional pharmacy services, care coordination, and all necessary supplies and equipment (drugs and nursing visits coded separately), per diem

S5498 Home infusion therapy, catheter care/maintenance, simple (single lumen), includes administrative services, professional pharmacy services, care coordination and all necessary supplies and equipment, (drugs and nursing visits coded separately), per diem

S5501 Home infusion therapy, catheter care/maintenance, complex (more than one lumen), includes administrative services, professional pharmacy services, care coordination, and all necessary supplies and equipment (drugs and nursing visits coded separately), per diem

S5502 Home infusion therapy, catheter care/maintenance, implanted access device, includes administrative services, professional pharmacy services, care coordination and all necessary supplies and equipment, (drugs and nursing visits coded separately), per diem (use this code for interim maintenance of vascular access not currently in use)

S5517 Home infusion therapy, all supplies necessary for restoration of catheter patency or declotting

S5518 Home infusion therapy, all supplies necessary for catheter repair

S5520 Home infusion therapy, all supplies (including catheter) necessary for a peripherally inserted central venous catheter (PICC) line insertion

S5521 Home infusion therapy, all supplies (including catheter) necessary for a midline catheter insertion

S5522 Home infusion therapy, insertion of peripherally inserted central venous catheter (PICC), nursing services only (no supplies or catheter included)

S5523 Home infusion therapy, insertion of midline central venous catheter, nursing services only (no supplies or catheter included)

☑ **S5550** Insulin, rapid onset, 5 units

☑ **S5551** Insulin, most rapid onset (Lispro or Aspart); 5 units

☑ **S5552** Insulin, intermediate acting (NPH or LENTE); 5 units

☑ **S5553** Insulin, long acting; 5 units

☑ **S5560** Insulin delivery device, reusable pen; 1.5 ml size

☑ **S5561** Insulin delivery device, reusable pen; 3 ml size

☑ **S5565** Insulin cartridge for use in insulin delivery device other than pump; 150 units

☑ **S5566** Insulin cartridge for use in insulin delivery device other than pump; 300 units

☑ **S5570** Insulin delivery device, disposable pen (including insulin); 1.5 ml size

☑ **S5571** Insulin delivery device, disposable pen (including insulin); 3 ml size

~~**S8004** Radioimmunopharmaceutical localization of targeted cells; whole body~~

S8030 Scleral application of tantalum ring(s) for localization of lesions for proton beam therapy

S8035 Magnetic source imaging

S8037 Magnetic resonance cholangiopancreatography (MRCP)

S8040 Topographic brain mapping

S8042 Magnetic resonance imaging (MRI), low-field

S8049 Intraoperative radiation therapy (single administration)

S8055 Ultrasound guidance for multifetal pregnancy reduction(s), technical component (only to be used when the physician doing the reduction procedure does not perform the ultrasound. Guidance is included in the CPT code for multifetal pregnancy reduction - 59866) Ⓜ ♀

S8075 Computer analysis of full-field digital mammogram and further physician review for interpretation, mammography (list separately in addition to code for primary procedure)

S8080 Scintimammography (radioimmunoscintigraphy of the breast), unilateral, including supply of radiopharmaceutical

S8085 Fluorine-18 fluorodeoxyglucose (F-18 FDG) imaging using dual-head coincidence detection system (non-dedicated PET scan)

S8092 Electron beam computed tomography (also known as Ultrafast CT, Cine CT)

S8093 Computed tomographic angiography, coronary arteries, with contrast material(s)

~~**S8095** Wig (for medically induced or congenital hair loss)~~ See code(s) A9282.

S8096 Portable peak flow meter

☑ **S8097** Asthma kit (including but not limited to portable peak expiratory flow meter, instructional video, brochure, and/or spacer)

S8100 Holding chamber or spacer for use with an inhaler or nebulizer; without mask

S8101 Holding chamber or spacer for use with an inhaler or nebulizer; with mask

S8110 Peak expiratory flow rate (physician services)

☑ **S8120** Oxygen contents, gaseous, 1 unit equals 1 cubic foot

☑ **S8121** Oxygen contents, liquid, 1 unit equals 1 pound

S8185 Flutter device

S8186 Swivel adaptor

☑ **S8189** Tracheostomy supply, not otherwise classified

S8190 Electronic spirometer (or microspirometer)

S8210 Mucus trap

S8260 Oral orthotic for treatment of sleep apnea, includes fitting, fabrication, and materials

S8262 Mandibular orthopedic repositioning device, each

S8265 Haberman Feeder for cleft lip/palate

● ☑ **S8270** Enuresis alarm, using auditory buzzer and/or vibration device

S8301 Infection control supplies, not otherwise specified

☑ **S8415** Supplies for home delivery of infant Ⓜ ♀

S8420 Gradient pressure aid (sleeve and glove combination), custom made

☑ **S8421** Gradient pressure aid (sleeve and glove combination), ready made

☑ **S8422** Gradient pressure aid (sleeve), custom made, medium weight

☑ **S8423** Gradient pressure aid (sleeve), custom made, heavy weight

☑ **S8424** Gradient pressure aid (sleeve), ready made

Special Coverage Instructions   Noncovered by Medicare   Carrier Discretion   ☑ Quantity Alert   ● New Code   ○ Reinstated Code   ▲ Revised Code

2006 HCPCS   1-9 ASC Groups   MED: Pub 100/NCD Reference   ♭ DMEPOS Paid   ⊘ SNF Excluded   **S Codes — 139**

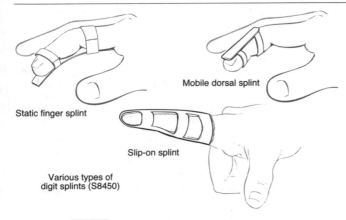

Mobile dorsal splint

Static finger splint

Slip-on splint

Various types of
digit splints (S8450)

☑ **S8425** Gradient pressure aid (glove), custom made, medium weight

☑ **S8426** Gradient pressure aid (glove), custom made, heavy weight

☑ **S8427** Gradient pressure aid (glove), ready made

☑ **S8428** Gradient pressure aid (gauntlet), ready made

☑ **S8429** Gradient pressure exterior wrap

☑ **S8430** Padding for compression bandage, roll

☑ **S8431** Compression bandage, roll

S8434 ~~Interim post operative orthotic device for upper extremity, custom made~~

☑ **S8450** Splint, prefabricated, digit (specify digit by use of modifier)

☑ **S8451** Splint, prefabricated, wrist or ankle

☑ **S8452** Splint, prefabricated, elbow

S8460 Camisole, postmastectomy

☑ **S8490** Insulin syringes (100 syringes, any size)

S8940 Equestrian/hippotherapy, per session

☑ **S8948** Application of a modality (requiring constant provider attendance) to one or more areas; low-level laser; each 15 minutes

S8950 Complex lymphedema therapy, each 15 minutes

S8990 Physical or manipulative therapy performed for maintenance rather than restoration

S8999 Resuscitation bag (for use by patient on artificial respiration during power failure or other catastrophic event)

S9001 Home uterine monitor with or without associated nursing services   Ⓜ♀

S9007 Ultrafiltration monitor

S9015 Automated EEG monitoring

S9022 Digital subtraction angiography (use in addition to CPT code for the procedure for further identification)

S9024 Paranasal sinus ultrasound

S9025 Omnicardiogram/cardiointegram

S9034 Extracorporeal shockwave lithotripsy for gallstones
If performed with ERCP, use CPT code 43265.

S9055 Procuren or other growth factor preparation to promote wound healing

S9056 Coma stimulation per diem

S9061 Home administration of aerosolized drug therapy (e.g., Pentamidine); administrative services, professional pharmacy services, care coordination, all necessary supplies and equipment (drugs and nursing visits coded separately), per diem

S9075 Smoking cessation treatment

S9083 Global fee urgent care centers

S9088 Services provided in an urgent care center (list in addition to code for service)

S9090 Vertebral axial decompression, per session

S9092 Canolith repositioning, per visit

S9097 Home visit for wound care

S9098 Home visit, phototherapy services (e.g., Bili-lite), including equipment rental, nursing services, blood draw, supplies, and other services, per diem

S9109 Congestive heart failure telemonitoring, equipment rental, including telescale, computer system and software, telephone connections, and maintenance, per month

S9117 Back school, per visit

☑ **S9122** Home health aide or certified nurse assistant, providing care in the home; per hour

☑ **S9123** Nursing care, in the home; by registered nurse, per hour (use for general nursing care only, not to be used when CPT codes 99500-99602 can be used)

☑ **S9124** Nursing care, in the home; by licensed practical nurse, per hour

☑ **S9125** Respite care, in the home, per diem

☑ **S9126** Hospice care, in the home, per diem

☑ **S9127** Social work visit, in the home, per diem

☑ **S9128** Speech therapy, in the home, per diem

☑ **S9129** Occupational therapy, in the home, per diem

S9131 Physical therapy; in the home, per diem

☑ **S9140** Diabetic management program, follow-up visit to non-MD provider

☑ **S9141** Diabetic management program, follow-up visit to MD provider

S9145 Insulin pump initiation, instruction in initial use of pump (pump not included)

S9150 Evaluation by ocularist

S9208 Home management of preterm labor, including administrative services, professional pharmacy services, care coordination, and all necessary supplies or equipment (drugs and nursing visits coded separately), per diem (do not use this code with any home infusion per diem code)   Ⓜ♀

S9209 Home management of preterm premature rupture of membranes (PPROM), including administrative services, professional pharmacy services, care coordination, and all necessary supplies or equipment (drugs and nursing visits coded separately), per diem (do not use this code with any home infusion per diem code)   Ⓜ♀

S9211 Home management of gestational hypertension, includes administrative services, professional pharmacy services, care coordination and all necessary supplies and equipment (drugs and nursing visits coded separately); per diem (do not use this code with any home infusion per diem code)   Ⓜ♀

| Special Coverage Instructions | Noncovered by Medicare | Carrier Discretion | ☑ Quantity Alert | ● New Code | ○ Reinstated Code | ▲ Revised Code |

140 — S Codes   Ⓐ Age   Ⓜ Maternity   ♀ Female Only   ♂ Male Only   Ⓐ-Ⓨ APC Status Indicator   *2006 HCPCS*

S9212 Home management of postpartum hypertension, includes administrative services, professional pharmacy services, care coordination, and all necessary supplies and equipment (drugs and nursing visits coded separately), per diem (do not use this code with any home infusion per diem code) ♀

S9213 Home management of preeclampsia, includes administrative services, professional pharmacy services, care coordination, and all necessary supplies and equipment (drugs and nursing services coded separately); per diem (do not use this code with any home infusion per diem code) Ⓜ ♀

S9214 Home management of gestational diabetes, includes administrative services, professional pharmacy services, care coordination, and all necessary supplies and equipment (drugs and nursing visits coded separately); per diem (do not use this code with any home infusion per diem code) Ⓜ ♀

S9325 Home infusion therapy, pain management infusion; administrative services, professional pharmacy services, care coordination, and all necessary supplies and equipment, (drugs and nursing visits coded separately), per diem (do not use this code with S9326, S9327 or S9328)

S9326 Home infusion therapy, continuous (24 hours or more) pain management infusion; administrative services, professional pharmacy services, care coordination and all necessary supplies and equipment (drugs and nursing visits coded separately), per diem

S9327 Home infusion therapy, intermittent (less than 24 hours) pain management infusion; administrative services, professional pharmacy services, care coordination, and all necessary supplies and equipment (drugs and nursing visits coded separately), per diem

S9328 Home infusion therapy, implanted pump pain management infusion; administrative services, professional pharmacy services, care coordination, and all necessary supplies and equipment (drugs and nursing visits coded separately), per diem

S9329 Home infusion therapy, chemotherapy infusion; administrative services, professional pharmacy services, care coordination, and all necessary supplies and equipment (drugs and nursing visits coded separately), per diem (do not use this code with S9330 or S9331)

S9330 Home infusion therapy, continuous (24 hours or more) chemotherapy infusion; administrative services, professional pharmacy services, care coordination, and all necessary supplies and equipment (drugs and nursing visits coded separately), per diem

S9331 Home infusion therapy, intermittent (less than 24 hours) chemotherapy infusion; administrative services, professional pharmacy services, care coordination, and all necessary supplies and equipment (drugs and nursing visits coded separately), per diem

☑ **S9335** Home therapy, hemodialysis; administrative services, professional pharmacy services, care coordination, and all necessary supplies and equipment (drugs and nursing services coded separately), per diem

S9336 Home infusion therapy, continuous anticoagulant infusion therapy (e.g., heparin), administrative services, professional pharmacy services, care coordination and all necessary supplies and equipment (drugs and nursing visits coded separately), per diem

S9338 Home infusion therapy, immunotherapy, administrative services, professional pharmacy services, care coordination, and all necessary supplies and equipment (drugs and nursing visits coded separately), per diem

S9339 Home therapy; peritoneal dialysis, administrative services, professional pharmacy services, care coordination and all necessary supplies and equipment (drugs and nursing visits coded separately), per diem

S9340 Home therapy; enteral nutrition; administrative services, professional pharmacy services, care coordination, and all necessary supplies and equipment (enteral formula and nursing visits coded separately), per diem

S9341 Home therapy; enteral nutrition via gravity; administrative services, professional pharmacy services, care coordination, and all necessary supplies and equipment (enteral formula and nursing visits coded separately), per diem

S9342 Home therapy; enteral nutrition via pump; administrative services, professional pharmacy services, care coordination, and all necessary supplies and equipment (enteral formula and nursing visits coded separately), per diem

S9343 Home therapy; enteral nutrition via bolus; administrative services, professional pharmacy services, care coordination, and all necessary supplies and equipment (enteral formula and nursing visits coded separately), per diem

S9345 Home infusion therapy, anti-hemophilic agent infusion therapy (e.g., factor VIII); administrative services, professional pharmacy services, care coordination, and all necessary supplies and equipment (drugs and nursing visits coded separately), per diem

S9346 Home infusion therapy, alpha-1-proteinase inhibitor (e.g., Prolastin); administrative services, professional pharmacy services, care coordination, and all necessary supplies and equipment (drugs and nursing visits coded separately), per diem

S9347 Home infusion therapy, uninterrupted, long-term, controlled rate intravenous or subcutaneous infusion therapy (e.g., Epoprostenol); administrative services, professional pharmacy services, care coordination, and all necessary supplies and equipment (drugs and nursing visits coded separately), per diem

S9348 Home infusion therapy, sympathomimetic/inotropic agent infusion therapy (e.g., Dobutamine); administrative services, professional pharmacy services, care coordination, all necessary supplies and equipment (drugs and nursing visits coded separately), per diem

S9349 Home infusion therapy, tocolytic infusion therapy; administrative services, professional pharmacy services, care coordination, and all necessary supplies and equipment (drugs and nursing visits coded separately), per diem Ⓜ ♀

Special Coverage Instructions   Noncovered by Medicare   Carrier Discretion   ☑ Quantity Alert   ● New Code   ○ Reinstated Code   ▲ Revised Code

2006 HCPCS   ❶-❾ ASC Groups   **MED:** Pub 100/NCD Reference   ♿ DMEPOS Paid   ⊘ SNF Excluded   **S Codes — 141**

S9351　Home infusion therapy, continuous anti-emetic infusion therapy; administrative services, professional pharmacy services, care coordination, all necessary supplies and equipment (drugs and nursing visits coded separately), per diem

S9353　Home infusion therapy, continuous insulin infusion therapy; administrative services, professional pharmacy services, care coordination, and all necessary supplies and equipment (drugs and nursing visits coded separately), per diem

S9355　Home infusion therapy, chelation therapy; administrative services, professional pharmacy services, care coordination, and all necessary supplies and equipment (drugs and nursing visits coded separately), per diem

S9357　Home infusion therapy, enzyme replacement intravenous therapy; (e.g., Imiglucerase); administrative services, professional pharmacy services, care coordination, and all necessary supplies and equipment (drugs and nursing visits coded separately), per diem

S9359　Home infusion therapy, anti-tumor necrosis factor intravenous therapy; (e.g., Infliximab); administrative services, professional pharmacy services, care coordination, and all necessary supplies and equipment (drugs and nursing visits coded separately), per diem

S9361　Home infusion therapy, diuretic intravenous therapy; administrative services, professional pharmacy services, care coordination, and all necessary supplies and equipment (drugs and nursing visits coded separately), per diem

S9363　Home infusion therapy, anti-spasmotic therapy; administrative services, professional pharmacy services, care coordination, and all necessary supplies and equipment (drugs and nursing visits coded separately), per diem

S9364　Home infusion therapy, total parenteral nutrition (TPN); administrative services, professional pharmacy services, care coordination, and all necessary supplies and equipment including standard TPN formula (lipids, specialty amino acid formulas, drugs other than in standard formula and nursing visits coded separately), per diem (do not use with home infusion codes S9365-S9368 using daily volume scales)

S9365　Home infusion therapy, total parenteral nutrition (TPN); 1 liter per day, administrative services, professional pharmacy services, care coordination, and all necessary supplies and equipment including standard TPN formula (lipids, specialty amino acid formulas, drugs other than in standard formula and nursing visits coded separately), per diem

S9366　Home infusion therapy, total parenteral nutrition (TPN); more than 1 liter but no more than 2 liters per day, administrative services, professional pharmacy services, care coordination, and all necessary supplies and equipment including standard TPN formula (lipids, specialty amino acid formulas, drugs other than in standard formula and nursing visits coded separately), per diem

S9367　Home infusion therapy, total parenteral nutrition (TPN); more than 2 liters but no more than 3 liters per day, administrative services, professional pharmacy services, care coordination, and all necessary supplies and equipment including standard TPN formula (lipids, specialty amino acid formulas, drugs other than in standard formula and nursing visits coded separately), per diem

S9368　Home infusion therapy, total parenteral nutrition (TPN); more than 3 liters per day, administrative services, professional pharmacy services, care coordination, and all necessary supplies and equipment including standard TPN formula (lipids, specialty amino acid formulas, drugs other than in standard formula and nursing visits coded separately), per diem

S9370　Home therapy, intermittent anti-emetic injection therapy; administrative services, professional pharmacy services, care coordination, and all necessary supplies and equipment (drugs and nursing visits coded separately), per diem

S9372　Home therapy; intermittent anticoagulant injection therapy (e.g., heparin); administrative services, professional pharmacy services, care coordination, and all necessary supplies and equipment (drugs and nursing visits coded separately), per diem (do not use this code for flushing of infusion devices with heparin to maintain patency)

S9373　Home infusion therapy, hydration therapy; administrative services, professional pharmacy services, care coordination, and all necessary supplies and equipment (drugs and nursing visits coded separately), per diem (do not use with hydration therapy codes S9374-S9377 using daily volume scales)

S9374　Home infusion therapy, hydration therapy; 1 liter per day, administrative services, professional pharmacy services, care coordination, and all necessary supplies and equipment (drugs and nursing visits coded separately), per diem

S9375　Home infusion therapy, hydration therapy; more than 1 liter but no more than 2 liters per day, administrative services, professional pharmacy services, care coordination, and all necessary supplies and equipment (drugs and nursing visits coded separately), per diem

S9376　Home infusion therapy, hydration therapy; more than 2 liters but no more than 3 liters per day, administrative services, professional pharmacy services, care coordination, and all necessary supplies and equipment (drugs and nursing visits coded separately), per diem

S9377　Home infusion therapy, hydration therapy; more than 3 liters per day, administrative services, professional pharmacy services, care coordination, and all necessary supplies (drugs and nursing visits coded separately), per diem

S9379　Home infusion therapy, infusion therapy, not otherwise classified; administrative services, professional pharmacy services, care coordination, and all necessary supplies and equipment (drugs and nursing visits coded separately), per diem

S9381　Delivery or service to high risk areas requiring escort or extra protection, per visit

S9401　Anticoagulation clinic, inclusive of all services except laboratory tests, per session

S9430　Pharmacy compounding and dispensing services

Special Coverage Instructions　　Noncovered by Medicare　　Carrier Discretion　　☑ Quantity Alert　　● New Code　　○ Reinstated Code　　▲ Revised Code

142 — S Codes　　Ⓐ Age　　Ⓜ Maternity　　♀ Female Only　　♂ Male Only　　Ⓐ-Ⓨ APC Status Indicator　　*2006 HCPCS*

S9434   Modified solid food supplements for inborn errors of metabolism

S9435   Medical foods for inborn errors of metabolism

S9436   Childbirth preparation/lamaze classes, nonphysician provider, per session   A ♀

S9437   Childbirth refresher classes, nonphysician provider, per session   A ♀

S9438   Cesarean birth classes, nonphysician provider, per session   A ♀

S9439   VBAC (vaginal birth after cesarean) classes, nonphysician provider, per session   A ♀

S9441   Asthma education, nonphysician provider, per session

S9442   Birthing classes, nonphysician provider, per session   A ♀

S9443   Lactation classes, nonphysician provider, per session   A ♀

S9444   Parenting classes, nonphysician provider, per session   A

S9445   Patient education, not otherwise classified, nonphysician provider, individual, per session

S9446   Patient education, not otherwise classified, nonphysician provider, group, per session

S9447   Infant safety (including CPR) classes, nonphysician provider, per session

S9449   Weight management classes, nonphysician provider, per session

S9451   Exercise classes, nonphysician provider, per session

S9452   Nutrition classes, nonphysician provider, per session

S9453   Smoking cessation classes, nonphysician provider, per session

S9454   Stress management classes, nonphysician provider, per session

S9455   Diabetic management program, group session

S9460   Diabetic management program, nurse visit

S9465   Diabetic management program, dietitian visit

S9470   Nutritional counseling, dietitian visit

S9472   Cardiac rehabilitation program, nonphysician provider, per diem

S9473   Pulmonary rehabilitation program, nonphysician provider, per diem

S9474   Enterostomal therapy by a registered nurse certified in enterostomal therapy, per diem

S9475   Ambulatory setting substance abuse treatment or detoxification services, per diem

☑ S9476   Vestibular rehabilitation program, nonphysician provider, per diem

S9480   Intensive outpatient psychiatric services, per diem

☑ S9482   Family stabilization services, per 15 minutes

S9484   Crisis intervention mental health services, per hour

S9485   Crisis intervention mental health services, per diem

S9490   Home infusion therapy, corticosteroid infusion; administrative services, professional pharmacy services, care coordination, and all necessary supplies and equipment (drugs and nursing visits coded separately), per diem

S9494   Home infusion therapy, antibiotic, antiviral, or antifungal therapy; administrative services, professional pharmacy services, care coordination, and all necessary supplies and equipment (drugs and nursing visits coded separately, per diem) (do not use this code with home infusion codes for hourly dosing schedules S9497-S9504)

S9497   Home infusion therapy, antibiotic, antiviral, or antifungal therapy; once every 3 hours; administrative services, professional pharmacy services, care coordination, and all necessary supplies and equipment (drugs and nursing visits coded separately), per diem

S9500   Home infusion therapy, antibiotic, antiviral, or antifungal therapy; once every 24 hours; administrative services, professional pharmacy services, care coordination, and all necessary supplies and equipment (drugs and nursing visits coded separately), per diem

S9501   Home infusion therapy, antibiotic, antiviral, or antifungal therapy; once every 12 hours; administrative services, professional pharmacy services, care coordination, and all necessary supplies and equipment (drugs and nursing visits coded separately), per diem

S9502   Home infusion therapy, antibiotic, antiviral, or antifungal therapy; once every 8 hours, administrative services, professional pharmacy services, care coordination, and all necessary supplies and equipment (drugs and nursing visits coded separately), per diem

S9503   Home infusion therapy, antibiotic, antiviral, or antifungal; once every 6 hours; administrative services, professional pharmacy services, care coordination, and all necessary supplies and equipment (drugs and nursing visits coded separately), per diem

S9504   Home infusion therapy, antibiotic, antiviral, or antifungal; once every 4 hours; administrative services, professional pharmacy services, care coordination, and all necessary supplies and equipment (drugs and nursing visits coded separately), per diem

S9529   Routine venipuncture for collection of specimen(s), single home bound, nursing home, or skilled nursing facility patient

S9537   Home therapy; hematopoietic hormone injection therapy (e.g., erythropoietin, G-CSF, GM-CSF); administrative services, professional pharmacy services, care coordination, and all necessary supplies and equipment (drugs and nursing visits coded separately), per diem

S9538   Home transfusion of blood product(s); administrative services, professional pharmacy services, care coordination and all necessary supplies and equipment (blood products, drugs, and nursing visits coded separately), per diem

S9542   Home injectable therapy, not otherwise classified, including administrative services, professional pharmacy services, care coordination, and all necessary supplies and equipment (drugs and nursing visits coded separately), per diem

S9558   Home injectable therapy; growth hormone, including administrative services, professional pharmacy services, care coordination, and all necessary supplies and equipment (drugs and nursing visits coded separately), per diem

Special Coverage Instructions   Noncovered by Medicare   Carrier Discretion   ☑ Quantity Alert   ● New Code   ○ Reinstated Code   ▲ Revised Code

2006 HCPCS   1-9 ASC Groups   MED: Pub 100/NCD Reference   ♿ DMEPOS Paid   Ⓢ SNF Excluded   S Codes — 143

S9559   Home injectable therapy, interferon, including administrative services, professional pharmacy services, care coordination, and all necessary supplies and equipment (drugs and nursing visits coded separately), per diem

S9560   Home injectable therapy; hormonal therapy (e.g., leuprolide, goserelin), including administrative services, professional pharmacy services, care coordination, and all necessary supplies and equipment (drugs and nursing visits coded separately), per diem

S9562   Home injectable therapy, palivizumab, including administrative services, professional pharmacy services, care coordination, and all necessary supplies and equipment (drugs and nursing visits coded separately), per diem

S9590   Home therapy, irrigation therapy (e.g., sterile irrigation of an organ or anatomical cavity); including administrative services, professional pharmacy services, care coordination, and all necessary supplies and equipment (drugs and nursing visits coded separately), per diem

S9810   Home therapy; professional pharmacy services for provision of infusion, specialty drug administration, and/or disease state management, not otherwise classified, per hour (do not use this code with any per diem code)

S9900   Services by authorized Christian Science practitioner for the process of healing, per diem; not to be used for rest or study; excludes inpatient services

S9970   Health club membership, annual

S9975   Transplant related lodging, meals and transportation, per diem

S9976   Lodging, per diem, not otherwise specified

S9977   Meals, per diem not otherwise specified

S9981   Medical records copying fee, administrative

S9982   Medical records copying fee, per page

S9986   Not medically necessary service (patient is aware that service not medically necessary)

S9988   Services provided as part of a Phase 1 clinical trial

S9989   Services provided outside of the United States of America (list in addition to code(s) for services(s))

S9990   Services provided as part of a Phase II clinical trial

S9991   Services provided as part of a Phase III clinical trial

S9992   Transportation costs to and from trial location and local transportation costs (e.g., fares for taxicab or bus) for clinical trial participant and one caregiver/companion

S9994   Lodging costs (e.g., hotel charges) for clinical trial participant and one caregiver/companion

S9996   Meals for clinical trial participant and one caregiver/companion

S9999   Sales tax

Special Coverage Instructions   Noncovered by Medicare   Carrier Discretion   ☑ Quantity Alert   ● New Code   ○ Reinstated Code   ▲ Revised Code

144 — S Codes   Ⓐ Age   Ⓜ Maternity   ♀ Female Only   ♂ Male Only   Ⓐ-Ⓨ APC Status Indicator   *2006 HCPCS*

NATIONAL T CODES ESTABLISHED FOR STATE MEDICAID AGENCIES *T1000-T9999*

The T codes are designed for use by Medicaid state agencies to establish codes for items for which there are no permanent national codes but for which codes are necessary to administer the Medicaid program (T codes are not accepted by Medicare but can be used by private insurers). This range of codes describes nursing and home health-related services, substance abuse treatment, and certain training-related procedures.

These codes are not valid for Medicare.

E		T1000	Private duty/independent nursing service(s) — licensed, up to 15 minutes
E		T1001	Nursing assessment/evaluation
E		T1002	RN services, up to 15 minutes
E		T1003	LPN/LVN services, up to 15 minutes
E		T1004	Services of a qualified nursing aide, up to 15 minutes
E		T1005	Respite care services, up to 15 minutes
E		T1006	Alcohol and/or substance abuse services, family/couple counseling
E		T1007	Alcohol and/or substance abuse services, treatment plan development and/or modification
E		T1009	Child sitting services for children of the individual receiving alcohol and/or substance abuse services
E		T1010	Meals for individuals receiving alcohol and/or substance abuse services (when meals not included in the program)
E		T1012	Alcohol and/or substance abuse services, skills development
E		T1013	Sign language or oral interpretive services, per 15 minutes
E		T1014	Telehealth transmission, per minute, professional services bill separately
E		T1015	Clinic visit/encounter, all-inclusive
E		T1016	Case management, each 15 minutes
E		T1017	Targeted case management, each 15 minutes
E		T1018	School-based individualized education program (IEP) services, bundled
E		T1019	Personal care services, per 15 minutes, not for an inpatient or resident of a hospital, nursing facility, ICF/MR or IMD, part of the individualized plan of treatment (code may not be used to identify services provided by home health aide or certified nurse assistant)
E		T1020	Personal care services, per diem, not for an inpatient or resident of a hospital, nursing facility, ICF/MR or IMD, part of the individualized plan of treatment (code may not be used to identify services provided by home health aide or certified nurse assistant)
E		T1021	Home health aide or certified nurse assistant, per visit
E		T1022	Contracted home health agency services, all services provided under contract, per day
E		T1023	Screening to determine the appropriateness of consideration of an individual for participation in a specified program, project or treatment protocol, per encounter
E		T1024	Evaluation and treatment by an integrated, specialty team contracted to provide coordinated care to multiple or severely handicapped children, per encounter ▲

E		T1025	Intensive, extended multidisciplinary services provided in a clinic setting to children with complex medical, physical, mental and psychosocial impairments, per diem ▲
E		T1026	Intensive, extended multidisciplinary services provided in a clinic setting to children with complex medical, physical, medical and psychosocial impairments, per hour ▲
E		T1027	Family training and counseling for child development, per 15 minutes
E		T1028	Assessment of home, physical and family environment, to determine suitability to meet patient's medical needs
E		T1029	Comprehensive environmental lead investigation, not including laboratory analysis, per dwelling
E		T1030	Nursing care, in the home, by registered nurse, per diem
E		T1031	Nursing care, in the home, by licensed practical nurse, per diem
E		T1502	Administration of oral, intramuscular and/or subcutaneous medication by health care agency/professional, per visit
E		T1999	Miscellaneous therapeutic items and supplies, retail purchases, not otherwise classified; identify product in remarks
E		T2001	Non-emergency transportation; patient attendant/escort
E		T2002	Non-emergency transportation; per diem
E		T2003	Non-emergency transportation; encounter/trip
E		T2004	Non-emergency transport; commercial carrier, multi-pass
E		T2005	Non-emergency transportation; stretcher van
		~~T2006~~	~~Ambulance response and treatment, no transport~~ See code(s) A0998.
E		T2007	Transportation waiting time, air ambulance and non-emergency vehicle, one-half (1/2) hour increments
E	☑	T2010	Preadmission screening and resident review (PASRR) level I identification screening, per screen
E		T2011	Preadmission screening and resident review (PASRR) level II evaluation, per evaluation
E	☑	T2012	Habilitation, educational; waiver, per diem
E	☑	T2013	Habilitation, educational, waiver; per hour
E	☑	T2014	Habilitation, prevocational, waiver; per diem
E	☑	T2015	Habilitation, prevocational, waiver; per hour
E	☑	T2016	Habilitation, residential, waiver; per diem
E	☑	T2017	Habilitation, residential, waiver; 15 minutes
E	☑	T2018	Habilitation, supported employment, waiver; per diem
E	☑	T2019	Habilitation, supported employment, waiver; per 15 minutes
E	☑	T2020	Day habilitation, waiver; per diem
E	☑	T2021	Day habilitation, waiver; per 15 minutes
E	☑	T2022	Case management, per month
E	☑	T2023	Targeted case management; per month
E		T2024	Service assessment/plan of care development, waiver
E		T2025	Waiver services; not otherwise specified (NOS)
E	☑	T2026	Specialized childcare, waiver; per diem

Special Coverage Instructions	Noncovered by Medicare	Carrier Discretion	☑ Quantity Alert	● New Code	○ Reinstated Code	▲ Revised Code

2006 HCPCS   **1-9** ASC Groups   **MED:** Pub 100/NCD Reference   ⅗ DMEPOS Paid   ⊘ SNF Excluded   **T Codes — 145**

National T Codes

T2027 — T5999

E ☑ **T2027** Specialized childcare, waiver; per 15 minutes

E **T2028** Specialized supply, not otherwise specified, waiver

E **T2029** Specialized medical equipment, not otherwise specified, waiver

E ☑ **T2030** Assisted living, waiver; per month

E ☑ **T2031** Assisted living; waiver, per diem

E ☑ **T2032** Residential care, not otherwise specified (NOS), waiver; per month

E ☑ **T2033** Residential care, not otherwise specified (NOS), waiver; per diem

E ☑ **T2034** Crisis intervention, waiver; per diem

E **T2035** Utility services to support medical equipment and assistive technology/devices, waiver

E ☑ **T2036** Therapeutic camping, overnight, waiver; each session

E ☑ **T2037** Therapeutic camping, day, waiver; each session

E ☑ **T2038** Community transition, waiver; per service

E ☑ **T2039** Vehicle modifications, waiver; per service

E ☑ **T2040** Financial management, self-directed, waiver; per 15 minutes

E ☑ **T2041** Supports brokerage, self-directed, waiver; per 15 minutes

E ☑ **T2042** Hospice routine home care; per diem

E ☑ **T2043** Hospice continuous home care; per hour

E ☑ **T2044** Hospice inpatient respite care; per diem

E ☑ **T2045** Hospice general inpatient care; per diem

E ☑ **T2046** Hospice long term care, room and board only; per diem

E ☑ **T2048** Behavioral health; long-term care residential (non-acute care in a residential treatment program where stay is typically longer than 30 days), with room and board, per diem

E ☑ **T2049** Non-emergency transportation; stretcher van, mileage; per mile

E **T2101** Human breast milk processing, storage and distribution only ♀

☑ **T4521** Adult sized disposable incontinence product, brief/diaper, small, each
MED: 100-3, 230.10

☑ **T4522** Adult sized disposable incontinence product, brief/diaper, medium, each
MED: 100-3, 230.10

☑ **T4523** Adult sized disposable incontinence product, brief/diaper, large, each
MED: 100-3, 230.10

☑ **T4524** Adult sized disposable incontinence product, brief/diaper, extra large, each
MED: 100-3, 230.10

☑ **T4525** Adult sized disposable incontinence product, protective underwear/pull-on, small size, each
MED: 100-3, 230.10

☑ **T4526** Adult sized disposable incontinence product, protective underwear/pull-on, medium size, each
MED: 100-3, 230.10

☑ **T4527** Adult sized disposable incontinence product, protective underwear/pull-on, large size, each
MED: 100-3, 230.10

☑ **T4528** Adult sized disposable incontinence product, protective underwear/pull-on, extra large size, each
MED: 100-3, 230.10

☑ **T4529** Pediatric sized disposable incontinence product, brief/diaper, small/medium size, each
MED: 100-3, 230.10

☑ **T4530** Pediatric sized disposable incontinence product, brief/diaper, large size, each
MED: 100-3, 230.10

☑ **T4531** Pediatric sized disposable incontinence product, protective underwear/pull-on, small/medium size, each
MED: 100-3, 230.10

☑ **T4532** Pediatric sized disposable incontinence product, protective underwear/pull-on, large size, each
MED: 100-3, 230.10

☑ **T4533** Youth sized disposable incontinence product, brief/diaper, each
MED: 100-3, 230.10

☑ **T4534** Youth sized disposable incontinence product, protective underwear/pull-on, each
MED: 100-3, 230.10

☑ **T4535** Disposable liner/shield/guard/pad/undergarment, for incontinence, each
MED: 100-3, 230.10

☑ **T4536** Incontinence product, protective underwear/pull-on, reusable, any size, each
MED: 100-3, 230.10

☑ **T4537** Incontinence product, protective underpad, reusable, bed size, each
MED: 100-3, 230.10

☑ **T4538** Diaper service, reusable diaper, each diaper
MED: 100-3, 230.10

☑ **T4539** Incontinence product, diaper/brief, reusable, any size, each
MED: 100-3, 230.10

☑ **T4540** Incontinence product, protective underpad, reusable, chair size, each
MED: 100-3, 230.10

☑ **T4541** Incontinence product, disposable underpad, large, each

☑ **T4542** Incontinence product, disposable underpad, small size, each

E **T5001** Positioning seat for persons with special orthopedic needs, for use in vehicles

E **T5999** Supply, not otherwise specified

| Special Coverage Instructions | Noncovered by Medicare | Carrier Discretion | ☑ Quantity Alert | ● New Code | ○ Reinstated Code | ▲ Revised Code |

146 — T Codes   Ⓐ Age   Ⓜ Maternity   ♀ Female Only   ♂ Male Only   Ⓐ-Ⓨ APC Status Indicator   *2006 HCPCS*

VISION SERVICES *V0000-V2999*

These V codes include vision-related supplies, including spectacles, lenses, contact lenses, prostheses, intraocular lenses, and miscellaneous lenses.

FRAMES

V codes fall under the jurisdiction of the DME regional contractor, unless incident to other services or otherwise noted.

Ⓐ   **V2020**   Frames, purchases   ♿⊘
           MED: 100-2, 15, 120

Ⓔ   **V2025**   Deluxe frame   ⊘
           MED: 100-4, 1, 30.3.5

SPECTACLE LENSES

See S0500-S0592 for temporary vision codes.

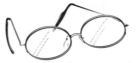

Monofocal spectacles (V2100-V2114)

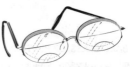

Trifocal spectacles (V2300-V2314)

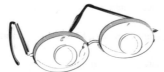

Low vision aids mounted to spectacles (V2610)

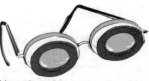

Telescopic or other compound lens fitted on spectacles as a low vision aid (V2615)

SINGLE VISION, GLASS, OR PLASTIC

Ⓐ ☑ **V2100** Sphere, single vision, plano to plus or minus 4.00, per lens ♿

Ⓐ ☑ **V2101** Sphere, single vision, plus or minus 4.12 to plus or minus 7.00d, per lens ♿

Ⓐ ☑ **V2102** Sphere, single vision, plus or minus 7.12 to plus or minus 20.00d, per lens ♿

Ⓐ ☑ **V2103** Spherocylinder, single vision, plano to plus or minus 4.00d sphere, 0.12 to 2.00d cylinder, per lens ♿

Ⓐ ☑ **V2104** Spherocylinder, single vision, plano to plus or minus 4.00d sphere, 2.12 to 4.00d cylinder, per lens ♿

Ⓐ ☑ **V2105** Spherocylinder, single vision, plano to plus or minus 4.00d sphere, 4.25 to 6.00d cylinder, per lens ♿

Ⓐ ☑ **V2106** Spherocylinder, single vision, plano to plus or minus 4.00d sphere, over 6.00d cylinder, per lens ♿

Ⓐ ☑ **V2107** Spherocylinder, single vision, plus or minus 4.25 to plus or minus 7.00 sphere, 0.12 to 2.00d cylinder, per lens ♿

Ⓐ ☑ **V2108** Spherocylinder, single vision, plus or minus 4.25d to plus or minus 7.00d sphere, 2.12 to 4.00d cylinder, per lens ♿

Ⓐ ☑ **V2109** Spherocylinder, single vision, plus or minus 4.25 to plus or minus 7.00d sphere, 4.25 to 6.00d cylinder, per lens ♿

Ⓐ ☑ **V2110** Spherocylinder, single vision, plus or minus 4.25 to 7.00d sphere, over 6.00d cylinder, per lens ♿

Ⓐ ☑ **V2111** Spherocylinder, single vision, plus or minus 7.25 to plus or minus 12.00d sphere, 0.25 to 2.25d cylinder, per lens ♿

Ⓐ ☑ **V2112** Spherocylinder, single vision, plus or minus 7.25 to plus or minus 12.00d sphere, 2.25d to 4.00d cylinder, per lens ♿

Ⓐ ☑ **V2113** Spherocylinder, single vision, plus or minus 7.25 to plus or minus 12.00d sphere, 4.25 to 6.00d cylinder, per lens ♿

Ⓐ ☑ **V2114** Spherocylinder, single vision sphere over plus or minus 12.00d, per lens ♿

Ⓐ ☑ **V2115** Lenticular (myodisc), per lens, single vision ♿

Ⓐ   **V2118** Aniseikonic lens, single vision ♿

Ⓐ   **V2121** Lenticular lens, per lens, single ♿
      MED: 100-2, 15, 120

Ⓐ   **V2199** Not otherwise classified, single vision lens

BIFOCAL, GLASS, OR PLASTIC

Ⓐ ☑ **V2200** Sphere, bifocal, plano to plus or minus 4.00d, per lens ♿

Ⓐ ☑ **V2201** Sphere, bifocal, plus or minus 4.12 to plus or minus 7.00d, per lens ♿

Ⓐ ☑ **V2202** Sphere, bifocal, plus or minus 7.12 to plus or minus 20.00d, per lens ♿

Ⓐ ☑ **V2203** Spherocylinder, bifocal, plano to plus or minus 4.00d sphere, 0.12 to 2.00d cylinder, per lens ♿

Ⓐ ☑ **V2204** Spherocylinder, bifocal, plano to plus or minus 4.00d sphere, 2.12 to 4.00d cylinder, per lens ♿

Ⓐ ☑ **V2205** Spherocylinder, bifocal, plano to plus or minus 4.00d sphere, 4.25 to 6.00d cylinder, per lens ♿

Ⓐ ☑ **V2206** Spherocylinder, bifocal, plano to plus or minus 4.00d sphere, over 6.00d cylinder, per lens ♿

Ⓐ ☑ **V2207** Spherocylinder, bifocal, plus or minus 4.25 to plus or minus 7.00d sphere, 0.12 to 2.00d cylinder, per lens ♿

Ⓐ ☑ **V2208** Spherocylinder, bifocal, plus or minus 4.25 to plus or minus 7.00d sphere, 2.12 to 4.00d cylinder, per lens ♿

Ⓐ ☑ **V2209** Spherocylinder, bifocal, plus or minus 4.25 to plus or minus 7.00d sphere, 4.25 to 6.00d cylinder, per lens ♿

Ⓐ ☑ **V2210** Spherocylinder, bifocal, plus or minus 4.25 to plus or minus 7.00d sphere, over 6.00d cylinder, per lens ♿

Ⓐ ☑ **V2211** Spherocylinder, bifocal, plus or minus 7.25 to plus or minus 12.00d sphere, 0.25 to 2.25d cylinder, per lens ♿

Ⓐ ☑ **V2212** Spherocylinder, bifocal, plus or minus 7.25 to plus or minus 12.00d sphere, 2.25 to 4.00d cylinder, per lens ♿

Ⓐ ☑ **V2213** Spherocylinder, bifocal, plus or minus 7.25 to plus or minus 12.00d sphere, 4.25 to 6.00d cylinder, per lens ♿

Ⓐ ☑ **V2214** Spherocylinder, bifocal, sphere over plus or minus 12.00d, per lens ♿

Ⓐ ☑ **V2215** Lenticular (myodisc), per lens, bifocal ♿

Ⓐ ☑ **V2218** Aniseikonic, per lens, bifocal ♿

Ⓐ ☑ **V2219** Bifocal seg width over 28mm ♿

Ⓐ ☑ **V2220** Bifocal add over 3.25d ♿

Ⓐ   **V2221** Lenticular lens, per lens, bifocal ♿
      MED: 100-2, 15, 120

Vision Services

V2299 — V2624

Ⓐ **V2299** Specialty bifocal (by report)
Pertinent documentation to evaluate medical appropriateness should be included when this code is reported.

TRIFOCAL, GLASS, OR PLASTIC

Ⓐ ☑ **V2300** Sphere, trifocal, plano to plus or minus 4.00d, per lens ♿

Ⓐ ☑ **V2301** Sphere, trifocal, plus or minus 4.12 to plus or minus 7.00d per lens ♿

Ⓐ ☑ **V2302** Sphere, trifocal, plus or minus 7.12 to plus or minus 20.00, per lens ♿

Ⓐ ☑ **V2303** Spherocylinder, trifocal, plano to plus or minus 4.00d sphere, 0.12 to 2.00d cylinder, per lens ♿

Ⓐ ☑ **V2304** Spherocylinder, trifocal, plano to plus or minus 4.00d sphere, 2.25 to 4.00d cylinder, per lens ♿

Ⓐ ☑ **V2305** Spherocylinder, trifocal, plano to plus or minus 4.00d sphere, 4.25 to 6.00 cylinder, per lens ♿

Ⓐ ☑ **V2306** Spherocylinder, trifocal, plano to plus or minus 4.00d sphere, over 6.00d cylinder, per lens ♿

Ⓐ ☑ **V2307** Spherocylinder, trifocal, plus or minus 4.25 to plus or minus 7.00d sphere, 0.12 to 2.00d cylinder, per lens ♿

Ⓐ ☑ **V2308** Spherocylinder, trifocal, plus or minus 4.25 to plus or minus 7.00d sphere, 2.12 to 4.00d cylinder, per lens ♿

Ⓐ ☑ **V2309** Spherocylinder, trifocal, plus or minus 4.25 to plus or minus 7.00d sphere, 4.25 to 6.00d cylinder, per lens ♿

Ⓐ ☑ **V2310** Spherocylinder, trifocal, plus or minus 4.25 to plus or minus 7.00d sphere, over 6.00d cylinder, per lens ♿

Ⓐ ☑ **V2311** Spherocylinder, trifocal, plus or minus 7.25 to plus or minus 12.00d sphere, 0.25 to 2.25d cylinder, per lens ♿

Ⓐ ☑ **V2312** Spherocylinder, trifocal, plus or minus 7.25 to plus or minus 12.00d sphere, 2.25 to 4.00d cylinder, per lens ♿

Ⓐ ☑ **V2313** Spherocylinder, trifocal, plus or minus 7.25 to plus or minus 12.00d sphere, 4.25 to 6.00d cylinder, per lens ♿

Ⓐ ☑ **V2314** Spherocylinder, trifocal, sphere over plus or minus 12.00d, per lens ♿

Ⓐ ☑ **V2315** Lenticular (myodisc), per lens, trifocal ♿

Ⓐ **V2318** Aniseikonic lens, trifocal ♿

Ⓐ ☑ **V2319** Trifocal seg width over 28 mm ♿

Ⓐ ☑ **V2320** Trifocal add over 3.25d ♿

Ⓐ **V2321** Lenticular lens, per lens, trifocal ♿
MED: 100-2, 15, 120

Ⓐ **V2399** Specialty trifocal (by report)
Pertinent documentation to evaluate medical appropriateness should be included when this code is reported.

VARIABLE ASPHERICITY LENS, GLASS, OR PLASTIC

Ⓐ ☑ **V2410** Variable asphericity lens, single vision, full field, glass or plastic, per lens ♿

Ⓐ ☑ **V2430** Variable asphericity lens, bifocal, full field, glass or plastic, per lens ♿

Ⓐ **V2499** Variable sphericity lens, other type

CONTACT LENS

If procedure code 92391 or 92396 is reported, recode with specific lens type listed below (per lens).

Ⓐ ☑ **V2500** Contact lens, PMMA, spherical, per lens ♿

Ⓐ ☑ **V2501** Contact lens, PMMA, toric or prism ballast, per lens ♿

Ⓐ ☑ **V2502** Contact lens, PMMA, bifocal, per lens ♿

Ⓐ ☑ **V2503** Contact lens, PMMA, color vision deficiency, per lens ♿

Ⓐ ☑ **V2510** Contact lens, gas permeable, spherical, per lens ♿

Ⓐ ☑ **V2511** Contact lens, gas permeable, toric, prism ballast, per lens ♿

Ⓐ ☑ **V2512** Contact lens, gas permeable, bifocal, per lens ♿

Ⓐ ☑ **V2513** Contact lens, gas permeable, extended wear, per lens ♿

Ⓐ ☑ **V2520** Contact lens, hydrophilic, spherical, per lens ♿
Hydrophilic contact lenses are covered by Medicare only for aphakic patients. Local contractor if incident to physician services.

MED: 100-3, 80.1; 100-3, 80.4

Ⓐ ☑ **V2521** Contact lens, hydrophilic, toric, or prism ballast, per lens
Hydrophilic contact lenses are covered by Medicare only for aphakic patients. Local contractor if incident to physician services.

MED: 100-3, 80.1; 100-3, 80.4

Ⓐ ☑ **V2522** Contact lens, hydrophilic, bifocal, per lens ♿
Hydrophilic contact lenses are covered by Medicare only for aphakic patients. Local contractor if incident to physician services.

MED: 100-3, 80.1; 100-3, 80.4

Ⓐ ☑ **V2523** Contact lens, hydrophilic, extended wear, per lens ♿
Hydrophilic contact lenses are covered by Medicare only for aphakic patients.

MED: 100-3, 80.1; 100-3, 80.4

Ⓐ ☑ **V2530** Contact lens, scleral, gas impermeable, per lens (for contact lens modification, see CPT Level I code 92325) ♿

Ⓐ ☑ **V2531** Contact lens, scleral, gas permeable, per lens (for contact lens modification, see CPT Level I code 92325) ♿
MED: 100-3, 80.5

Ⓐ **V2599** Contact lens, other type ⊘
Local contractor if incident to physician services.

VISION AIDS

If procedure code 92392 is reported, recode with specific systems below.

Ⓐ **V2600** Hand held low vision aids and other nonspectacle mounted aids ⊘

Ⓐ **V2610** Single lens spectacle mounted low vision aids ⊘

Ⓐ **V2615** Telescopic and other compound lens system, including distance vision telescopic, near vision telescopes and compound microscopic lens system ⊘

PROSTHETIC EYE

Ⓐ **V2623** Prosthetic eye, plastic, custom ♿
MED: 100-2, 15, 120

Ⓐ **V2624** Polishing/resurfacing of ocular prosthesis ♿

A		V2625	Enlargement of ocular prosthesis	ᴆ
A		V2626	Reduction of ocular prosthesis	ᴆ
A		V2627	Scleral cover shell	ᴆ

A scleral shell covers the cornea and the anterior sclera. Medicare covers a scleral shell when it is prescribed as an artificial support to a shrunken and sightless eye or as a barrier in the treatment of severe dry eye.

MED: 100-3, 80.5

A		V2628	Fabrication and fitting of ocular conformer	ᴆ
A		V2629	Prosthetic eye, other type	⊘

INTRAOCULAR LENSES

N		V2630	Anterior chamber intraocular lens	⊘

The IOL must be FDA-approved for reimbursement. Medicare payment for an IOL is included in the payment for ASC facility services. Medicare jurisdiction: local contractor.

MED: 100-2, 15, 120

N		V2631	Iris supported intraocular lens	⊘

The IOL must be FDA-approved for reimbursement. Medicare payment for an IOL is included in the payment for ASC facility services. Medicare jurisdiction: local contractor.

MED: 100-2, 15, 120

N		V2632	Posterior chamber intraocular lens	⊘

The IOL must be FDA-approved for reimbursement. Medicare payment for an IOL is included in the payment for ASC facility services. Medicare jurisdiction: local contractor.

MED: 100-2, 15, 120

MISCELLANEOUS

A	☑	V2700	Balance lens, per lens	ᴆ
		V2702	Deluxe lens feature	

MED: 100-2, 15, 120

A	☑	V2710	Slab off prism, glass or plastic, per lens	ᴆ
A	☑	V2715	Prism, per lens	ᴆ
A	☑	V2718	Press-on lens, Fresnel prism, per lens	ᴆ
A	☑	V2730	Special base curve, glass or plastic, per lens	ᴆ
A	☑	V2744	Tint, photochromatic, per lens	ᴆ

MED: 100-2, 15, 120

A	☑	V2745	Addition to lens; tint, any color, solid, gradient or equal, excludes photochromatic, any lens material, per lens	ᴆ

MED: 100-2, 15, 120

A	☑	V2750	Antireflective coating, per lens	ᴆ

MED: 100-2, 15, 120

A	☑	V2755	U-V lens, per lens	ᴆ

MED: 100-2, 15, 120

E		V2756	Eye glass case	⊘
A	☑	V2760	Scratch resistant coating, per lens	ᴆ
B	☑	V2761	Mirror coating, any type, solid, gradient or equal, any lens material, per lens	

MED: 100-2, 15, 120

A	☑	V2762	Polarization, any lens material, per lens	ᴆ

MED: 100-2, 15, 120

A	☑	V2770	Occluder lens, per lens	ᴆ
A	☑	V2780	Oversize lens, per lens	ᴆ
B	☑	V2781	Progressive lens, per lens	⊘

A	☑	V2782	Lens, index 1.54 to 1.65 plastic or 1.60 to 1.79 glass, excludes polycarbonate, per lens	ᴆ

MED: 100-2, 15, 120

A	☑	V2783	Lens, index greater than or equal to 1.66 plastic or greater than or equal to 1.80 glass, excludes polycarbonate, per lens	ᴆ

MED: 100-2, 15, 120

A	☑	V2784	Lens, polycarbonate or equal, any index, per lens	ᴆ

MED: 100-2, 15, 120

F		V2785	Processing, preserving and transporting corneal tissue	⊘

Medicare jurisdiction: local contractor.

A	☑	V2786	Specialty occupational multifocal lens, per lens	ᴆ

MED: 100-2, 15, 120

●	E	V2788	Presbyopia correcting function of intraocular lens	
	N	V2790	Amniotic membrane for surgical reconstruction, per procedure	⊘

Medicare jurisdiction: local contractor.

A		V2797	Vision supply, accessory and/or service component of another HCPCS vision code	⊘
A		V2799	Vision service, miscellaneous	⊘

Determine if an alternative HCPCS Level II or a CPT code better describes the service being reported. This code should be used only if a more specific code is unavailable.

HEARING SERVICES *V5000-V5999*

This range of codes describes hearing tests and related supplies and equipment, speech-language pathology screenings, and repair of augmentative communicative system.

Hearing services fall under the jurisdiction of the local contractor unless incidental or otherwise noted.

E		V5008	Hearing screening	⊘

MED: 100-2, 16, 90

E		V5010	Assessment for hearing aid	⊘
E		V5011	Fitting/orientation/checking of hearing aid	⊘
E		V5014	Repair/modification of a hearing aid	⊘
E		V5020	Conformity evaluation	⊘
E		V5030	Hearing aid, monaural, body worn, air conduction	⊘
E		V5040	Hearing aid, monaural, body worn, bone conduction	⊘
E		V5050	Hearing aid, monaural, in the ear	⊘
E		V5060	Hearing aid, monaural, behind the ear	⊘
E		V5070	Glasses, air conduction	⊘
E		V5080	Glasses, bone conduction	⊘
E		V5090	Dispensing fee, unspecified hearing aid	⊘
E		V5095	Semi-implantable middle ear hearing prosthesis	

Use this code for Vibrant Soundbridge Implantable Middle Ear Prosthesis.

E		V5100	Hearing aid, bilateral, body worn	⊘
E		V5110	Dispensing fee, bilateral	⊘
E		V5120	Binaural, body	⊘
E		V5130	Binaural, in the ear	⊘
E		V5140	Binaural, behind the ear	⊘
E		V5150	Binaural, glasses	⊘
E		V5160	Dispensing fee, binaural	⊘
E		V5170	Hearing aid, CROS, in the ear	⊘

Special Coverage Instructions   Noncovered by Medicare   Carrier Discretion   ☑ Quantity Alert   ● New Code   ○ Reinstated Code   ▲ Revised Code

2006 HCPCS   ❶-❾ ASC Groups   MED: Pub 100/NCD Reference   ᴆ DMEPOS Paid   ⊘ SNF Excluded   **V Codes — 149**

Hearing Services

V5180 — V5364

E	V5180	Hearing aid, CROS, behind the ear	⊘
E	V5190	Hearing aid, CROS, glasses	⊘
E	V5200	Dispensing fee, CROS	⊘
E	V5210	Hearing aid, BICROS, in the ear	⊘
E	V5220	Hearing aid, BICROS, behind the ear	⊘
E	V5230	Hearing aid, BICROS, glasses	⊘
E	V5240	Dispensing fee, BICROS	⊘
E	V5241	Dispensing fee, monaural hearing aid, any type	
E	V5242	Hearing aid, analog, monaural, CIC (completely in the ear canal)	
E	V5243	Hearing aid, analog, monaural, ITC (in the canal)	
E	V5244	Hearing aid, digitally programmable analog, monaural, CIC	
E	V5245	Hearing aid, digitally programmable, analog, monaural, ITC	
E	V5246	Hearing aid, digitally programmable analog, monaural, ITE (in the ear)	
E	V5247	Hearing aid, digitally programmable analog, monaural, BTE (behind the ear)	
E	V5248	Hearing aid, analog, binaural, CIC	
E	V5249	Hearing aid, analog, binaural, ITC	
E	V5250	Hearing aid, digitally programmable analog, binaural, CIC	
E	V5251	Hearing aid, digitally programmable analog, binaural, ITC	
E	V5252	Hearing aid, digitally programmable, binaural, ITE	
E	V5253	Hearing aid, digitally programmable, binaural, BTE	
E	V5254	Hearing aid, digital, monaural, CIC	
E	V5255	Hearing aid, digital, monaural, ITC	
E	V5256	Hearing aid, digital, monaural, ITE	
E	V5257	Hearing aid, digital, monaural, BTE	
E	V5258	Hearing aid, digital, binaural, CIC	
	V5259	Hearing aid, digital, binaural, ITC	
	V5260	Hearing aid, digital, binaural, ITE	

	V5261	Hearing aid, digital, binaural, BTE
	V5262	Hearing aid, disposable, any type, monaural
☑	V5263	Hearing aid, disposable, any type, binaural
☑	V5264	Ear mold/insert, not disposable, any type
☑	V5265	Ear mold/insert, disposable, any type
☑	V5266	Battery for use in hearing device
☑	V5267	Hearing aid supplies/accessories
☑	V5268	Assistive listening device, telephone amplifier, any type
	V5269	Assistive listening device, alerting, any type
	V5270	Assistive listening device, television amplifier, any type
	V5271	Assistive listening device, television caption decoder
	V5272	Assistive listening device, TDD
	V5273	Assistive listening device, for use with cochlear implant
	V5274	Assistive listening device, not otherwise specified
	V5275	Ear impression, each
	V5298	Hearing aid, not otherwise classified
B	V5299	Hearing service, miscellaneous

Determine if an alternative HCPCS Level II or a CPT code better describes the service being reported. This code should be used only if a more specific code is unavailable.

MED: 100-2, 16, 90

SPEECH-LANGUAGE PATHOLOGY SERVICES

E	V5336	Repair/modification of augmentative communicative system or device (excludes adaptive hearing aid)	⊘

Medicare jurisdiction: DME regional contractor.

E	V5362	Speech screening
E	V5363	Language screening
E	V5364	Dysphagia screening

APPENDIX 1 — TABLE OF DRUGS

INTRODUCTION AND DIRECTIONS

The *HCPCS 2006* Table of Drugs is designed to quickly and easily direct the user to drug names and their corresponding codes. Both generic and brand or trade names are alphabetically listed in the "Drug Name" column of the table. The associated A, C, J, K, Q, or S code is given only for the generic name of the drug.

The "Amount" column lists the stated amount for the referenced generic drug as provided by CMS. "Up to" listings are inclusive of all quantities up to and including the listed amount. All other listings are for the amount of the drug as listed. The editors recognize that the availability of some drugs in the quantities listed is dependent on many variables beyond the control of the clinical ordering clerk. The availability in your area of regularly used drugs in the most cost-effective quantities should be relayed to your third-party payers.

The "Route of Administration" column addresses the most common methods of delivering the referenced generic drug as described in current pharmaceutical literature. The official definitions for Level II drug codes generally describe administration other than by oral method. Therefore, with a handful of exceptions, oral-delivered options for most drugs are omitted from the Route of Administration column. The following abbreviations and listings are used in the Route of Administration column:

IA — Intra-arterial administration

IM — Intramuscular administration

INH — Administration by inhaled solution

INJ — Injection not otherwise specified

IT — Intrathecal

IV — Intravenous administration

MICRO — Microcurie

ORAL — Administered orally

OTH — Other routes of administration

SC — Subcutaneous administration

VAR — Various routes of administration

Intravenous administration includes all methods, such as gravity infusion, injections, and timed pushes. When several routes of administration are listed, the first listing is simply the first, or most common, method as described in current reference literature. The "VAR" posting denotes various routes of administration and is used for drugs that are commonly administered into joints, cavities, tissues, or topical applications, in addition to other parenteral administrations. Listings posted with "OTH" alert the user to other administration methods, such as suppositories or catheter injections.

Please be reminded that the Table of Drugs, as well as all HCPCS Level II national definitions and listings, constitutes a post-treatment medical reference for billing purposes only. Although the editors have exercised all normal precautions to ensure the accuracy of the table and related material, the use of any of this information to select medical treatment is entirely inappropriate.

Table of Drugs

Drug Name	Unit	Route	Code
10% LMD	500 ML	IV	J7100
5% DEXTROSE/NORMAL SALINE	5%	VAR	J7042
5% DEXTROSE/WATER	500 ML	IV	J7060
ABARELIX	10 MG	IM	J0128
ABBOKINASE	250,000 IU	IV	J3365
ABBOKINASE	5,000 IU	IV	J3364
ABCIXIMAB	10 MG	IV	J0130
ABELCENT	50 MG	IV	J0285
ABRAXANE	1 MG	IV	J9264
ACCUNEB CONCENTRATED	1 MG	INH	J7611
ACCUNEB	1 MG	INH	J7613
ACELLULAR SKIN SUBSTITUTE	PER 16 SQ CM	OTH	C9221
ACETADOTE	1 G	INH	J7608
ACETADOTE	100 MG	IV	J0132
ACETAZOLAMIDE SODIUM	500 MG	IM, IV	J1120
ACETYLCYSTEINE	1 G	INH	J7608
ACOVA	5 MG	INJ	C9121
ACTHREL	1 MCG	IV	J0795
ACTIMMUNE	0.25 MG	SC	J1830
ACTIMMUNE	3 MU	SC	J9216
ACTIVASE	1 MG	IV	J2997
ACUTECT	PER DOSE	IV	A9504
ACYCLOVIR SODIUM	50 MG	INJ	J0133
ACYCLOVIR	5 MG	IV	J0133
ADAGEN	25 IU	IM	J2504
ADALIMUMAB	20 MG	INJ	J0135
ADBEON	4 MG	IM, IV	J0704
ADENOCARD	6 MG	IV	J0150
ADENOSCAN	30 MG	IV	J0152
ADENOSINE	30 MG	IV	J0152
ADENOSINE	6 MG	IV	J0150
ADRENALIN CHLORIDE	1 MG	IM, IV, SC	J0170
ADRENALIN	1 MG	IM, IV, SC	J0170
ADRIAMYCIN	10 MG	IV	J9000
ADRUCIL	500 MG	IV	J9190
AEROBID	1 MG	INH	J7641
AGALSIDASE BETA	1 MG	IV	J0180
AGGRASTAT	12.5 MG	IM, IV	J3246
A-HYDROCORT	100 MG	IV, IM, SC	J1720
ALATROFLOXACIN MESYLATE	100 MG	IV	J0200
ALBUTEROL CONCENETRATED FORM	1 MG	INH	J7611
ALBUTEROL UNIT DOSE FORM	1 MG	INH	J7613
ALDESLEUKIN	1 VIAL	IV	J9015
ALDOMET	250 MG	IV	J0210
ALDURAZYME	0.1 MG	IV	J1931
ALEFACEPT	0.5 MG	IV, IM	J0215
ALFERON N	250,000 IU	IM	J9215
ALGLUCERASE	10 U	IV	J0205
ALIMTA	10 MG	IV	J9305
ALKERAN	2 MG	ORAL	J8600
ALKERAN	50 MG	IV	J9245
ALOXI	25 MCG	IV	J2469
ALPHA 1 - PROTEINASE INHIBITOR — HUMAN	10 MG	IV	J0256
ALPHANATE	PER IU	IV	J7190
ALPHANINE SD	PER IU	IV	J7193
ALPHANINE SD	PER IU	IV	J7194
ALPROSTADIL	1.25 MCG	INJ	J0270
ALPROSTADIL	EA	OTH	J0275

Drug Name	Unit	Route	Code
ALTEPLASE RECOMBINANT	1 MG	IV	J2997
ALUPENT	10 MG	INH	J7668
AMANTADINE HYDROCHLORIDE (BRAND NAME)	100 MG	ORAL	G9033
AMANTADINE HYDROCHLORIDE (GENERIC)	100 MG	ORAL	G9017
AMBISOME	10 MG	IV	J0289
AMCORT	5 MG	IM	J3302
AMERGAN	12.5 MG	ORAL	Q0169
A-METHAPRED	125 MG	IM, IV	J2930
A-METHAPRED	40 MG	IM, IV	J2920
AMEVIVE	0.5 MG	IV, IM	J0215
AMICAR	5 G	INJ	S0017
AMIFOSTINE	500 MG	IV	J0207
AMIKACIN SULFATE	100 MG	IM, IV	J0278
AMIKIN	100 MG	IM, IV	S0072
AMINOCAPROIC ACID	5 G	INJ	J0278
AMINOPHYLLIN/AMINOPHYLLINE	250 MG	IV	J0280
AMIODARONE HCL	30 MG	IV	J0282
AMITRIPTYLINE HCL	20 MG	IM	J1320
AMMONIA N-13	PER DOSE	IV	A9526
AMOBARBITAL	125 MG	IM, IV	J0300
AMPHOCIN	50 MG	IV	J0285
AMPHOTEC	10 MG	IV	J0288
AMPHOTERICIN B CHOLESTERYL SULFATE COMPLEX	10 MG	IV	J0288
AMPHOTERICIN B LIPID COMPLEX	10 MG	IV	J0287
AMPHOTERICIN B LIPOSOME	10 MG	IV	J0289
AMPHOTERICIN B	50 MG	IV	J0285
AMPICILLIN SODIUM	500 MG	IM, IV	J0290
AMPICILLIN SODIUM/SULBACTAM SODIUM	1.5 G	IM, IV	J0295
AMYTAL	125 MG	IM, IV	J0300
ANABOLIN LA 100	100 MG	IM	J2321
ANASTROZOLE	1 MG	ORAL	S0170
ANCEF	500 MG	IV, IM	J0690
ANDRO LA 200	200 MG	IM	J3130
ANDROLONE-D 100	100 MG	IM	J2321
ANDRONAQ 50	50 MG	IM	J3140
ANDROPOSITORY 100	100 MG	IM	J3120
ANECTINE	20 MG	IM, IV	J0330
ANERGAN 25	50 MG	IM, IV	J2550
ANERGAN 50	50 MG	IM, IV	J2550
ANGIOMAX	1 MG	INJ	J0583
ANISTREPLASE	30 U	IV	J0350
ANTAGON	75 IU	IV, SC	S0132
ANTIFLEX	60 MG	IV, IM	J2360
ANTIHEMOPHILIC FACTOR HUMAN METHOD M MONOCLONAL PURIFIED	PER IU	IV	J7192
ANTIHEMOPHILIC FACTOR PORCINE	PER IU	IV	J7191
ANTI-INHIBITOR	PER IU	IV	J7198
ANTINAUS	50 MG	IM, IV	J2550
ANTITHROMBIN III	PER IU	IV	J7195
ANTI-THYMOCYTE GLOBULIN,EQUINE	250 MG	OTH	J7504
ANTIZOL	15 MG	IV	J1451
ANZEMET	10 MG	IV	J1260
ANZEMET	100 MG	ORAL	Q0180
ANZEMET	50 MG	ORAL	S0174
APLIGRAF	SQ CM	OTH	J7340
APOMORPHINE HYDROCHLORIDE	1 MG	SC	S0167

Drug Name	Unit	Route	Code
APREPITANT, ORAL, 5 MG	5 MG	ORAL	J8501
APROTININ	10,000 KIU	IV	J0365
AQUAMEPHYTON	1 MG	IM, SC, IV	J3430
ARA-C	100 MG	SC, IV	J9100
ARALEN	UP TO 250 MG	IV, IM, SC	J0390
ARAMINE	10 MG	IV, IM, SC	J0380
ARANESP, ESRD USE	1 MCG	SC, IV	J0882
ARANESP, NON-ESRD USE	1 MCG	SC, IV	J0881
AREDIA	30 MG	IV	J2430
ARGATROBAN	30 MG	IV	J2430
ARGATROBAN	5 MG	IV	C9121
ARIMIDEX	1 MG	ORAL	S0170
ARISTOCORT	5 MG	IM	J3302
ARISTOCORTE FORTE	5 MG	IM	J3302
ARISTOCORTE INTRALESIONAL	5 MG	OTH	J3302
ARISTOSPAN	5 MG	VAR	J3303
ARIXTRA	0.5 MG	INJ	J1652
AROMASIN	25 MG	ORAL	S0156
ARRESTIN	200 MG	IM	J3250
ARSENIC TRIOXIDE	1 MG	IV	J9017
ASPARAGINASE	10,000 U	VAR	J9020
ASTRAMORPH PF	10 MG	IM, IV, SC	J2275
ATGAM	250 MG	OTH	J7504
ATIVAN	2 MG	IM, IV	J2060
ATROPEN	0.3 MG	IV, IM, SC	J0460
ATROPINE SULFATE	0.3 MG	IV, IM, SC	J0460
ATROPINE	PER MG	INH	J7636
ATROVENT	PER MG	INH	J7644
AUROTHIOGLUCOSE	50 MG	IM	J2910
AUTOPLEX T	PER IU	IV	J7198
AVASTIN	10 MG	IV	J9035
AVELOX	100 MG	INJ	J2280
AVONEX	11 MCG	IM	Q3025
AVONEX	33 MCG	IM	J1825
AZACITIDINE	1 MG	SC	J9025
AZACTAM	500 MG	IV	S0073
AZASAN	50 MG	ORAL	J7500
AZATHIOPRINE SODIUM	100 MG	OTH	J7501
AZATHIOPRINE	100 MG	OTH	J7501
AZATHIOPRINE	50 MG	ORAL	J7500
AZITHROMYCIN	500 MG	IV	J0456
AZMACORT CONCENTRATED	PER MG	INH	J7683
AZMACORT	PER MG	INH	J7684
AZTREONAM	500 MG	IV	S0073
AZTREONAM	PER MG	INH	S0143
BACLOFEN	10 MG	IT	J0475
BACLOFEN	50 MCG	OTH	J0476
BACTERIOSTATIC WATER	5%	VAR	J7051
BACTOCILL	250 MG	IM, IV	J2700
BACTRAMYCIN	300 MG	IV	J2010
BACTRIM IV	10 ML	IV	S0039
BAL	100 MG	IM	J0470
BANFLEX	60 MG	IV, IM	J2360
BASILIXIMAB	20 MG	IV	J0480
BAYGAM	1 CC	IM	J1460
BAYRHO D	50 MCG	IM	J2788
BAYRHO-D	100 IU	IM	J2792
BAYRHO-D	300 MCG	IM	J2790

Drug Name	Unit	Route	Code
BAYTET	250 U	IM	J1670
BCG VACCINE LIVE	PER VIAL	IV	J9031
BEBULIN VH	PER IU	IV	J7194
BECAPLERMIN GEL 0.01%	0.5 G	OTH	S0157
BECLOMETHASONE	1 MG	INH	J7622
BECLOVENT	1 MG	INH	J7622
BECONASE	1 MG	INH	J7622
BENA-D 10	50 MG	IV, IM	J1200
BENA-D 50	50 MG	IV, IM	J1200
BENADRYL	50 MG	IV, IM	J1200
BENAHIST 10	50 MG	IV, IM	J1200
BENAHIST 50	50 MG	IV, IM	J1200
BENEFIX	PER IU	IV	J7195
BENOJECT-10	50 MG	IV, IM	J1200
BENOJECT-50	50 MG	IV, IM	J1200
BENTYL	20 MG	IM	J0500
BENZTROPINE MESYLATE	1 MG	IM, IV	J0515
BERUBIGEN	1,000 MCG	SC, IM	J3420
BETA-2	1 MG	INH	J7648
BETALIN 12	1,000 MCG	SC, IM	J3420
BETAMETHASONE ACETATE AND BETAMETHASONE SODIUM PHOSPHATE	3 MG, OF EACH	IM	J0702
BETAMETHASONE SODIUM PHOSPHATE	4 MG	IM, IV	J0704
BETAMETHASONE	1 MG	INH	J7624
BETASERON	0.25 MG	SC	J1830
BETHANECHOL CHLORIDE, MYOTONACHOL OR URECHOLINE	5 MG	SC	J0520
BEVACIZUMAB	10 MG	IV	J9035
BEVACIZUMAB	100 MG	IV	S0116
BEXXAR DIAGNOSTIC	STUDY DOSE		A9544
BEXXAR THERAPEUTIC	TX DOSE	IV	A9545
BICILLIN CR 900/300	1,200,000 U	IM, IV	J0540
BICILLIN CR 900/300	2,400,000 U	IM, IV	J0550
BICILLIN CR	1,200,000 U	IM	J0540
BICILLIN CR	600,000 U	IM	J0530
BICILLIN LA	1,200,000 U	IM	J0570
BICILLIN LA	2,400,000 U	INJ	J0580
BICILLIN LA	600,000 U	IM	J0560
BICNU	100 MG	IV	J9050
BIOCLATE	PER IU	IV	J7192
BIOTROPIN	1 MG	SC	J2941
BITOLTEROL MESYLATE	PER MG	INH	J7629
BITOLTEROL MESYLATE, CONCENTRATED	PER MG	INH	J7628
BIVALIRUDIN	1 MG	INJ	J0583
BLENOXANE	15 U	IM, IV, SC	J9040
BLEOMYCIN LYOPHILLIZED	15 U	IM, IV, SC	J9040
BLEOMYCIN SULFATE	15 U	IM, IV, SC	J9040
BORTEZOMIB	0.1 MG	INJ	J9041
BOTOX	1 U	IM	J0585
BOTULINUM TOXIN TYPE A	1 U	OTH	J0585
BOTULINUM TOXIN TYPE B	100 U	OTH	J0587
BRAVELLE	75 IU	IM	J3355
BRETHINE CONCENTRATED	PER MG	INH	J7680
BRETHINE	1 MG	SC, IV	J3105
BRETHINE	PER MG	INH	J7681
BRETYLIUM TOSYLATE	1 EA		J3490
BRICANYL CONCENTRATED	PER MG	INH	J7680
BRICANYL SUBCUTANEOUS	1 MG	SC	J3105
BRICANYL	PER MG	INH	J7681

Drug Name	Unit	Route	Code
BROM-A-COT	10 MG	IM, SC, IV	J0945
BROMPHENIRAMINE MALEATE	10 MG	IM, SC, IV	J0945
BRONCHO SALINE	5 CC	VAR	J7051
BUDESONIDE	0.25 MG	INH	J7633
BUDESONIDE	5 MG	INH	J7626
BUMETANIDE	0.5 MG	IM, IV	S0171
BUMEX	0.5 MG	IM, IV	S0171
BUPIVACAINE HCL	30 ML	INJ	S0020
BUPRENEX	0.1 MG	INJ	J0592
BUPRENORPHINE HCL	0.1 MG	INJ	J0592
BUPROPION HCL	150 MG	ORAL	S0106
BUSULFAN	2 MG	ORAL	J8510
BUSULFAN	6 MG	IV	C1178
BUSULFEX	2 MG	ORAL	J8510
BUSULFEX	6 MG	IV	C1178
BUTORPHANOL TARTRATE	2 MG	IM, IV	J0595
BUTORPHANOL TARTRATE	25 MG	OTH	S0012
CABERGOLINE	0.25 MG	ORAL	J8515
CAFCIT	5 MG	IV	J0706
CAFFEINE CITRATE	5 MG	IV	J0706
CALCIJEX	0.1 MCG	IM	J0636
CALCIMAR	UP TO 400 U	SC, IM	J0630
CALCITONIN SALMON	400 U	SC, IM	J0630
CALCITRIOL	0.1 MCG	IM	J0636
CALCITROL	0.25 MCG	ORAL	S0161
CALCIUM CHLORIDE	1 EA		J3490
CALCIUM DISODIUM VERSENATE	1,000 MG	IV, SC, IM	J0600
CALCIUM GLUCONATE	10 ML	IV	J0610
CALCIUM GLYCEROPHOSPHATE AND CALCIUM LACTATE	10 ML	IM, SC	J0620
CAMPATH	10 MG	INJ	J9010
CAMPTOSAR	20 MG	IV	J9206
CANCIDAS	5 MG	IV	J0637
CAPECITABINE	150 MG	ORAL	J8520
CAPROMAB PENDETIDE	PER DOSE	IV	A9507
CARBACOT	10 ML	IV, IM	J2800
CARBOCAINE	10 ML	VAR	J0670
CARBOPLATIN	50 MG	IV	J9045
CARDIOGEN 82	60 MCI	IV	A9555
CARDIOLITE	PER DOSE	IV	A9500
CARIMUNE	1 GM	IV	J1563
CARMUSTINE	100 MG	IV	J9050
CARNITOR	1 G	IV	J1955
CARTICEL		OTH	J7330
CASPOFUNGIN ACETATE	5 MG	IV	J0637
CATAPRES	1 MG	OTH	J0735
CATHFLO	1 MG	IV	J2997
CAVERJECT	1.25 MCG	INJ	J0270
CEA-SCAN	25 MCI	IV	A9549
CEENU	10 MG	ORAL	S0178
CEFAZOLIN SODIUM	500 MG	IV, IM	J0690
CEFEPIME HCL	500 MG	IV	J0692
CEFIZOX	500 MG	IV, IM	J0715
CEFOBID	1 G	IV	S0021
CEFOPERAZONE SODIUM	1 G	IV	S0021
CEFOTAN	500 MG	IM, IV	S0074
CEFOTAXIME SODIUM	1 GM	IV, IM	J0698
CEFOTETAN DISODIUM	500 MG	IM. IV	S0074
CEFOXITIN SODIUM	1 GM	IV, IM	J0694

Drug Name	Unit	Route	Code
CEFOXITIN	1 GM	IV, IM	J0694
CEFTAZIDIME	500 MG	IM, IV	J0713
CEFTIZOXIME SODIUM	500 MG	IV, IM	J0715
CEFTRIAXONE SODIUM	250 MG	IV, IM	J0696
CEFTRIAXONE	250 MG	IV, IM	J0696
CEFUROXIME SODIUM STERILE	750 MG	IM, IV	J0697
CEFUROXIME	750 MG	IM, IV	J0697
CELESTONE SOLUSPAN	3 MG	IM	J0702
CELLCEPT	250 MG	ORAL	J7517
CENACORT A-40	10 MG	IM	J3301
CENACORT FORTE	5 MG	IM	J3302
CEPHALOTHIN SODIUM	1 G	IM, IV	J1890
CEPTAZ	500 MG	IM, IV	J0713
CEREBRYX	50 MG	INJ	Q2009
CEREBRYX	750 MG	IM	S0078
CEREDASE	10 U	IV	J0205
CERETEC	PER DOSE	IV	A9521
CEREZYME	1 U	IV	J1785
CERUBIDINE	10 MG	IV	J9150
CETUXIMAB	10 MG	INJ	J9055
CHLORAMBUCIL	2 MG	ORAL	S0172
CHLORAMPHENICOL SODIUM SUCCINATE	1 G	IV	J0720
CHLORDIAZEPOXIDE HCL	100 MG	IM, IV	J1990
CHLOROMYCETIN	1 G	INJ	J0720
CHLOROPROCAINE HCL	30 ML	VAR	J2400
CHLOROTHIAZIDE SODIUM	500 MG	IV	J1205
CHLORPROMAZINE HCL	10 MG	ORAL	Q0171
CHLORPROMAZINE HCL	25 MG	ORAL	Q0172
CHLORPROMAZINE HCL	50 MG	IM, IV	J3230
CHORIONIC GONADOTROPIN	1,000 USP U	IM	J0725
CHROMIC PHOSPHATE P32	PER MCI	IV	A9564
CHROMITOPE	250 MICRO	IV	A9553
CHROMIUM CR-51 SODIUM IOTHALAMATE, DIAGNOSTIC	10 MICRO	IV	A9553
CIDOFOVIR	375 MG	IV	J0740
CILASTATIN SODIUM	250 MG	IV, IM	J0743
CIMETIDINE HCL	300 MG	IV	S0023
CIMETIDINE HYDROCHLORIDE	1 EA		J3490
CIPRO	200 MG	IV	J0744
CIPROFLOXACIN FOR INTRAVENOUS INFUSION	200 MG	IV	J0744
CISPLATIN	10 MG	IV	J9060
CLADRIBINE	1 MG	IV	J9065
CLAFORAN	1 GM	IV, IM	J0698
CLAVULANATE POTASSIUM/TICARCILLIN DISODIUM	1 EA		J3490
CLEOCIN PHOSPHATE	300 MG	IV	S0077
CLINAGEN LA	UP TO 40 MG	IM	J0970
CLINDAMYCIN PHOSPHATE	300 MG	IV	S0077
CLOFARABINE	1 MG	IV	J9027
CLOLAR	1 MG	IV	J9027
CLONIDINE HCL	1 MG	OTH	J0735
CLOSTRIDIUM BOTULINUM TOXIN	1 U	OTH	J0585
CLOZAPINE	25 MG	ORAL	S0136
CLOZARIL	25 MG	ORAL	S0136
COBAL	1,000 MCG	IM, SC	J3420
COBALT CO-57 CYNOCOBALAMIN, DIAGNOSTIC	1 MICRO	ORAL	A9559
COBATOPE 57	1 MICRO	ORAL	A9559

Drug Name	Unit	Route	Code
COBEX	1,000 MCG	SC, IM	J3420
CODEINE PHOSPHATE	30 MG	IM, IV, SC	J0745
COGENTIN	1 MG	IM, IV	J0515
COGNEX	10 MG	ORAL	S0014
COLCHICINE	1 MG	IV	J0760
COLHIST	10 MG	IM, SC, IV	J0945
COLISTIMETHATE SODIUM	150 MG	IM, IV	J0770
COLISTIMETHATE SODIUM	PER MG	INH	S0142
COLLAGEN-GLYCOSAMINOGLYCAN SKIN SUBSTITUTE	PER SQ CM	OTH	J7343
COLY-MYCIN M	150 MG	IM, IV	J0770
COMPAZINE	10 MG	IM, IV	J0780
COMPAZINE	10 MG	ORAL	Q0165
COMPAZINE	5 MG	ORAL	Q0164
COMPAZINE	5 MG	ORAL	S0183
CONTRACEPTIVE SUPPLY, HORMONE CONTAINING PATCH	EACH	OTH	J7304
COPAXONE	20 MG	INJ	J1595
COPPER T MODEL TCU380A IUD COPPER WIRE/COPPER COLLAR	EA	OTH	J7300
CORDARONE	30 MG	IV	J0282
CORTASTAT LA	1 MG	IM	J1094
CORTASTAT	1 MG	IM, IV, OTH	J1100
CORTICORELIN OVINE TRIFLUTATE	1 MCG	IV	J0795
CORTICOTROPIN	40 U	IV, IM, SC	J0800
CORTIMED	80 MG	IM	J1040
CORTROSYN	0.25 MG	IM, IV	J0835
CORVERT	1 MG	IV	J1742
COSMEGEN	0.5 MG	IV	J9120
COSYNTROPIN	0.25 MG	IM, IV	J0835
COTOLONE	1 ML	IM	J2650
COTOLONE	5 MG	ORAL	J7510
CROMOLYN SODIUM	10 MG	INH	J7631
CRYSTAL B12	1,000 MCG	IM, SC	J3420
CRYSTICILLIN 300 A.S.	600,000 UNITS	IM, IV	J2510
CRYSTICILLIN 600 A.S.	600,000 UNITS	IM, IV	J2510
CUBICIN	1 MG	IV	J0878
CYANO	1,000 MCG	IM, SC	J3420
CYANOCOBALAMIN COBALT 58/57	1 MICRO	IV	A9546
CYANOCOBALAMIN COBALT CO-57	1 MICRO	ORAL	A9559
CYANOCOBALAMIN	1,000 MCG	IM, SC	J3420
CYCLOPHOSPHAMIDE LYOPHILIZED	1 G	IV	J9096
CYCLOPHOSPHAMIDE LYOPHILIZED	100 MG	IV	J9093
CYCLOPHOSPHAMIDE LYOPHILIZED	2 G	IV	J9097
CYCLOPHOSPHAMIDE LYOPHILIZED	200 MG	IV	J9094
CYCLOPHOSPHAMIDE LYOPHILIZED	500 MG	IV	J9095
CYCLOPHOSPHAMIDE	1 G	IV	J9091
CYCLOPHOSPHAMIDE	100 MG	IV	J9070
CYCLOPHOSPHAMIDE	2 G	IV	J9092
CYCLOPHOSPHAMIDE	200 MG	IV	J9080
CYCLOPHOSPHAMIDE	25 MG	ORAL	J8530
CYCLOPHOSPHAMIDE	500 MG	IV	J9090
CYCLOSPORINE	100 MG	ORAL	J7502
CYCLOSPORINE	25 MG	ORAL	J7515
CYCLOSPORINE	250 MG	OTH	J7516
CYTARABINE LIPOSOME	10 MG	IT	J9098
CYTARABINE	100 MG	SC, IV	J9100
CYTARABINE	500 MG	SC, IV	J9110
CYTOGAM	PER VIAL	IV	J0850

Drug Name	Unit	Route	Code
CYTOMEGALOVIRUS IMMUNE GLOB	PER VIAL	IV	J0850
CYTOSAR-U	100 MG	SC, IV	J9100
CYTOSAR-U	500 MG	SC, IV	J9110
CYTOVENE	500 MG	IV	J1570
CYTOXAN LYOPHILIZED	1 G	IV	J9096
CYTOXAN LYOPHILIZED	100 MG	IV	J9093
CYTOXAN LYOPHILIZED	2 G	IV	J9097
CYTOXAN LYOPHILIZED	200 MG	IV	J9094
CYTOXAN LYOPHILIZED	500 MG	IV	J9095
CYTOXAN	1 G	IV	J9091
CYTOXAN	100 MG	IV	J9070
CYTOXAN	2 G	IV	J9092
CYTOXAN	200 MG	IV	J9080
CYTOXAN	25 MG	ORAL	J8530
CYTOXAN	500 MG	IV	J9090
D.H.E. 45	1 MG	IM, IV	J1110
DACARBAZINE	100 MG	IV	J9130
DACARBAZINE	200 MG	IV	J9140
DACLIZUMAB	25 MG	OTH	J7513
DACTINOMYCIN	0.5 MG	IV	J9120
DALALONE LA	1 MG	IM	J1094
DALALONE	1 MG	IM, IV, OTH	J1100
DALTEPARIN SODIUM	2,500 IU	SC	J1645
DANTROLENE SODIUM	1 EA		J3490
DAPTOMYCIN	1 MG	INJ	J0878
DARBEPOETIN ALFA, ESRD USE	1 MCG	SC, IV	J0882
DARBEPOETIN ALFA, NON-ESRD USE	1 MCG	SC, IV	J0881
DAUNORUBICIN CITRATE	10 MG	IV	J9151
DAUNORUBICIN HCL	10 MG	IV	J9150
DAUNOXOME	10 MG	IV	J9151
DDAVP	1 MCG	IV, SC	J2597
DECADRON LA	1 MG	IM	J1094
DECADRON PHOSPHATE	1 MG	IM, IV, OTH	J1100
DECADRON	0.25 MG	ORAL	J8540
DECA-DURABOLIN	100 MG	IM	J2321
DECA-DURABOLIN	200 MG	IM	J2322
DECA-DURABOLIN	50 MG	IM	J2320
DECELLURIZED SKIN SUBSTITUTE	1 CC	OTH	C9222
DECOLONE-100	100 MG	IM	J2321
DECOLONE-50	50 MG	IM	J2320
DEFEROXAMINE MESYLATE	500 MG	IM, SC, IV	J0895
DEFINITY	1 ML	INJ	Q9957
DELATEST	100 MG	IM	J3120
DELATESTRYL	100 MG	IM	J3120
DELATESTRYL	200 MG	IM	J3130
DELESTROGEN	10 MG	IM	J1380
DELESTROGEN	20 MG	IM	J1390
DELESTROGEN	UP TO 40 MG	IM	J0970
DELTA-CORTEF	5 MG	ORAL	J7510
DELTASONE	5 MG	ORAL	J7506
DELTASONE	5 MG	OTH	J7506
DEMADEX	10 MG	IV	J3265
DEMEROL	100 MG	IM, IV, SC	J2175
DENILEUKIN DIFTITOX	300 MCG	INJ	J9160
DEPANDRATE	1 CC, 200 MG	IM	J1080
DEPANDROGYN	1 ML	IM	J1060
DEPGYNOGEN	UP TO 5 MG	IM	J1000
DEPHENACEN-50	50 MG	IM, IV	J1200

Drug Name	Unit	Route	Code
DEPMEDALONE	40 MG	IM	J1030
DEPMEDALONE	80 MG	IM	J1040
DEPOCYT	10 MG	IT	J9098
DEPO-ESTRADIOL CYPIONATE	UP TO 5 MG	IM	J1000
DEPOGEN	UP TO 5 MG	IM	J1000
DEPO-MEDROL	20 MG	IM	J1020
DEPO-MEDROL	40 MG	IM	J1030
DEPO-MEDROL	80 MG	IM	J1040
DEPO-PROVERA	150 MG	IM	J1055
DEPO-PROVERA	50 MG	IM	J1051
DEPO-TESTADIOL	1 ML	IM	J1060
DEPO-TESTOSTERONE CYPIONATE	UP TO 100 MG	IM	J1070
DEPO-TESTOSTERONE	1 CC, 200 MG	IM	J1080
DEPO-TESTOSTERONE	UP TO 100 MG	IM	J1070
DEPTESTROGEN	UP TO 100 MG	IM	J1070
DERMAGRAFT	SQ CM	OTH	J7342
DERMAL AND EPIDERMAL, TISSUE OF NON-HUMAN ORIGIN, WITH OR WITHOUT OTHER BIOENGINEERED OR PROCESSED ELEMENTS, WITHOUT METABOLICALLY ACTIVE ELEMENTS	PER SQ CM	EA	J7343
DERMAL TISSUE, OF HUMAN ORIGIN, WITH OR WITHOUT OTHER BIOENGINEERED OR PROCESSED ELEMENTS, WITH METABOLICALLY ACTIVE ELEMENTS	PER SQ CM	EA	J7342
DERMAL TISSUE, OF HUMAN ORIGIN, WITH OR WITHOUT OTHER BIOENGINEERED OR PROCESSED ELEMENTS, WITHOUT METABOLICALLY ACTIVE ELEMENTS	PER SQ CM	EA	J7344
DESFERAL	500 MG	IM, SC, IV	J0895
DESMOPRESSIN ACETATE	1 MCG	IV, SC	J2597
DEXAMETHASONE ACETATE ANHYDROUS	1 MG	IM	J1094
DEXAMETHASONE ACETATE	1 MG	IM	J1094
DEXAMETHASONE SODIUM PHOSPHATE	1 MG	IM, IV, OTH	J1100
DEXAMETHASONE	0.25 MG	ORAL	J8540
DEXAMETHASONE	PER MG	INH	J7637
DEXAMETHASONE	PER MG	INH	J7638
DEXONE LA	1 MG	IM	J1094
DEXONE	0.25 MG	ORAL	J8540
DEXRAZOXANE HYDROCHLORIDE	250 MG	IV	J1190
DEXRAZOXANE	250 MG	IV	J1190
DEXTRAN 40	500 ML	IV	J7100
DEXTROAMPHETAMINE SULFATE	5 MG	ORAL	S0160
DEXTROSE	500 ML	IV	J7060
DEXTROSE/SODIUM CHLORIDE	5%	VAR	J7042
DEXTROSE/THEOPHYLLINE	40 MG	IV	J2810
DIALYSIS/STRESS VITAMINS	100 CAPS	ORAL	S0194
DIAMOX	500 MG	IM, IV	J1120
DIASTAT	5 MG	IV, IM	J3360
DIAZEPAM	5 MG	IV, IM	J3360
DIAZOXIDE	300 MG	IV	J1730
DICYCLOMINE HCL	20 MG	IM	J0500
DIDANOSINE (DDI)	25 MG	ORAL	S0137
DIDRONEL	300 MG	IV	J1436
DIETHYLSTILBESTROL DIPHSPHATE	250 MG	INJ	J9165
DIFLUCAN	200 MG	IV	J1450
DIGIBIND	VIAL	IV	J1162
DIGIFAB	VIAL	IV	J1162
DIGOXIN IMMUNE FAB	VIAL	IV	J1162

Drug Name	Unit	Route	Code
DIGOXIN	0.5 MG	IM, IV	J1160
DIHYDROERGOTAMINE MESYLATE	1 MG	IM, IV	J1110
DILANTIN	50 MG	IM, IV	J1165
DILAUDID	250 MG	OTH	S0092
DILAUDID	4 MG	SC, IM, IV	J1170
DILOR	500 MG	IM	J1180
DILTIAZEM HYDROCHLORIDE	1 EA		J3490
DIMENHYDRINATE	50 MG	IM, IV	J1240
DIMERCAPROL	100 MG	IM	J0470
DIMINE	50 MG	IV, IM	J1200
DINATE	50 MG	IM, IV	J1240
DIOVAL 40	10 MG	IM	J1380
DIOVAL 40	20 MG	IM	J1390
DIOVAL XX	10 MG	IM	J1380
DIOVAL XX	20 MG	IM	J1390
DIOVAL	10 MG	IM	J1380
DIOVAL	20 MG	IM	J1390
DIPHENHYDRAMINE HCL	50 MG	IV, IM	J1200
DIPHENHYDRAMINE HCL	50 MG	ORAL	Q0163
DIPYRIDAMOLE	10 MG	IV	J1245
DISOTATE	150 MG	IV	J3520
DIURIL SODIUM	500 MG	IV	J1205
DIURIL	500 MG	IV	J1205
DIZAC	5 MG	IV, IM	J3360
DMSA KIT	PER VIAL	IV	C1201
DMSA	VIAL	IV	C1201
DMSO, DIMETHYL SULFOXIDE	50%, 50 ML	OTH	J1212
DOBUTAMINE HCL	250 MG	IV	J1250
DOBUTREX	250 MG	IV	J1250
DOCETAXEL	20 MG	IV	J9170
DOLASETRON MESYLATE	10 MG	IV	J1260
DOLASETRON MESYLATE	100 MG	ORAL	Q0180
DOLASETRON MESYLATE	50 MG	ORAL	S0174
DOLOPHINE HCL	10 MG	IM, SC	J1230
DOLOPHINE	5 MG	ORAL	S0109
DOMMANATE	50 MG	IM, IV	J1240
DOPAMINE HCL	40 MG	IV	J1265
DORNASE ALPHA	PER MG	INH	J7639
DOSTINEX	0.25 MG	ORAL	J8515
DOXERCALCIFEROL	1 MG	IV	J1270
DOXIL	10 MG	IV	J9001
DOXORUBICIN HCL	10 MG	IV	J9000
DRAMAMINE	50 MG	IM, IV	J1240
DRAMILIN	50 MG	IM, IV	J1240
DRAMOCEN	50 MG	IM, IV	J1240
DRAMOJECT	50 MG	IM, IV	J1240
DRONABINAL	2.5 MG	ORAL	Q0167
DRONABINAL	5 MG	ORAL	Q0168
DROPERIDOL AND FENTANYL CITRATE	2 ML	IM, IV	J1810
DROPERIDOL	5 MG	IM, IV	J1790
DROXIA	500 MG	ORAL	S0176
DTIC-DOME	100 MG	IV	J9130
DTIC-DOME	200 MG	IV	J9140
DUO-SPAN II	1 ML	IM	J1060
DUO-SPAN	1 ML	IM	J1060
DURACILLIN A.S.	600,000 UNITS	IM, IV	J2510
DURACLON	1 MG	OTH	J0735
DURAGEN-10	10 MG	IM	J1380

APPENDIX 1 — TABLE OF DRUGS

Drug Name	Unit	Route	Code	Drug Name	Unit	Route	Code
DURAGEN-10	20 MG	IM	J1390	ESTRADIOL L.A. 40	20 MG	IM	J1390
DURAGEN-20	10 MG	IM	J1380	ESTRADIOL L.A.	10 MG	IM	J1380
DURAGEN-20	20 MG	IM	J1390	ESTRADIOL L.A.	20 MG	IM	J1390
DURAGEN-40	10 MG	IM	J1380	ESTRADIOL VALERATE	10 MG	IM	J1380
DURAGEN-40	20 MG	IM	J1390	ESTRADIOL VALERATE	20 MG	IM	J1390
DURAMORPH	10 MG	IM, IV, SC	J2275	ESTRADIOL VALERATE	UP TO 40 MG	IM	J0970
DURAMORPH	500 MG	OTH	S0093	ESTRAGYN	1 MG	IV, IM	J1435
DURATHATE-200	100 MG	IM	J3130	ESTRA-L 20	10 MG	IM	J1380
DURO CORT	80 MG	IM	J1040	ESTRA-L 20	20 MG	IM	J1390
DYMENATE	50 MG	IM, IV	J1240	ESTRA-L 40	10 MG	IM	J1380
DYPHYLLINE	500 MG	IM	J1180	ESTRA-L 40	20 MG	IM	J1390
ECHOCARDIOGRAM IMAGE ENHANCER	1 ML	INJ	Q9956	ESTRO-A	1 MG	IV, IM	J1435
ECHOCARDIOGRAM IMAGE ENHANCER	1 ML	IV	Q9955	ESTROGEN CONJUGATED	25 MG	IV, IM	J1410
EDETATE CALCIUM DISODIUM	1,000 MG	IV, SC, IM	J0600	ESTRONE	1 MG	IV, IM	J1435
EDETATE DISODIUM	150 MG	IV	J3520	ESTRONOL	1 MG	IM, IV	J1435
EDEX	1.25 MCG	INJ	J0270	ETANERCEPT	25 MG	IM, IV	J1438
EDROPHONIUM CHLORIDE	1 EA		J3490	ETHAMOLIN	100 MG	IV	J1430
EFALIZUMAB	125 MG	INJ	S0162	ETHANOLAMINE OLEATE	100 MG	IV	J1430
ELAVIL	20 MG	IM	J1320	ETHYOL	500 MG	IV	J0207
ELIGARD	1 MG	IM	J9218	ETIDRONATE DISODIUM	300 MG	IV	J1436
ELIGARD	7.5 MG	IM	J9217	ETOPOSIDE	10 MG	IV	J9181
ELITEK	50 MCG	IM	J2783	ETOPOSIDE	100 MG	IV	J9182
ELLENCE	2 MG	INJ	J9178	ETOPOSIDE	50 MG	ORAL	J8560
ELLIOTT'S B SOLUTION	PER ML	IV, IT	J9175	EULEXIN	125 MG	ORAL	S0175
ELOXATIN	0.5 MG	INJ	J9263	EVERONE	100 MG	IM	J3120
ELSPAR	10,000 U	VAR	J9020	EVERONE	100 MG	IM	J3130
EMEND	5 MG	ORAL	J8501	EXMESTANE	25 MG	ORAL	S0156
EMINASE	30 U	IV	J0350	FABRAZYME	1 MG	IV	J0180
ENBREL	25 MG	IM, IV	J1438	FACTOR IX NON-RECOMBINANT	PER IU	IV	J7193
ENDOXAN-ASTA	1 G	IV	J9091	FACTOR IX RECOMBINANT	PER IU	IV	J7195
ENDOXAN-ASTA	100 MG	IV	J9070	FACTOR IX+ COMPLEX	PER IU	IV	J7194
ENDOXAN-ASTA	200 MG	IV	J9080	FACTOR VIIA RECOMBINANT	1.2 MG	IV	J7189
ENDOXAN-ASTA	500 MG	IV	J9090	FACTOR VIII PORCINE	PER IU	IV	J7191
ENDRATE	150 MG	IV	J3520	FACTOR VIII RECOMBINANT	PER IU	IV	J7192
ENOVIL	20 MG	IM	J1320	FACTOR VIII, HUMAN	PER IU	IV	J7190
ENOXAPARIN SODIUM	10 MG	SC	J1650	FACTREL	100 MCG	SC, IV	J1620
EPINEPHRINE HCL	1 MG	VAR	J0170	FAMOTIDINE	20 MG	INJ	S0028
EPINEPHRINE	1 MG	IM, IV, SC, VAR	J0170	FASTODEX	25 MG	INJ	J9395
EPIPEN	0.3 MG	IM	J0170	FDG	STUDY DOSE		A9552
EPIRUBICIN HCL	2 MG	IV	J9178	FEIBA-VH AICC	PER IU	IV	J7198
EPOETIN ALFA, ESRD USE	1,000 U	SC, IV	J0886	FENTANYL CITRATE	0.1 MG	IM, IV	J3010
EPOETIN ALFA, NON-ESRD USE	1,000 U	SC, IV	J0885	FERRLECIT	12.5 MG	IV	J2916
EPOGEN, ESRD USE	1,000 U	SC, IV	J0886	FERTINEX	75 IU	SC	J3355
EPOGEN, NON-ESRD USE	1,000 U	SC, IV	J0885	FILGRASTIM	300 MCG	SC, IV	J1440
EPOPROSTENOL STERILE DILUTANT	50 ML	IV	S0155	FILGRASTIM	480 MCG	SC, IV	J1441
EPOPROSTENOL	0.5 MG	IV	J1325	FINASTERIDE	5 MG	ORAL	S0138
EPTIFIBATIDE	5 MG	IM, IV	J1327	FLAGYL	500 MG	INJ	S0030
ERBITUX	10 MG	IV	J9055	FLEBOGAMMA	1 CC	IM	J1460
ERGAMISOL	50 MG	ORAL	S0177	FLEBOGAMMA	1 G	IV	J1563
ERGONOVINE MALEATE	0.2 MG	IM, IV	J1330	FLEXOJECT	60 MG	IV, IM	J2360
ERTAPENEM SODIUM	500 MG	IM, IV	J1335	FLEXON	60 MG	IV, IM	J2360
ERYTHROCIN LACTOBIONATE	500 MG	IV	J1364	FLOLAN	0.5 MG	IV	J1325
ESMOLOL HYDROCHLORIDE	1 EA		J3490	FLOLAN	50 ML	IV	S0155
ESTONE AQUEOUS	1 MG	IM, IV	J1435	FLOXIN IV	400 MG	IV	S0034
ESTRADIOL CYPIONATE	UP TO 5 MG	INJ	J1000	FLOXURIDINE	500 MG	IV	J9200
ESTRADIOL L.A. 20	10 MG	IM	J1380	FLUCONAZOLE	200 MG	IV	J1450
ESTRADIOL L.A. 20	20 MG	IM	J1390	FLUDARA	50 MG	IV	J9185
ESTRADIOL L.A. 40	10 MG	IM	J1380	FLUDARABINE PHOSPHATE	50 MG	IV	J9185

Table of Drugs

Drug Name	Unit	Route	Code
FLUDEOXYGLUCOSE F18	STUDY DOSE	IV	A9552
FLUNISOLIDE	1 MG	INH	J7641
FLUOCINOLONE ACETONIDE	0.59 MG	OTH	C9225
FLUORODEOXYGLUCOSE F-18 FDG, DIAGNOSTIC	45 MCI	IV	A9552
FLUOROURACIL	500 MG	IV	J9190
FLUPHENAZINE DECANOATE	25 MG	INJ	J2680
FLUTAMIDE	125 MG	ORAL	S0175
FOLEX PFS	5 MG	IV, IM, IT, IA	J9250
FOLEX PFS	50 MG	IV, IM, IT, IA	J9260
FOLEX	5 MG	IV, IM, IT, IA	J9250
FOLEX	50 MG	IV, IM, IT, IA	J9260
FOLLISTIM	75 IU	INJ	S0128
FOLLITROPIN ALFA	75 IU	SC	S0126
FOLLITROPIN BETA	75 IU	INJ	S0128
FOMEPIZOLE	15 MG	IV	J1451
FOMIVIRSEN SODIUM	1.65 MG	OTH	J1452
FONDAPARINUX SODIUM	0.5 MG	INJ	J1652
FORMOTEROL	12 MCG	INH	J7640
FORTAZ	500 MG	IM, IV	J0713
FORTEO	10 MCG	INJ	J3110
FORTOVASE	200 MG	ORAL	S0140
FOSCARNET SODIUM	1,000 MG	IV	J1455
FOSCAVIR	1,000 MG	IV	J1455
FOSPHENYTOIN SODIUM	750 MG	IM	S0078
FOSPHENYTOIN	50 MG	INJ	Q2009
FRAGMIN	2,500 IU	SC	J1645
FUDR	500 MG	IV	J9200
FULVESTRANT	25 MG	INJ	J9395
FUNGIZONE	50 MG	IV	J0285
FUROCOT	20 MG	IM, IV	J1940
FUROMIDE M.D.	20 MG	IM, IV	J1940
FUROSEMIDE	20 MG	IM, IV	J1940
GADOLINIUM-BASED MAGNETIC RESONANCE CONTRAST AGENT	PER ML	IV	Q9952
GALLIUM GA-67	PER MCI	IV	A9556
GALLIUM NITRATE	1 MG	INJ	J1457
GALSULFASE	5 MG	IV	C9224
GAMASTAN	1 CC	IM	J1460
GAMASTAN	10 CC	IM	J1550
GAMASTAN	2 CC	IM	J1470
GAMASTAN	3 CC	IM	J1480
GAMASTAN	4 CC	IM	J1490
GAMASTAN	5 CC	IM	J1500
GAMASTAN	6 CC	IM	J1510
GAMASTAN	7 CC	IM	J1520
GAMASTAN	8 CC	IM	J1530
GAMASTAN	9 CC	IM	J1540
GAMASTAN	OVER 10 CC	IM	J1560
GAMIMMUNE N	500 MG	IV	J1567
GAMMA GLOBULIN	1 CC	IM	J1460
GAMMA GLOBULIN	10 CC	IM	J1550
GAMMA GLOBULIN	2 CC	IM	J1470
GAMMA GLOBULIN	3 CC	IM	J1480
GAMMA GLOBULIN	4 CC	IM	J1490
GAMMA GLOBULIN	5 CC	IM	J1500
GAMMA GLOBULIN	6 CC	IM	J1510
GAMMA GLOBULIN	7 CC	IM	J1520
GAMMA GLOBULIN	8 CC	IM	J1530

Drug Name	Unit	Route	Code
GAMMA GLOBULIN	9 CC	IM	J1540
GAMMA GLOBULIN	OVER 10 CC	IM	J1560
GAMMAGARD S/D	500 MG	IV	J1566
GAMMAR P	500 MG	IV	J1566
GAMMAR	1 CC	IM	J1460
GAMMAR	10 CC	IM	J1550
GAMMAR	2 CC	IM	J1470
GAMMAR	3 CC	IM	J1480
GAMMAR	4 CC	IM	J1490
GAMMAR	5 CC	IM	J1500
GAMMAR	6 CC	IM	J1510
GAMMAR	7 CC	IM	J1520
GAMMAR	8 CC	IM	J1530
GAMMAR	9 CC	IM	J1540
GAMMAR	OVER 10 CC	IM	J1560
GAMULIN RH	300 MCG	IM	J2790
GAMUNEX	500 MG	IV	J1567
GANCICLOVIR SODIUM	500 MG	IV	J1570
GANCICLOVIR	4.5 MG	OTH	J7310
GANITE	1 MG	INJ	J1457
GARAMYCIN	80 MG	IM, IV	J1580
GASTROCROM	10 MG	INH	J7631
GATIFLOXACIN	10 MG	IV	J1590
GEFITINIB	250 MG	ORAL	J8565
GEMCITABINE HCL	200 MG	IV	J9201
GEMTUZUMAB	5 MG	IV	J9300
GEMZAR	200 MG	IV	J9201
GENARC	PER IU	IV	J7192
GENGRAF	100 MG	ORAL	J7502
GENGRAF	25 MG	ORAL	J7515
GENOTROPIN MINIQUICK	1 MG	SC	J2941
GENOTROPIN NUTROPIN	1 MG	SC	J2941
GENOTROPIN	1 MG	SC	J2941
GENTAMICIN SULFATE	80 MG	IM, IV	J1580
GENTAMICIN	80 MG	IM, IV	J1580
GENTRAN 75	500 ML	IV	J7110
GENTRAN	500 ML	IV	J7100
GEODON	10 MG	INJ	J3486
GEREF	1MCG	SC	Q0515
GESTERONE	50 MG	IM	J2675
GESTRIN	50 MG	IM	J2675
GLATIRAMER ACETATE	20 MG	INJ	J1595
GLEEVEC	100 MG	ORAL	S0088
GLOFIL-125	10 MICRO	IV	A9554
GLUCAGEN	1 MG	SC, IM, IV	J1610
GLUCAGON	1 MG	SC, IM, IV	J1610
GLUCOTOPE	STUDY DOSE	IV	A9552
GLYCOPYRROLATE	1 MG	INH	J7643
GOLD SODIUM THIOMALATE	50 MG	IM	J1600
GONADORELIN HCL	100 MCG	SC, IV	J1620
GONAL-F	75 IU	SC	S0126
GOSERELIN ACETATE	3.6 MG	SC	J9202
GRAFTJACKET REGULAR MATRIX	PER 16 SQ CM	OTH	C9221
GRAFTJACKET SOFT TISSUE MATRIX	1 CC	OTH	C9222
GRANISETRON HCL	1 MG	IV	S0091
GRANISETRON HCL	1 MG	ORAL	Q0166
GRANISETRON HCL	100 MCG	IV	J1626
GYNOGEN L.A. 10	10 MG	IM	J1380

Drug Name	Unit	Route	Code
GYNOGEN L.A. 10	20 MG	IM	J1390
GYNOGEN L.A. 20	10 MG	IM	J1380
GYNOGEN L.A. 20	20 MG	IM	J1390
GYNOGEN L.A. 40	10 MG	IM	J1380
GYNOGEN L.A. 40	20 MG	IM	J1390
GYNOGEN LA	20 MG	IM	J1390
H.P. ACTHAR	40 U	VAR	J0800
HALDOL DECANOATE	50 MG	IM	J1631
HALDOL	5 MG	IM, IV	J1630
HALOPERIDOL	5 MG	IM, IV	J1630
HAVID	0.375 MG	ORAL	S0141
HECTOROL	1 MG	IV	J1270
HELIXATE	PER IU	IV	J7192
HEMIN	1 MG	IV	J1640
HEMOFIL-M	PER IU	IV	J7190
HEP LOCK	10 U	IV	J1642
HEPARIN SODIUM	1,000 U	IV, SC	J1644
HEPARIN SODIUM	10 U	IV	J1642
HERCEPTIN	10 MG	IV	J9355
HEXADROL	0.25 MG	ORAL	J8540
HIGH OSMOLAR CONTRAST MATERIAL, UP TO 149 MG/ML IODINE CONCENTRATION	PER ML	IV	Q9958
HIGH OSMOLAR CONTRAST MATERIAL, UP TO 150-199 MG/ML IODINE CONCENTRATION	PER ML	IV	Q9959
HIGH OSMOLAR CONTRAST MATERIAL, UP TO 200-249 MG/ML IODINE CONCENTRATION	PER ML	IV	Q9960
HIGH OSMOLAR CONTRAST MATERIAL, UP TO 250-299 MG/ML IODINE CONCENTRATION	PER ML	IV	Q9961
HIGH OSMOLAR CONTRAST MATERIAL, UP TO 300-349 MG/ML IODINE CONCENTRATION	PER ML	IV	Q9962
HIGH OSMOLAR CONTRAST MATERIAL, UP TO 350-399 MG/ML IODINE CONCENTRATION	PER ML	IV	Q9963
HIGH OSMOLAR CONTRAST MATERIAL, UP TO 400 OR GREATER MG/ML IODINE CONCENTRATION	PER ML	IV	Q9964
HISTERLIN ACETATE	10 MG	INJ	J1675
HISTERLIN IMPLANT	50 MG	OTH	J9225
HISTERONE 100	50 MG	IM	J3140
HISTERONE 50	50 MG	IM	J3140
HISTINE B	10 MG	INJ	J0945
HUMALOG	5 U	SC	J1815
HUMALOG	5 U	SC	S5551
HUMALOG	50 U	SC	J1817
HUMATROPE	1 MG	SC	J2941
HUMEGON	75 IU	IM	S0122
HUMIRA	20 MG	INJ	J0135
HUMULIN R U-500	5 U	SC	J1815
HUMULIN R	5 U	SC	J1815
HUMULIN	5 U	SC	J1815
HUMULIN	50 U	SC	J1817
HYLAN G-F 20	16 MG	OTH	J7320
HYALGAN	1 MG	OTH	J7318
HYALGAN	20-25 MG	OTH	J7317
HYALGAN	30 MG	OTH	C9220
HYALURONAN	1 MG	OTH	J7318

Drug Name	Unit	Route	Code
HYALURONIDASE	150 UNITS	VAR	J3470
HYATE C	PER IU	IV	J7191
HYBOLIN DECANOATE	100 MG	IM	J2321
HYBOLIN DECANOATE	50 MG	IM	J2320
HYCAMTIN	4 MG	IV	J9350
HYDRALAZINE HCL	20 MG	IV, IM	J0360
HYDRATE	50 MG	IM, IV	J1240
HYDREA	500 MG	ORAL	S0176
HYDROCORTISONE ACETATE	25 MG	IV, IM, SC	J1700
HYDROCORTISONE SODIUM PHOSPHATE	50 MG	IV, IM, SC	J1710
HYDROCORTISONE SODIUM SUCCINATE	100 MG	IV, IM, SC	J1720
HYDROCORTONE PHOSPHATE	50 MG	SC, IM, IV	J1710
HYDROMORPHONE HCL	4 MG	SC, IM, IV	J1170
HYDROMORPHONE HYDROCHLORIDE	250 MG	OTH	S0092
HYDROXOCOBALAMIN	1,000 MCG	IM, SC	J3420
HYDROXYCOBAL	1,000 MCG	IM, SC	J3420
HYDROXYUREA	500 MG	ORAL	S0176
HYDROXYZINE HCL	25 MG	IM	J3410
HYDROXYZINE PAMOATE	25 MG	ORAL	Q0177
HYLAN G-F 20	16 MG	IA	J7320
HYOSCYAMINE SULFATE	0.25 MG	SC, IM, IV	J1980
HYPERSTAT	300 MG	IV	J1730
HYPRHO-D	300 MCG	IM	J2790
HYPRHO-D	50 MCG	IM	J2788
HYREXIN	50 MG	IV, IM	J1200
HYZINE	25 MG	IM	J3410
HYZINE-50	25 MG	IM	J3410
I-131 TOSITUMOMAB DIAGNOSTIC	PER DOSE	IV	A9544
I-131 TOSITUMOMAB THERAPEUTIC	PER DOSE	IV	A9545
IBRITUMOMAB TUXETAN	5 MCI	IV	A9542
IBUTILIDE FUMARATE	1 MG	IV	J1742
IDAMYCIN PFS	5 MG	IV	J9211
IDAMYCIN	5 MG	IV	J9211
IDARUBICIN HCL	5 MG	IV	J9211
IFEX	1 G	IV	J9208
IFOSFAMIDE	1 G	IV	J9208
IL-2	1 VIAL	IV	J9015
ILETIN II NPH PORK	50 U	SC	J1817
ILETIN II REGULAR PORK	5 U	SC	J1815
ILETIN	5 UNITS	SC	J1815
ILOPROST INHALATION SOLUTION	20 MG	INH	Q4080
IMAGENT	1 MG	IV	Q9955
IMATINIB	100 MG	ORAL	S0088
IMIGLUCERASE	1 U	IV	J1785
IMITREX	6 MG	SC	J3030
IMMUNE GLOBULIN LYOPHILIZED	500 MG	IV	J1566
IMMUNE GLOBULIN NONLYOPHILIZED	500 MG	IV	J1567
IMURAN	100 MG	OTH	J7501
IMURAN	50 MG	ORAL	J7500
IN-111 SATUMOMAB PENDETIDE	PER DOSE	IV	A4642
INAPSINE	5 MG	IM, IV	J1790
INDERAL	1 MG	IV	J1800
INDIUM IN-111 IBRITUMOMAB TIUXETAN, DIAGNOSTIC	5 MCI	IV	A9542
INDIUM IN-111 OXYQUINOLINE	0.5 MCI	IV	A9547
INDIUM IN-111 PENTETREOTIDE	PER MCI	IV	A9565
INFERGEN	1 MCG	SC	J9212
INFLIXIMAB	100 MG	IV	J1745
INFUMORPH PRESERVATIVE FREE	100 MG	IM, IV, SC	J2271

Drug Name	Unit	Route	Code
INFUMORPH	10 MG	IM, IV, SC	J2270
INFUMORPH	10 MG	OTH	J2275
INNOHEP	1,000 IU	SC	J1655
INNOVAR	2 ML	IM, IV	J1810
INSULIN LISPRO	5 U	SC	J1815
INSULIN LISPRO	5 U	SC	S5551
INSULIN PURIFIED REGULAR PORK	5 U	SC	J1815
INSULIN	5 U	SC	J1815
INSULIN	50 U	SC	J1817
INTAL	10 MG	INH	J7631
INTEGRA BILAYER MATRIX	PER SQ CM	OTH	J3743
INTEGRILIN	5 MG	IM, IV	J1327
INTERFERON ALFA-2A	3,000,000 U	SC, IM	J9213
INTERFERON ALFA-2B	1,000,000 U	SC, IM	J9214
INTERFERON ALFACON-1	1 MCG	SC	J9212
INTERFERON ALFA-N3	250,000 IU	IM	J9215
INTERFERON BETA-1A	11 MCG	IM	Q3025
INTERFERON BETA-1A	11 MCG	SC	Q3026
INTERFERON BETA-1A	33 MCG	IM	J1825
INTERFERON BETA-1B	0.25 MG	SC	J1830
INTERFERON, ALFA-2A, RECOMBINANT	3,000,000 U	SC, IM	J9213
INTERFERON, ALFA-2B, RECOMBINANT	1,000,000 U	SC, IM	J9214
INTERFERON, ALFA-N3, (HUMAN LEUKOCYTE DERIVED)	250,000 IU	IM	J9215
INTERFERON, GAMMA 1-B	3 MU	SC	J9216
INTERLUEKIN	1 VIAL	IV	J9015
INTRON A	1,000,000 U	SC, IM	J9214
INTROPIN	40 MG	IV	J1265
INVANZ	500 MG	IM, IV	J1335
INVIRASE	200 MG	ORAL	S0140
IOBENGUANE SULFATE I-131	0.5 MCI	IV	A9508
IODINE 1-123 SODIUM IODIDE CAPSULE(S) DIAGNOSTIC	100 MICRO	ORAL	A9516
IODINE 1-123 SODIUM IODIDE CAPSULE(S) THERAPEUTIC	MCI	ORAL	A9517
IODINE 1-125 SERUM ALBUMIN, DIAGNOSTIC	10 MICRO	IV	A9554
IODINE 1-125 SODIUM IOTHALAMATE, DIAGNOSTIC	10 MICRO	IV	A9554
IODINE 1-131 IODINATED SERIUM ALBUMIN, DIAGNOSTIC	PER 5 MICRO	ORAL	A9524
IODINE 1-131 SERUM ALBUMIN, DIAGNOSTIC	5 MICRO	IV	A9532
IODINE 1-131 SODIUM IODIDE CAPSULE(S) DIAGNOSTIC	PER MCI	ORAL	A9528
IODINE 1-131 SODIUM IODIDE SOLUTION, DIAGNOSTIC	PER MCI	ORAL	A9529
IODINE 1-131 SODIUM IODIDE SOLUTION, THERAPEUTIC	PER MCI	ORAL	A9530
IODINE 1-131 SODIUM IODIDE, DIAGNOSTIC	100 MICRO	IV	A9531
IODINE 1-131 TOSITUMOMAB, DIAGNOSTIC	PER STUDY DOSE	IV	A9544
IODINE 1-131 TOSITUMOMAB, THERAPEUTIC	PER STUDY DOSE	IV	A9545
IODOTOPE	PER MCI	ORAL	A9528
ION-BASED MAGNETIC RESONANCE CONTRAST AGENT	PER ML	IV	Q9953
IOTHALAMATE SODIUM I-125	STUDY DOSE	IV	A9554
IPRATROPIUM BROMIDE	1 MG	INH	J7644
IRESSA	250 MG	ORAL	J8565

Drug Name	Unit	Route	Code
IRINOTECAN	20 MG	IV	J9206
IRON DEXTRAN 165	50 MG	IM, IV	J1751
IRON DEXTRAN 237	50 MG	IM, IV	J1752
IRON SUCROSE	1 MG	IV	J1756
ISOCAINE	10 ML	VAR	J0670
ISOETHARINE HCL	1 MG	INH	J7649
ISOPROTERENOL HCL CONCENTRATED	1 MG	INH	J7659
ISUPREL HCL	PER MG	INH	J7658
ISUPREL	1 MG	INH	J7659
ITRACONAZOLE	50 MG	IV	J1835
IVEEGAM	500 MG	IV	J1566
JENAMICIN	80 MG	IM, IV	J1580
KABIKINASE	250,000 IU	IV	J2995
KANAMYCIN	500 MG	IM, IV	J1840
KANTREX	500 MG	IM, IV	J1840
KANTREX	75 MG	IM, IV	J1850
KEFLIN	1 G	IM, IV	J1890
KEFZOL	500 MG	IV, IM	J0690
KENAJECT-40	10 MG	IM	J3301
KENALOG-10	10 MG	IM	J3301
KENALOG-40	10 MG	IM	J3301
KEPIVANC	50 MCG	INJ	J2425
KESTRONE	1 MG	IV, IM	J1435
KETOROLAC TROMETHAMINE	15 MG	IM, IV	J1885
KEY-PRED 25	1 ML	IM	J2650
KEY-PRED 50	1 ML	IM	J2650
K-FLEX	60 MG	IV, IM	J2360
KINEVAC	5 MCG	INJ	J2805
KLEBCIL	500 MG	IM, IV	J1840
KLEBCIL	75 MG	IM, IV	J1850
KOATE-DVI	PER IU	IV	J7190
KOGENATE	PER IU	IV	J7190
KOGENATE	PER IU	IV	J7192
KONAKION	1 MG	SC, IM, IV	J3430
KONYNE 80	PER IU	IV	J7195
KONYNE	PER IU	IV	J7194
KYTRIL	1 MG	IV	S0091
KYTRIL	1 MG	ORAL	Q0166
KYTRIL	100 MCG	IV	J1626
L.A.E. 20	10 MG	IM	J1380
L.A.E. 20	20 MG	IM	J1390
LANOXIN	0.5 MG	IM, IV	J1160
LANTUS	50 U	SC	J1817
LARONIDASE	0.1 MG	IV	J1931
LASIX	20 MG	IM, IV	J1940
L-CARNITINE	1 G	IV	J1955
LENTE ILETIN I	5 U	SC	J1815
LEPIRUDIN	50 MG	IV	J1945
LEUCOVORIN CALCIUM	50 MG	IM, IV	J0640
LEUKERAN	2 MG	ORAL	S0172
LEUKINE	50 MCG	IV	J2820
LEUPROLIDE ACETATE (FOR DEPOT SUSPENSION)	3.75 MG	IM	J1950
LEUPROLIDE ACETATE DEPOT	7.5 MG	IM	J9217
LEUPROLIDE ACETATE IMPLANT	65 MG	OTH	J9219
LEUPROLIDE ACETATE	1 MG	IM	J9218
LEUPROLIDE ACETATE	7.5 MG	IM	J9217
LEUSTATIN	1 MG	IV	J9065
LEVALBUTEROL CONCENTRATED FORM	0.5 MG	INH	J7612

Drug Name	Unit	Route	Code
LEVALBUTEROL UNIT FORM	0.5 MG	INH	J7614
LEVAMISOLE HCL	50 MG	ORAL	S0177
LEVAQUIN	1 G	IV	J1956
LEVOCARNITINE	1 G	IV	J1955
LEVO-DROMORAN	2 MG	SC, IV	J1960
LEVOFLOXACIN	1 G	IV	J1956
LEVONORGESTREL	52 MG	OTH	J7302
LEVORPHANOL TARTRATE	2 MG	SC, IV	J1960
LEVOXYL	5 MG	ORAL	J7506
LEVSIN	0.25 MG	SC, IM, IV	J1980
LIBRIUM	100 MG	IM, IV	J1990
LIDOCAINE HCL	10 MG	IV	J2001
LINCOCIN HCL	300 MG	IV	J2010
LINEZOLID	200 MG	IV	J2020
LIORESAL INTRATHECAL REFILL	50 MCG	IT	J0476
LIORESAL	10 MG	IT	J0475
LIQUAEMIN SODIUM	1,000 UNITS	SC, IV	J1644
LIQUID PRED SYRUP	5 MG	OTH	J7506
LISPRO-PFC	50 U	SC	J1817
LOMUSTINE	10 MG	ORAL	S0178
LONITEN	10 MG	ORAL	S0139
LORAZEPAM	2 MG	IM, IV	J2060
LOVENOX	10 MG	SC	J1650
LOW OSMOLAR CONTRAST MATERIAL, 400 OR GREATER MG/ML IODINE CONCENTRATION	PER ML	IV	Q9951
LOW OSMOLAR CONTRAST MATERIAL, UP TO 150-199 MG/ML IODINE CONCENTRATION	PER ML	IV	Q9946
LOW OSMOLAR CONTRAST MATERIAL, UP TO 200-249 MG/ML IODINE CONCENTRATION	PER ML	IV	Q9947
LOW OSMOLAR CONTRAST MATERIAL, UP TO 250-299 MG/ML IODINE CONCENTRATION	PER ML	IV	Q9948
LOW OSMOLAR CONTRAST MATERIAL, UP TO 300-349 MG/ML IODINE CONCENTRATION	PER ML	IV	Q9949
LOW OSMOLAR CONTRAST MATERIAL, UP TO 350-399 MG/ML IODINE CONCENTRATION	PER ML	IV	Q9950
L-PHENYLALANINE MUSTARD	50 MG	IV	J9245
LUFYLLIN	500 MG	IM	J1180
LUMINAL SODIUM	120 MG	IM, IV	J2560
LUNELLE	5 MG/25 MG	IM	J1056
LUPRON DEPOT	3.75 MG	INJ	J1950
LUPRON DEPOT	7.5 MG	IM	J9217
LUPRON IMPLANT	65 MG	OTH	J9219
LUPRON	1 MG	IM	J9218
LUPRON	7.5 MG	IM	J9217
LUTREPULSE	100 MCG	SC, IV	J1620
LYMPHOCYTE IMMUNE GLOBULIN, ANTITHYMOCYTE GLOBULIN, EQUINE	250 MG	OTH	J7504
LYMPHOCYTE IMMUNE GLOBULIN, ANTITHYMOCYTE GLOBULIN, RABBIT	25 MG	OTH	J7511
MACUGEN	0.3 MG	OTH	J2503
MACUGEN	0.3 MG	OTH	S0198
MAG SUL	500 MG	IV	J3475
MAG-3	STUDY DOSE	IV	A9562
MAGNESIUM SULFATE	10 MG	IV	J3475

Drug Name	Unit	Route	Code
MAGNETIC RESONANCE CONTRAST AGENT	PER ML	ORAL	Q9954
MANNITOL	25% IN 50 ML	IV	J2150
MARCAINE HCL	30 ML	INJ	S0200
MARINOL	2.5 MG	ORAL	Q0167
MARINOL	5 MG	ORAL	Q0168
MARMINE	50 MG	IM, IV	J1240
MATULANE	50 MG	ORAL	S0182
MAXIPIME	500 MG	IV	J0692
MECHLORETHAMINE HYDROCHLORIDE	10 MG	IV	J9230
MEDIHALER-ISO CONCENTRATED	PER MG	INH	J7658
MEDIHALER-ISO	PER MG	INH	J7659
MEDROL	4 MG	ORAL	J7509
MEDROXYPROGESTERONE ACETATE	150 MG	IM	J1055
MEDROXYPROGESTERONE ACETATE	50 MG	IM	J1051
MEDROXYPROGESTERONE ACETATE/ ESTRADIOL CYPIONATE	5 MG/25 MG	IM	J1056
MEFOXIN	1 G	IV	J0694
MEGACE	20 MG	ORAL	S0179
MEGESTROL ACETATE	20 MG	ORAL	S0179
MELPHALAN HCL	2 MG	ORAL	J8600
MELPHALAN HCL	50 MG	IV	J9245
MENADIONE	1 MG	IM, SC, IV	J3430
MENOTROPINS	75 IU	SC, IM, IV	S0122
MEPERGAN	50 MG	IM, IV	J2180
MEPERIDINE AND PROMETHAZINE HCL	50 MG	IM, IV	J2180
MEPERIDINE HCL	100 MG	IM, IV, SC	J2175
MEPIVACAINE HCL	10 ML	VAR	J0670
MERCAPTOPURINE	50 MG	ORAL	S0108
MERITATE	150 MG	IV	J3520
MEROPENEM	100 MG	INJ	J2185
MERREM	100 MG	INJ	J2185
MESNA	200 MG	IV	J9209
MESNEX	200 MG	IV	J9209
METAPREL	10 MG	INH	J7668
METARAMINOL BITARTRATE	10 MG	IV, IM, SC	J0380
METASTRON STRONTIUM 89 CHLORIDE	PER MCI	IV	A9600
METATRACE	STUDY DOSE	IV	A9552
METHACHOLINE CHLORIDE	1 MG	INH	J7674
METHADONE HCL	10 MG	IM, SC	J1230
METHADONE	5 MG	ORAL	S0109
METHERGINE	0.2 MG	IM, IV	J2210
METHOCARBAMOL	10 ML	IV, IM	J2800
METHOTREXATE LPF	5 MG	IV, IM, IT, IA	J9250
METHOTREXATE LPF	50 MG	IV, IM, IT, IA	J9260
METHOTREXATE SODIUM	2.5 MG	ORAL	J8610
METHOTREXATE SODIUM	5 MG	IV, IM, IT, IA	J9250
METHOTREXATE SODIUM	50 MG	IV, IM, IT, IA	J9260
METHOTREXATE	5 MG	IV, IM, IT, IA	J9250
METHOTREXATE	50 MG	IV, IM, IT, IA	J9260
METHYLCOTOLONE	80 MG	IM	J1040
METHYLDOPA HCL	250 MG	IV	J0210
METHYLDOPATE HCL	5 MG	IV	J0210
METHYLENE BLUE	1 ML	INJ	A9535
METHYLERGONOVINE MALEATE	0.2 MG	IM, IV	J2210
METHYLPRED	4 MG	ORAL	J7509
METHYLPREDNISOLONE ACETATE	20 MG	IM	J1020
METHYLPREDNISOLONE ACETATE	40 MG	IM	J1030
METHYLPREDNISOLONE ACETATE	80 MG	IM	J1040

Drug Name	Unit	Route	Code
METHYLPREDNISOLONE	125 MG	IM, IV	J2930
METHYLPREDNISOLONE	4 MG	ORAL	J7509
METHYLPREDNISOLONE	UP TO 40 MG	IM, IV	J2920
METOCLOPRAMIDE	10 MG	IV	J2765
METRODIN	75 IU	IM	J3355
METRONIDAZOLE	500 MG	INJ	S0030
MIACALCIN	400 U	SC, IM	J0630
MIBG	0.5 MCI	IV	A9508
MIDAZOLAM HCI	1 MG	IM, IV	J2250
MILRINONE LACTATE	5 MG	IV	J2260
MINOXIDIL	10 MG	ORAL	S0139
MIO REL	60 MG	IV, IM	J2360
MIRENA	52 MG	OTH	J7302
MISOPROSTOL	200 MG	ORAL	S0191
MITHRACIN	2,500 MCG	IV	J9270
MITOMYCIN	20 MG	IV	J9290
MITOMYCIN	40 MG	IV	J9291
MITOMYCIN	5 MG	IV	J9280
MITOXANA	1 G	IV	J9208
MITOXANTRONE HYDROCHLORIDE	5 MG	IV	J9293
MONARC-M	PER IU	IV	J7190
MONOCLATE-P	PER IU	IV	J7190
MONONINE	PER IU	IV	J7193
MORPHINE SULFATE	10 MG	IM, IV, SC	J2270
MORPHINE SULFATE	100 MG	IM, IV, SC	J2271
MORPHINE SULFATE	500 MG	OTH	S0093
MORPHINE SULFATE, PRESERVATIVE FREE, STERILE SOLUTION	10 MG	IM, IV, SC	J2275
MOXIFLOXACIN	100 MG	INJ	J2280
MPI INDIUM DTPA	0.5 MCI	IV	A9548
MS CONTIN	500 MG	OTH	S0093
MUCOMYST	1 G	INH	J7608
MUCOSIL	PER G	INH	J7608
MUROMONAB-CD3	5 MG	OTH	J7505
MUSE	EA	OTH	J0275
MUSTARGEN	10 MG	IV	J9230
MUTAMYCIN	20 MG	IV	J9290
MUTAMYCIN	40 MG	IV	J9291
MUTAMYCIN	5 MG	IV	J9280
MYCOPHENOLATE MOFETIL	250 MG	ORAL	J7517
MYCOPHENOLIC ACID	180 MG	ORAL	J7518
MYFORTIC DELAYED RELEASE	180 MG	ORAL	J7518
MYLERAN	2 MG	ORAL	J8510
MYLOCEL	500 MG	ORAL	S0176
MYLOTARG	5 MG	IV	J9300
MYOBLOC	100 U	IM	J0587
MYOCHRYSINE	50 MG	IM	J1600
MYOLIN	60 MG	IV, IM	J2360
MYOPHEN	60 MG	IV, IM	J2360
MYOVIEW	PER DOSE	IV	A9502
NAFCILLIN SODIUM	1 EA		J3490
NAFCILLIN SODIUM	2 GM	INJ	S0032
NAGLAZYME	5 MG	IV	C9224
NALBUPHINE HCL	10 MG	IM, IV, SC	J2300
NALLPEN	2 GM	INJ	S0032
NALOXONE HCL	1 MG	IM, IV, SC	J2310
NANDROBOLIC L.A.	100 MG	IM	J2321
NANDROLONE DECANOATE	100 MG	IM	J2321
NANDROLONE DECANOATE	200 MG	IM	J2322

Drug Name	Unit	Route	Code
NANDROLONE DECANOATE	50 MG	IM	J2320
NARCAN	1 MG	IM, IV, SC	J2310
NAROPIN	1 MG	INJ	J2795
NASALCROM	10 MG	INH	J7631
NATALIZUMAB	1 MG	INJ	Q4079
NATRECOR	0.1 MG	IV	J2325
NATURAL ESTROGENIC SUBSTANCE	1 MG	IM, IV	J1410
NAVELBINE	10 MG	IV	J9390
ND-STAT	10 MG	IM, SC, IV	J0945
NEBCIN	80 MG	IM, IV	J3260
NEBUPENT	300 MG	IM, IV	S0080
NEBUPENT	300 MG	INH	J2545
NEMBUTAL SODIUM	120 MG	IM, IV	J2560
NEMBUTAL SODIUM	50 MG	IM, IV, OTH	J2515
NEO SYNEPHRINE HCL	1 ML	SC, IM, IV	J2370
NEOCYTEN	60 MG	IV, IM	J2360
NEO-DURABOLIC	100 MG	IM	J2321
NEO-DURABOLIC	200 MG	IM	J2322
NEO-DURABOLIC	50 MG	IM	J2320
NEORAL	25 MG	ORAL	J7515
NEORAL	250 MG	ORAL	J7516
NEOSAR	1 G	IV	J9091
NEOSAR	100 MG	IV	J9070
NEOSAR	2 G	IV	J9092
NEOSAR	200 MG	IV	J9080
NEOSAR	500 MG	IV	J9090
NEOSTIGMINE METHYLSULFATE	250 MG	IM, IV	J2710
NEOTECT	STUDY DOSE	IV	A9536
NESACAINE	30 ML	VAR	J2400
NESACAINE-MPF	30 ML	VAR	J2400
NESIRITIDE	0.1 MG	IV	J2325
NEULASTA	6 MG	SC, SQ	J2505
NEUMEGA	5 MG	SC	J2355
NEUPOGEN	300 MCG	SC, IV	J1440
NEUPOGEN	480 MCG	SC, IV	J1441
NEUROLITE	25 MCI	IV	A9557
NEUTREXIN	25 MG	IV	J3305
NEUTROSPEC	25 MCI	IV	A9566
NIPENT	10 MG	IV	J9268
NITROGEN N-13 AMMONIA, DIAGNOSTIC	PER STUDY DOSE, UP TO 40 MCI	INJ	A9526
NITROGLYCERIN	1 EA		J3490
NOC DRUGS, INHALATION SOLUTION ADMINISTERED THROUGH DME	1 EA		J7699
NOLVADEX	10 MG	ORAL	S0187
NOLVADEX	10 MG	ORAL	S0187
NORDITROPIN	1 MG	SC	J2941
NORDYL	50 MG	IV, IM	J1200
NORFLEX	60 MG	IV, IM	J2360
NORMAL SALINE	2 ML	IV	J2912
NORPLANT	EA	OTH	J7306
NORZINE	10 MG	IM	J3280
NOT OTHERWISE CLASSIFIED, ANTINEOPLASTIC DRUGS			J9999
NOVANTRONE	5 MG	IV	J9293
NOVAREL	1,000 USP U	IM	J0725
NOVO NORDISK	5 UNITS	SC	J1815
NOVOLIN R	5 U	SC	J1815

APPENDIX 1 — TABLE OF DRUGS

Drug Name	Unit	Route	Code	Drug Name	Unit	Route	Code
NOVOLIN	50 U	SC	J1817	PARAGARD T380A	EA	OTH	J7300
NOVOLOG	50 U	SC	J1817	PARAPLANTIN	50 MG	IV	J9045
NOV-ONXOL	30 MG	IV	J9265	PARICALCITOL	1 MCG	IV, IM	J2501
NOVOSEVEN	1.0 MG	IV	J7189	PEDIAPRED	5 MG	ORAL	J7510
NPH	5 UNITS	SC	J1815	PEGADEMASE BOVINE	25 IU	IM	J2504
NUBAIN	10 MG	IM, IV, SC	J2300	PEGAPTANIB SODIUM	0.3 MG	OTH	J2503
NUMORPHAN H.P.	1 MG	IV, SC, IM	J2410	PEGAPTANIB SODIUM	0.3 MG	OTH	S0198
NUMORPHAN	1 MG	IV, SC, IM	J2410	PEGASPARGASE	PER VIAL	IM, IV	J9266
NUTRI-TWELVE	1,000 MCG	IM, SC	J3420	PEGASYS	10 MCG	SC	S0146
NUTROPIN A.Q.	1 MG	SC	J2941	PEGFILGRASTIM	6 MG	SC	J2505
NUTROPIN	1 MG	SC	J2941	PEGINTERFERON ALFA-2A	180 MCG	IV	S0145
NUVARING VAGINAL RING	EA	OTH	J7303	PEG-INTRON	180 MCG	SC	S0145
OCATMIDE PFS	10 MG	IV	J2765	PEGYLATED INTERFERON ALFA-2A	180 MCG	SC	S0145
OCTAFLUOROPROPANE MICROSPHERES	PER ML	INJ	Q9956	PEGYLATED INTERFERON ALFA-2B	10 MCG	SC	S0146
OCTAGAM IMMUNE GLOBULIN	1 GM	IV	J1563	PEMETREXED	10 MG	IV	J9305
OCTREOSCAN	PER MCI	IV	A9565	PEN G BENZ/PEN G PROCAINE	600,000 U	IM	J0530
OCTREOTIDE ACETATE DEPOT	1 MG	IM	J2353	PENICILLIN G BENZATHINE AND PENICILLIN G PROCAINE	1,200,000 U	IM	J0540
OCTREOTIDE, NON-DEPOT FORM	25 MCG	SC, IV	J2354	PENICILLIN G BENZATHINE	1,200,000 U	IM	J0570
O-FLEX	60 MG	IV, IM	J2360	PENICILLIN G BENZATHINE	2,400,000 U	INJ	J0580
OFLOXACIN	400 MG	IV	S0034	PENICILLIN G BENZATHINE	600,000 U	IM	J0560
OLANZAPINE	2.5 MG	IM	S0166	PENICILLIN G POTASSIUM	600,000 U	IM, IV	J2540
OMALIZUMAB	5 MG	SC	J2357	PENICILLIN G PROCAINE	600,000 U	IM, IV	J2510
ONCASPAR	PER VIAL	IM, IV	J9266	PENTACARINAT	300 MG	IM, IV	S0080
ONCOSCINT	PER DOSE	IV	A4642	PENTACARINAT	300 MG	INH	J2545
ONCOVIN	1 MG	IV	J9370	PENTAM 300	300 MG	IM, IV	S0080
ONCOVIN	2 MG	IV	J9375	PENTAM	300 MG	INJ	J2545
ONCOVIN	5 MG	IV	J9380	PENTAMIDINE ISETHIONATE	300 MG	IM, IV	S0080
ONDANSETRON HCL	4 MG	ORAL	S0181	PENTAMIDINE ISETHIONATE	300 MG	INH	J2545
ONDANSETRON HCL	8 MG	ORAL	Q0179	PENTASPAN	100 ML	IV	J2513
ONDANSETRON HYDROCHLORIDE	1 MG	IV	J2405	PENTASTARCH 10% SOLUTION	100 ML	IV	J2513
ONTAK	300 MCG	INJ	J9160	PENTAZOCINE	30 MG	IM, SC, IV	J3070
ONXOL	30 MG	IV	J9265	PENTOBARBITAL SODIUM	50 MG	IM, IV, OTH	J2515
OPRELVEKIN	5 MG	SC	J2355	PENTOSTATIN	10 MG	IV	J9268
OPTISON	PER ML	INJ	Q9956	PEPCID	20 MG	INJ	S0028
ORCEL	PER SQ CM	OTH	J7340	PERFLEXANE LIPID MICROSPHERE	PER ML	INJ	Q9955
ORPHENADRINE CITRATE	60 MG	IV, IM	J2360	PERFLUTREN LIPID MICROSPHERE	PER ML	INJ	Q9957
ORPHENATE	60 MG	IV, IM	J2360	PERGONAL	75 IU	IM	S0122
ORTHOCLONE OKT3	5 MG	OTH	J7505	PERMAPEN	600,000	IM	J0560
ORTHOVISC	30 MG	OTH	J7318	PERMAPEN	>1,200,000 U	IM	J0570
OSELTAMIVIR PHOSPHATE (BRAND NAME)	75 MG	ORAL	G9035	PERMAPEN	> 2,400,000 U	INJ	J0580
OSELTAMIVIR PHOSPHATE (GENERIC)	75 MG	ORAL	G9019	PERPHENAZINE	4 MG	ORAL	Q0175
OSMITROL	25% IN 50 ML	IV	J2150	PERPHENAZINE	5 MG	IM, IV	J3310
OXACILLIN SODIUM	250 MG	IM, IV	J2700	PERSANTINE	10 MG	IV	J1245
OXALIPLATIN	0.5 MG	INJ	J9263	PFIZERPEN A.S.	600,000 UNITS	IM, IV	J2510
OXYMORPHONE HCL	1 MG	IV, SC, IM	J2410	PHENAZINE 25	50 MG	IM, IV	J2550
OXYTETRACYCLINE HCL	50 MG	IM	J2460	PHENAZINE 50	50 MG	IM, IV	J2550
OXYTOCIN	10 U	IV, IM	J2590	PHENERGAN	12.5 MG	ORAL	Q0169
PACIS BCG	VIAL	OTH	J9031	PHENERGAN	50 MG	IM, IV	J2550
PACLITAXEL PROTEIN-BOUND PARTICLES	1 MG	IV	J9264	PHENOBARBITAL SODIUM	120 MG	IM, IV	J2560
PACLITAXEL	30 MG	IV	J9265	PHENTOLAMINE MESYLATE	5 MG	IM, IV	J2760
PALIVIZUMAB	50 MG	IM	C9003	PHENYLEPHRINE HCL	1 ML	SC, IM, IV	J2370
PALONOSETRON HCL	25 MCG	IV	J2469	PHENYTOIN SODIUM	50 MG	IM, IV	J1165
PAMIDRONATE DISODIUM	30 MG	IV	J2430	PHOSPHOCOL (P32)	PER MCI	IV	A9563
PANGLOBULIN	1 G	IV	J1563	PHOTOFRIN	75 MG	IV	J9600
PANHEMATIN	1 MG	IV	J1640	PHYTONADIONE	1 MG	IM, SC, IV	J3430
PANTOPRAZOLE SODIUM	40 MG	IV	S0164	PIPERACILLIN SODIUM	500 MG	IM, IV	S0081
PANTOPRAZOLE SODIUM	PER VIAL	INJ	C9113	PIPERACILLIN SODIUM/TAZOBACTAM SODIUM	1 G/1.125 GM	IV	J2543
PAPAVERINE HCL	60 MG	IV, IM	J2440				

Table of Drugs

Drug Name	Unit	Route	Code
PIPRACIL	500 MG	IM, IV	S0081
PITOCIN	10 U	IV, IM	J2590
PLATINOL AQ	10 MG	IV	J9060
PLATINOL AQ	50 MG	IV	J9062
PLENAXIS	10 MG	IM	J0128
PLICAMYCIN	2,500 MCG	IV	J9270
PNEUMOCOCCAL CONJUGATE	EA	IM	S0195
PNEUMOVAX II	EA	IM	S0195
POLOCAINE	10 ML	VAR	J0670
POLYGAM S/D	500 MG	IV	J1566
POLYGAM	500 MG	IV	J1566
POLY-L-LACTIC ACID	1 ML	SC	S0196
PORFIMER SODIUM	75 MG	IV	J9600
PORK INSULIN	5 UNITS	SC	J1815
POTASSIUM CHLORIDE	2 MEQ	IV	J3480
PRALIDOXIME CHLORIDE	1 MG	IV, IM, SC	J2730
PREDACORT	1 ML	IM	J2650
PREDALONE-50	1 ML	IM	J2650
PREDCOR-25	1 ML	IM	J2650
PREDCOR-50	1 ML	IM	J2650
PREDICORT-50	1 ML	IM	J2650
PREDNICOT	5 ML	ORAL	J7506
PREDNISOLONE ACETATE	1 ML	IM	J2650
PREDNISOLONE	5 MG	ORAL	J7510
PREDNISONE	5 MG	ORAL	J7506
PREDNORAL	5 MG	ORAL	J7510
PREDOJECT-50	1 ML	IM	J2650
PREDONE	5 MG	ORAL	J7506
PREGNYL	1,000 USP U	IM	J0725
PRELONE	5 MG	ORAL	J7510
PREMARIN	25 MG	IV, IM	J1410
PRENATAL VITAMINS	30 TABS	ORAL	S0197
PRIALT	1 MCG	IV	J2278
PRI-ANDRIOL LA	50 MG	IM	J2320
PRIMACOR	5 MG	IV	J2260
PRIMAXIN	250 MG	IV, IM	J0743
PRIMESTRIN AQUEOUS	1 MG	IM, IV	J1410
PRI-METHYLATE	80 MG	IM	J1040
PRISCOLINE HCL	25 MG	IV	J2670
PROCAINAMIDE HCL	1 G	IM, IV	J2690
PROCARBAZINE HCL	50 MG	ORAL	S0182
PROCHLOPERAZINE MALEATE	10 MG	ORAL	Q0165
PROCHLOPERAZINE MALEATE	5 MG	ORAL	Q0164
PROCHLOPERAZINE MALEATE	5 MG	ORAL	S0183
PROCHLORPERAZINE MALEATE	10 MG	ORAL	Q0165
PROCHLORPERAZINE MALEATE	5 MG	ORAL	Q0164
PROCHLORPERAZINE	10 MG	IM, IV	J0780
PROCRIT, ESRD USE	1,000 U	SC, IV	J0886
PROCRIT, NON-ESRD USE	1,000 U	SC, IV	J0885
PROFILNINE HEAT-TREATED	PER IU	IV	J7194
PROFILNINE SD	PER IU	IV	J7194
PROFONIX	PER VIAL	INJ	C9113
PROGESTERONE	50 MG	IM	J2675
PROGRAF	1 MG	ORAL	J7507
PROGRAF	5 MG	OTH	J7525
PROKINE	50 MCG	IV	J2820
PROLASTIN	10 MG	IV	J0256
PROLEUKIN	1 VIAL	VAR	J9015

Drug Name	Unit	Route	Code
PROLIXIN DECANOATE	25 MG	INJ	J2680
PROMAZINE HCL	25 MG	IM	J2950
PROMETHAZINE HCL	12.5 MG	ORAL	Q0169
PROMETHAZINE HCL	50 MG	IM, IV	J2550
PRONESTYL	1 G	IM, IV	J2690
PROPECIA	5 MG	ORAL	S0138
PROPLEX SX-T	PER IU	IV	J7194
PROPLEX T	PER IU	IV	J7194
PROPLEX T	PER IU	IV	J7195
PROPRANOLOL HCL	1 MG	IV	J1800
PROREX	50 MG	IM, IV	J2550
PROSCAR	5 MG	ORAL	S0138
PROSTAPHLIN	250 MG	IM, IV	J2700
PROSTASCINT	PER DOSE	IV	A9507
PROSTIGMIN	0.5 MG	IM, IV	J2710
PROSTIN VR	1.25 MCG	INJ	J0270
PROTAMINE SULFATE	10 MG	IV	J2720
PROTEINASE INHIBITOR (HUMAN)	10 MG	IV	J0256
PROTHAZINE	50 MG	IM, IV	J2550
PROTIRELIN	250 MCG	IV	J2725
PROTONIX IV	40 MG	IV	S0164
PROTONIX	40 MG	IV	S0164
PROTOPAM CHLORIDE	1 G	SC, IM, IV	J2730
PROTROPIN	1 MG	INJ	J2940
PROVENTIL CONCENTRATED	1 MG	INH	J7611
PROVENTIL	1 MG	INH	J7613
PROVOCHOLINE POWDER	1 MG	INH	J7674
PROZINE-50	25 MG	IM	J2950
PULMICORT RESPULES	0.25-0.50 MG	INH	J7626
PULMICORT	0.25 MG	INH	J7633
PULMOZYME	1 MG	INH	J7639
PURINETHOL	50 MG	ORAL	S0108
PYRIDOXINE HCL	100 MG	INJ	J3415
QUADRAMET	50 MCI	IV	A9605
QUELICIN	20 MG	IM, IV	J0330
QUINUPRISTIN/DALFOPRISTIN	500 MG	IV	J2770
RANITIDINE HCL	25 MG	INJ	J2780
RAPAMUNE	1 MG	ORAL	J7520
RAPTIVA	125 MG	INJ	S0162
RASBURICASE	50 MCG	IM	J2783
REBETRON KIT	1,000,000 UNITS	SC, IM	J9214
REBIF	11 MCG	SC	Q3026
REBIF	33 MCG	SC	J1825
RECOMBINATE	PER IU	IV	J7192
REDISOL	1,000 MCG	SC. IM	J3420
REFACTO	PER IU	IV	J7192
REFLUDAN	50 MG	IM, IV	J1945
REGITINE	5 MG	IM, IV	J2760
REGLAN	10 MG	IV	J2765
REGRANEX GEL	0.5 G	OTH	J0157
REGRANEX GEL	0.5 G	OTH	S0157
REGULAR INSULIN	5 UNITS	SC	J1815
RELAXIN	10 ML	IV, IM	J2800
RELEFACT TRH	250 MCG	IV	J2725
RELION NOVOLIN	50 U	SC	J1817
RELION	5 U	SC	J1815
REMICADE	10 MG	IV	J1745
REMODULIN	1 MG	SC	J3285

APPENDIX 1 — TABLE OF DRUGS

Drug Name	Unit	Route	Code
REODULIN	1 MG	SC	J3285
REOPRO	10 MG	IV	J0130
REPRONEX	75 IU	SC, IM, IV	S0122
RESP SYNCYTIAL VIR IMMUNE GLOB	50 MG	IV	J1565
RESPIGAM	50 MG	IV	J1565
RESPIROL CONCENTRATED	1 MG	INH	J7611
RESPIROL	1 MG	INH	J7613
RETAVASE	18.1 MG	IV	J2993
RETEPLASE	18.1 MG	IV	J2993
RETROVIR	10 MG	IV	J3485
RETROVIR	100 MG	ORAL	S0104
RHEOMACRODEX	500 ML	IV	J7100
RHEUMATREX DOSE PACK	2.5 MG	ORAL	J8610
RHO D IMMUNE GLOBULIN	100 IU	IV	J2792
RHO D IMMUNE GLOBULIN	50 MCG	IM	J2788
RHOGAM	300 MCG	IM	J2790
RHOGAM	50 MCG	IM	J2788
RHOPHYLAC	100 IU	IV	J2792
RHOPHYLAC	300 MCG	IM	J2790
RIFAMPIN	1 EA		J3490
RIMANTADINE HYDROCHLORIDE (GENERIC)	100 MG	ORAL	G9020
RIMANTADINE HYDROCHLORIDE	100 MG	ORAL	G9036
RIMSO	50 ML	OTH	J1212
RINGERS LACTATE INFUSION	1,000 ML	VAR	J7120
RISPERDAL COSTA LONG ACTING	0.5 MG	INJ	J2794
RISPERIDONE, LONG ACTING	0.5 MG	IM	J2794
RITUXAN	100 MG	IV	J9310
RITUXIMAB	100 MG	IV	J9310
ROBAXIN	10 ML	IV, IM	J2800
ROBINUL	1 MG	INH	J7643
ROCEPHIN	250 MG	IV, IM	J0696
ROFERON-A	3,000,000 U	SC, IM	J9213
ROPIVACAINE HYDROCHLORIDE	1 MG	INJ	J2795
RUBEX	10 MG	IV	J9000
RUBIDIUM RB-82	60 MCI	IV	A9555
RUBRAMIN PC	1,000 MCG	SC, IM	J3420
RUBRATOPE 57	1 MCI	ORAL	A9559
SAIZEN SOMATROPIN RDNA ORIGIN	1 MG	SC	J2941
SAIZEN	1 MG	SC	J2941
SAMARIUM LEXIDRONAMM	50 MCI	IV	A9605
SANDIMMUNE	100 MG	ORAL	J7502
SANDIMMUNE	25 MG	ORAL	J7515
SANDIMMUNE	250 MG	OTH	J7516
SANDOGLOBULIN	1 G	IV	J1563
SANDOSTATIN LAR	1 MG	IM	J2353
SANDOSTATIN	25 MCG	SC, IV	J2354
SANGCYA	100 MG	ORAL	J7502
SANO-DROL	40 MG	IM	J1030
SANO-DROL	80 MG	IM	J1040
SAQUINAVIR	200 MG	ORAL	S0140
SARGRAMOSTIM (GM-CSF)	50 MCG	IV	J2820
SECRETIN, SYNTHETIC, HUMAN	1 MCG	IV	J2850
SENSORCAINE	30 ML	INJ	S0200
SEPTRA IV	10 ML	IV	S0039
SERMORELIN ACETATE	1 MCG	IV	Q0515
SEROSTIM RDNA ORIGIN	1 MG	SC	J2941
SEROSTIM	1 MG	SC	J2941
SILDENAFIL CITRATE	25 MG	ORAL	S0090

Drug Name	Unit	Route	Code
SIMULECT	20 MG	IV	J0480
SINCALIDE	5 MCG	INJ	J2805
SIROLIMUS	1 MG	ORAL	J7520
SMZ-TMP	10 ML	IV	S0039
SODIUM CHLORIDE	2 ML	IV	J2912
SODIUM CHLORIDE	5 CC	VAR	J7051
SODIUM CHROMATE CR51	250 MICRO	INJ	A9553
SODIUM FERRIC GLUCONATE COMPLEX IN SUCROSE	12.5 MG	IV	J2916
SODIUM HYALURONATE	1 MG	OTH	J7318
SODIUM HYALURONATE	20-25 MG	OTH	J7317
SODIUM HYALURONATE	30 MG	OTH	C9220
SODIUM IODIDE I-131 CAPSULE DIAGNOSTIC	PER MCI	ORAL	A9528
SODIUM IODIDE I-131 CAPSULE THERAPEUTIC	PER MCI	ORAL	A9517
SODIUM IODIDE I-131 SOLUTION THERAPEUTIC	PER MCI	ORAL	A9530
SODIUM PHOSPHATE P32	PER MCI	IV	A9563
SOLGANAL	50 MG	IM	J2910
SOLU-CORTEF	100 MG	IV, IM, SC	J1720
SOLU-MEDROL	125 MG	IM, IV	J2930
SOLU-MEDROL	40 MG	IM, IV	J2920
SOMATREM	1 MG	INJ	J2940
SOMATROPIN	1 MG	SC	J2941
SPARINE	25 MG	IM	J2950
SPECTINOMYCIN DIHYDROCHLORIDE	2 G	IM	J3320
SPORANOX	50 MG	IV	J1835
STADOL NS	25 MG	OTH	S0012
STADOL	1 MG	IM, IV	J0595
STERAPRED	5 MG	ORAL	J7506
STERILE SALINE OR WATER	5 CC	VAR	J7051
STILPHOSTROL	250 MG	INJ	J9165
STREPTASE	250,000 IU	IV	J2995
STREPTOKINASE	250,000 IU	IV	J2995
STREPTOMYCIN	1 G	IM	J3000
STREPTOZOCIN	1 GM	IV	J9320
STRONTIUM 89 CHLORIDE	PER MCI	IV	A9600
SUBLIMAZE	0.1 MG	IM, IV	J3010
SUCCINYLCHOLINE CHLORIDE	20 MG	IM, IV	J0330
SULFA MAG	500 MG	IV	J3475
SULFAMETHOXAZOLE AND TRIMETHOPRIM	10 ML	IV	S0039
SULFUTRIM	10 ML	IV	S0039
SUMATRIPTAN SUCCINATE	6 MG	SC	J3030
SUPARTZ	1 MG	OTH	J7318
SUPARTZ	20-25 MG	OTH	J7317
SUPARTZ	30 MG	OTH	C9220
SUPPRELIN	10 MG	INJ	J1675
SUS-PHRINE	UP TO 1 ML	VAR	J0170
SYNAGIS	50 MG	IM	C9003
SYNERCID	500 MG	IV	J2770
SYNTOCINON	10 UNITS	IV	J2590
SYNVISC	16 MG	IA	J7320
SYREX	2 ML	IV	J2912
SYTOBEX	1,000 MCG	SC, IM	J3420
TACRINE HCL	10 MG	ORAL	S0014
TACROLIMUS	1 MG	ORAL	J7507
TACROLIMUS	5 MG	OTH	J7525

Drug Name	Unit	Route	Code
TAGAMET HCL	300 MG	IV	S0023
TALWIN	30 MG	IM, SC, IV	J3070
TAMOSIFEN CITRATE	10 MG	ORAL	S0187
TAMOXIFEN CITRATE	10 MG	ORAL	S0187
TAXOL	30 MG	IV	J9265
TAXOTERE	20 MG	IV	J9170
TAZICEF	500 MG	IM, IV	J0713
TEBAMIDE	250 MG	ORAL	Q0173
TECHNESCAN FANOLESOMAB	STUDY DOSE	IV	A9566
TECHNESCAN MAG3	STUDY DOSE	IV	A9562
TECHNESCAN	PER MCI	IV	A9512
TECHNETIUM 99 OXIDRONATE	30 MCI	IV	A9561
TECHNETIUM SESTAMBI	PER DOSE	IV	A9500
TECHNETIUM TC 99 MACROAGGREGATED ALBUMIN	10 MCI	IV	A9540
TECHNETIUM TC 99 MEBROFENIN	15 MCI	IV	A9537
TECHNETIUM TC 99 PENTETATE	25 MCI	IV	A9539
TECHNETIUM TC 99 PYROPHOSPHATE	25 MCI	IV	A9538
TECHNETIUM TC 99 SUCCIMER	10 MCI	IV	A9551
TECHNETIUM TC 99 SULFUR COLLOID	20 MCI	IV	A9541
TECHNETIUM TC 99M BICISATE	25 MCI	IV	A9557
TECHNETIUM TC 99M FANOLESOMAB	25 MCI	IV	A9566
TECHNETIUM TC 99M LABELED RED BLOOD CELLS	30 MCI	IV	A9560
TECHNETIUM TC 99M MERTIATIDE	15 MCI	IV	A9562
TECHNETIUM TC 99M PENTETATE	75 MCI	INH	A9539
TECHNETIUM TC 99M SODIUM GLUCEPATATE	25 MCI	IV	A9550
TECHNETIUM TC 99M APCITIDE	PER DOSE	IV	A9504
TECHNETIUM TC 99M DEPREOTIDE	35 MCI	IV	A9536
TECHNETIUM TC 99M EXAMETAZIME	25 MCI	IV	A9521
TECHNETIUM TC 99M ACRCITUMOMAB	25 MCI	IV	A9549
TECHNETIUM TC 99M TETROFOSMIN	PER DOSE	IV	A9502
TEMODAR	100 MG	ORAL	J8700
TEMOZOLOMIDE	100 MG	ORAL	J8700
TENECTEPLASE	50 MG	INJ	J3100
TENIPOSIDE	50 MG	IV	Q2017
TEQUIN	10 MG	IV	J1590
TERBUTALINE SULFATE	1 MG	INH	J7681
TERBUTALINE SULFATE	1 MG	SC, IV	J3105
TERIPARATIDE	10 MCG	INJ	J3110
TERRAMYCIN	50 MG	IM	J2460
TESTAQUA	50 MG	IM	J3140
TESTERONE	50 MG	IM	J3140
TESTEX	50 MG	IM	J3150
TESTOJECT-50	50 MG	IM	J3140
TESTONE LA 100	100 MG	IM	J3120
TESTONE LA 200	100 MG	IM	J3130
TESTOSTERONE AQUEOUS	50 MG	IM	J3140
TESTOSTERONE CYPIONATE & ESTRADIOL CYPIONATE	1 ML	IM	J1060
TESTOSTERONE CYPIONATE	1 CC, 200 MG	IM	J1080
TESTOSTERONE CYPIONATE	UP TO 100 MG	IM	J1070
TESTOSTERONE ENANTHATE & ESTRADIOL VALERATE	UP TO 1 CC	IM	J0900
TESTOSTERONE ENANTHATE	100 MG	IM	J3120
TESTOSTERONE ENANTHATE	200 MG	IM	J3130
TESTOSTERONE PELLET	75 MG	OTH	S0189
TESTOSTERONE PROPIONATE	100 MG	IM	J3150

Drug Name	Unit	Route	Code
TESTOSTERONE SUSPENSION	50 MG	IM	J3140
TESTRIIN PA	100 MG	IM	J3130
TESTRO AQ	50 MG	IM	J3140
TETANUS IMMUNE GLOBULIN	250 U	IM	J1670
TETRACYCLINE HCL	250 MG	IV	J0120
T-GEN	250 MG	ORAL	Q0173
THALLOUS CHLORIDE TL-201	PER MCI	IV	A9505
THALLOUS CHLORIDE USP	PER MCI	IV	A9505
THALLOUS CHLORIDE	PER MCI	IV	A9505
THEELIN AQUEOUS	1 MG	IM, IV	J1435
THEOPHYLLINE	40 MG	IV	J2810
THERACYS	PER VIAL	IV	J9031
THIAMINE HCL	100 MG	INJ	J3411
THIETHYLPERAZINE MALEATE	10 MG	IM	J3280
THIETHYLPERAZINE MALEATE	10 MG	ORAL	Q0174
THIMAZIDE	250 MG	ORAL	Q0173
THIOPLEX	15 MG	IV	J9340
THIOTEPA	15 MG	IV	J9340
THORAZINE	10 MG	ORAL	Q0171
THORAZINE	25 MG	ORAL	Q0172
THORAZINE	50 MG	IM, IV	J3230
THROMBATE III	PER IU	IV	J7197
THYMOGLOBULIN	25 MG	OTH	J7511
THYPINONE	250 MCG	IV	J2725
THYREL TRH	250 MCG	IV	J2725
THYROGEN	0.9 MG	IM, SC	J3240
THYROTROPIN ALPHA	0.9 MG	IM, SC	J3240
THYTROPAR	0.9 MG	SC, IM	J3240
TICARCILLIN DISODIUM AND CLAVULANATE	3.1 G	IV	S0040
TICE BCG	VIAL	OTH	J9031
TICON	200 MG	IM	J3250
TICON	250 MG	ORAL	Q0173
TIGAN	200 MG	IM	J3250
TIJECT-20	200 MG	IM	J3250
TIMENTIN	3.1 G	IV	S0040
TINZAPARIN	1,000 IU	SC	J1655
TIROFIBAN HCL	0.25 MG	IM, IV	J3246
TIROFIBAN HYDROCHLORIDE	12.5 MG	IM, IV	J3246
TNKASE	50 MG	INJ	J3100
TOBI	300 MG	INH	J7682
TOBRAMYCIN SULFATE	80 MG	IM, IV	J3260
TOBRAMYCIN	300 MG	INH	J7682
TOLAZOLINE HCL	25 MG	IV	J2670
TOPOSAR	10 MG	IV	J9181
TOPOSAR	100 MG	IV	J9182
TOPOTECAN	4 MG	IV	J9350
TORADOL IV/IM	15 MG	IM, IV	J1885
TORECAN	10 MG	IM	J3280
TORECAN	10 MG	ORAL	Q0174
TORNALATE CONCENTRATE	PER MG	INH	J7628
TORNALATE	PER MG	INH	J7629
TORSEMIDE	10 MG	IV	J3265
TOSITUMOMAB DIAGNOSTIC	PER DOSE	IV	A9544
TOSITUMOMAB THERAPEUTIC	PER DOSE	IV	A9545
TRANSCYTE	PER 247 SQ CM	OTH	J7340
TRASTUZUMAB	10 MG	IV	J9355
TRASYLOL	10,000 KIU	IV	J0365
TRELSTAR DEPOT PLUS DEBIOCLIP KIT	3.75 MG	IM	J3315

APPENDIX 1 — TABLE OF DRUGS

Drug Name	Unit	Route	Code
TRELSTAR DEPOT	3.75 MG	INJ	J3315
TRELSTAR LA	3.75 MG	INJ	J3315
TREPROSTINIL	1 MG	SC	J3285
TRETINOIN	5 G	OTH	S0117
TRIAM-A	10 MG	IM	J3301
TRIAMCINOLONE ACETONIDE	10 MG	IM	J3301
TRIAMCINOLONE DIACETATE	5 MG	IM	J3302
TRIAMCINOLONE HEXACETONIDE	5 MG	VAR	J3303
TRIAMCINOLONE	1 MG	INH	J7684
TRIBAN	250 MG	ORAL	Q0173
TRI-KORT	10 MG	IM	J3301
TRILAFON	5 MG	IM, IV	J3310
TRILIFON	4 MG	ORAL	Q0175
TRILOG	10 MG	IM	J3301
TRILONE	5 MG	IM	J3302
TRIMETHOBENZAMIDE HCL	200 MG	IM	J3250
TRIMETHOBENZAMIDE HCL	250 MG	ORAL	Q0173
TRIMETREXATE GLUCURONATE	25 MG	IV	J3305
TRIPTORELIN PAMOATE	3.75 MG	IM	J3315
TRISENOX	1 MG	IV	J9017
TROBICIN	2 G	IM	J3320
TROVAN IV	100 MG	IV	J0200
TRUXADRYL	50 MG	IV, IM	J1200
TRYPTANOL	20 MG	IM	J1320
TYPE A BOTOX	1 U	OTH	J0585
TYSABRI	1 MG	IV	Q4079
ULTRALENTE	5 UNITS	SC	J1815
ULTRATAG	30 MCI	IV	A9560
UNASYN	1.5 G	IM, IV	J0295
UNCLASSIFIED BIOLOGICS			J3590
UNIPEN	2 GM	INJ	S0032
UREA	40 G	IV	J3350
UREAPHIL	40 G	IV	J3350
UROFOLLITROPIN	75 IU	SC	J3355
UROKINASE	250,000 IU	IV	J3365
UROKINASE	5,000 IU	IV	J3364
VALERGEN	10 MG	IM	J1380
VALERGEN	20 MG	IM	J1390
VALIUM	5 MG	IV, IM	J3360
VALRUBICIN	200 MG	OTH	J9357
VALSTAR	200 MG	OTH	J9357
VANCOLET	500 MG	IM, IV	J3370
VANCOMYCIN HCL	500 MG	IV, IM	J3370
VANTAS	1 EA		J3490
VAROCIN	500 MG	IM, IV	J3370
VELBAN	1 MG	IV	J9360
VELCADE	0.1 MG	IV	J9041
VELOSULIN BR	5 U	SC	J1815
VELOSULIN	5 UNITS	SC	J1815
VENOFER	1 MG	IV	J1756
VENOGLOBULIN-S	1 G	IV	J1563
VENTOLIN CONCENTRATED	1 MG	INH	J7611
VENTOLIN	1 MG	INH	J7613
VEPESID	10 MG	IV	J9181
VEPESID	100 MG	IV	J9182
VEPESID	50 MG	ORAL	J8560
VERSED	1 MG	IM, IV	J2250
VERTEPORFIN	0.1 MG	IV	J3396

Drug Name	Unit	Route	Code
VFEND	200 MG	INJ	J3465
V-GAN 25	50 MG	IM, IV	J2550
V-GAN 50	50 MG	IM, IV	J2550
VIAGRA	25 MG	ORAL	S0090
VIDAZA	1 MG	SC	J9025
VIDEX	25 MG	ORAL	S0137
VINBLASTINE SULFATE	1 MG	IV	J9360
VINCASAR PFS	1 MG	IV	J9370
VINCASAR PFS	2 MG	IV	J9375
VINCRISTINE SULFATE	1 MG	IV	J9370
VINCRISTINE SULFATE	2 MG	IV	J9375
VINORELBINE TARTRATE	10 MG	IV	J9390
VIRILON	1 CC, 200 MG	IM	J1080
VISTAJECT-25	25 MG	IM	J3410
VISTARIL	25 MG	IM	J3410
VISTARIL	25 MG	ORAL	Q0177
VISTIDE	375 MG	IV	J0740
VISUDYNE	0.1 MG	IV	J3396
VITAMIN B-12 CYANOCOBALAMIN	1,000 MCG	IM, SC	J3420
VITRASERT	4.5 MG	OTH	J7310
VITRAVENE	1.65 MG	OTH	J1452
VON WILLEBRAND FACTOR COMPLEX, HUMAN	IU	IV	J7188
VORICONAZOLE	200 MG	INJ	J3465
VUMON	50 MG	IV	Q2017
WEHAMINE	50 MG	IM, IV	J1240
WEHDRYL	50 MG	IM, IV	J1200
WELBUTRIN SR	150 MG	ORAL	S0106
WINRHO SDF	100 IU	IV	J2792
WYCILLIN	600,000 U	IM, IV	J2510
WYDASE	150 UNITS	VAR	J3470
XELODA	150 MG	ORAL	J8520
XELODA	500 MG	ORAL	J8521
XENON XE-133	10 MCI	OTH	A9558
XOLAIR	5 MG	SC	J2357
XOPENENEX CONCENTRATED	0.5 MG	INH	J7612
XOPENEX	0.5 MG	INH	J7614
XYLOCAINE	10 MG	IV	J2001
YTTRIUM 90 IBRITUMOMAB TIUXETAN	TX DOSE	IV	A9543
ZALCITABINE (DDC)	0.375 MG	ORAL	S0141
ZANAMIVIR (BRAND NAME)	10 MG	INH	G9034
ZANAMIVIR (GENERIC)	10 MG	INH	G9018
ZANOSAR	1 GM	IV	J9320
ZANTAC	25 MG	INJ	J2780
ZEMAIRA	10 MG	IV	J0256
ZEMPLAR	1 MCG	IV, IM	J2501
ZENAPAX	25 MG	OTH	J7513
ZETRAN	5 MG	IM, IV	J3360
ZEVALIN DIAGNOSTIC	TX DOSE	IV	A9542
ZEVALIN THERAPEUTIC	TX DOSE	IV	A9543
ZICONOTIDE	1 MCG	IT	J2278
ZIDOVUDINE	10 MG	IV	J3485
ZIDOVUDINE	100 MG	ORAL	S0104
ZINECARD	250 MG	IV	J1190
ZIPRASIDONE MESYLATE	10 MG	INJ	J3486
ZITHROMAX	1 G	ORAL	Q0144
ZITHROMAX	500 MG	IV	J0456
ZOFRAN	1 MG	IV	J2405
ZOFRAN	4 MG	ORAL	S0181

Table of Drugs

Drug Name	Unit	Route	Code
ZOFRAN	8 MG	ORAL	Q0179
ZOLADEX	3.6 MG	SC	J9202
ZOLEDRONIC ACID	1 MG	INJ	J3487
ZOMETA	1 MG	INJ	J3487
ZORBTIVE	1 MG	SC	J2941
ZOSYN	1 G/1.125 GM	IV	J2543
ZOVIRAX	5 MG	IV	J0133
ZOVIRAX	50 MG	IV	S0071
ZYPREXA	2.5 MG	IM	S0166
ZYVOX	200 MG	IV	J2020

Drug Name	Unit	Route	Code
UNCLASSIFIED DRUGS			
ALLOPURINOL SODIUM	300 MG	IV	J9999
ALOPRIM	300 MG	IV	J9999
ARIMIDEX	1 EA		J8999
ATROPINE SULFATE/EDROPHONIUM CHLORIDE	1 EA		J3490
AZTREONAM	1 EA		J3490
BREVITAL SODIUM	1 EA		J3490
BUMETANIDE	1 EA		J3490
CEENU	1 EA		J8999
CIMETIDINE HCL	1 EA		J3490
DIPRIVAN	1 EA		J3490
FAMOTIDINE	1 EA		J3490
GONAL-F	1 EA		J3490
GRAFTJACKET GEL	1 EA		J3490
HETASTARCH-NACL	1 EA		J3490
INAMRINONE LACTATE	1 EA		J3490
KETAMINE HCL	1 EA		J3490
KINERET	1 EA		J3490
LABETALOL HCL	1 EA		J3490
LEUKERAN	1 EA		J8999
LYSODREN	1 EA	ORAL	J8999
METOPROLOL TARTRATE	1 EA		J3490
METRONIDAZOLE IN NACL	1 EA		J3490
MITOTANE	1 EA	ORAL	J8999
MORRHUATE SODIUM	1 EA		J3490
NABI-HB (HUMAN)	1 ML	INJ	C9105
PEGINTERFERON ALFA-2A	1 EA		J3490
POTASSIUM ACETATE	1 EA		J3490
PRESCRIPTION DRUG, ORAL, CHEMOTHERAPEUTIC, NOS	1 EA		J8999
PRESCRIPTION DRUG, ORAL, NON CHEMOTHERAPEUTIC, NOS	1 EA		J8499
PROPOFOL	1 EA		J3490
PROPOFOL	1 EA		J3490
PROTONIX	1 EA		J3490
RESECTISOL	1 EA		J7799
SMZ-TMP	10 ML	IV	S0039
SODIUM ACETATE	1 EA		J3490
SODIUM BICARBONATE, 8.4%	1 EA		J3490

APPENDIX 2 — MODIFIERS

A1	Dressing for one wound
A2	Dressing for two wounds
A3	Dressing for three wounds
A4	Dressing for four wounds
A5	Dressing for five wounds
A6	Dressing for six wounds
A7	Dressing for seven wounds
A8	Dressing for eight wounds
A9	Dressing for nine or more wounds
AA	Anesthesia services performed personally by anesthesiologist
AD	Medical supervision by a physician: more than four concurrent anesthesia procedures
AE	Registered dietician
AF	Specialty physician
AG	Primary physician
AH	Clinical psychologist
AJ	Clinical social worker
AK	Non-participating physician
AM	Physician, team member service
AP	Determination of refractive state was not performed in the course of diagnostic ophthalmological examination
AQ	Physician providing a service in an unlisted health professional shortage area (HPSA)
AR	Physician provider services in a physician scarcity area
AS	Physician assistant, nurse practitioner, or clinical nurse specialist services for assistant at surgery
AT	Acute treatment (this modifier should be used when reporting service 98940, at 98941, 98942)
AU	Item furnished in conjunction with a urological, ostomy, or tracheostomy supply
AV	Item furnished in conjunction with a prosthetic device, prosthetic or orthotic
AW	Item furnished in conjunction with a surgical dressing
AX	Item furnished in conjunction with dialysis services
BA	Item furnished in conjunction with parenteral enteral nutrition (pen) services
BL	Special acquisition of blood and blood products
BO	Orally administered nutrition, not by feeding tube
BP	The beneficiary has been informed of the purchase and rental options and has elected to purchase the item
BR	The beneficiary has been informed of the purchase and rental options and has elected to rent the item
BU	The beneficiary has been informed of the purchase and rental options and after 30 days has not informed the supplier of his/her decision
CA	Procedure payable only in the inpatient setting when performed emergently on an outpatient who expires prior to admission
CB	Service ordered by a renal dialysis facility (RDF) physician as part of the ESRD beneficiary's dialysis

	benefit, is not part of the composite rate, and is separately reimbursable
CC	Procedure code change (use 'CC' when the procedure code submitted was changed either for administrative reasons or because an incorrect code was filed)
CD	AMCC test has been ordered by an ESRD facility or MCP physician that is part of the composite rate and is not separately billable
CE	AMCC test has been ordered by an ESRD facility or MCP physician that is a composite rate test but is beyond the normal frequency covered under the rate and is separately reimbursable based on medical necessity
CF	AMCC test has been ordered by an ESRD facility or MCP physician that is not part of the composite rate and is separately billable
CR	Catastrophe/disaster related
E1	Upper left, eyelid
E2	Lower left, eyelid
E3	Upper right, eyelid
E4	Lower right, eyelid
EJ	Subsequent claims for a defined course of therapy, e.g., EPO, sodium hyaluronate, infliximab
EM	Emergency reserve supply (for ESRD benefit only)
EP	Service provided as part of Medicaid early periodic screening diagnosis and treatment (EPSDT) program
ET	Emergency services
EY	No physician or other licensed health care provider order for this item or service
F1	Left hand, second digit
F2	Left hand, third digit
F3	Left hand, fourth digit
F4	Left hand, fifth digit
F5	Right hand, thumb
F6	Right hand, second digit
F7	Right hand, third digit
F8	Right hand, fourth digit
F9	Right hand, fifth digit
FA	Left hand, thumb
FB	Item provided without cost to provider, supplier or practitioner (examples, but not limited to: covered under warranty, replaced due to defect, free samples)
FP	Service provided as part of family planning program
G1	Most recent URR reading of less than 60
G2	Most recent URR reading of 60 to 64.9
G3	Most recent URR reading of 65 to 69.9
G4	Most recent URR reading of 70 to 74.9
G5	Most recent URR reading of 75 or greater
G6	ESRD patient for whom less than six dialysis sessions have been provided in a month
G7	Pregnancy resulted from rape or incest or pregnancy certified by physician as life threatening
G8	Monitored anesthesia care (MAC) for deep complex, complicated, or markedly invasive surgical procedure
G9	Monitored anesthesia care for patient who has history of severe cardio-pulmonary condition

Modifiers

GA	Waiver of liability statement on file
GB	Claim being re-submitted for payment because it is no longer covered under a global payment demonstration
GC	This service has been performed in part by a resident under the direction of a teaching physician
GE	This service has been performed by a resident without the presence of a teaching physician under the primary care exception
GF	Non-physician (e.g. nurse practitioner (NP), certified registered nurse anaesthetist (CRNA), certified registered nurse (CRN), clinical nurse specialist (CNS), physician assistant (PA) services in a critical access hospital
GG	Performance and payment of a screening mammogram and diagnostic mammogram on the same patient, same day
GH	Diagnostic mammogram converted from screening mammogram on same day
GJ	"Opt out" physician or practitioner emergency or urgent service
GK	Actual item/service ordered by physician, item associated with GA or GZ modifier
GL	Medically unnecessary upgrade provided instead of standard item, no charge, no advance beneficiary notice (ABN)
GM	Multiple patients on one ambulance trip
GN	Services delivered under an outpatient speech language pathology plan of care
GO	Services delivered under an outpatient occupational therapy plan of care
GP	Services delivered under an outpatient physical therapy plan of care
GQ	Via asynchronous telecommunications system
GR	This service was performed in whole or in part by a resident in a department of veterans affairs medical center or clinic, supervised in accordance with VA policy
GS	Dosage of EPO or darbepoietin alfa has been reduced 25% of preceeding month's dosage
GT	Via interactive audio and video telecommunication systems
GV	Attending physician not employed or paid under arrangement by the patient's hospice provider
GW	Service not related to the hospice patient's terminal condition
GX	Service not covered by Medicare
GY	Item or service statutorily excluded or does not meet the definition of any Medicare benefit
GZ	Item or service expected to be denied as not reasonable and necessary
H9	Court-ordered
HA	Child/adolescent program
HB	Adult program, non-geriatric
HC	Adult program, geriatric
HD	Pregnant/parenting women's program
HE	Mental Health Program
HF	Substance abuse program
HG	Opioid addiction treatment program
HH	Integrated mental health/substance abuse program
HI	Integrated mental health and mental retardation/developmental disabilities program
HJ	Employee assistance program
HK	Specialized mental health programs for high-risk populations
HL	Intern
HM	Less than bachelor degree level
HN	Bachelors degree level
HO	Masters degree level
HP	Doctoral level
HQ	Group setting
HR	Family/couple with client present
HS	Family/couple without client present
HT	Multi-disciplinary team
HU	Funded by child welfare agency
HV	Funded state addictions agency
HW	Funded by state mental health agency
HX	Funded by county/local agency
HY	Funded by juvenile justice agency
HZ	Funded by criminal justice agency
J1	Competitive acquisition program no-pay submission for a prescription number
J2	Competitive acquisition program, restocking of emergency drugs after emergency administration
J3	Competitive acquisition program (CAP), drug not available through cap as written, reimbursed under average sales price methodology
JW	Drug amount discarded/not administered to any patient
K0	Lower extremity prosthesis functional level 0 - does not have the ability or potential to ambulate or transfer safely with or without assistance and a prosthesis does not enhance their quality of life or mobility
K1	Lower extremity prosthesis functional level 1 - has the ability or potential to use a prosthesis for transfers or ambulation on level surfaces at fixed cadence. Typical of the limited and unlimited household ambulatory
K2	Lower extremity prosthesis functional level 2 - has the ability or potential for ambulation with the ability to traverse low level environmental barriers such as curbs, stairs or uneven surfaces. Typical of the limited community ambulator
K3	Lower extremity prosthesis functional level 3 - has the ability or potential for ambulation with variable cadence. Typical of the community ambulator who has the ability to transverse most environmental barriers and may have vocational, therapeutic, or exercise activity that demands prosthetic utilization beyond simple locomotion
K4	Lower extremity prosthesis functional level 4 - has the ability or potential for prosthetic ambulation that exceeds the basic ambulation skills, exhibiting high

	impact, stress, or energy levels, typical of the prosthetic demands of the child, active adult, or athlete
KA	Add on option/accessory for wheelchair
KB	Beneficiary requested upgrade for ABN, more than 4 modifiers identified on claim
KC	Replacement of special power wheelchair interface
KD	Drug or biological infused through DME
KF	Item designated by FDA as Class III device
KH	DMEPOS item, initial claim, purchase or first month rental
KI	DMEPOS item, second or third month rental
KJ	DMEPOS item, parenteral enteral nutrition (PEN) pump or capped rental, months four to fifteen
KM	Replacement of facial prosthesis including new impression/moulage
KN	Replacement of facial prosthesis using previous master model
KO	Single drug unit dose formulation
KP	First drug of a multiple drug unit dose formulation
KQ	Second or subsequent drug of a multiple drug unit dose formulation
KR	Rental item, billing for partial month
KS	Glucose monitor supply for diabetic beneficiary not treated with insulin
KX	Specific required documentation on file
KZ	New coverage not implemented by managed care
LC	Left circumflex coronary artery
LD	Left anterior descending coronary artery
LL	Lease/rental (use the 'LL' modifier when DME equipment rental is to be applied against the purchase price)
LR	Laboratory round trip
LS	FDA-monitored intraocular lens implant
LT	Left side (used to identify procedures performed on the left side of the body)
MS	Six month maintenance and servicing fee for reasonable and necessary parts and labor which are not covered under any manufacturer or supplier warranty
NR	New when rented (use the 'NR' modifier when DME which was new at the time of rental is subsequently purchased)
NU	New equipment
P1	A normal healthy patient
P2	A patient with mild systemic disease
P3	A patient with severe systemic disease
P4	A patient with severe systemic disease that is a constant threat to life
P5	A moribund patient who is not expected to survive without the operation
P6	A declared brain-dead patient whose organs are being removed for donor purposes
PL	Progressive addition lenses
Q2	HCFA/ORD demonstration project procedure/service

Q3	Live kidney donor surgery and related services
Q4	Service for ordering/referring physician qualifies as a service exemption
Q5	Service furnished by a substitute physician under a reciprocal billing arrangement
Q6	Service furnished by a locum tenens physician
Q7	One class A finding
Q8	Two class B findings
Q9	One class B and two class C findings
QA	FDA investigational device exemption
QB	Physician providing service in a rurual HPSA
QC	Single channel monitoring
QD	Recording and storage in solid state memory by a digital recorder
QE	Prescribed amount of oxygen is less than 1 liter per minute (lpm)
QF	Prescribed amount of oxygen exceeds 4 liters per minute (lpm) and portable oxygen is prescribed
QG	Prescribed amount of oxygen is greater than 4 liters per minute(lpm)
QH	Oxygen conserving device is being used with an oxygen delivery system
QJ	Services/items provided to a prisoner or patient in state or local custody, however the state or local government, as applicable, meets the requirements in 42 cfr 411.4 (b)
QK	Medical direction of two, three, or four concurrent anesthesia procedures involving qualified individuals
QL	Patient pronounced dead after ambulance called
QM	Ambulance service provided under arrangement by a provider of services
QN	Ambulance service furnished directly by a provider of services
QP	Documentation is on file showing that the laboratory test(s) was ordered individually or ordered as a CPT-recognized panel other than automated profile codes 80002-80019, G0058, G0059, and G0060
QR	Item or service provided in a Medicare specified study
QS	Monitored anesthesia care service
QT	Recording and storage on tape by an analog tape recorder
QV	Item or service provided as routine care in a Medicare qualifying clinical trial
QW	CLIA waived test
QX	CRNA service: with medical direction by a physician
QY	Medical direction of one certified registered nurse anesthetist (CRNA) by an anesthesiologist
QZ	CRNA service: without medical direction by a physician
RC	Right coronary artery
RD	Drug provided to beneficiary, but not administered incident-to
RP	Replacement and repair RP may be used to indicate replacement of DME, orthotic and prosthetic devices which have been in use for sometime. The claim shows the code for the part, followed by the 'RP' modifier and the charge for the part

RR	Rental (use the 'RR' modifier when DME is to be rented)
RT	Right side (used to identify procedures performed on the right side of the body)
SA	Nurse practitioner rendering service in collaboration with a physician
SB	Nurse midwife
SC	Medically necessary service or supply
SD	Services provided by registered nurse with specialized, highly technical home infusion training
SE	State and/or federally-funded programs/services
SF	Second opinion ordered by a professional review organization (PRO) per section 9401, p.l. 99-272 (100% reimbursement - no Medicare deductible or coinsurance)
SG	Ambulatory surgical center (ASC) facility service
SH	Second concurrently administered infusion therapy
SJ	Third or more concurrently administered infusion therapy
SK	Member of high risk population (use only with codes for immunization)
SL	State supplied vaccine
SM	Second surgical opinion
SN	Third surgical opinion
SQ	Item ordered by home health
SS	Home infusion services provided in the infusion suite of the IV therapy provider
ST	Related to trauma or injury
SU	Procedure performed in physician's office (to denote use of facility and equipment)
SV	Pharmaceuticals delivered to patient's home but not utilized
SW	Services provided by a certified diabetic educator
SY	Persons who are in close contact with member of high-risk population (use only with codes for immunization)
T1	Left foot, second digit
T2	Left foot, third digit
T3	Left foot, fourth digit
T4	Left foot, fifth digit
T5	Right foot, great toe
T6	Right foot, second digit
T7	Right foot, third digit
T8	Right foot, fourth digit
T9	Right foot, fifth digit
TA	Left foot, great toe
TC	Technical component. Under certain circumstances, a charge may be made for the technical component alone. Under those circumstances the technical component charge is identified by adding modifier 'TC' to the usual procedure number. technical component charges are institutional charges and not billed separately by physicians. However, portable x-ray suppliers only bill for technical component and should utilize modifier TC. The charge data from portable x-ray suppliers will then be used to build customary and prevailing profiles

TD	RN
TE	LPN/LVN
TF	Intermediate level of care
TG	Complex/high tech level of care
TH	Obstetrical treatment/services, prenatal or postpartum
TJ	Program group, child and/or adolescent
TK	Extra patient or passenger, non-ambulance
TL	Early intervention/individualized family service plan (IFSP)
TM	Individualized education program (IEP)
TN	Rural/outside providers' customary service area
TP	Medical transport, unloaded vehicle
TQ	Basic life support transport by a volunteer ambulance provider
TR	School-based individualized education program (IEP) services provided outside the public school district responsible for the student
TS	Follow-up service
TT	Individualized service provided to more than one patient in same setting
TU	Special payment rate, overtime
TV	Special payment rates, holidays/weekends
TW	Back-up equipment
U1	Medicaid level of care 1, as defined by each state
U2	Medicaid level of care 2, as defined by each state
U3	Medicaid level of care 3, as defined by each state
U4	Medicaid level of care 4, as defined by each state
U5	Medicaid level of care 5, as defined by each state
U6	Medicaid level of care 6, as defined by each state
U7	Medicaid level of care 7, as defined by each state
U8	Medicaid level of care 8, as defined by each state
U9	Medicaid level of care 9, as defined by each state
UA	Medicaid level of care 10, as defined by each state
UB	Medicaid level of care 11, as defined by each state
UC	Medicaid level of care 12, as defined by each state
UD	Medicaid level of care 13, as defined by each state
UE	Used durable medical equipment
UF	Services provided in the morning
UG	Services provided in the afternoon
UH	Services provided in the evening
UJ	Services provided at night
UK	Services provided on behalf of the client to someone other than the client (collateral relationship)
UN	Two patients served
UP	Three patients served
UQ	Four patients served
UR	Five patients served
US	Six or more patients served
VP	Aphakic patient

APPENDIX 3 — ABBREVIATIONS AND ACRONYMS

HCPCS ABBREVIATIONS AND ACRONYMS

The following abbreviations and acronyms are used in the HCPCS descriptions:

/	or
<	less than
<=	less than equal to
>	greater than
>=	greater than equal to
AC	alternating current
AFO	ankle-foot orthosis
AICC	anti-inhibitor coagulant complex
AK	above the knee
AKA	above knee amputation
ALS	advanced life support
AMP	ampule
ART	artery
ART	Arterial
ASC	ambulatory surgery center
ATT	attached
A-V	Arteriovenous
AVF	arteriovenous fistula
BICROS	bilateral routing of signals
BK	below the knee
BLS	basic life support
BP	blood pressure
BTE	behind the ear (hearing aid)
CAPD	continuous ambulatory peritoneal dialysis
Carb	carbohydrate
CBC	complete blood count
cc	cubic centimeter
CCPD	continuous cycling peritoneal analysis
CHF	congestive heart failure
CIC	completely in the canal (hearing aid)
CIM	Coverage Issue Manual
Clsd	closed
cm	centimeter
CMN	certificate of medical necessity
CMS	Centers for Medicare and Medicaid Services
CMV	Cytomegalovirus
Conc	concentrate
Conc	concentrated
Cont	continuous
CP	clinical psychologist
CPAP	continuous positive airway pressure
CPT	Current Procedural Terminology
CRF	chronic renal failure
CRNA	certified registered nurse anesthetist
CROS	contralateral routing of signals
CSW	clinical social worker
CT	computed tomography

CTLSO	cervical-thoracic-lumbar-sacral orthosis
cu	cubic
DC	direct current
DI	diurnal rhythm
Dx	diagnosis
DLI	donor leukocyte infusion
DME	durable medical equipment
DMEPOS	Durable Medical Equipment, Prosthestics, Orthotics and Other Supplies
DMERC	durable medical equipment regional carrier
DR	diagnostic radiology
DX	diagnostic
e.g.	for example
Ea	each
ECF	extended care facility
EEG	electroencephalogram
EKG	electrocardiogram
EMG	electromyography
EO	elbow orthosis
EP	electrophysiologic
EPO	epoetin alfa
EPSDT	early periodic screening, diagnosis and treatment
ESRD	end-stage renal disease
Ex	extended
Exper	experimental
Ext	external
F	french
FDA	Food and Drug Administration
FDG-PET	Positron emission with tomography with 18 fluorodeoxyglucose
Fem	female
FO	finger orthosis
FPD	fixed partial denture
Fr	french
ft	foot
G-CSF	filgrastim (granulocyte colony-stimulating factor)
gm	gram (g)
H_2O	water
HCl	hydrochloric acid, hydrochloride
HCPCS	Healthcare Common Procedural Coding System
HCT	hematocrit
HFO	hand-finger orthosis
HHA	home health agency
HI	high
HI-LO	high-low
HIT	home infusion therapy
HKAFO	hip-knee-ankle foot orthosis
HLA	human leukocyte antigen
HMES	heat and moisture exchange system
HNPCC	hereditary non-polyposis colorectal cancer
HO	hip orthosis
HPSA	health professional shortage area

ip	interphalangeal	NMES	neuromuscular electrical stimulation
I-131	Iodine 131	NOC	not otherwise classified
ICF	intermediate care facility	NOS	not otherwise specified
ICU	intensive care facility	O_2	oxygen
IM	intramuscular	OBRA	Omnibus Budget Reconciliation Act
in	inch	OMT	osteopathic manipulation therapy
INF	infusion	OPPS	outpatient prospective payment system
INH	inhalation solution	OSA	obstructive sleep apnea
INJ	injection	Ost	ostomy
IOL	intraocular lens	OTH	other routes of administration
IPD	intermittent peritoneal dialysis	oz	ounce
IPPB	intermittent positive pressure breathing	PA	physician's assistant
IT	intrathecal administration	PAR	parenteral
ITC	in the canal (hearing aid)	PCA	patient controlled analgesia
ITE	in the ear (hearing aid)	PCH	pouch
IU	international units	PEN	parenteral and enteral nutrition
IV	intravenous	PENS	percutaneous electrical nerve stimulation
IVF	in vitro fertilization	PET	positron emission tomography
KAFO	knee-ankle-foot orthosis	PHP	pre-paid health plan
KO	knee orthosis	PHP	physician hospital plan
KOH	potassium hydroxide	PI	paramedic intercept
L	left	PICC	peripherally inserted central venous catheter
LASIK	laser in situ keratomileusis	PKR	photorefractive keratotomy
LAUP	laser assisted uvulopalatoplasty	Pow	powder
lbs	pounds	PRK	photoreactive keratectomy
LDL	low density lipoprotein	PRO	peer review organization
Lo	low	PSA	prostate specific antigen
LPM	liters per minute	PTB	patellar tendon bearing
LPN/LVN	Licensed Practical Nurse/Licensed Vocational Nurse	PTK	phototherapeutic keratectomy
LSO	lumbar-sacral orthosis	PVC	polyvinyl chloride
mp	metacarpophalangeal	R	right
mcg	microgram	Repl	replace
mCi	millicurie	RN	registered nurse
MCM	Medicare Carriers Manual	RP	retrograde pyelogram
MCP	metacarparpophalangeal joint	Rx	prescription
MCP	monthly capitation payment	SACH	solid ankle, cushion heel
mEq	milliequivalent	SC	subcutaneous
MESA	microsurgical epididymal sperm aspiration	SCT	specialty care transport
mg	milligram	SEO	shoulder-elbow orthosis
mgs	milligrams	SEWHO	shoulder-elbow-wrist-hand orthosis
MHT	megahertz	SEXA	single energy x-ray absorptiometry
ml	milliliter	SGD	speech generating device
mm	millimeter	SGD	sinus rhythm
mmHg	millimeters of Mercury	SM	samarium
MRA	magnetic resonance angiography	SNCT	sensory nerve conduction test
MRI	magnetic resonance imaging	SNF	skilled nursing facility
NA	sodium	SO	sacroilliac othrosis
NCI	National Cancer Institute	SO	shoulder orthosis
NEC	not elsewhere classified	Sol	solution
NG	nasogastric	SQ	square
NH	nursing home	SR	screen

ST	standard		U	unit
ST	sustained release		VAR	various routes of administration
Syr	syrup		w	with
TABS	tablets		w/	with
Tc	Technetium		w/o	with or without
Tc 99m	technetium isotope		WAK	wearable artificial kidney
TENS	transcutaneous electrical nerve stimulator		wc	wheelchair
THKAO	thoracic-hip-knee-ankle orthosis		WHFO	wrist-hand-finger orthotic
TLSO	thoracic-lumbar-sacral-orthosis		Wk	week
TM	temporomandibular		w/o	without
TMJ	temporomandibular joint		Xe	xenon (isotope mass of xenon 133)
TPN	total parenteral nutrition			

APPENDIX 4 — PUB 100/NCD REFERENCES

REVISIONS TO THE CMS MANUAL SYSTEM

The Centers for Medicare and Medicaid Services (CMS) initiated its long awaited transition from a paper-based manual system to a Web-based system on October 1, 2003, which updates and restructures all manual instructions. The new system, called the online CMS Manual system, combines all of the various program instructions into an electronic manual, which can be found at http://www.cms.hhs.gov/manuals.

Effective September 30, 2003, the former method of publishing program memoranda (PMs) to communicate program instructions was replaced by the following four templates:

- One-time notification
- Manual revisions
- Business requirement
- Confidential requirements

The Office of Strategic Operations and Regulatory Affairs (OSORA), Division of Issuances, will continue to communicate advanced program instructions to the regions and contractor community every Friday as it currently does. These instructions will also contain a transmittal sheet to identify changes pertaining to a specific manual, requirement, or notification.

The Web-based system has been organized by functional area (e.g., eligibility, entitlement, claims processing, benefit policy, program integrity) in an effort to eliminate redundancy within the manuals, simplify the updating process, and make CMS program instructions available in a more timely manner. The initial release will include Pub. 100, Pub. 100-02, Pub. 100-03, Pub. 100-04, Pub. 100-05, Pub. 100-09, Pub. 100-15, and Pub. 100-20.

The Web-based system contains the functional areas included in the table below:

Publication #	Title
Pub. 100	Introduction
Pub. 100-1	Medicare General Information, Eligibility, and Entitlement
Pub. 100-2	Medicare Benefit Policy (basic coverage rules)
Pub. 100-3	Medicare National Coverage Determinations (national coverage decisions)
Pub. 100-4	Medicare Claims Processing (includes appeals, contractor interface with CWF, and MSN)
Pub. 100-5	Medicare Secondary Payer
Pub. 100-6	Medicare Financial Management (includes Intermediary Desk Review and Audit)
Pub. 100-7	Medicare State Operations
Pub. 100-8	Medicare Program Integrity
Pub. 100-9	Medicare Contractor Beneficiary and Provider Communications
Pub. 100-10	Medicare Quality Improvement Organization
Pub. 100-11	Reserved
Pub. 100-12	State Medicaid
Pub. 100-13	Medicaid State Children's Health Insurance Program
Pub. 100-14	Medicare End Stage Renal Disease Network
Pub. 100-15	Medicare State Buy-In
Pub. 100-16	Medicare Managed Care
Pub. 100-17	Medicare Business Partners Systems Security
Pub. 100-18	Medicare Business Partners Security Oversight
Pub. 100-19	Demonstrations
Pub. 100-20	One-Time Notification

Table of Contents

The table below shows the paper-based manuals used to construct the Web-based system. Although this is just an overview, CMS is in the process of developing detailed crosswalks to guide you from a specific section of the old manuals to the appropriate area of the new manual, as well as to show how the information in each section was derived.

Paper-Based Manuals	Internet-Only Manuals
Pub. 06—Medicare Coverage Issues	Pub. 100-01—Medicare General Information, Eligibility, and Entitlement
Pub. 09—Medicare Outpatient Physical Therapy	Pub. 100-02—Medicare Benefit Policy

Pub. 10—Medicare Hospital	Pub. 100-03—Medicare National Coverage Determinations
Pub. 11—Medicare Home Health Agency	Pub. 100-04—Medicare Claims Processing
Pub. 12—Medicare Skilled Nursing Facility	Pub. 100-05—Medicare Secondary Payer
Pub. 13—Medicare Intermediary Manual, Parts 1, 2, 3, and 4	Pub. 100-06—Medicare Financial Management
Pub. 14—Medicare Carriers Manual, Parts 1, 2, 3, and 4	Pub. 100-08—Medicare Program Integrity
Pub. 21—Medicare Hospice	Pub. 100-09—Medicare Contractor Beneficiary and Provider Communications
Pub. 27—Medicare Rural Health Clinic and Federally Qualified Health Center	
Pub. 29--Medicare Renal Dialysis Facility	

Program Memoranda
Pub. 60A—Intermediaries
Pub. 60B—Carriers
Pub. 60AB—Intermediaries/Carriers
NOTE: Information derived from Pub. 06 to Pub. 60AB was used to develop Pub. 100-01 to Pub. 100-09 for the Internet-only manual.

Pub. 19—Medicare Peer Review	Pub. 100-10—Medicare Quality Organization Improvement Organization
Pub. 07—Medicare State Operations	Pub. 100-07—Medicare State Operations
Pub. 45—State Medicaid	Pub. 100-12—State Medicaid
Pub. 81—Medicare End Stage Renal Disease	Pub. 100-13—Medicaid State Children's Health Insurance Program
Pub. 24—Medicare State Buy-In	Pub. 100-14—Medicare End Stage Renal Disease Network Organizations Network Organizations
Pub. 75—Health Maintenance Organization/Competitive Medical Plan Care	Pub. 100-15—Medicare State Buy-In
Pub. 76—Health Maintenance Organization/Competitive Medical Plan (PM)	Pub. 100-16—Medicare Managed
Pub. 77—Manual for Federally Qualified Health Maintenance Organizations	Pub. 100-17—Business Partners Systems Security
Pub. 13—Medicare Intermediaries Manual, Part 2	Pub. 100-18—Business Partners Security Oversight
Pub. 14—Medicare Carriers Manual, Part 2	Pub 100-19—Demonstrations
Pub. 13—Medicare Intermediaries Manual, Part 2	Pub 100-20—One-Time
Pub. 14—Medicare Carriers Manual, Part 2	
Demonstrations (PMs)	
Program instructions that impact multiple manuals or have no manual impact.	

NATIONAL COVERAGE DETERMINATIONS MANUAL

The National Coverage Determinations Manual (NCD), which is the electronic replacement for the Coverage Issues Manual (CIM), is organized according to categories such as diagnostic services, supplies, and medical procedures. The table of contents lists each category and subject within that category. A revision transmittal sheet will identify any new material and recap the changes as well as provide an effective date for the change and any background information. At any time, one can refer to a transmittal indicated on the page of the manual to view this information.

By the time it is complete, the book will contain two chapters. Chapter 1 includes a description of national coverage determinations that have been made by CMS. When available, chapter 2 will contain a list of HCPCS codes related to each coverage determination. To make the manual easier to use, it is organized in accordance with CPT category sequences. Where there is no national coverage determination that affects a particular CPT category, the category is listed as reserved in the table of contents.

The following table is the crosswalk of the NCD to the CIM. However, at this time, many of the NCD policies are not yet available. The CMS Web site also contains a crosswalk of the CIM to the NCD.

MEDICARE BENEFIT POLICY MANUAL

The Medicare Benefit Policy Manual replaces current Medicare general coverage instructions that are not national coverage determinations. As a general rule, in the past these instructions have been found in chapter II of the Medicare Carriers Manual, the Medicare Intermediary Manual, other provider manuals, and program memoranda. New

Appendixes

instructions will be published in this manual. As new transmittals are included they will be identified.

On the CMS Web site, a crosswalk from the new manual to the source manual is provided with each chapter and may be accessed from the chapter table of contents. In addition, the crosswalk for each section is shown immediately under the section heading.

The list below is the table of contents for the Medicare Benefit Policy Manual:

MCM/CIM CROSSWALK TO PUB 100 REFERENCE

MCM	PUB 100
15022	100-4,12,70; 100-4,13,20; 100-4,13,90
15360	100-4,12,30.4
2049	100-2,15,50
2070.1	100-1,5,90.2; 100-2,15,80.1; 100-4,16,10; 100-4,16,10.1; 100-4,16,110.4
2070.4	100-4,13,90
2079	100-2,15,100
2130	100-2,15,120
2136	100-2,15,150
2210	100-2,15,230
2300	100-2,16,10
2320	100-2,16,90
2323	100-2,15,290
2455	100-1,3,20.5; 100-1,3,20.5.2; 100-1,3,20.5.3
3045.4	100-4,1,30.3.5
3324	100-4,20,100.2.2
4120	100-2,15,290
4182	100-4,18,50
4270	100-4,8,70; 100-4,8,80; 100-4,8,90; 100-4,8,90.1; 100-4,8,90.3.2; 100-4,8,130
4270.1	100-4,8,90.1
4450	100-4,20,100.2.2
4471.2	100-2,15,50.5
5249	100-4,8,120.1

CIM	NCD
20.9	100-3,20.9
210.3	100-3,210.3
35-10	100-3,20.29
35-101	100-3,130.5; 100-3,130.6; 100-3,230.1; 100-3,160.2; 100-3,40.5
35-102	100-3,270.1
35-13	100-3,150.7
35-20	100-3,130.5; 100-3,130.6; 100-3,230.1; 100-3,160.2; 100-3,40.5
35-22.2	100-3,130.5; 100-3,130.6; 100-3,230.1; 100-3,160.2; 100-3,40.5
35-22.3	100-3,130.5; 100-3,130.6; 100-3,230.1; 100-3,160.2; 100-3,40.5
35-26	100-3,130.5; 100-3,130.6; 100-3,230.1; 100-3,160.2; 100-3,40.5
35-27	100-3,30.1; 100-3,30.1.1
35-27.1	100-3,30.1; 100-3,30.1.1
35-30	100-3,110.8
35-31	100-3,130.5; 100-3,130.6; 100-3,230.1; 100-3,160.2; 100-3,40.5
35-34	100-3,20.23
35-46	100-3,160.7.1
35-47	100-3,140.2
35-48	100-3,150.2
35-5	100-3,30.8
35-64	100-3,20.21
35-65	100-3,100.6
35-66	100-3,130.5; 100-3,130.6; 100-3,230.1; 100-3,160.2; 100-3,40.5
35-74	100-3,20.20
35-77	100-3,160.12
35-81	100-3,130.5; 100-3,130.6; 100-3,230.1; 100-3,160.2; 100-3,40.5
35-82	100-3,260.3
35-98	100-3,270.1
45-10	100-3,30.7
45-16	100-3,110.2
45-19	100-3,280.13
45-20	100-3,20.22
45-22	100-3,260.7
45-23	100-3,230.12
45-25	100-3,160.13
45-32	100-3,230.19
45-4	100-3,150.6
45-7	100-3,80.1; 100-3,80.4
50-1	100-3,20.8.1; 100-3,20.8
50-10	100-3,230.6
50-15	100-3,20.15
50-2	100-3,110.3
50-20	100-3,190.2
50-24	100-3,190.6
50-26	100-3,260.6
50-34	100-3,300.1
50-36	100-3,220.6
50-4	100-3,230.5
50-42	100-3,20.19
50-44	100-3,150.3
50-50	100-3,20.24
50-55	100-3,210.1
50-57	100-3,160.23
50-8.1	100-3,70.2.1
55-1	100-3,230.7
60-11	100-3,40.2
60-14	100-3,280.14
60-15	100-3,280.5
60-16	100-3,280.6
60-17	100-3,240.4
60-18	100-3,280.7
60-19	100-3,280.8
60-20	100-3,280.13
60-21	100-3,240.5
60-23	100-3,50.1
60-24	100-3,230.8
60-25	100-3,270.2
60-3	100-3,280.2
60-4	100-3,240.2
60-5	100-3,280.9
60-6	100-3,280.3
60-7	100-3,20.8.2
60-8	100-3,280.4
60-9	100-3,280.1
65-1	100-3,80.1; 100-3,80.4
65-10	100-3,180.2
65-11	100-3,230.16
65-14	100-3,50.3
65-16	100-3,50.4
65-17	100-3,230.17
65-3	100-3,80.5
65-4	100-3,160.6
65-5	100-3,50.2
65-6	100-3,20.8.1; 100-3,20.8
65-8	100-3,160.7
65-9	100-3,230.10
70-1	100-3,280.11
70-2	100-3,280.12
80.2.1	100-3,80.2
80.3.1	100-3,80.3

PUB 100 REFERENCES

Pub. 100-1, Chapter 3, Section 20.5
Blood Deductibles (Part A and Part B)

Program payment may not be made for the first 3 pints of whole blood or equivalent units of packed red cells received under Part A and Part B combined in a calendar year. However, blood processing (e.g., administration, storage) is not subject to the deductible.

The blood deductibles are in addition to any other applicable deductible and coinsurance amounts for which the patient is responsible.

The deductible applies only to the first 3 pints of blood furnished in a calendar year, even if more than one provider furnished blood.

Pub. 100-1, Chapter 3, Section 20.5.2
Part B Blood Deductible

Blood is furnished on an outpatient basis or is subject to the Part B blood deductible and is counted toward the combined limit. It should be noted that payment for blood may be made to the hospital under Part B only for blood furnished in an outpatient setting. Blood is not covered for inpatient Part B services.

Pub. 100-1, Chapter 3, Section 20.5.3
Items Subject to Blood Deductibles

The blood deductibles apply only to whole blood and packed red cells. The term whole blood means human blood from which none of the liquid or cellular components have been removed. Where packed red cells are furnished, a unit of packed red cells is considered equivalent to a pint of whole blood. Other components of blood such as platelets, fibrinogen, plasma, gamma globulin, and serum albumin are not subject to the blood deductible. However, these components of blood are covered as biologicals.

Refer to Pub. 100-04, Medicare Claims Processing Manual, chapter 4, §231 regarding billing for blood and blood products under the Hospital Outpatient Prospective Payment System (OPPS).

Pub. 100-1, Chapter 5, Section 90.2
Laboratory Defined

Laboratory means a facility for the biological, microbiological, serological, chemical, immuno-hematological, hematological, biophysical, cytological, pathological, or other examination of materials derived from the human body for the purpose of providing information for the diagnosis, prevention, or treatment of any disease or impairment of, or the assessment of the health of, human beings. These examinations also include procedures to determine, measure, or otherwise describe the presence or absence of various substances or organisms in the body. Facilities only collecting or preparing specimens (or both) or only serving as a mailing service and not performing testing are not considered laboratories.

Pub. 100-2, Chapter 10, Section 10.1
Vehicle and Crew Requirement

B3-2120.1, A3-3114, HO-236.1

Pub. 100-2, Chapter 10, Section 20
Coverage Guidelines for Ambulance Service Claims

B3-2125

Payment may be made for expenses incurred by a patient for ambulance service provided conditions l, 2, and 3 in the left-hand column have been met. The right-hand column indicates the documentation needed to establish that the condition has been met.

Conditions	Review Action
1. Patient was transported by an approved supplier of ambulance services.	1. Ambulance supplier is listed in the table of approved ambulance companies (§10.1.3)
2. The patient was suffering from an illness or injury, which contraindicated transportation by other means. (§10.2)	2. (a) The contractor presumes the requirement was met if the submitted documentation indicates that the patient:

- Was transported in an emergency situation, e.g., as a result of an accident, injury or acute illness, or
- Needed to be restrained to prevent injury to the beneficiary or others; or
- Was unconscious or in shock; or
- Required oxygen or other emergency treatment during transport to the nearest appropriate facility; or
- Exhibits signs and symptoms of acute respiratory distress or cardiac distress such as shortness of breath or chest pain; or
- Exhibits signs and symptoms that indicate the possibility of acute stroke; or
- Had to remain immobile because of a fracture that had not been set or the possibility of a fracture; or
- Was experiencing severe hemorrhage; or
- Could be moved only by stretcher; or
- Was bed-confined before and after the ambulance trip.

(b)

In the absence of any of the conditions listed in (a) above additional documentation should be obtained to establish medical need where the evidence indicates the existence of the circumstances listed below:

(i) Patient's condition would not ordinarily require movement by stretcher, or

(ii) The individual was not admitted as a hospital inpatient (except in accident cases), or

(iii) The ambulance was used solely because other means of transportation were unavailable, or

(iv) The individual merely needed assistance in getting from his room or home to a vehicle.

(c) Where the information indicates a situation not listed in 2(a) or 2(b) above, refer the case to your supervisor.

3. The patient was transported from and to points listed below.	3. Claims should show the ZIP code of the point of pickup.
(a) From patient's residence (or other place where need arose) to hospital or skilled nursing facility.	(a) i. Condition met if trip began within the institution's service area as shown in the carrier's locality guide ii. Condition met where the trip began outside the institution's service area if the institution was the nearest one with appropriate facilities.

NOTE: A patient's residence is the place where he or she makes his/her home and dwells permanently, or for an extended period of time. A skilled nursing facility is one, which is listed in the Directory of Medical Facilities as a participating SNF or as an institution which meets §1861(j)(1) of the Act.

NOTE: A claim for ambulance service to a participating hospital or skilled nursing facility should not be denied on the grounds that there is a nearer nonparticipating institution having appropriate facilities.

(b) Skilled nursing facility to a hospital or hospital to a skilled nursing facility.	(b) (i) Condition met if the ZIP code of the pickup point is within the service area of the destination as shown in the carrier's locality guide. (ii) Condition met where the ZIP code of the pickup point is outside the service area of the destination if the destination institution was the nearest appropriate facility.
(c) Hospital to hospital or skilled nursing facility to skilled nursing facility.	(c) Condition met if the discharging institution was not an appropriate facility and the admitting institution was the nearest appropriate facility.
(d) From a hospital or skilled nursing facility to patient's residence.	(d) (i) Condition met if patient's residence is within the institution's service area as shown in the carrier's locality guide. (ii) Condition met where the patient's residence is outside the institution's service area if the institution was the nearest appropriate facility.
(e) Round trip for hospital or	(e) Condition met if the reasonable and necessary

participating skilled nursing facility inpatients to the nearest hospital or nonhospital treatment facility.

diagnostic or therapeutic service required by patient's condition is not available at the institution where the beneficiary is an inpatient.

NOTE: Ambulance service to a physician's office or a physician-directed clinic is not covered. See §10.3.7 above, where a stop is made at a physician's office en route to a hospital and §10.3.3 for additional exceptions.)

4. Ambulance services involving hospital admissions in Canada or Mexico are covered (Medicare Claims Processing Manual, Chapter 1, "General Billing Requirements, " §§10.1.3.) if the following conditions are met:

(a) The foreign hospitalization has been determined to be covered; and

(b) The ambulance service meets the coverage requirements set forth in §§10-10.3. If the foreign hospitalization has been determined to be covered on the basis of emergency services (See the Medicare Claims Processing Manual, Chapter 1, "General Billing Requirements," §10.1.3), the necessity requirement (§10.2) and the destination requirement (§10.3) are considered met.

5. The carrier will make partial payment for otherwise covered ambulance service, which exceeded limits defined in item 6. The carrier will base the payment on the amount payable had the patient been transported:

(a) From the pickup point to the nearest appropriate facility, or

(b) From the nearest appropriate facility to the beneficiary's residence where he or she is being returned home from a distant institution.

Pub. 100-2, Chapter 11, Section 130.1
Inpatient Dialysis in Nonparticipating Hospitals

A3-3173.3

Emergency inpatient dialysis services provided by a nonparticipating U.S. hospital are covered if the requirements in §130 above are met.

Pub. 100-2, Chapter 15, Section 50
Drugs and Biologicals

B3-2049, A3-3112.4.B, HO-230.4.B

The Medicare program provides limited benefits for outpatient drugs. The program covers drugs that are furnished "incident to" a physician's service provided that the drugs are not usually self-administered by the patients who take them.

Generally, drugs and biologicals are covered only if all of the following requirements are met:

They meet the definition of drugs or biologicals (see §50.1);

They are of the type that are not usually self-administered. (see §50.2);

They meet all the general requirements for coverage of items as incident to a physician's services (see §§50.1 and 50.3);

They are reasonable and necessary for the diagnosis or treatment of the illness or injury for which they are administered according to accepted standards of medical practice (see §50.4);

They are not excluded as noncovered immunizations (see §50.4.4.2); and

They have not been determined by the FDA to be less than effective. (See §§50.4.4).

Medicare Part B does generally not cover drugs that can be self-administered, such as those in pill form, or are used for self-injection. However, the statute provides for the coverage of some self-administered drugs. Examples of self-administered drugs that are covered include blood-clotting factors, drugs used in immunosuppressive therapy, erythropoietin for dialysis patients, osteoporosis drugs for certain homebound patients, and certain oral cancer drugs. (See §110.3 for coverage of drugs, which are necessary to the effective use of Durable Medical Equipment (DME) or prosthetic devices.)

Pub. 100-2, Chapter 15, Section 50.2
Determining Self-Administration of Drug or Biological

AB-02-072, AB-02-139, B3-2049.2

The Medicare program provides limited benefits for outpatient prescription drugs. The program covers drugs that are furnished "incident to" a physician's service provided that the drugs are not usually self-administered by the patients who take them. Section 112 of the Benefits, Improvements & Protection Act of 2000 (BIPA) amended sections 1861(s)(2)(A) and 1861(s)(2)(B) of the Act to redefine this exclusion. The prior statutory language referred to those drugs "which cannot be self-administered." Implementation of the BIPA provision requires interpretation of the phrase "not usually self-administered by the patient".

A. Policy

Fiscal intermediaries and carriers are instructed to follow the instructions below when applying the exclusion for drugs that are usually self-administered by the patient. Each individual contractor must make its own individual determination on each drug. Contractors must continue to apply the policy that not only the drug is medically reasonable and necessary for any individual claim, but also that the route of administration is medically reasonable and necessary. That is, if a drug is available in both oral and injectable forms, the injectable form of the drug must be medically reasonable and necessary as compared to using the oral form.

For certain injectable drugs, it will be apparent due to the nature of the condition(s) for which they are administered or the usual course of treatment for those conditions, they are, or are not, usually self-administered. For example, an injectable drug used to treat migraine headaches is usually self-administered. On the other hand, an injectable drug, administered at the same time as chemotherapy, used to treat anemia secondary to chemotherapy is not usually self-administered.

B. Administered

The term "administered" refers only to the physical process by which the drug enters the patient's body. It does not refer to whether the process is supervised by a medical professional (for example, to observe proper technique or side-effects of the drug). Only injectable (including intravenous) drugs are eligible for inclusion under the "incident to" benefit. Other routes of administration including, but not limited to, oral drugs, suppositories, topical medications are all considered to be usually self-administered by the patient.

C. Usually

For the purposes of applying this exclusion, the term "usually" means more than 50 percent of the time for all Medicare beneficiaries who use the drug. Therefore, if a drug is self-administered by more than 50 percent of Medicare beneficiaries, the drug is excluded from coverage and the contractor may not make any Medicare payment for it. In arriving at a single determination as to whether a drug is usually self-administered, contractors should make a separate determination for each indication for a drug as to whether that drug is usually self-administered.

After determining whether a drug is usually self-administered for each indication, contractors should determine the relative contribution of each indication to total use of the drug (i.e., weighted average) in order to make an overall determination as to whether the drug is usually self-administered. For example, if a drug has three indications, is not self-administered for the first indication, but is self administered for the second and third indications, and the first indication makes up 40 percent of total usage, the second indication makes up 30 percent of total usage, and the third indication makes up 30 percent of total usage, then the drug would be considered usually self-administered.

Reliable statistical information on the extent of self-administration by the patient may not always be available. Consequently, CMS offers the following guidance for each contractor's consideration in making this determination in the absence of such data:

1. Absent evidence to the contrary, presume that drugs delivered intravenously are not usually self-administered by the patient.

2. Absent evidence to the contrary, presume that drugs delivered by intramuscular injection are not usually self-administered by the patient. (Avonex, for example, is delivered by intramuscular injection, not usually self-administered by the patient.) The contractor may consider the depth and nature of the particular intramuscular injection in applying this presumption. In applying this presumption, contractors should examine the use of the particular drug and consider the following factors:

3. Absent evidence to the contrary, presume that drugs delivered by subcutaneous injection are self-administered by the patient. However, contractors should examine the use of the particular drug and consider the following factors:

A. **Acute Condition** - Is the condition for which the drug is used an acute condition If so, it is less likely that a patient would self-administer the drug. If the condition were longer term, it would be more likely that the patient would self-administer the drug.

B. **Frequency of Administration** - How often is the injection given For example, if the drug is administered once per month, it is less likely to be self-administered by the patient. However, if it is administered once or more per week, it is likely that the drug is self-administered by the patient.

In some instances, carriers may have provided payment for one or perhaps several doses of a drug that would otherwise not be paid for because the drug is usually self-administered. Carriers may have exercised this discretion for limited coverage, for example, during a brief time when the patient is being trained under the supervision of a physician in the proper technique for self-administration. Medicare will no longer pay for such doses. In addition, contractors may no longer pay for any drug when it is administered on an outpatient emergency basis, if the drug is excluded because it is usually self-administered by the patient.

D. Definition of Acute Condition

For the purposes of determining whether a drug is usually self-administered, an acute condition means a condition that begins over a short time period, is likely to be of short duration and/or the expected course of treatment is for a short, finite interval. A course of treatment consisting of scheduled injections lasting less than two weeks, regardless of frequency or route of administration, is considered acute. Evidence to support this may include Food and Drug administration (FDA) approval language, package inserts, drug compendia, and other information.

E. By the Patient

The term "by the patient" means Medicare beneficiaries as a collective whole. The carrier includes only the patients themselves and not other individuals (that is, spouses, friends, or other care-givers are not considered the patient). The determination is based on whether the drug is self-administered by the patient a majority of the time that the drug is used on an outpatient basis by Medicare beneficiaries for medically necessary indications. The carrier ignores all instances when the drug is administered on an inpatient basis.

The carrier makes this determination on a drug-by-drug basis, not on a beneficiary-by-beneficiary basis. In evaluating whether beneficiaries as a collective whole self-administer, individual beneficiaries who do not have the capacity to self-administer any drug due to a condition other than the condition for which they are taking the drug in question are not considered. For example, an individual afflicted with paraplegia or advanced dementia would not have the capacity to self-administer any injectable drug, so such individuals would not be included in the population upon which the determination for self-administration by the patient was based. Note that some individuals afflicted with a less severe stage of an otherwise debilitating condition would be included in the population upon which the determination for "self-administered by the patient" was based; for example, an early onset of dementia.

F. Evidentiary Criteria

Contractors are only required to consider the following types of evidence: peer reviewed medical literature, standards of medical practice, evidence-based practice guidelines, FDA approved label, and package inserts. Contractors may also consider other evidence submitted by interested individuals or groups subject to their judgment.

Contractors should also use these evidentiary criteria when reviewing requests for making a determination as to whether a drug is usually self-administered, and requests for reconsideration of a pending or published determination.

Please note that prior to the August 1, 2002, one of the principal factors used to determine whether a drug was subject to the self-administered exclusion was whether the FDA label contained instructions for self-administration. However, CMS notes that under the new standard, the fact that the FDA label includes instructions for self-administration is not, by itself, a determining factor that a drug is subject to this exclusion.

G. Provider Notice of Noncovered Drugs

Contractors must describe on their Web site the process they will use to determine whether a drug is usually self-administered and thus does not meet the "incident to" benefit category. Contractors must publish a list of the injectable drugs that are subject to the self-administered exclusion on their Web site, including the data and rationale that led to the determination. Contractors will report the workload associated with developing new coverage statements in CAFM 21208.

Contractors must provide notice 45 days prior to the date that these drugs will not be covered. During the 45-day time period, contractors will maintain existing medical review and payment procedures. After the 45-day notice, contractors may deny payment for the drugs subject to the notice.

Contractors must not develop local medical review policies (LMRPs) for this purpose because further elaboration to describe drugs that do not meet the 'incident to' and the 'not usually self-administered' provisions of the statute are unnecessary. Current LMRPs based solely on these provisions must be withdrawn. LMRPs that address the self-administered exclusion and other information may be reissued absent the self-administered drug exclusion material. Contractors will report this workload in CAFM 21206. However, contractors may continue to use and write LMRPs to describe reasonable and necessary uses of drugs that are not usually self-administered.

H. Conferences Between Contractors

Contractors' Medical Directors may meet and discuss whether a drug is usually self-administered without reaching a formal consensus. Each contractor uses its discretion as to whether or not it will participate in such discussions. Each contractor must make its own individual determinations, except that fiscal intermediaries may, at their discretion, follow the determinations of the local carrier with respect to the self-administered exclusion.

I. Beneficiary Appeals

If a beneficiary's claim for a particular drug is denied because the drug is subject to the "self-administered drug" exclusion, the beneficiary may appeal the denial. Because it is a "benefit category" denial and not a denial based on medical necessity, an Advance Beneficiary Notice (ABN) is not required. A "benefit category" denial (i.e., a denial based on the fact that there is no benefit category under which the drug may be covered) does not trigger the financial liability protection provisions of Limitation On Liability (under §1879 of the Act). Therefore, physicians or providers may charge the beneficiary for an excluded drug.

J. Provider and Physician Appeals

A physician accepting assignment may appeal a denial under the provisions found in Chapter 29 of the Medicare Claims Processing Manual.

K. Reasonable and Necessary

Carriers and fiscal intermediaries will make the determination of reasonable and necessary with respect to the medical appropriateness of a drug to treat the patient's condition. Contractors will continue to make the determination of whether the intravenous or injection form of a drug is appropriate as opposed to the oral form. Contractors will also continue to make the determination as to whether a physician's office visit was reasonable and necessary. However, contractors should not make a determination of whether it was reasonable and necessary for the patient to choose to have his or her drug administered in the physician's office or outpatient hospital setting. That is, while a physician's office

visit may not be reasonable and necessary in a specific situation, in such a case an injection service would be payable.

L. Reporting Requirements

Each carrier and intermediary must report to CMS, every September 1 and March 1, its complete list of injectable drugs that the contractor has determined are excluded when furnished incident to a physician's service on the basis that the drug is usually self-administered. The CMS anticipates that contractors will review injectable drugs on a rolling basis and publish their list of excluded drugs as it is developed. For example, contractors should not wait to publish this list until every drug has been reviewed. Contractors must send their exclusion list to the following e-mail address: drugdata@cms.hhs.gov a template that CMS will provide separately, consisting of the following data elements in order:

1. Carrier Name
2. State
3. Carrier ID#
4. HCPCS
5. Descriptor
6. Effective Date of Exclusion
7. End Date of Exclusion
8. Comments

Any exclusion list not provided in the CMS mandated format will be returned for correction.

To view the presently mandated CMS format for this report, open the file located at:

http://cms.hhs.gov/manuals/pm_trans/AB02_139a.zip

Pub. 100-2, Chapter 15, Section 50.4
Reasonableness and Necessity

B3-2049.4

Pub. 100-2, Chapter 15, Section 50.4.2
Unlabeled Use of Drug

B3-2049.3

An unlabeled use of a drug is a use that is not included as an indication on the drug's label as approved by the FDA. FDA approved drugs used for indications other than what is indicated on the official label may be covered under Medicare if the carrier determines the use to be medically accepted, taking into consideration the major drug compendia, authoritative medical literature and/or accepted standards of medical practice. In the case of drugs used in an anti-cancer chemotherapeutic regimen, unlabeled uses are covered for a medically accepted indication as defined in §50.5.

These decisions are made by the contractor on a case-by-case basis.

Pub. 100-2, Chapter 15, Section 50.5
Self-Administered Drugs and Biologicals

B3-2049.5

Medicare Part B does not cover drugs that are usually self-administered by the patient unless the statute provides for such coverage. The statute explicitly provides coverage, for blood clotting factors, drugs used in immunosuppressive therapy, erythropoietin for dialysis patients, certain oral anti-cancer drugs and anti-emetics used in certain situations.

Pub. 100-2, Chapter 15, Section 50.5.5
Hemophilia Clotting Factors

A3-3112.4.B.2, HO-230.4.B.2

Section 1861(s)(2)(I) of the Act provides Medicare coverage of blood clotting factors for hemophilia patients competent to use such factors to control bleeding without medical supervision, and items related to the administration of such factors. Hemophilia, a blood disorder characterized by prolonged coagulation time, is caused by deficiency of a factor in plasma necessary for blood to clot. For purposes of Medicare Part B coverage, hemophilia encompasses the following conditions:

- Factor VIII deficiency (classic hemophilia);
- Factor IX deficiency (also termed plasma thromboplastin component (PTC) or Christmas factor deficiency); and
- Von Willebrand's disease.

Claims for blood clotting factors for hemophilia patients with these diagnoses may be covered if the patient is competent to use such factors without medical supervision.

The amount of clotting factors determined to be necessary to have on hand and thus covered under this provision is based on the historical utilization pattern or profile developed by the contractor for each patient. It is expected that the treating source, e.g., a family physician or comprehensive hemophilia diagnostic and treatment center, have such information. From this data, the contractor is able to anticipate and make reasonable projections concerning the quantity of clotting factors the patient will need over a specific period of time. Unanticipated occurrences involving extraordinary events, such as automobile accidents or inpatient hospital stays, will change this base line data and should be appropriately considered. In addition, changes in a patient's medical needs over a period of time require adjustments in the profile.

Pub. 100-2, Chapter 15, Section 80.1
Clinical Laboratory Services

B3-2070.1

Section 1833 and 1861 of the Act provides for payment of clinical laboratory services under Medicare Part B. Clinical laboratory services involve the biological, microbiological, serological, chemical, immunohematological, hematological, biophysical, cytological, pathological, or other examination of materials derived from the human body for the diagnosis, prevention, or treatment of a disease or assessment of a medical condition. Laboratory services must meet all applicable requirements of the Clinical Laboratory Improvement Amendments of 1988 (CLIA), as set forth at 42 CFR part 493. Section 1862(a)(1)(A) of the Act provides that Medicare payment may not be made for services that are not reasonable and necessary. Clinical laboratory services must be ordered and used promptly by the physician who is treating the beneficiary as described in 42 CFR 410.32(a), or by a qualified nonphysician practitioner, as described in 42 CFR 410.32(a)(3).

See the Medicare Claims Processing Manual Chapter 16 for related claims processing instructions.

Pub. 100-2, Chapter 15, Section 100
Surgical Dressings, Splints, Casts, and Other Devices Used for Reductions of Fractures and Dislocations

B3-2079, A3-3110.3, HO-228.3,

Surgical dressings are limited to primary and secondary dressings required for the treatment of a wound caused by, or treated by, a surgical procedure that has been performed by a physician or other health care professional to the extent permissible under State law. In addition, surgical dressings required after debridement of a wound are also covered, irrespective of the type of debridement, as long as the debridement was reasonable and necessary and was performed by a health care professional acting within the scope of his/her legal authority when performing this function. Surgical dressings are covered for as long as they are medically necessary.

Primary dressings are therapeutic or protective coverings applied directly to wounds or lesions either on the skin or caused by an opening to the skin. Secondary dressing materials that serve a therapeutic or protective function and that are needed to secure a primary dressing are also covered. Items such as adhesive tape, roll gauze, bandages, and disposable compression material are examples of secondary dressings. Elastic stockings, support hose, foot coverings, leotards, knee supports, surgical leggings, gauntlets, and pressure garments for the arms and hands are examples of items that are not ordinarily covered as surgical dressings. Some items, such as transparent film, may be used as a primary or secondary dressing.

If a physician, certified nurse midwife, physician assistant, nurse practitioner, or clinical nurse specialist applies surgical dressings as part of a professional service that is billed to Medicare, the surgical dressings are considered incident to the professional services of the health care practitioner. (See §§60.1, 180, 190, 200, and 210.) When surgical dressings are not covered incident to the services of a health care practitioner and are obtained by the patient from a supplier (e.g., a drugstore, physician, or other health care practitioner that qualifies as a supplier) on an order from a physician or other health care professional authorized under State law or regulation to make such an order, the surgical dressings are covered separately under Part B.

Splints and casts, and other devices used for reductions of fractures and dislocations are covered under Part B of Medicare. This includes dental splints.

Pub. 100-2, Chapter 15, Section 110
Durable Medical Equipment - General

B3-2100, A3-3113, HO-235, HHA-220

Expenses incurred by a beneficiary for the rental or purchases of durable medical equipment (DME) are reimbursable if the following three requirements are met:

- The equipment meets the definition of DME (§110.1);
- The equipment is necessary and reasonable for the treatment of the patient's illness or injury or to improve the functioning of his or her malformed body member (§110.1); and
- The equipment is used in the patient's home.

The decision whether to rent or purchase an item of equipment generally resides with the beneficiary, but the decision on how to pay rests with CMS. For some DME, program payment policy calls for lump sum payments and in others for periodic payment. Where covered DME is furnished to a beneficiary by a supplier of services other than a provider of services, the DMERC makes the reimbursement. If a provider of services furnishes the equipment, the intermediary makes the reimbursement. The payment method is identified in the annual fee schedule update furnished by CMS.

The CMS issues quarterly updates to a fee schedule file that contains rates by HCPCS code and also identifies the classification of the HCPCS code within the following categories.

Category Code	Definition
IN	Inexpensive and Other Routinely Purchased Items

Category Code	Definition
FS	Frequently Serviced Items
CR	Capped Rental Items
OX	Oxygen and Oxygen Equipment
OS	Ostomy, Tracheostomy & Urological Items
SD	Surgical Dressings
PO	Prosthetics & Orthotics
SU	Supplies
TE	Transcutaneous Electrical Nerve Stimulators

The DMERCs, carriers, and intermediaries, where appropriate, use the CMS files to determine payment rules. See the Medicare Claims Processing Manual, Chapter 20, "Durable Medical Equipment, Surgical Dressings and Casts, Orthotics and Artificial Limbs, and Prosthetic Devices," for a detailed description of payment rules for each classification.

Payment may also be made for repairs, maintenance, and delivery of equipment and for expendable and nonreusable items essential to the effective use of the equipment subject to the conditions in §110.2.

See the Medicare Benefit Policy Manual, Chapter 11, "End Stage Renal Disease," for hemodialysis equipment and supplies.

Pub. 100-2, Chapter 15, Section 110.1
Definition of Durable Medical Equipment

B3-2100.1, A3-3113.1, HO-235.1, HHA-220.1, B3-2100.2, A3-3113.2, HO-235.2, HHA-220.2

Durable medical equipment is equipment which:

- Can withstand repeated use;
- Is primarily and customarily used to serve a medical purpose;
- Generally is not useful to a person in the absence of an illness or injury; and
- Is appropriate for use in the home.

All requirements of the definition must be met before an item can be considered to be durable medical equipment.

The following describes the underlying policies for determining whether an item meets the definition of DME and may be covered.

A. Durability

An item is considered durable if it can withstand repeated use, i.e., the type of item that could normally be rented. Medical supplies of an expendable nature, such as incontinent pads, lambs wool pads, catheters, ace bandages, elastic stockings, surgical facemasks, irrigating kits, sheets, and bags are not considered "durable" within the meaning of the definition. There are other items that, although durable in nature, may fall into other coverage categories such as supplies, braces, prosthetic devices, artificial arms, legs, and eyes.

B. Medical Equipment

Medical equipment is equipment primarily and customarily used for medical purposes and is not generally useful in the absence of illness or injury. In most instances, no development will be needed to determine whether a specific item of equipment is medical in nature. However, some cases will require development to determine whether the item constitutes medical equipment. This development would include the advice of local medical organizations (hospitals, medical schools, medical societies) and specialists in the field of physical medicine and rehabilitation. If the equipment is new on the market, it may be necessary, prior to seeking professional advice, to obtain information from the supplier or manufacturer explaining the design, purpose, effectiveness and method of using the equipment in the home as well as the results of any tests or clinical studies that have been conducted.

1. Equipment Presumptively Medical

Items such as hospital beds, wheelchairs, hemodialysis equipment, iron lungs, respirators, intermittent positive pressure breathing machines, medical regulators, oxygen tents, crutches, canes, trapeze bars, walkers, inhalators, nebulizers, commodes, suction machines, and traction equipment presumptively constitute medical equipment. (Although hemodialysis equipment is covered as a prosthetic device (§120), it also meets the definition of DME, and reimbursement for the rental or purchase of such equipment for use in the beneficiary's home will be made only under the provisions for payment applicable to DME. See the Medicare Benefit Policy Manual, Chapter 11, "End Stage Renal Disease," §30.1, for coverage of home use of hemodialysis.) NOTE: There is a wide variety in types of respirators and suction machines. The DMERC's medical staff should determine whether the apparatus specified in the claim is appropriate for home use.

2. Equipment Presumptively Nonmedical

Equipment which is primarily and customarily used for a nonmedical purpose may not be considered "medical" equipment for which payment can be made under the medical insurance program. This is true even though the item has some remote medically related use. For example, in the case of a cardiac patient, an air conditioner might possibly be used to lower room temperature to reduce fluid loss in the patient and to restore an environment conducive to maintenance of the proper fluid balance. Nevertheless, because the primary and customary use of an air conditioner is a nonmedical one, the air conditioner cannot be deemed to be medical equipment for which payment can be made.

Other devices and equipment used for environmental control or to enhance the environmental setting in which the beneficiary is placed are not considered covered DME. These include, for example, room heaters, humidifiers, dehumidifiers, and electric air cleaners. Equipment which basically serves comfort or convenience functions or is primarily for the convenience of a person caring for the patient, such as elevators, stairway elevators, and posture chairs, do not constitute medical equipment. Similarly, physical fitness equipment (such as an exercycle), first-aid or precautionary-type equipment (such as preset portable oxygen units), self-help devices (such as safety grab bars), and training equipment (such as Braille training texts) are considered nonmedical in nature.

3. Special Exception Items

Specified items of equipment may be covered under certain conditions even though they do not meet the definition of DME because they are not primarily and customarily used to serve a medical purpose and/or are generally useful in the absence of illness or injury. These items would be covered when it is clearly established that they serve a therapeutic purpose in an individual case and would include:

a. Gel pads and pressure and water mattresses (which generally serve a preventive purpose) when prescribed for a patient who had bed sores or there is medical evidence indicating that they are highly susceptible to such ulceration; and

b. Heat lamps for a medical rather than a soothing or cosmetic purpose, e.g., where the need for heat therapy has been established.

In establishing medical necessity for the above items, the evidence must show that the item is included in the physician's course of treatment and a physician is supervising its use.

NOTE: The above items represent special exceptions and no extension of coverage to other items should be inferred

C. Necessary and Reasonable

Although an item may be classified as DME, it may not be covered in every instance. Coverage in a particular case is subject to the requirement that the equipment be necessary and reasonable for treatment of an illness or injury, or to improve the functioning of a malformed body member. These considerations will bar payment for equipment which cannot reasonably be expected to perform a therapeutic function in an individual case or will permit only partial therapeutic function in an individual case or will permit only partial payment when the type of equipment furnished substantially exceeds that required for the treatment of the illness or injury involved.

See the Medicare Claims Processing Manual, Chapter 1, "General Billing Requirements;" §60, regarding the rules for providing advance beneficiary notices (ABNs) that advise beneficiaries, before items or services actually are furnished, when Medicare is likely to deny payment for them. ABNs allow beneficiaries to make an informed consumer decision about receiving items or services for which they may have to pay out-of-pocket and to be more active participants in their own health care treatment decisions.

1. Necessity for the Equipment

Equipment is necessary when it can be expected to make a meaningful contribution to the treatment of the patient's illness or injury or to the improvement of his or her malformed body member. In most cases the physician's prescription for the equipment and other medical information available to the DMERC will be sufficient to establish that the equipment serves this purpose.

2. Reasonableness of the Equipment

Even though an item of DME may serve a useful medical purpose, the DMERC or intermediary must also consider to what extent, if any, it would be reasonable for the Medicare program to pay for the item prescribed. The following considerations should enter into the determination of reasonableness:

1. Would the expense of the item to the program be clearly disproportionate to the therapeutic benefits which could ordinarily be derived from use of the equipment

2. Is the item substantially more costly than a medically appropriate and realistically feasible alternative pattern of care

3. Does the item serve essentially the same purpose as equipment already available to the beneficiary

3. Payment Consistent With What is Necessary and Reasonable

Where a claim is filed for equipment containing features of an aesthetic nature or features of a medical nature which are not required by the patient's condition or where there exists a reasonably feasible and medically appropriate alternative pattern of care which is less costly than the equipment furnished, the amount payable is based on the rate for the equipment or alternative treatment which meets the patient's medical needs.

The acceptance of an assignment binds the supplier-assignee to accept the payment for the medically required equipment or service as the full charge and the supplier-assignee cannot charge the beneficiary the differential attributable to the equipment actually furnished.

4. Establishing the Period of Medical Necessity

Generally, the period of time an item of durable medical equipment will be considered to be medically necessary is based on the physician's estimate of the time that his or her patient will need the equipment. See the Medicare Program Integrity Manual, Chapters 5 and 6, for medical review guidelines.

D. Definition of a Beneficiary's Home

For purposes of rental and purchase of DME a beneficiary's home may be his/her own dwelling, an apartment, a relative's home, a home for the aged, or some other type of institution. However, an institution may not be considered a beneficiary's home if it:

- Meets at least the basic requirement in the definition of a hospital, i.e., it is primarily engaged in providing by or under the supervision of physicians, to inpatients, diagnostic and therapeutic services for medical diagnosis, treatment, and care of injured, disabled, and sick persons, or rehabilitation services for the rehabilitation of injured, disabled, or sick persons; or

- Meets at least the basic requirement in the definition of a skilled nursing facility, i.e., it is primarily engaged in providing to inpatients skilled nursing care and related services for patients who require medical or nursing care, or rehabilitation services for the rehabilitation of injured, disabled, or sick persons.

Thus, if an individual is a patient in an institution or distinct part of an institution which provides the services described in the bullets above, the individual is not entitled to have separate Part B payment made for rental or purchase of DME. This is because such an institution may not be considered the individual's home. The same concept applies even if the patient resides in a bed or portion of the institution not certified for Medicare.

If the patient is at home for part of a month and, for part of the same month is in an institution that cannot qualify as his or her home, or is outside the U.S., monthly payments may be made for the entire month. Similarly, if DME is returned to the provider before the end of a payment month because the beneficiary died in that month or because the equipment became unnecessary in that month, payment may be made for the entire month.

Pub. 100-2, Chapter 15, Section 110.2
Repairs, Maintenance, Replacement, and Delivery

Under the circumstances specified below, payment may be made for repair, maintenance, and replacement of medically required DME, including equipment which had been in use before the user enrolled in Part B of the program. However, do not pay for repair, maintenance, or replacement of equipment in the frequent and substantial servicing or oxygen equipment payment categories. In addition, payments for repair and maintenance may not include payment for parts and labor covered under a manufacturer's or supplier's warranty.

A. Repairs

To repair means to fix or mend and to put the equipment back in good condition after damage or wear. Repairs to equipment which a beneficiary owns are covered when necessary to make the equipment serviceable. However, do not pay for repair of previously denied equipment or equipment in the frequent and substantial servicing or oxygen equipment payment categories. If the expense for repairs exceeds the estimated expense of purchasing or renting another item of equipment for the remaining period of medical need, no payment can be made for the amount of the excess. (See subsection C where claims for repairs suggest malicious damage or culpable neglect.)

Since renters of equipment recover from the rental charge the expenses they incur in maintaining in working order the equipment they rent out, separately itemized charges for repair of rented equipment are not covered. This includes items in the frequent and substantial servicing, oxygen equipment, capped rental, and inexpensive or routinely purchased payment categories which are being rented.

A new Certificate of Medical Necessity (CMN) and/or physician's order is not needed for repairs.

For replacement items, see Subsection C below.

B. Maintenance

Routine periodic servicing, such as testing, cleaning, regulating, and checking of the beneficiary's equipment, is not covered. The owner is expected to perform such routine maintenance rather than a retailer or some other person who charges the beneficiary. Normally, purchasers of DME are given operating manuals which describe the type of servicing an owner may perform to properly maintain the equipment. It is reasonable to expect that beneficiaries will perform this maintenance. Thus, hiring a third party to do such work is for the convenience of the beneficiary and is not covered. However, more extensive maintenance which, based on the manufacturers' recommendations, is to be performed by authorized technicians, is covered as repairs for medically necessary equipment which a beneficiary owns. This might include, for example, breaking down sealed components and performing tests which require specialized testing equipment not available to the beneficiary. Do not pay for maintenance of purchased items that require frequent and substantial servicing or oxygen equipment.

Since renters of equipment recover from the rental charge the expenses they incur in maintaining in working order the equipment they rent out, separately itemized charges for maintenance of rented equipment are generally not covered. Payment may not be made for maintenance of rented equipment other than the maintenance and servicing fee established for capped rental items. For capped rental items which have reached the 15-month rental cap, contractors pay claims for maintenance and servicing fees after 6 months have passed from the end of the final paid rental month or from the end of the period the item is no longer covered under the supplier's or manufacturer's warranty, whichever is later. See the Medicare Claims Processing Manual, Chapter 20, "Durable Medical Equipment, Prosthetics and Orthotics, and Supplies (DMEPOS)," for additional instruction and an example.

A new CMN and/or physician's order is not needed for covered maintenance.

C. Replacement

Replacement refers to the provision of an identical or nearly identical item. Situations involving the provision of a different item because of a change in medical condition are not addressed in this section.

Equipment which the beneficiary owns or is a capped rental item may be replaced in cases of loss or irreparable damage. Irreparable damage refers to a specific accident or to a natural disaster (e.g., fire, flood). A physician's order and/or new Certificate of Medical Necessity (CMN), when required, is needed to reaffirm the medical necessity of the item.

Irreparable wear refers to deterioration sustained from day-to-day usage over time and a specific event cannot be identified. Replacement of equipment due to irreparable wear takes into consideration the reasonable useful lifetime of the equipment. If the item of equipment has been in continuous use by the patient on either a rental or purchase basis for the equipment's useful lifetime, the beneficiary may elect to obtain a new piece of equipment. Replacement may be reimbursed when a new physician order and/or new CMN, when required, is needed to reaffirm the medical necessity of the item.

The reasonable useful lifetime of durable medical equipment is determined through program instructions. In the absence of program instructions, carriers may determine the reasonable useful lifetime of equipment, but in no case can it be less than 5 years. Computation of the useful lifetime is based on when the equipment is delivered to the beneficiary, not the age of the equipment. Replacement due to wear is not covered during the reasonable useful lifetime of the equipment. During the reasonable useful lifetime, Medicare does cover repair up to the cost of replacement (but not actual replacement) for medically necessary equipment owned by the beneficiary. (See subsection A.)

Charges for the replacement of oxygen equipment, items that require frequent and substantial servicing or inexpensive or routinely purchased items which are being rented are not covered.

Cases suggesting malicious damage, culpable neglect, or wrongful disposition of equipment should be investigated and denied where the DMERC determines that it is unreasonable to make program payment under the circumstances. DMERCs refer such cases to the program integrity specialist in the RO.

D. Delivery

Payment for delivery of DME whether rented or purchased is generally included in the fee schedule allowance for the item. See Pub. 100-04, Medicare Claims Processing Manual, Chapter 20, "Durable Medical Equipment, Prosthetics and Orthotics, and Supplies (DMEPOS)," for the rules that apply to making reimbursement for exceptional cases.

Pub. 100-2, Chapter 15, Section 110.3
Coverage of Supplies and Accessories

B3-2100.5, A3-3113.4, HO-235.4, HHA-220.5

Payment may be made for supplies, e.g., oxygen, that are necessary for the effective use of durable medical equipment. Such supplies include those drugs and biologicals which must be put directly into the equipment in order to achieve the therapeutic benefit of the durable medical equipment or to assure the proper functioning of the equipment, e.g., tumor chemotherapy agents used with an infusion pump or heparin used with a home dialysis system. However, the coverage of such drugs or biologicals does not preclude the need for a determination that the drug or biological itself is reasonable and necessary for treatment of the illness or injury or to improve the functioning of a malformed body member.

In the case of prescription drugs, other than oxygen, used in conjunction with durable medical equipment, prosthetic, orthotics, and supplies (DMEPOS) or prosthetic devices, the entity that dispenses the drug must furnish it directly to the patient for whom a prescription is written. The entity that dispenses the drugs must have a Medicare supplier number, must possess a current license to dispense prescription drugs in the State in which the drug is dispensed, and must bill and receive payment in its own name. A supplier that is not the entity that dispenses the drugs cannot purchase the drugs used in conjunction with DME for resale to the beneficiary. Reimbursement may be made for replacement of essential accessories such as hoses, tubes, mouthpieces, etc., for necessary DME, only if the beneficiary owns or is purchasing the equipment.

Pub. 100-2, Chapter 15, Section 120
Prosthetic Devices

B3-2130, A3-3110.4, HO-228.4, A3-3111, HO-229

A. General

Prosthetic devices (other than dental) which replace all or part of an internal body organ (including contiguous tissue), or replace all or part of the function of a permanently inoperative or malfunctioning internal body organ are covered when furnished on a physician's order. This does not require a determination that there is no possibility that the patient's condition may improve sometime in the future. If the medical record, including the judgment of the attending physician, indicates the condition is of long and indefinite duration, the test of permanence is considered met. (Such a device may also be covered under §60.I as a supply when furnished incident to a physician's service.)

Examples of prosthetic devices include artificial limbs, parenteral and enteral (PEN) nutrition, cardiac pacemakers, prosthetic lenses (see subsection B), breast prostheses (including a surgical brassiere) for postmastectomy patients, maxillofacial devices, and devices which replace all or part of the ear or nose. A urinary collection and retention system with or without a tube is a prosthetic device replacing bladder function in case of permanent urinary incontinence. The foley catheter is also considered a prosthetic device when ordered for a patient with permanent urinary incontinence. However, chucks, diapers, rubber sheets, etc., are supplies that are not covered under this provision. Although hemodialysis equipment is a prosthetic device, payment for the rental or purchase of such equipment in the home is made only for use under the provisions for payment applicable to durable medical equipment.

An exception is that if payment cannot be made on an inpatient's behalf under Part A, hemodialysis equipment, supplies, and services required by such patient could be covered under Part B as a prosthetic device, which replaces the function of a kidney. See the Medicare Benefit Policy Manual, Chapter 11, "End Stage Renal Disease," for payment for hemodialysis equipment used in the home. See the Medicare Benefit Policy Manual, Chapter 1, "Inpatient Hospital Services," §10, for additional instructions on hospitalization for renal dialysis.

NOTE: Medicare does not cover a prosthetic device dispensed to a patient prior to the time at which the patient undergoes the procedure that makes necessary the use of the device. For example, the carrier does not make a separate Part B payment for an intraocular lens (IOL) or pacemaker that a physician, during an office visit prior to the actual surgery, dispenses to the patient for his or her use. Dispensing a prosthetic device in this manner raises health and safety issues. Moreover, the need for the device cannot be clearly established until the procedure that makes its use possible is successfully performed. Therefore, dispensing a prosthetic device in this manner is not considered reasonable and necessary for the treatment of the patient's condition.

Colostomy (and other ostomy) bags and necessary accouterments required for attachment are covered as prosthetic devices. This coverage also includes irrigation and flushing equipment and other items and supplies directly related to ostomy care, whether the attachment of a bag is required.

Accessories and/or supplies which are used directly with an enteral or parenteral device to achieve the therapeutic benefit of the prosthesis or to assure the proper functioning of the device may also be covered under the prosthetic device benefit subject to the additional guidelines in the Medicare National Coverage Determinations Manual.

Covered items include catheters, filters, extension tubing, infusion bottles, pumps (either food or infusion), intravenous (I.V.) pole, needles, syringes, dressings, tape, Heparin Sodium (parenteral only), volumetric monitors (parenteral only), and parenteral and enteral nutrient solutions. Baby food and other regular grocery products that can be blenderized and used with the enteral system are not covered. Note that some of these items, e.g., a food pump and an I.V. pole, qualify as DME. Although coverage of the enteral and parenteral nutritional therapy systems is provided on the basis of the prosthetic device benefit, the payment rules relating to lump sum or monthly payment for DME apply to such items.

The coverage of prosthetic devices includes replacement of and repairs to such devices as explained in subsection D.

Finally, the Benefits Improvement and Protection Act of 2000 amended §1834(h)(1) of the Act by adding a provision (1834 (h)(1)(G)(i)) that requires Medicare payment to be made for the replacement of prosthetic devices which are artificial limbs, or for the replacement of any part of such devices, without regard to continuous use or useful lifetime restrictions if an ordering physician determines that the replacement device, or replacement part of such a device, is necessary.

Payment may be made for the replacement of a prosthetic device that is an artificial limb, or replacement part of a device if the ordering physician determines that the replacement device or part is necessary because of any of the following:

1. A change in the physiological condition of the patient;
2. An irreparable change in the condition of the device, or in a part of the device; or
3. The condition of the device, or the part of the device, requires repairs and the cost of such repairs would be more than 60 percent of the cost of a replacement device, or, as the case may be, of the part being replaced.

This provision is effective for items replaced on or after April 1, 2001. It supersedes any rule that that provided a 5-year or other replacement rule with regard to prosthetic devices.

B. Prosthetic Lenses

The term "internal body organ" includes the lens of an eye. Prostheses replacing the lens of an eye include post-surgical lenses customarily used during convalescence from eye surgery in which the lens of the eye was removed. In addition, permanent lenses are also covered when required by an individual lacking the organic lens of the eye because of surgical removal or congenital absence. Prosthetic lenses obtained on or after the beneficiary's date of entitlement to supplementary medical insurance benefits may be covered even though the surgical removal of the crystalline lens occurred before entitlement.

1. Prosthetic Cataract Lenses

One of the following prosthetic lenses or combinations of prosthetic lenses furnished by a physician (see §30.4 for coverage of prosthetic lenses prescribed by a doctor of optometry) may be covered when determined to be reasonable and necessary to restore essentially the vision provided by the crystalline lens of the eye:

Prosthetic bifocal lenses in frames;

Prosthetic lenses in frames for far vision, and prosthetic lenses in frames for near vision; or

APPENDIX 4 — PUB100/NCD REFERENCES

When a prosthetic contact lens(es) for far vision is prescribed (including cases of binocular and monocular aphakia), make payment for the contact lens(es) and prosthetic lenses in frames for near vision to be worn at the same time as the contact lens(es), and prosthetic lenses in frames to be worn when the contacts have been removed.

Lenses which have ultraviolet absorbing or reflecting properties may be covered, in lieu of payment for regular (untinted) lenses, if it has been determined that such lenses are medically reasonable and necessary for the individual patient.

Medicare does not cover cataract sunglasses obtained in addition to the regular (untinted) prosthetic lenses since the sunglasses duplicate the restoration of vision function performed by the regular prosthetic lenses.

2. Payment for Intraocular Lenses (IOLs) Furnished in Ambulatory Surgical Centers (ASCs)

Effective for services furnished on or after March 12, 1990, payment for intraocular lenses (IOLs) inserted during or subsequent to cataract surgery in a Medicare certified ASC is included with the payment for facility services that are furnished in connection with the covered surgery.

Refer to the Medicare Claims Processing Manual, Chapter 14, "Ambulatory Surgical Centers," for more information.

3. Limitation on Coverage of Conventional Lenses

One pair of conventional eyeglasses or conventional contact lenses furnished after each cataract surgery with insertion of an IOL is covered.

C. Dentures

Dentures are excluded from coverage. However, when a denture or a portion of the denture is an integral part (built-in) of a covered prosthesis (e.g., an obturator to fill an opening in the palate), it is covered as part of that prosthesis.

D. Supplies, Repairs, Adjustments, and Replacement

Supplies are covered that are necessary for the effective use of a prosthetic device (e.g., the batteries needed to operate an artificial larynx). Adjustment of prosthetic devices required by wear or by a change in the patient's condition is covered when ordered by a physician. General provisions relating to the repair and replacement of durable medical equipment in §110.2 for the repair and replacement of prosthetic devices are applicable. (See the Medicare Benefit Policy Manual, Chapter 16, "General Exclusions from Coverage," §40.4, for payment for devices replaced under a warranty.) Replacement of conventional eyeglasses or contact lenses furnished in accordance with §120.B.3 is not covered.

Necessary supplies, adjustments, repairs, and replacements are covered even when the device had been in use before the user enrolled in Part B of the program, so long as the device continues to be medically required.

Pub. 100-2, Chapter 15, Section 130
Leg, Arm, Back, and Neck Braces, Trusses, and Artificial Legs, Arms, and Eyes

B3-2133, A3-3110.5, HO-228.5, AB-01-06 dated 1/18/01

These appliances are covered under Part B when furnished incident to physicians' services or on a physician's order. A brace includes rigid and semi-rigid devices which are used for the purpose of supporting a weak or deformed body member or restricting or eliminating motion in a diseased or injured part of the body. Elastic stockings, garter belts, and similar devices do not come within the scope of the definition of a brace. Back braces include, but are not limited to, special corsets, e.g., sacroiliac, sacrolumbar, dorsolumbar corsets, and belts. A terminal device (e.g., hand or hook) is covered under this provision whether an artificial limb is required by the patient. Stump stockings and harnesses (including replacements) are also covered when these appliances are essential to the effective use of the artificial limb.

Adjustments to an artificial limb or other appliance required by wear or by a change in the patient's condition are covered when ordered by a physician.

Adjustments, repairs and replacements are covered even when the item had been in use before the user enrolled in Part B of the program so long as the device continues to be medically required.

Pub. 100-2, Chapter 15, Section 140
Therapeutic Shoes for Individuals with Diabetes

B3-2134

Coverage of therapeutic shoes (depth or custom-molded) along with inserts for individuals with diabetes is available as of May 1, 1993. These diabetic shoes are covered if the requirements as specified in this section concerning certification and prescription are fulfilled. In addition, this benefit provides for a pair of diabetic shoes even if only one foot suffers from diabetic foot disease. Each shoe is equally equipped so that the affected limb, as well as the remaining limb, is protected. Claims for therapeutic shoes for diabetics are processed by the Durable Medical Equipment Regional Carriers (DMERCs).

Therapeutic shoes for diabetics are not DME and are not considered DME nor orthotics, but a separate category of coverage under Medicare Part B. (See §1861(s)(12) and §1833(o) of the Act.)

A. Definitions

The following items may be covered under the diabetic shoe benefit:

1. Custom-Molded Shoes

Custom-molded shoes are shoes that:

Are constructed over a positive model of the patient's foot;

Are made from leather or other suitable material of equal quality;

Have removable inserts that can be altered or replaced as the patient's condition warrants; and

Have some form of shoe closure.

2. Depth Shoes

Depth shoes are shoes that:

Have a full length, heel-to-toe filler that, when removed, provides a minimum of 3/16 inch of additional depth used to accommodate custom-molded or customized inserts;

Are made from leather or other suitable material of equal quality;

Have some form of shoe closure; and

Are available in full and half sizes with a minimum of three widths so that the sole is graded to the size and width of the upper portions of the shoes according to the American standard last sizing schedule or its equivalent. (The American standard last sizing schedule is the numerical shoe sizing system used for shoes sold in the United States.)

3. Inserts

Inserts are total contact, multiple density, removable inlays that are directly molded to the patient's foot or a model of the patient's foot and that are made of a suitable material with regard to the patient's condition.

B. Coverage

1. Limitations

For each individual, coverage of the footwear and inserts is limited to one of the following within one calendar year:

No more than one pair of custom-molded shoes (including inserts provided with such shoes) and two additional pairs of inserts; or

No more than one pair of depth shoes and three pairs of inserts (not including the noncustomized removable inserts provided with such shoes).

2. Coverage of Diabetic Shoes and Brace

Orthopedic shoes, as stated in the Medicare Claims Processing Manual, Chapter 20, "Durable Medical Equipment, Surgical Dressings and Casts, Orthotics and Artificial Limbs, and Prosthetic Devices," generally are not covered. This exclusion does not apply to orthopedic shoes that are an integral part of a leg brace. In situations in which an individual qualifies for both diabetic shoes and a leg brace, these items are covered separately. Thus, the diabetic shoes may be covered if the requirements for this section are met, while the brace may be covered if the requirements of §130 are met.

3. Substitution of Modifications for Inserts

An individual may substitute modification(s) of custom-molded or depth shoes instead of obtaining a pair(s) of inserts in any combination. Payment for the modification(s) may not exceed the limit set for the inserts for which the individual is entitled. The following is a list of the most common shoe modifications available, but it is not meant as an exhaustive list of the modifications available for diabetic shoes:

Rigid Rocker Bottoms - These are exterior elevations with apex positions for 51 percent to 75 percent distance measured from the back end of the heel. The apex is a narrowed or pointed end of an anatomical structure. The apex must be positioned behind the metatarsal heads and tapered off sharply to the front tip of the sole. Apex height helps to eliminate pressure at the metatarsal heads. Rigidity is ensured by the steel in the shoe. The heel of the shoe tapers off in the back in order to cause the heel to strike in the middle of the heel;

Roller Bottoms (Sole or Bar) - These are the same as rocker bottoms, but the heel is tapered from the apex to the front tip of the sole;

Metatarsal Bars - An exterior bar is placed behind the metatarsal heads in order to remove pressure from the metatarsal heads. The bars are of various shapes, heights, and construction depending on the exact purpose;

Wedges (Posting) - Wedges are either of hind foot, fore foot, or both and may be in the middle or to the side. The function is to shift or transfer weight bearing upon standing or during ambulation to the opposite side for added support, stabilization, equalized weight distribution, or balance; and

Offset Heels - This is a heel flanged at its base either in the middle, to the side, or a combination, that is then extended upward to the shoe in order to stabilize extreme positions of the hind foot.

Other modifications to diabetic shoes include, but are not limited to flared heels, Velcro closures, and inserts for missing toes.

4. Separate Inserts

Inserts may be covered and dispensed independently of diabetic shoes if the supplier of the shoes verifies in writing that the patient has appropriate footwear into which the insert can be placed. This footwear must meet the definitions found above for depth shoes and custom-molded shoes.

C. Certification

The need for diabetic shoes must be certified by a physician who is a doctor of medicine or a doctor of osteopathy and who is responsible for diagnosing and treating the patient's diabetic systemic condition through a comprehensive plan of care. This managing physician must:

Document in the patient's medical record that the patient has diabetes;

Certify that the patient is being treated under a comprehensive plan of care for diabetes, and that the patient needs diabetic shoes; and

Document in the patient's record that the patient has one or more of the following conditions:

o Peripheral neuropathy with evidence of callus formation;

o History of pre-ulcerative calluses;

o History of previous ulceration;

o Foot deformity;

o Previous amputation of the foot or part of the foot; or

o Poor circulation.

D. Prescription

Following certification by the physician managing the patient's systemic diabetic condition, a podiatrist or other qualified physician who is knowledgeable in the fitting of diabetic shoes and inserts may prescribe the particular type of footwear necessary.

E. Furnishing Footwear

The footwear must be fitted and furnished by a podiatrist or other qualified individual such as a pedorthist, an orthotist, or a prosthetist. The certifying physician may not furnish the diabetic shoes unless the certifying physician is the only qualified individual in the area. It is left to the discretion of each carrier to determine the meaning of "in the area."

Pub. 100-2, Chapter 15, Section 150
Dental Services

B3-2136

As indicated under the general exclusions from coverage, items and services in connection with the care, treatment, filling, removal, or replacement of teeth or structures directly supporting the teeth are not covered. "Structures directly supporting the teeth" means the periodontium, which includes the gingivae, dentogingival junction, periodontal membrane, cementum of the teeth, and alveolar process.

In addition to the following, see Pub 100-1, the Medicare General Information, Eligibility, and Entitlement Manual, Chapter 5, Definitions and Pub 3, the Medicare National Coverage Determinations Manual for specific services which may be covered when furnished by a dentist. If an otherwise noncovered procedure or service is performed by a dentist as incident to and as an integral part of a covered procedure or service performed by the dentist, the total service performed by the dentist on such an occasion is covered.

EXAMPLE 1:

The reconstruction of a ridge performed primarily to prepare the mouth for dentures is a noncovered procedure. However, when the reconstruction of a ridge is performed as a result of and at the same time as the surgical removal of a tumor (for other than dental purposes), the totality of surgical procedures is a covered service.

EXAMPLE 2:

Medicare makes payment for the wiring of teeth when this is done in connection with the reduction of a jaw fracture.

The extraction of teeth to prepare the jaw for radiation treatment of neoplastic disease is also covered. This is an exception to the requirement that to be covered, a noncovered procedure or service performed by a dentist must be an incident to and an integral part of a covered procedure or service performed by the dentist. Ordinarily, the dentist extracts the patient's teeth, but another physician, e.g., a radiologist, administers the radiation treatments.

When an excluded service is the primary procedure involved, it is not covered, regardless of its complexity or difficulty. For example, the extraction of an impacted tooth is not covered. Similarly, an alveoplasty (the surgical improvement of the shape and condition of the alveolar process) and a frenectomy are excluded from coverage when either of these procedures is performed in connection with an excluded service, e.g., the preparation of the mouth for dentures. In a like manner, the removal of a torus palatinus (a bony protuberance of the hard palate) may be a covered service. However, with rare exception, this surgery is performed in connection with an excluded service, i.e., the preparation of the mouth for dentures. Under such circumstances, Medicare does not pay for this procedure.

Dental splints used to treat a dental condition are excluded from coverage under 1862(a)(12) of the Act. On the other hand, if the treatment is determined to be a covered medical condition (i.e., dislocated upper/lower jaw joints), then the splint can be covered.

Whether such services as the administration of anesthesia, diagnostic x-rays, and other related procedures are covered depends upon whether the primary procedure being performed by the dentist is itself covered. Thus, an x-ray taken in connection with the reduction of a fracture of the jaw or facial bone is covered. However, a single x-ray or x-ray survey taken in connection with the care or treatment of teeth or the periodontium is not covered.

Medicare makes payment for a covered dental procedure no matter where the service is performed. The hospitalization or nonhospitalization of a patient has no direct bearing on the coverage or exclusion of a given dental procedure.

Payment may also be made for services and supplies furnished incident to covered dental services. For example, the services of a dental technician or nurse who is under the direct supervision of the dentist or physician are covered if the services are included in the dentist's or physician's bill.

Pub. 100-2, Chapter 15, Section 230
Practice of Physical Therapy, Occupational Therapy, and Speech-Language Pathology

Pub. 100-2, Chapter 15, Section 290
Foot Care

A3-3158, B3-2323, HO-260.9, B3-4120.1

A. Treatment of Subluxation of Foot

Subluxations of the foot are defined as partial dislocations or displacements of joint surfaces, tendons ligaments, or muscles of the foot. Surgical or nonsurgical treatments undertaken for the sole purpose of correcting a subluxated structure in the foot as an isolated entity are not covered.

However, medical or surgical treatment of subluxation of the ankle joint (talo-crural joint) is covered. In addition, reasonable and necessary medical or surgical services, diagnosis, or treatment for medical conditions that have resulted from or are associated with partial displacement of structures is covered. For example, if a patient has osteoarthritis that has resulted in a partial displacement of joints in the foot, and the primary treatment is for the osteoarthritis, coverage is provided

B. Exclusions from Coverage

The following foot care services are generally excluded from coverage under both Part A and Part B. (See §290.F and §290.G for instructions on applying foot care exclusions.)

1. Treatment of Flat Foot

The term "flat foot" is defined as a condition in which one or more arches of the foot have flattened out. Services or devices directed toward the care or correction of such conditions, including the prescription of supportive devices, are not covered.

2. Routine Foot Care

Except as provided above, routine foot care is excluded from coverage. Services that normally are considered routine and not covered by Medicare include the following:

The cutting or removal of corns and calluses;

The trimming, cutting, clipping, or debriding of nails; and

Other hygienic and preventive maintenance care, such as cleaning and soaking the feet, the use of skin creams to maintain skin tone of either ambulatory or bedfast patients, and any other service performed in the absence of localized illness, injury, or symptoms involving the foot.

3. Supportive Devices for Feet

Orthopedic shoes and other supportive devices for the feet generally are not covered. However, this exclusion does not apply to such a shoe if it is an integral part of a leg brace, and its expense is included as part of the cost of the brace. Also, this exclusion does not apply to therapeutic shoes furnished to diabetics.

C. Exceptions to Routine Foot Care Exclusion

1. Necessary and Integral Part of Otherwise Covered Services

Incertain circumstances, services ordinarily considered to be routine may be covered if they are performed as a necessary and integral part of otherwise covered services, such as diagnosis and treatment of ulcers, wounds, or infections.

2. Treatment of Warts on Foot

The treatment of warts (includingplantar warts) on the foot is covered to the same extent as services provided for the treatment of warts located elsewhere on the body.

3. Presence of Systemic Condition

The presence of a systemic condition such as metabolic, neurologic, or peripheral vascular disease may require scrupulous foot care by a professional that in the absence of such condition(s) would be considered routine (and, therefore, excluded from coverage). Accordingly, foot care that would otherwise be considered routine may be covered when systemic condition(s) result in severe circulatory embarrassment or areas of diminished sensation in the individual's legs or feet. (See subsection A.

In these instances, certain foot care procedures that otherwise are considered routine (e.g., cutting or removing corns and calluses, or trimming, cutting, clipping, or debriding nails) may pose a hazard when performed by a nonprofessional person on patients with such systemic conditions. (See §290.G for procedural instructions.)

4. Mycotic Nails

In the absence of a systemic condition, treatment of mycotic nails may be covered.

The treatment of mycotic nails for an ambulatory patient is covered only when the physician attending the patient's mycotic condition documents that (1) there is clinical evidence of mycosis of the toenail, and (2) the patient has marked limitation of ambulation, pain, or secondary infection resulting from the thickening and dystrophy of the infected toenail plate.

The treatment of mycotic nails for a nonambulatory patient is covered only when the physician attending the patient's mycotic condition documents that (1) there is clinical evidence of mycosis of the toenail, and (2) the patient suffers from pain or secondary infection resulting from the thickening and dystrophy of the infected toenail plate.

For the purpose of these requirements, documentation means any written information that is required by the carrier in order for services to be covered. Thus, the information submitted with claims must be substantiated by information found in the patient's medical record. Any information, including that contained in a form letter, used for documentation purposes is subject to carrier verification in order to ensure that the information adequately justifies coverage of the treatment of mycotic nails.

D. Systemic Conditions That Might Justify Coverage

Although not intended as a comprehensive list, the following metabolic, neurologic, and peripheral vascular diseases (with synonyms in parentheses) most commonly represent the underlying conditions that might justify coverage for routine foot care.

Diabetes mellitus *

Arteriosclerosis obliterans (A.S.O., arteriosclerosis of the extremities, occlusive peripheral arteriosclerosis)

Buerger's disease (thromboangiitis obliterans)

Chronic thrombophlebitis *

Peripheral neuropathies involving the feet -

Associated with malnutrition and vitamin deficiency *

• Malnutrition (general, pellagra)

• Alcoholism

• Malabsorption (celiac disease, tropical sprue)

• Pernicious anemia

Associated with carcinoma *

Associated with diabetes mellitus *

Associated with drugs and toxins *

Associated with multiple sclerosis *

Associated with uremia (chronic renal disease) *

Associated with traumatic injury

Associated with leprosy or neurosyphilis

Associated with hereditary disorders

• Hereditary sensory radicular neuropathy

• Angiokeratoma corporis diffusum (Fabry's)

• Amyloid neuropathy

When the patient's condition is one of those designated by an asterisk (*), routine procedures are covered only if the patient is under the active care of a doctor of medicine or osteopathy who documents the condition.

E. Supportive Devices for Feet

Orthopedic shoes and other supportive devices for the feet generally are not covered. However, this exclusion does not apply to such a shoe if it is an integral part of a leg brace, and its expense is included as part of the cost of the brace. Also, this exclusion does not apply to therapeutic shoes furnished to diabetics.

F. Presumption of Coverage

In evaluating whether the routine services can be reimbursed, a presumption of coverage may be made where the evidence available discloses certain physical and/or clinical findings consistent with the diagnosis and indicative of severe peripheral involvement. For purposes of applying this presumption the following findings are pertinent:

Class A Findings

Nontraumatic amputation of foot or integral skeletal portion thereof.

Class B Findings

Absent posterior tibial pulse;

Advanced trophic changes as: hair growth (decrease or absence) nail changes (thickening) pigmentary changes (discoloration) skin texture (thin, shiny) skin color (rubor or redness) (Three required); and

Absent dorsalis pedis pulse.

Class C Findings

Claudication;

Temperature changes (e.g., cold feet);

Edema;

Paresthesias (abnormal spontaneous sensations in the feet); and

Burning.

The presumption of coverage may be applied when the physician rendering the routine foot care has identified:

1. A Class A finding;

2. Two of the Class B findings; or

3. One Class B and two Class C findings.

Cases evidencing findings falling short of these alternatives may involve podiatric treatment that may constitute covered care and should be reviewed by the intermediary's medical staff and developed as necessary.

For purposes of applying the coverage presumption where the routine services have been rendered by a podiatrist, the contractor may deem the active care requirement met if the claim or other evidence available discloses that the patient has seen an M.D. or D.O. for treatment and/or evaluation of the complicating disease process during the 6-month period prior to the rendition of the routine-type services. The intermediary may also accept the podiatrist's statement that the diagnosing and treating M.D. or D.O. also concurs with the podiatrist's findings as to the severity of the peripheral involvement indicated.

Services ordinarily considered routine might also be covered if they are performed as a necessary and integral part of otherwise covered services, such as diagnosis and treatment of diabetic ulcers, wounds, and infections.

G. Application of Foot Care Exclusions to Physician's Services

The exclusion of foot care is determined by the nature of the service. Thus, payment for an excluded service should be denied whether performed by a podiatrist, osteopath, or a doctor of medicine, and without regard to the difficulty or complexity of the procedure.

When an itemized bill shows both covered services and noncovered services not integrally related to the covered service, the portion of charges attributable to the noncovered services should be denied. (For example, if an itemized bill shows surgery for an ingrown toenail and also removal of calluses not necessary for the performance of toe surgery, any additional charge attributable to removal of the calluses should be denied.)

In reviewing claims involving foot care, the carrier should be alert to the following exceptional situations:

1. Payment may be made for incidental noncovered services performed as a necessary and integral part of, and secondary to, a covered procedure. For example, if trimming of toenails is required for application of a cast to a fractured foot, the carrier need not allocate and deny a portion of the charge for the trimming of the nails. However, a separately itemized charge for such excluded service should be disallowed. When the primary procedure is covered the administration of anesthesia necessary for the performance of such procedure is also covered.

2. Payment may be made for **initial** diagnostic services performed in connection with a specific symptom or complaint if it seems likely that its treatment would be covered even though the resulting diagnosis may be one requiring only noncovered care.

The name of the M.D. or D.O. who diagnosed the complicating condition must be submitted with the claim. In those cases, where active care is required, the approximate date the beneficiary was last seen by such physician must also be indicated.

NOTE: Section 939 of P.L. 96-499 removed "warts" from the routine foot care exclusion effective July 1, 1981.

Relatively few claims for routine-type care are anticipated considering the severity of conditions contemplated as the basis for this exception. Claims for this type of foot care should not be paid in the absence of convincing evidence that nonprofessional performance of the service would have been hazardous for the beneficiary because of an underlying systemic disease. The mere statement of a diagnosis such as those mentioned in §D above does not of itself indicate the severity of the condition. Where development is indicated to verify diagnosis and/or severity the carrier should follow existing claims processing practices which may include review of carrier's history and medical consultation as well as physician contacts.

The rules in §290.F concerning presumption of coverage also apply.

Codes and policies for routine foot care and supportive devices for the feet are not exclusively for the use of podiatrists. These codes must be used to report foot care services regardless of the specialty of the physician who furnishes the services. Carriers must instruct physicians to use the most appropriate code available when billing for routine foot care.

Pub. 100-2, Chapter 16, Section 10
General Exclusions From Coverage

A3-3150, HO-260, HHA-232, B3-2300

No payment can be made under either the hospital insurance or supplementary medical insurance program for certain items and services, when the following conditions exist:

- Not reasonable and necessary (§20);
- No legal obligation to pay for or provide (§40);
- Paid for by a governmental entity (§50);

- Not provided within United States (§60);
- Resulting from war (§70);
- Personal comfort (§80);
- Routine services and appliances (§90);
- Custodial care (§110);
- Cosmetic surgery (§120);
- Charges by immediate relatives or members of household (§130);
- Dental services (§140);
- Paid or expected to be paid under workers' compensation (§150);
- Nonphysician services provided to a hospital inpatient that were not provided directly or arranged for by the hospital (§170);
- Services Related to and Required as a Result of Services Which are not Covered Under Medicare (§180);
- Excluded foot care services and supportive devices for feet (§30); or
- Excluded investigational devices (See Chapter 14, §30).

Pub. 100-2, Chapter 16, Section 20
Services Not Reasonable and Necessary

A3-3151, HO-260.1, B3-2303, AB-00-52 - 6/00

Items and services which are not reasonable and necessary for the diagnosis or treatment of illness or injury or to improve the functioning of a malformed body member are not covered, e.g., payment cannot be made for the rental of a special hospital bed to be used by the patient in their home unless it was a reasonable and necessary part of the patient's treatment. See also §80.

A health care item or service for the purpose of causing, or assisting to cause, the death of any individual (assisted suicide) is not covered. This prohibition does not apply to the provision of an item or service for the purpose of alleviating pain or discomfort, even if such use may increase the risk of death, so long as the item or service is not furnished for the specific purpose of causing death.

Pub. 100-2, Chapter 16, Section 90
Routine Services and Appliances

A3-3157, HO-260.7, B3-2320, R-1797A3 - 5/00

Routine physical checkups; eyeglasses, contact lenses, and eye examinations for the purpose of prescribing, fitting, or changing eyeglasses; eye refractions by whatever practitioner and for whatever purpose performed; hearing aids and examinations for hearing aids; and immunizations are not covered.

The routine physical checkup exclusion applies to (a) examinations performed without relationship to treatment or diagnosis for a specific illness, symptom, complaint, or injury; and (b) examinations required by third parties such as insurance companies, business establishments, or Government agencies.

If the claim is for a diagnostic test or examination performed solely for the purpose of establishing a claim under title IV of Public Law 91-173, "Black Lung Benefits," the service is not covered under Medicare and the claimant should be advised to contact their Social Security office regarding the filing of a claim for reimbursement under the "Black Lung" program.

The exclusions apply to eyeglasses or contact lenses, and eye examinations for the purpose of prescribing, fitting, or changing eyeglasses or contact lenses for refractive errors. The exclusions do not apply to physicians' services (and services incident to a physicians' service) performed in conjunction with an eye disease, as for example, glaucoma or cataracts, or to post-surgical prosthetic lenses which are customarily used during convalescence from eye surgery in which the lens of the eye was removed, or to permanent prosthetic lenses required by an individual lacking the organic lens of the eye, whether by surgical removal or congenital disease. Such prosthetic lens is a replacement for an internal body organ - the lens of the eye. (See the Medicare Benefit Policy Manual, Chapter 15, "Covered Medical and Other Health Services," §120.)

Expenses for all refractive procedures, whether performed by an ophthalmologist (or any other physician) or an optometrist and without regard to the reason for performance of the refraction, are excluded from coverage.

A - Immunizations

Vaccinations or inoculations are excluded as immunizations unless they are either

- Directly related to the treatment of an injury or direct exposure to a disease or condition, such as antirabies treatment, tetanus antitoxin or booster vaccine, botulin antitoxin, antivenin sera, or immune globulin.(In the absence of injury or direct exposure, preventive immunization (vaccination or inoculation) against such diseases as smallpox, polio, diphtheria, etc., is not covered.); or
- Specifically covered by statute, as described in the Medicare Benefit Policy Manual, Chapter 15, "Covered Medical and Other Health Services," §50.

B - Antigens

Prior to the Omnibus Reconciliation Act of 1980, a physician who prepared an antigen for a patient could not be reimbursed for that service unless the physician also administered the antigen to the patient. Effective January 1, 1981, payment may be made for a reasonable supply of antigens that have been prepared for a particular patient even though they have not been administered to the patient by the same physician who prepared them if:

- The antigens are prepared by a physician who is a doctor of medicine or osteopathy, and
- The physician who prepared the antigens has examined the patient and has determined a plan of treatment and a dosage regimen.

A reasonable supply of antigens is considered to be not more than a 12-week supply of antigens that has been prepared for a particular patient at any one time. The purpose of the reasonable supply limitation is to assure that the antigens retain their potency and effectiveness over the period in which they are to be administered to the patient. (See the Medicare Benefit Policy Manual, Chapter 15, "Covered Medical and Other Health Services," §50.4.4.2)

Pub. 100-2, Chapter 16, Section 140
Dental Services Exclusion

A3-3162, HO-260.13, B3-2336

Items and services in connection with the care, treatment, filling, removal, or replacement of teeth, or structures directly supporting the teeth are not covered. Structures directly supporting the teeth mean the periodontium, which includes the gingivae, dentogingival junction, periodontal membrane, cementum, and alveolar process. However, payment may be made for certain other services of a dentist. (See the Medicare Benefit Policy Manual, Chapter 15, "Covered Medical and Other Health Services," §150.)

The hospitalization or nonhospitalization of a patient has no direct bearing on the coverage or exclusion of a given dental procedure.

When an excluded service is the primary procedure involved, it is not covered regardless of its complexity or difficulty. For example, the extraction of an impacted tooth is not covered. Similarly, an alveoplasty (the surgical improvement of the shape and condition of the alveolar process) and a frenectomy are excluded from coverage when either of these procedures is performed in connection with an excluded service, e.g., the preparation of the mouth for dentures. In like manner, the removal of the torus palatinus (a bony protuberance of the hard palate) could be a covered service. However, with rare exception, this surgery is performed in connection with an excluded service, i.e., the preparation of the mouth for dentures. Under such circumstances, reimbursement is not made for this purpose.

The extraction of teeth to prepare the jaw for radiation treatments of neoplastic disease is also covered. This is an exception to the requirement that to be covered, a noncovered procedure or service performed by a dentist must be an incident to and an integral part of a covered procedure or service performed by the dentist. Ordinarily, the dentist extracts the patient's teeth, but another physician, e.g., a radiologist, administers the radiation treatments.

Whether such services as the administration of anesthesia, diagnostic x-rays, and other related procedures are covered depends upon whether the primary procedure being performed by the dentist is covered. Thus, an x-ray taken in connection with the reduction of a fracture of the jaw or facial bone is covered. However, a single x-ray or x-ray survey taken in connection with the care or treatment of teeth or the periodontium is not covered.

See also the Medicare Benefit Policy Manual, Chapter 1, "Inpatient Hospital Services," §70, and Chapter 15, "Covered Medical and Other Health Services," §150 for additional information on dental services.

Pub. 100-3, Section 20.8
Cardiac Pacemakers

Cardiac pacemakers are covered as prosthetic devices under the Medicare program, subject to the following conditions and limitations. While cardiac pacemakers have been covered under Medicare for many years, there were no specific guidelines for their use other than the general Medicare requirement that covered services be reasonable and necessary for the treatment of the condition. Services rendered for cardiac pacing on or after the effective dates of this instruction are subject to these guidelines, which are based on certain assumptions regarding the clinical goals of cardiac pacing. While some uses of pacemakers are relatively certain or unambiguous, many other uses require considerable expertise and judgment.

Consequently, the medical necessity for permanent cardiac pacing must be viewed in the context of overall patient management. The appropriateness of such pacing may be conditional on other diagnostic or therapeutic modalities having been undertaken. Although significant complications and adverse side effects of pacemaker use are relatively rare, they cannot be ignored when considering the use of pacemakers for dubious medical conditions, or marginal clinical benefit.

These guidelines represent current concepts regarding medical circumstances in which permanent cardiac pacing may be appropriate or necessary. As with other areas of medicine, advances in knowledge and techniques in cardiology are expected. Consequently, judgments about the medical necessity and acceptability of new uses for cardiac pacing in new classes of patients may change as more more conclusive evidence becomes available. This instruction applies only to permanent cardiac pacemakers, and does not address the use of temporary, non-implanted pacemakers.

The two groups of conditions outlined below deal with the necessity for cardiac pacing for patients in general. These are intended as guidelines in assessing the medical necessity for pacing therapies, taking into account the particular circumstances in each case. However, as a general rule, the two groups of current medical concepts may be viewed as representing:

Group I: Single-Chamber Cardiac Pacemakers – a) conditions under which single chamber pacemaker claims may be considered covered without further claims development; and b) conditions under which single-chamber pacemaker claims would be denied unless further claims development shows that they fall into the covered category, or special medical circumstances exist of the sufficiency to convince the contractor that the claim should be paid.

Group II: Dual-Chamber Cardiac Pacemakers - a) conditions under which dual-chamber pacemaker claims may be considered covered without further claims development, and b) conditions under which dual-chamber pacemaker claims would be denied unless further claims development shows that they fall into the covered categories for single- and dual-chamber pacemakers, or special medical circumstances exist sufficient to convince the contractor that the claim should be paid.

CMS opened the NCD on Cardiac Pacemakers to afford the public an opportunity to comment on the proposal to revise the language contained in the instruction. The revisions transfer the focus of the NCD from the actual pacemaker implantation procedure itself to the reasonable and necessary medical indications that justify cardiac pacing. This is consistent with our findings that pacemaker implantation is no longer considered routinely harmful or an experimental procedure.

Group I: Single-Chamber Cardiac Pacemakers (Effective March 16, 1983)

A. Nationally Covered Indications

Conditions under which cardiac pacing is generally considered acceptable or necessary, provided that the conditions are chronic or recurrent and not due to transient causes such as acute myocardial infarction, drug toxicity, or electrolyte imbalance. (In cases where there is a rhythm disturbance, if the rhythm disturbance is chronic or recurrent, a single episode of a symptom such as syncope or seizure is adequate to establish medical necessity.)

1. Acquired complete (also referred to as third-degree) AV heart block.
2. Congenital complete heart block with severe bradycardia (in relation to age), or significant physiological deficits or significant symptoms due to the bradycardia.
3. Second-degree AV heart block of Type II (i.e., no progressive prolongation of P-R interval prior to each blocked beat. P-R interval indicates the time taken for an impulse to travel from the atria to the ventricles on an electrocardiogram).
4. Second-degree AV heart block of Type I (i.e., progressive prolongation of P-R interval prior to each blocked beat) with significant symptoms due to hemodynamic instability associated with the heart block.
5. Sinus bradycardia associated with major symptoms (e.g., syncope, seizures, congestive heart failure); or substantial sinus bradycardia (heart rate less than 50) associated with dizziness or confusion. The correlation between symptoms and bradycardia must be documented, or the symptoms must be clearly attributable to the bradycardia rather than to some other cause.
6. In selected and few patients, sinus bradycardia of lesser severity (heart rate 50-59) with dizziness or confusion. The correlation between symptoms and bradycardia must be documented, or the symptoms must be clearly attributable to the bradycardia rather than to some other cause.
7. Sinus bradycardia is the consequence of long-term necessary drug treatment for which there is no acceptable alternative when accompanied by significant symptoms (e.g., syncope, seizures, congestive heart failure, dizziness or confusion). The correlation between symptoms and bradycardia must be documented, or the symptoms must be clearly attributable to the bradycardia rather than to some other cause.
8. Sinus node dysfunction with or without tachyarrhythmias or AV conduction block (i.e., the bradycardia-tachycardia syndrome, sino-atrial block, sinus arrest) when accompanied by significant symptoms (e.g., syncope, seizures, congestive heart failure, dizziness or confusion).
9. Sinus node dysfunction with or without symptoms when there are potentially life-threatening ventricular arrhythmias or tachycardia secondary to the bradycardia (e.g., numerous premature ventricular contractions, couplets, runs of premature ventricular contractions, or ventricular tachycardia).
10. Bradycardia associated with supraventricular tachycardia (e.g., atrial fibrillation, atrial flutter, or paroxysmal atrial tachycardia) with high-degree AV block which is unresponsive to appropriate pharmacological management and when the bradycardia is associated with significant symptoms (e.g., syncope, seizures, congestive heart failure, dizziness or confusion).
11. The occasional patient with hypersensitive carotid sinus syndrome with syncope due to bradycardia and unresponsive to prophylactic medical measures.
12. Bifascicular or trifascicular block accompanied by syncope which is attributed to transient complete heart block after other plausible causes of syncope have been reasonably excluded.
13. Prophylactic pacemaker use following recovery from acute myocardial infarction during which there was temporary complete (third-degree) and/or Mobitz Type II second-degree AV block in association with bundle branch block.
14. In patients with recurrent and refractory ventricular tachycardia, "overdrive pacing" (pacing above the basal rate) to prevent ventricular tachycardia.

(Effective May 9, 1985)

15. Second-degree AV heart block of Type I with the QRS complexes prolonged.

B. Nationally Noncovered Indications

Conditions which, although used by some physicians as a basis for permanent cardiac pacing, are considered unsupported by adequate evidence of benefit and therefore should not generally be considered appropriate uses for single-chamber pacemakers in the absence of the above indications. Contractors should review claims for pacemakers with these indications to determine the need for further claims development prior to denying the claim, since additional claims development may be required. The object of such further development is to establish whether the particular claim actually meets the conditions in a) above. In claims where this is not the case or where such an event appears unlikely, the contractor may deny the claim

1. Syncope of undetermined cause.
2. Sinus bradycardia without significant symptoms.
3. Sino-atrial block or sinus arrest without significant symptoms.
4. Prolonged P-R intervals with atrial fibrillation (without third-degree AV block) or with other causes of transient ventricular pause.
5. Bradycardia during sleep.
6. Right bundle branch block with left axis deviation (and other forms of fascicular or bundle branch block) without syncope or other symptoms of intermittent AV block).
7. Asymptomatic second-degree AV block of Type I unless the QRS complexes are prolonged or electrophysiological studies have demonstrated that the block is at or beyond the level of the His bundle (a component of the electrical conduction system of the heart).

Effective October 1, 2001

8. Asymptomatic bradycardia in post-mycardial infarction patients about to initiate long-term beta-blocker drug therapy.

Group II: Dual-Chamber Cardiac Pacemakers – (Effective May 9, 1985)

A. Nationally Covered Indications

Conditions under dual-chamber cardiac pacing are considered acceptable or necessary in the general medical community unless conditions 1 and 2 under Group II. B., are present:

1. Patients in who single-chamber (ventricular pacing) at the time of pacemaker insertion elicits a definite drop in blood pressure, retrograde conduction, or discomfort.
2. Patients in whom the pacemaker syndrome (atrial ventricular asynchrony), with significant symptoms, has already been experienced with a pacemaker that is being replaced.
3. Patients in whom even a relatively small increase in cardiac efficiency will importantly improve the quality of life, e.g., patients with congestive heart failure despite adequate other medical measures.
4. Patients in whom the pacemaker syndrome can be anticipated, e.g., in young and active people, etc.

Dual-chamber pacemakers may also be covered for the conditions, as listed in Group I. A., if the medical necessity is sufficiently justified through adequate claims development. Expert physicians differ in their judgments about what constitutes appropriate criteria for dual-chamber pacemaker use. The judgment that such a pacemaker is warranted in the patient meeting accepted criteria must be based upon the individual needs and characteristics of that patient, weighing the magnitude and likelihood of anticipated benefits against the magnitude and likelihood of disadvantages to the patient.

B. Nationally Noncovered Indications

Whenever the following conditions (which represent overriding contraindications) are present, dual-chamber pacemakers are not covered:

1. Ineffective atrial contractions (e.g., chronic atrial fibrillation or flutter, or giant left atrium.
2. Frequent or persistent supraventricular tachycardias, except where the pacemaker is specifically for the control of the tachycardia.
3. A clinical condition in which pacing takes place only intermittently and briefly, and which is not associated with a reasonable likelihood that pacing needs will become prolonged, e.g., the occasional patient with hypersensitive carotid sinus syndrome with syncope due to bradycardia and unresponsive to prophylactic medical measures.
4. Prophylactic pacemaker use following recovery from acute myocardial infarction during which there was temporary complete (third-degree) and/or Type II second-degree AV block in association with bundle branch block.

C. Other

All other indications for dual-chamber cardiac pacing for which CMS has not specifically indicated coverage remain nationally noncovered, ecept for Category B IDE clinical trails, or as routine costs of dual-chamber cardiac pacing associated with clinical trials, in accordance with section 310.1 of the NCD Manual..

(This NCD last reviewed June 2004.)

Pub. 100-3, Section 20.8.1
Cardiac Pacemaker Evaluation Services

Medicare covers a variety of services for the post-implant follow-up and evaluation of implanted cardiac pacemakers. The following guidelines are designed to assist contractors in identifying and processing claims for such services.

NOTE: These new guidelines are limited to lithium battery-powered pacemakers, because mercury-zinc battery-powered pacemakers are no longer being manufactured and virtually all have been replaced by lithium units. Contractors still receiving claims for monitoring such units should continue to apply the guidelines published in 1980 to those units until they are replaced.

One fact of which contractors should be aware is that many dual-chamber units may be programmed to pace only the ventricles; this may be done either at the time the pacemaker is implanted or at some time afterward. In such cases, a dual-chamber unit, when programmed or reprogrammed for ventricular pacing, should be treated as a single-chamber pacemaker in applying screening guidelines.

The decision as to how often any patient's pacemaker should be monitored is the responsibility of the patient's physician who is best able to take into account the condition and circumstances of the individual patient. These may vary over time, requiring modifications of the frequency with which the patient should be monitored. In cases where monitoring is done by some entity other than the patient's physician, such as a commercial monitoring service or hospital outpatient department, the physician's prescription for monitoring is required and should be periodically renewed (at least annually) to assure that the frequency of monitoring is proper for the patient. When a patient is monitored both during clinica visits and transtelephonically, the contractor should be sure to include frequency data on both ypes of monitoring in evaluating the reasonableness of the frequency of monitoring services received by the patient.

Since there are over 200 pacemaker models in service at any given point, and a variety of patient conditions that give rise to the need for pacemakers, the question of the appropriate frequency of monitorings is a complex one. Nevertheless, it is possible to develop guidelines within which the vast majority of pacemaker monitorings will fall and contractors should do this, using their own data and experience, as well as the frequency guidelines which follow, in order to limit extensive claims development to those cases requiring special attention.

Pub. 100-3, Section 20.8.2
Self-Contained Pacemaker Monitors

Self-contained pacemaker monitors are accepted devices for monitoring cardiac pacemakers. Accordingly, program payment may be made for the rental or purchase of either of the following pacemaker monitors when it is prescribed by a physician for a patient with a cardiac pacemaker:

A. Digital Electronic Pacemaker Monitor.--This device provides the patient with an instantaneous digital readout of his pacemaker pulse rate. Use of this device does not involve professional services until there has been a change of five pulses (or more) per minute above or below the initial rate of the pacemaker; when such change occurs, the patient contacts his physician.

B. Audible/Visible Signal Pacemaker Monitor.--This device produces an audible and visible signal which indicates the pacemaker rate. Use of this device does not involve professional services until a change occurs in these signals; at such time, the patient contacts his physician.

NOTE: The design of the self-contained pacemaker monitor makes it possible for the patient to monitor his pacemaker periodically and minimizes the need for regular visits to the outpatient department of the provider.

Therefore, documentation of the medical necessity for pacemaker evaluation in the outpatient department of the provider should be obtained where such evaluation is employed in addition to the self-contained pacemaker monitor used by the patient in his home.

Pub. 100-3, Section 20.9
Artificial Hearts and Related Devices

A. Covered Indications

1. Post-cardiotomy (effective for services performed on or after October 18, 1993)

Post-cardiotomy is the period following open-heart surgery. VADs used for support of blood circulation post-cardiotomy are covered only if they have received approval from the Food and Drug Administration (FDA) for that purpose, and the VADs are used according to the FDA-approved labeling instructions.

2. Bridge-to-Transplant (effective for services performed on or after January 22, 1996)

VADs used for bridge-to-transplant are covered only if they have received approval from the FDA for that purpose, and the VADs are used according to the FDA-approved labeling instructions. All of the following criteria must be fulfilled in order for Medicare coverage to be provided for a VAD used as a bridge-to-transplant:

    a. The patient is approved and listed as a candidate for heart transplantation by a Medicare-approved heart transplant center; and,

    b. The implanting site, if different than the Medicare-approved transplant center, must receive written permission from the Medicare-approved heart transplant center under which the patient is listed prior to implantation of the VAD.

The Medicare-approved heart transplant center should make every reasonable effort to transplant patients on such devices as soon as medically reasonable. Ideally, the Medicare-approved heart transplant centers should determine patient-specific timetables for transplantation, and should not maintain such patients on VADs if suitable hearts become available.

3. Destination Therapy (effective for services performed on or after October 1, 2003)

Destination therapy is for patients that require permanent mechanical cardiac support. VADs used for destination therapy are covered only if they have received approval from the FDA for that purpose, and the device is used according to the FDA-approved labeling instructions. VADs are covered for patients who have chronic end-stage heart failure (New York Heart Association Class IV end-stage left ventricular failure for at least 90 days with a life expectancy of less than 2 years), are not candidates for heart transplantation, and meet **all** of the following conditions:

    a. The patient's Class IV heart failure symptoms have failed to respond to optimal medical management, including dietary salt restriction, diuretics, digitalis, beta-blockers, and ACE inhibitors (if tolerated) for at least 60 of the last 90 days;

    b. The patient has a left ventricular ejection fraction (LVEF) < 25%;

    c. The patient has demonstrated functional limitation with a peak oxygen consumption of < 12 ml/kg/min; **or** the patient has a continued need for intravenous inotropic therapy owing to symptomatic hypotension, decreasing renal function, or worsening pulmonary congestion; **and**

    d. The patient has the appropriate body size > to support the VAD implantation.

In addition, the Centers for Medicare & Medicaid Services (CMS) has determined that VAD implantation as destination therapy is reasonable and necessary only when the procedure is performed in a Medicare-approved heart transplant facility that, between January 1, 2001, and September 30, 2003, implanted at least 15 VADs as a bridge-to-transplant or as destination therapy. These devices must have been approved by the FDA for destination therapy or as a bridge-to-transplant, or have been implanted as part of an FDA investigational device exemption (IDE) trial for one of these two indications. VADs implanted for other investigational indications or for support of blood circulation post-cardiotomy do not satisfy the volume requirement for this purpose. Since the relationship between volume and outcomes has not been well-established for VAD use, facilities that have minimal deficiencies in meeting this standard may apply and include a request for an exception based upon additional factors. Some of the factors CMS will consider are geographic location of the center, number of destination procedures performed, and patient outcomes from VAD procedures completed.

Also, this facility must be an active, continuous member of a national, audited registry that requires submission of health data on all VAD destination therapy patients from the date of implantation throughout the remainder of their lives. This registry must have the ability to accommodate data related to any device approved by the FDA for destination therapy regardless of manufacturer. The registry must also provide such routine reports as may be specified by CMS, and must have standards for data quality and timeliness of data submissions such that hospitals failing to meet them will be removed from membership. CMS believes that the registry sponsored by the International Society for Heart and Lung Transplantation is an example of a registry that meets these characteristics.

Hospitals also must have in place staff and procedures that ensure that prospective VAD recipients receive all information necessary to assist them in giving appropriate informed consent for the procedure so that they and their families are fully aware of the aftercare requirements and potential limitations, as well as benefits, following VAD implantation.

CMS plans to develop accreditation standards for facilities that implant VADs and, when implemented, VAD implantation will be considered reasonable and necessary only at accredited facilities.

A list of facilities eligible for Medicare reimbursement for VADs as destination therapy will be maintained on our website and available at www.cms.hhs.gov/coverage/lvadfacility.asp. In order to be placed on this list, facilities must submit a letter to the Director, Coverage and Analysis Group, 7500 Security Blvd, Mailstop C1-09-06, Baltimore, MD 21244. This letter must be received by CMS within 90 days of the issue date on this transmittal. The letter must include the following information

- Facility's name and complete address;
- Facility's Medicare provider number;
- List of all implantations between Jan. 1, 2001, and Sept. 30, 2003, with the following information:
  - Date of implantation;
  - Indication for implantation (only destination and bridge-to-transplant can be reported; post-cardiotomy VAD implants are not to be included),
  - Device name and manufacturer, and,
  - Date of device removal and reason (e.g., transplantation, recovery, device malfunction), or date and cause of patient's death;
- Point-of-contact for questions with telephone number
- Registry to which patient information will be submitted; **and**
- Signature of a senior facility administrative official.

Facilities not meeting the minimal standards and requesting exception should, in addition to supplying the information above, include the factors that they deem critical in requesting the exception to the standards.

CMS will review the information contained in the above letters. When the review is complete, all necessary information is received, and criteria are met, CMS will include the name of the newly Medicare-approved facility on the CMS web site. No reimbursement for destination therapy will be made for implantations performed before the date the facility is added to the CMS web site. Each newly approved facility will also receive a formal letter from CMS stating the official approval date it was added to the list.

B. Noncovered Indications (effective for services performed on or after May 19, 1986)

1.Artificial Heart

Since there is no authoritative evidence substantiating the safety and effectiveness of a VAD used as a replacement for the human heart, Medicare does not cover this device when used as an artificial heart.

2. All other indications for the use of VADs not otherwise listed remain noncovered, except in the context of Category B IDE clinical trials (42 CFR 405) or as a routine cost in clinical trials defined under section 310.1 of the NCD manual (old CIM 30-1).

(This NCD last reviewed October 2003.)

Pub. 100-3, Section 20.15
Electrocardiographic Services

Reimbursement may be made under Part B for electrocardiographic (EKG) services rendered by a physician or incident to his/her services or by an approved laboratory or an approved supplier of portable X-ray services. Since there is no coverage for EKG services of any type rendered on a screening basis or as part of a routine examination, the claim must indicate the signs and symptoms or other clinical reason necessitating the services.

A separate charge by an attending or consulting physician for EKG interpretation is allowed only when it is the normal practice to make such charge in addition to the regular office visit charge. No payment is made for EKG interpretations by individuals other than physicians.

On a claim involving EKG services furnished by a laboratory or portable x-ray supplier, identify the physician ordering the service and, when the charge includes both the taking of the tracing and its interpretation, include the identity of the physician making the interpretation. No separate bill for the services of a physician is paid unless it is clear that he/she was the patient's attending physician or was acting as a consulting physician. The taking of an EKG in an emergency, i.e., when the patient is or may be experiencing what is commonly referred to as a heart attack, is covered as a laboratory service or a diagnostic service by a portable X-ray supplier only when the evidence shows that a physician was in attendance at the time the service was performed or immediately thereafter.

The documentation required in the various situations mentioned above must be furnished not only when the laboratory or portable X-ray supplier bills the patient or carrier for its service, but also when such a facility bills the attending physician who, in turn, bills the patient or carrier for the EKG services.(In addition to the evidence required to document the claim, the laboratory or portable x-ray supplier must maintain in its records the referring physician 's written order and the identity of the employee taking the tracing.)

Long Term EKG Monitoring, also referred to as long-term EKG recording, Holter recording, or dynamic electrocardiography, is a diagnostic procedure which provides a continuous record of the electrocardiographic activity of a patient's heart while he is engaged in his daily activities.

The basic components of the long-term EKG monitoring systems are a sensing element, the design of which may provide either for the recording of electrocardiographic information on magnetic tape or for detecting significant variations in rate or rhythm as they occur, and a component for either graphically recording the electrocardiographic data or for visual or computer assisted analysis of the information recorded on magnetic tape. The long-term EKG permits the examination in the ambulant or potentially ambulant patient of as many as 70,000 heartbeats in a 12-hour recording while the standard EKG which is obtained in the recumbent position, yields information on only 50 to 60 cardiac cycles and provides only a limited data base on which diagnostic judgments may be made.

Many patients with cardiac arrhythmias are unaware of the presence of an irregularity in heart rhythm. Due to the transient nature of many arrhythmias and the short intervals in which the rhythm of the heart is observed by conventional standard EKG techniques, the offending arrhythmias can go undetected. With the extended examination provided by the long-term EKG, the physician is able not only to detect but also to classify various types of rhythm disturbances and waveform abnormalities and note the frequency of their occurrence. The knowledge of the reaction of the heart to daily activities with respect to rhythm, rate, conduction disturbances, and changes are of great assistance in directing proper therapy and

This modality is valuable in both inpatient and outpatient diagnosis and therapy. Long-term monitoring of ambulant or potentially ambulant inpatients provides significant potential for reducing the length of stay for post-coronary infarct patients in the intensive care setting and may result in earlier discharge from the hospital with greater assurance of safety to the patients. The indications for the use of this technique, noted below, are similar for both inpatients and outpatients.

The long-term EKG has proven effective in detecting transient episodes of cardiac dysrhythmia and in permitting the correlation of these episodes with cardiovascular symptomatology.It is also useful for patients who have symptoms of obscure etiology

suggestive of cardiac arrhythmia.Examples of such symptoms include palpitations, chest pain, dizziness, light-headedness, near syncope, syncope, transient ischemic episodes, dyspnea, and shortness of breath.

This technique would also be appropriate at the time of institution of any arrhythmic drug therapy and may be performed during the course of therapy to evaluate response.It is also appropriate for evaluating a change of dosage and may be indicated shortly before and after the discontinuation of anti-arrhythemic medication.The therapeutic response to a drug whose duration of action and peak of effectiveness is defined in hours cannot be properly assessed by examining 30-40 cycles on a standard EKG rhythm strip.The knowledge that all patients placed on anti-arrhythmic medication do not respond to therapy and the known toxicity of anti-arrhythmic agents clearly indicate that proper assessment should be made on an individual basis to determine whether medication should be continued and at what dosage level.

The long-term EKG is also valuable in the assessment of patients with coronary artery disease. It enables the documentation of etiology of such symptoms as chest pain and shortness of breath.Since the standard EKG is often normal during the intervals between the episodes of precordial pain, it is essential to obtain EKG information while the symptoms are occurring. The long-term EKG has enabled the correlation of chest symptoms with the objective evidence of ST-segment abnormalities.It is appropriate for patients who are recovering from an acute mycardial infarction or coronary insufficiency before and after discharge from the hospital, since it is impossible to predict which of these patients is subject to ventricular arrhythmias on the basis of the presence or absence of rhythm disturbances during the period of initial coronary care. The long-term EKG enables the physician to identify patients who are at a higher risk of dying suddenly in the period following an acute myocardial infarction.It may also be reasonable and necessary where the high-risk patient with known cardiovascular disease advances to a substantially higher level of activity which might trigger increased or new types of arrhythmias necessitating treatment. Such a high-risk case would be one in which there is documentation that acute phase arrhythmias have not totally disappeared during the period of convalescence.

The use of the long-term EKG for routine assessment of pacemaker function can no longer be justified (see §20.8.1). Its use for the patient with an internal pacemaker would be covered only when he has symptoms suggestive of arrhythmia not revealed by the standard EKG or rhythm strip.

These guidelines are intended as a general outline of the circumstances under which the use of this diagnostic procedure would be warranted. Each patient receiving a long-term EKG should be evaluated completely, prior to performance of this diagnostic study. A complete history and physical examination should be obtained and the referring physician should review the indications for use of the long-term EKG.

The performance of a long-term EKG does not necessarily require the prior performance of a standard EKG. Nor does the demonstration of a normal standard EKG preclude the need for a long- term EKG. Finally, the demonstration of an abnormal standard EKG does not obviate the need for a long-term EKG if there is suspicion that the dysrhythmia is transient in nature.

A period of recording of up to 24 hours would normally be adequate to detect most transient arrhythmias and provide essential diagnostic information. The medical necessity for longer periods of monitoring must be documented.

Medical documentation for adjudicating claims for the use of the long-term EKG should be similar to other EKG services, X-ray services, and laboratory procedures. Generally, a statement of the diagnostic impression of the referring physician with an indication of the patient's relevant signs and symptoms should be sufficient for purposes of making a determination regarding the reasonableness and medical necessity for the use of this procedure. However, the intermediaries or carriers should require whatever additional documentation their medical consultants deem necessary to properly adjudicate the individual claim where the information submitted is not adequate.

It should be noted that the recording device furnished to the patient is simply one component of the diagnostic system and a separate charge for it will not be recognized under the durable medical equipment benefit.

Patient-Activated EKG Recorders, distributed under a variety of brand names, permit the patient to record an EKG upon manifestation of symptoms, or in response to a physician's order (e.g., immediately following strong exertion).Most such devices also permit the patient to simultaneously voice-record in order to describe symptoms and/or activity. In addition, some of these devices permit transtelephonic transmission of the recording to a physician's office, clinic, hospital, etc., having a decoder/recorder for review and analysis, thus eliminating the need to physically transport the tape. Some of these devices also permit a "time sampling" mode of operation. However, the "time sampling" mode is not covered--only the patient-activated mode of operation, when used for the indications described below, is covered at this time.

Services in connection with patient-activated EKG recorders are covered when used as an alternative to the long-term EKG monitoring (described above) for similar indications--detecting and characterizing symptomatic arrhythmias, regulation of anti-arrhythmic drug therapy, etc. Like long- term EKG monitoring, use of these devices is covered for evaluating patients with symptoms of obscure etiology suggestive of cardiac arrhythmia such as palpitations, chest pain, dizziness, lightheadedness, near syncope, syncope, transient ischemic episodes, dyspnea and shortness of breath.

As with long-term EKG monitors, patient-activated EKG recorders may be useful for both inpatient and outpatient diagnosis and therapy.While useful for assessing some post-coronary infarct patients in the hospital setting, these devices should not, however, be covered for outpatient monitoring of recently discharged post-infarct patients.

Computer Analyzed Electrocardiograms-Computer interpretation of EKG's is recognized as a valid and effective technique which will improve the quality and availability of cardiology services. Reimbursement may be made for such computer interpretation when furnished in the setting and under the circumstances required for coverage of other electrocardiographic services. Where either a laboratory's or a portable x-ray supplier's charge for EKG services includes the physician review and certification of the printout as well as the computer interpretation, the certifying physician must be identified on the HCFA-1490 before the entire charge can be considered a reimbursable charge. Where the laboratory's (or portable x-ray supplier's) reviewing physician is not identified, the carrier should conclude that no professional component is involved and make its charge determination accordingly. If the supplying laboratory (or portable x-ray supplier when supplied by such a facility) does not include professional review and certification of the hard copy, a charge by the patient's physician may be recognized for the service. In any case the charge for the physician component should be substantially less than that for physician interpretation of the conventional EKG tracing in view of markedly reduced demand on the physician's time where computer interpretation is involved. Considering the unit cost reduction expected of this innovation, the total charge for the complete EKG service (taking of tracing and interpretation) when computer interpretation is employed should never exceed that considered reasonable for the service when physician interpretation is involved.

Transtelephonic Electrocardiographic Transmissions (Formerly Referred to as EKG Telephone Reporter Systems) is extended to include the use of transtelephonic electrocardiographic (EKG) transmissions as a diagnostic service for the indications described below, when performed with equipment meeting the standards described below, subject to the limitations and conditions specified below. Coverage is further limited to the amounts payable with respect to the physician's service in interpreting the results of such transmissions, including charges for rental of the equipment. The device used by the beneficiary is part of a total diagnostic system and is not considered durable medical equipment.

1. Covered Uses

The use of transtelephonic EKGs is covered for the following uses:

- To detect, characterize, and document symptomatic transient arrhythmias;
- To overcome problems in regulating antiarrhythmic drug dosage;
- To carry out early posthospital monitoring of patients discharged after myocardial infarction; (only if 24-hour coverage is provided, see 4. below).

Since cardiology is a rapidly changing field, some uses other than those specified above may be covered if, in the judgment of the contractor's medical consultants, such a use was justifiable in the particular case. The enumerated uses above represent uses for which a firm coverage determination has been made, and for which contractors may make payment without extensive claims development or review.

2. Specifications for Devices

The devices used by the patient are highly portable (usually pocket-sized) and detect and convert the normal EKG signal so that it can be transmitted via ordinary telephone apparatus to a receiving station. At the receiving end, the signal is decoded and transcribed into a conventional EKG. There are numerous devices available which transmit EKG readings in this fashion. For purposes of Medicare coverage, however, the transmitting devices must meet at least the following criteria:

- They must be capable of transmitting EKG Leads, I, II, or III;
- These lead transmissions must be sufficiently comparable to readings obtained by a conventional EKG to permit proper interpretation of abnormal cardiac rhythms.

3. Potential for Abuse - Need for Screening Guidelines

While the use of these devices may often compare favorably with more costly alternatives, this is the case only where the information they contribute is actively utilized by a knowledgeable practitioner as part of overall medical management of the patient. Consequently, it is vital that contractors be aware of the potential for abuse of these devices, and adopt necessary screening and physician education policies to detect and halt potentially abusive situations. For example, use of these devices to diagnose and treat suspected arrhythmias as a routine substitute for more conventional methods of diagnosis, such as a careful history, physical examination, and standard EKG and rhythm strip would not be appropriate. Moreover, contractors should require written justification for use of such devices in excess of 30 consecutive days in cases involving detection of transient arrhythmias.

Contractors may find it useful to review claims for these devices with a view toward detecting patterns of practice which may be useful in developing schedules which may be adopted for screening such claims in the future.

4. Twenty-four Hour Coverage

No payment may be made for the use of these devices to carry out early posthospital monitoring of patients discharged after myocardial infarction unless provision is made for 24 hour coverage in the manner described below.

Twenty-four hour coverage means that there must be, at the monitoring site (or sites) an experienced EKG technician receiving calls; tape recording devices do not meet this requirement. Further, such technicians should have immediate access to a physician, and

have been instructed in when and how to contact available facilities to assist the patient in case of emergencies.

Pub. 100-3, Section 20.19
Ambulatory Blood Pressure Monitoring

ABPM must be performed for at least 24 hours to meet coverage criteria.

ABPM is only covered for those patients with suspected white coat hypertension. Suspected white coat hypertension is defined as

1) office blood pressure >140/90 mm Hg on at least three separate clinic/office visits with two separate measurements made at each visit;

2) at least two documented blood pressure measurements taken outside the office which are <140/90 mm Hg; and

3) no evidence of end-organ damage.

The information obtained by ABPM is necessary in order to determine the appropriate management of the patient. ABPM is not covered for any other uses. In the rare circumstance that ABPM needs to be performed more than once in a patient, the qualifying criteria described above must be met for each subsequent ABPM test.

For those patients that undergo ABPM and have an ambulatory blood pressure of <135/85 with no evidence of end-organ damage, it is likely that their cardiovascular risk is similar to that of normotensives. They should be followed over time. Patients for which ABPM demonstrates a blood pressure of >135/85 may be at increased cardiovascular risk, and a physician may wish to consider antihypertensive therapy.

Pub. 100-3, Section 20.20
External Counterpulsation (ECP) for Severe Angina

Although ECP devices are cleared by the Food and Drug Administration (FDA) for use in treating a variety of cardiac conditions, including stable or unstable angina pectoris, acute myocardial infarction and cardiogenic shock, the use of this device to treat cardiac conditions other than stable angina pectoris is not covered, since only that use has developed sufficient evidence to demonstrate its medical effectiveness. Non-coverage of hydraulic versions of these types of devices remains in force.

Coverage is provided for the use of ECP for patients who have been diagnosed with disabling angina (Class III or Class IV, Canadian Cardiovascular Society Classification or equivalent classification) who, in the opinion of a cardiologist or cardiothoracic surgeon, are not readily amenable to surgical intervention, such as PTCA or cardiac bypass because:

1. Their condition is inoperable, or at high risk of operative complications or post-operative failure;
2. Their coronary anatomy is not readily amenable to such procedures; or
3. They have co-morbid states which create excessive risk.

A full course of therapy usually consists of 35 one-hour treatments, which may be offered once or twice daily, usually 5 days per week. The patient is placed on a treatment table where their lower trunk and lower extremities are wrapped in a series of three compressive air cuffs which inflate and deflate in synchronization with the patient's cardiac cycle.

During diastole the three sets of air cuffs are inflated sequentially (distal to proximal) compressing the vascular beds within the muscles of the calves, lower thighs and upper thighs. This action results in an increase in diastolic pressure, generation of retrograde arterial blood flow and an increase in venous return. The cuffs are deflated simultaneously just prior to systole, which produces a rapid drop in vascular impedance, a decrease in ventricular workload and an increase in cardiac output.

The augmented diastolic pressure and retrograde aortic flow appear to improve myocardial perfusion, while systolic unloading appears to reduce cardiac workload and oxygen requirements. The increased venous return coupled with enhanced systolic flow appears to increase cardiac output. As a result of this treatment, most patients experience increased time until onset of ischemia, increased exercise tolerance, and a reduction in the number and severity of anginal episodes. Evidence was presented that this effect lasted well beyond the immediate post-treatment phase, with patients symptom-free for several months to two years.

This procedure must be done under direct supervision of a physician.

Pub. 100-3, Section 20.21
Chelation Therapy for Treatment of Atherosclerosis

The application of chelation therapy using ethylenediamine-tetra-acetic acid (EDTA) for the treatment and prevention of atherosclerosis is controversial. There is no widely accepted rationale to explain the beneficial effects attributed to this therapy. Its safety is questioned and its clinical effectiveness has never been established by well designed, controlled clinical trials. It is not widely accepted and practiced by American physicians. EDTA chelation therapy for atherosclerosis is considered experimental. For these reasons, EDTA chelation therapy for the treatment or prevention of atherosclerosis is not covered.

Some practitioners refer to this therapy as chemoendarterectomy and may also show a diagnosis other than atherosclerosis, such as arteriosclerosis or calcinosis. Claims employing such variant terms should also be denied under this section.

Pub. 100-3, Section 20.22
Ethylenediamine-Tetra-Acetic (EDTA) Chelation Therapy for Treatment of Atherosclerosis

The use of EDTA as a chelating agent to treat atherosclerosis, arteriosclerosis, calcinosis, or similar generalized condition not listed by the FDA as an approved use is not covered. Any such use of EDTA is considered experimental.

Pub. 100-3, Section 20.23
Fabric Wrapping of Abdominal Aneurysms

Fabric wrapping of abdominal aneurysms is not a covered Medicare procedure. This is a treatment for abdominal aneurysms which involves wrapping aneurysms with cellophane or fascia lata. This procedure has not been shown to prevent eventual rupture. In extremely rare instances, external wall reinforcement may be indicated when the current accepted treatment (excision of the aneurysm and reconstruction with synthetic materials) is not a viable alternative, but external wall reinforcement is not fabric wrapping. Accordingly, fabric wrapping of abdominal aneurysms is not considered reasonable and necessary within the meaning of §1862(a)(1) of the Act.

Pub. 100-3, Section 20.24
Displacement Cardiography

A.-Cardiokymography

Cardiokymography is covered for services rendered on or after October 12, 1998.

Cardiokymography is a covered service only when it is used as an adjunct to electrocardiographic stress testing in evaluating coronary artery disease and only when the following clinical indications are present:

- For male patients, atypical angina pectoris or nonischemic chest pain; or
- For female patients, angina, either typical or atypical.

B. Photokymography-NOT COVERED

Photokymography remains excluded from coverage

Pub. 100-3, Section 20.29
Hyperbaric Oxygen Therapy

A. Covered Conditions.--Program reimbursement for HBO therapy will be limited to that which is administered in a chamber (including the one man unit) and is limited to the following conditions:
  1. Acute carbon monoxide intoxication, (ICD-9-CM diagnosis 986).
  2. Decompression illness, (ICD-9-CM diagnosis 993.2, 993.3).
  3. Gas embolism, (ICD-9-CM diagnosis 958.0, 999.1).
  4. Gas gangrene, (ICD-9-CM diagnosis 0400).
  5. Acute traumatic peripheral ischemia. HBO therapy is a valuable adjunctive treatment to be used in combination with accepted standard therapeutic measures when loss of function, limb, or life is threatened. (ICD-9-CM diagnosis 902.53, 903.01, 903.1, 904.0, 904.41.)
  6. Crush injuries and suturing of severed limbs. As in the previous conditions, HBO therapy would be an adjunctive treatment when loss of function, limb, or life is threatened. (ICD-9-CM diagnosis 927.00-927.03, 927.09-927.11, 927.20-927.21, 927.8-927.9, 928.00-928.01, 928.10-928.11, 928.20-928.21, 928.3, 928.8-928.9, 929.0, 929.9, 996.90- 996.99.)
  7. Progressive necrotizing infections (necrotizing fasciitis), (ICD-9-CM diagnosis 728.86).
  8. Acute peripheral arterial insufficiency, (ICD-9-CM diagnosis 444.21, 444.22, 81).
  9. Preparation and preservation of compromised skin grafts (not for primary management of wounds), (ICD-9CM diagnosis 996.52; excludes artificial skin graft).
  10. Chronic refractory osteomyelitis, unresponsive to conventional medical and surgical management, (ICD-9-CM diagnosis 730.10-730.19).
  11. Osteoradionecrosis as an adjunct to conventional treatment, (ICD-9-CM diagnosis 526.89).
  12. Soft tissue radionecrosis as an adjunct to conventional treatment, (ICD-9-CM diagnosis 990).
  13. Cyanide poisoning, (ICD-9-CM diagnosis 987.7, 989.0).
  14. Actinomycosis, only as an adjunct to conventional therapy when the disease process is refractory to antibiotics and surgical treatment, (ICD-9-CM diagnosis 039.0-039.4, 039.8, 039.9).
  15. Diabetic wounds of the lower extremities in patients who meet the following three criteria:
    a. Patient has type I or type II diabetes and has a lower extremity wound that is due to diabetes;
    b. Patient has a wound classified as Wagner grade III or higher; and
    c. Patient has failed an adequate course of standard wound therapy.

The use of HBO therapy is covered as adjunctive therapy only after there are no measurable signs of healing for at least 30 –days of treatment with standard wound therapy and must be used in addition to standard wound care. Standard wound care in patients with diabetic wounds includes: assessment of a patient's vascular status and correction of any vascular problems in the affected limb if possible, optimization of nutritional status, optimization of glucose control, debridement by any means to remove devitalized tissue, maintenance of a clean, moist bed of granulation tissue with appropriate moist dressings, appropriate off-loading, and

necessary treatment to resolve any infection that might be present. Failure to respond to standard wound care occurs when there are no measurable signs of healing for at least 30 consecutive days. Wounds must be evaluated at least every 30 days during administration of HBO therapy. Continued treatment with HBO therapy is not covered if measurable signs of healing have not been demonstrated within any 30-day period of treatment.

B. Noncovered Conditions.--All other indications not specified under §35-10(A) are not covered under the Medicare program. No program payment may be made for any conditions other than those listed in §35-10 (A).

No program payment may be made for HBO in the treatment of the following conditions:
  1. Cutaneous, decubitus, and stasis ulcers.
  2. Chronic peripheral vascular insufficiency.
  3. Anaerobic septicemia and infection other than clostridial.
  4. Skin burns (thermal).
  5. Senility.
  6. Myocardial infarction.
  7. Cardiogenic shock.
  8. Sickle cell anemia.
  9. Acute thermal and chemical pulmonary damage, i.e., smoke inhalation with pulmonary insufficiency.
  10. Acute or chronic cerebral vascular insufficiency.
  11. Hepatic necrosis.
  12. Aerobic septicemia.
  13. Nonvascular causes of chronic brain syndrome (Pick's disease, Alzheimer's disease, Korsakoff's disease).
  14. Tetanus.
  15. Systemic aerobic infection.
  16. Organ transplantation.
  17. Organ storage.
  18. Pulmonary emphysema.
  19. Exceptional blood loss anemia.
  20. Multiple Sclerosis.
  21. Arthritic Diseases.
  22. Acute cerebral edema.
C. Topical Application of Oxygen.

This method of administering oxygen does not meet the definition of HBO therapy as stated above. Also, its clinical efficacy has not been established. Therefore, no Medicare reimbursement may be made for the topical application of oxygen.

Pub. 100-3, Section 30.1
Biofeedback Therapy

Biofeedback therapy is covered under Medicare only when it is reasonable and necessary for the individual patient for muscle re-education of specific muscle groups or for treating pathological muscle abnormalities of spasticity, incapacitating muscle spasm, or weakness, and more conventional treatments (heat, cold, massage, exercise, support) have not been successful. This therapy is not covered for treatment of ordinary muscle tension states or for psychosomatic conditions. (See the Medicare Benefit Policy Manual, Chapter 15, for general coverage requirements about physical therapy requirements.)

Pub. 100-3, Section 30.1.1
Biofeedback Therapy for the Treatment of Urinary Incontinence

This policy applies to biofeedback therapy rendered by a practitioner in an office or other facility setting.

Biofeedback is covered for the treatment of stress and/or urge incontinence in cognitively intact patients who have failed a documented trial of pelvic muscle exercise (PME)training. Biofeedback is not a treatment, per se, but a tool to help patients learn how to perform PME. Biofeedback-assisted PME incorporates the use of an electronic or mechanical device to relay visual and/or auditory evidence of pelvic floor muscle tone, in order to improve awareness of pelvic floor musculature and to assist patients in the performance of PME.

A failed trial of PME training is defined as no clinically significant improvement in urinary incontinence after completing 4 weeks of an ordered plan of pelvic muscle exercises to increase periurethral muscle strength.

Contractors may decide whether or not to cover biofeedback as an initial treatment modality.

Home use of biofeedback therapy is not covered.

Pub. 100-3, Section 30.7
Laetrile and Related Substances

The FDA has determined that neither Laetrile nor any other drug called by the various terms mentioned above, nor any other product which might be characterized as a "nitriloside" is generally recognized (by experts qualified by scientific training and experience to evaluate the safety and effectiveness of drugs) to be safe and effective for any therapeutic use. Therefore, use of this drug cannot be considered to be reasonable and necessary within the meaning of §1862(a)(1) of the Act and program payment may not be made for its use or any services furnished in connection with its administration.

A hospital stay only for the purpose of having laetrile (or any other drug called by the terms mentioned above) administered is not covered. Also, program payment may not be made

Appendixes

for laetrile (or other drug noted above) when it is used during the course of an otherwise covered hospital stay, since the FDA has found such drugs to not be safe and effective for any therapeutic purpose.

Pub. 100-3, Section 30.8
Cellular Therapy

Accordingly, cellular therapy is not considered reasonable and necessary within the meaning of section 1862(a)(1) of the law.

Pub. 100-3, Section 40.2
Home Blood Glucose Monitors

There are several different types of blood glucose monitors that use reflectance meters to determine blood glucose levels. Medicare coverage of these devices varies, both with respect to the type of device and the medical condition of the patient for whom the device is prescribed.

Reflectance colorimeter devices used for measuring blood glucose levels in clinical settings are not covered as durable medical equipment for use in the home because their need for frequent professional re-calibration makes them unsuitable for home use. However, some types of blood glucose monitors which use a reflectance meter specifically designed for home use by diabetic patients may be covered as durable medical equipment, subject to the conditions and limitations described below.

Accordingly, coverage of home blood glucose monitors is limited to patients meeting the following conditions.

- The patient has been diagnosed as having diabetes;
- The patient's physician states that the patient is capable of being trained to tuse the particular device prescribed in an appropriate manner. In some cases, the patient may not be able to perform this function, but a responsible individual can be trained to use the equipment and monitor the patient to assure that th intended effect is achieved. This is permissible if the record is properly documented by the patient's physician; and
- The device is designed for home rather that clinical use.

There is also a blood glucose monitoring system designed especially for use by those with visual impairments. The monitors used in such systems are identical in terms of reliability and sensitivity to the standard blood glucose monitors described above. They differ by having such features as voice synthesizers, automatic timers, and specially designed arrangements of supplies and materials to enable the visually impaired to use the equipment without assistance.

These special blood glucose monitoring systems are covered under Medicare if the following conditions are met:

- The patient and device meet the three conditions listed above for coverage of standard home blood glucose monitors; and
- The patient's physician certifies that he or she has a visual impairment severe enough to require use of this special monitoring system.

The additional features and equipment of these special systems justify a higher reimbursement amount than allowed for standard blood glucose monitors. Separately identify claims for such devices and establish a separate reimbursement amount for them. For those carriers using HCPCS, the procedure code and definition is E0609--Blood Glucose Monitor--with special features (e.g., voice synthesizers, automatic timer).

Pub. 100-3, Section 40.5
Treatment of Obesity

B. Nationally Covered Indications

Service performed in connection with the treatment of obesity are covered by medicare when such servcies are an integral and necessary aprt of a course of treatment for diseases such as hypothryroidism, Cushing's disease, hypothalamic lesions, cardiovascular diseases, respiratory diseases, diabetes, and hypertension.

C. Nationally Noncovered Indications

1. The treatment of obesity unrelated to such a medical condition (see section B above) is not considered reasonable and necessary and is not covered under the Medicare program.
2. Supplemented fasting is not covered under the Medicare program as a general treatment for obesity (see section D below for discretionary local coverage).

D.Other

Where weight loss is necessary before surgery in order to ameliorate the complications posed by obesity when it coexists with pathological conditions such as cardiac and respiratory diseases, diabetes, or hypertension (and other more conservative techniques to achieve this end are not regarded as appropriate), supplemented fasting with adequate monitoring of the patient is eligible for local coverage determination through individual contractor discretion. The risks associated with the achievement of rapid weight loss must be carefully balanced against the risk posed by the condition requiring the surgical treatment.

(This NCD last reviewed September 2004.)

Cross-reference §100.1, 100.8, 100.11

Pub. 100-3, Section 50.1
Speech Generating Devices

Effective January 1, 2001, augmentative and alternative communication devices or communicators, which are hereafter referred to as "speech generating devices" are now considered to fall within the DME benefit category established by §1861(n) of the Social Security Act. They may be covered if the contractor's medical staff determines that the patient suffers from a severe speech impairment and that the medical condition warrants the use of a device based on the following definitions.

Pub. 100-3, Section 50.2
Electronic Speech Aids
Electronic speech aids are covered under Part B as prosthetic devices when the patient has had a laryngectomy or his larynx is permanently inoperative.

Pub. 100-3, Section 50.3
Cochlear Implantation

B. Nationally Covered Indications

1. Effective for services performed on or after April 4, 2005, cochlear implantation may be covered for treatment of bilateral pre- or -post- linguistic, sensorineural, moderate-to-profound hearing loss in individuals who demonstrate limited benefit from amplification. Limited benefit from amplification is defined by test scores of les than or equal to 40% correct in the best aided listening condition on tape recorded tests of open-set sentence cognition. Medicare coverage is provided only for those patients who meet all of the following selection guidelines.

- Diagnosis of bilateral severe-to-profound sensorineural hearing impairment with limited benefit from appropriate hearing (or vibrotactile) aids;
- Cognitive ability to use auditory clues and a willingness to undergo an extended program of rehabilitation;
- Freedom from middle ear infection, an accessible cochlear lumen that is structurally suited to implantation, and freedom from lesions in the auditory nerve and acoustic areas of the central nervous system;
- No contraindications to surgery; and
- The device must be used in accordance withe the FDA-approved labeling.

2. Effective for services performed on or after April 4, 2005, cochlear implantation may be covered for individuals meeting the selection guidelines above and with hearing test scores of greater than 40% and less than or equal to 60% only when the provider is participating in, and patients are enrolled in, either an FDA-approved category B investigational device exemption clinical trial as defined at 42 CFR 405.201, a trial under the Centers for Medicare & Medicaid (CMS) Clinical Trial Policy as defined at section 310.1 of the National Coverage Determinations Manual, or a prospective, controlled comparative trial approved by CMS as consistent with the evidentiary requirements for National Coverage Analyses and meeting specific quality standards.

C. Nationally Noncovered Indications

Medicare beneficiaries not meeting all of the coverage criteria for cochlear iimplantation listed are deemed not eligible for Medicare coverage under section 1862(a)(1)(A) of the Social Security Act.

D. Other

All other indications for cochlear implantation not otherwise indicated as nationally covered on non-covered above remain at local contractor discretion.

Pub. 100-3, Section 50.4
Tracheostomy Speaking Valve
A trachea tube has been determined to satisfy the definition of a prosthetic device, and the tracheostomy speaking valve is an add on to the trachea tube which may be considered a medically necessary accessory that enhances the function of the tube. In other words, it makes the system a better prosthesis. As such, a tracheostomy speaking valve is covered as an element of the trachea tube which makes the tube more effective.

Pub. 100-3, Section 70.2.1
Services Provided for the Diagnosis and Treatment of Diabetic Sensory Neuropathy with Loss of Protective Sensation (AKA Diabetic Peripheral Neuropathy)

Diabetic sensory neuropathy with LOPS is a localized illness of the feet and falls within the regulation's exception to the general exclusionary rule [see 42 CFR §411.15(l)(1)(i)]. Foot exams for people with diabetic sensory neuropathy with LOPS are reasonable and necessary to allow for early intervention in serious complications that typically afflict diabetics with the disease.

Effective for services furnished on or after July 1, 2002, Medicare covers, as a physician service, an evaluation (examination and treatment) of the feet no more often than every six months for individuals with a documented diagnosis of diabetic sensory neuropathy and LOPS, as long as the beneficiary has not seen a foot care specialist for some other reason in the interim. LOPS shall be diagnosed through sensory testing with the 5.07 monofilament using established guidelines, such as those developed by the National Institute of Diabetes and Digestive and Kidney Diseases guidelines. Five sites should be tested on the plantar surface of each foot, according to the National Institute of Diabetes and Digestive and Kidney Diseases guidelines. The areas must be tested randomly since the loss of protective sensation may be patchy in distribution, and the patient may get clues if the test is done rhythmically. Heavily callused areas should be avoided. As suggested by the American Podiatric Medicine Association, an absence of sensation at two or more sites out of 5 tested on either foot when tested with the 5.07 Semmes-Weinstein monofilament must be present and documented to diagnose peripheral neuropathy with loss of protective sensation.

A. The examination includes:

1) a patient history, and

2) a physical examination that must consist of at least the following elements:
   a. visual inspection of forefoot and hindfoot (including toe web spaces);
   b. evaluation of protective sensation;
   c. evaluation of foot structure and biomechanics;
   d. evaluation of vascular status and skin integrity;
   e. evaluation of the need for special footwear; and

3) patient education.

B. Treatment includes, but is not limited to:

1) local care of superficial wounds;

2) debridement of corns and calluses; and

3) trimming and debridement of nails.

The diagnosis of diabetic sensory neuropathy with LOPS should be established and documented prior to coverage of foot care. Other causes of peripheral neuropathy should be considered and investigated by the primary care physician prior to initiating or referring for foot care for persons with LOPS.

Pub. 100-3, Section 80.1
Hydrophilic Contact Lens For Corneal Bandage

Payment may be made under §1861(s)(2) of the Act for a hydrophilic contact les approved by the Food and Drug Administration (FDA) and used as a supply incident to a pphysician's service. Payment for the lens is included in the payment for the physician's service to which the lens is incident. Contractors are authorized to accept an FDA letter of approval or other FDA published material as evidence of FDA approval. (See §80.4 of the NCD Manual for coverage of a hydrophilic contact lens as prosthetic device.)

Pub. 100-3, Section 80.2
Ocular Photodynamic Therapy

OPT is only covered when used in conjunction with verteporfin.

Effective July 1, 2001, OPT with verteporfin was approved for a diagnosis of neovascular AMD with predominately classic subfoveal choroidal neovascularization (CNV) lesions (where the area of classic CNV occupies >= 50% of the area of the entire lesion) at the initial visit as determined by a fluorescein angiogram.

On October 17, 2001, CMS announced its "intent to cover" OPT with verteporfin for AMD patients with occult and no classic subfoveal CNV as determined by a fluorescein angiogram. The October 17, 2001, decision was never implemented.

On March 28, 2002, after thorough review and reconsideration of the October 17, 2001, intent to cover policy, CMS determined that the current noncoverage policy for OPT for verteporfin for AMD patients with occult and no classic subfoveal CNV as determined by a fluorescein angiogram should remain in effect.

Effective August 20, 2002, CMS issued a noncovered instruction for OPT with verteporfin for AMD patients with occult and no classic subfoveal CNV as determined by a fluorescein angiogram.

Covered Indications

Effective April 1, 2004, OPT with verteporfin continues to be approved for a diagnosis of neovascular AMD with predominately classic subfoveal CNV lesions (where the area of classic CNV occupies >= 50% of the area of the entire lesion) at the initial visit as determined by a fluorescein angiogram. (CNV lesions are comprised of classic and/or occult components.) Subsequent follow-up visits require a fluorescein angiogram prior to treatment. There are no requirements regarding visual acuity, lesion size, and number of re-treatments when treating predominantly classic lesions.

In addition, after thorough review and reconsideration of the August 20, 2002, noncoverage policy, CMS determines that the evidence is adequate to conclude that OPT with verteporfin is reasonable and necessary for treating:

1. Subfoveal occult with no classic CNV associated with AMD; and,
2. Subfoveal minimally classic CNV (where the area of classic CNV occupies <50% of the area of the entire lesion) associated with AMD.

The above 2 indications are considered reasonable and necessary only when:

1. The lesions are small (4 disk areas or less in size) at the time of initial treatment or within the 3 months prior to initial treatment; and,
2. The lesions have shown evidence of progression within the 3 months prior to initial treatment. Evidence of progression must be documented by deterioration of visual acuity (at least 5 letters on a standard eye examination chart), lesion growth (an increase in at least 1 disk area), or the appearance of blood associated with the lesion.

Noncovered Indications

Other uses of OPT with verteporfin to treat AMD not already addressed by CMS will continue to be noncovered. These include, but are not limited to, the following AMD indications:

- Juxtafoveal or extrafoveal CNV lesions (lesions outside the fovea),
- Inability to obtain a fluorescein angiogram,
- Atrophic or "dry" AMD.

Other

OPT with verteporfin for other ocular indications, such as pathologic myopia or presumed ocular histoplasmosis syndrome, continue to be eligible for local coverage determinations through individual contractor discretion.

(This NCD last reviewed March 2004.)

Pub. 100-3, Section 80.3
Verteporfin

Covered Indications

Effective April 1, 2004, OPT with verteporfin is covered for patients with a diagnosis of neovascular age-related macular degeneration (AMD) with:

- Predominately classic subfoveal choroidal neovascularization (CNV) lesions (where the area of classic CNV occupies >= 50% of the area of the entire lesion) at the initial visit as determined by a fluorescein angiogram. (CNV lesions are comprised of classic and/or occult components.) Subsequent follow-up visits require a fluorescein angiogram prior to treatment. There are no requirements regarding visual acuity, lesion size, and number of retreatments when treating predominantly classic lesions.
- Subfoveal occult with no classic associated with AMD.
- Subfoveal minimally classic CNV CNV (where the area of classic CNV occupies <50% of the area of the entire lesion) associated with AMD.

The above 2 indications are considered reasonable and necessary only when:

1. The lesions are small (4 disk areas or less in size) at the time of initial treatment or within the 3 months prior to initial treatment; and,
2. The lesions have shown evidence of progression within the 3 months prior to initial treatment. Evidence of progression must be documented by deterioration of visual acuity (at least 5 letters on a standard eye examination chart), lesion growth (an increase in at least 1 disk area), or the appearance of blood associated with the lesion.

Noncovered Indications

Other uses of OPT with verteporfin to treat AMD not already addressed by CMS will continue to be noncovered. These include, but are not limited to, the following AMD indications: juxtafoveal or extrafoveal CNV lesions (lesions outside the fovea), inability to obtain a fluorescein angiogram, or atrophic or "dry" AMD.

Other

OPT with verteporfin for other ocular indications, such as pathologic myopia or presumed ocular histoplasmosis syndrome, continue to be eligible for local coverage determinations through individual contractor discretion.

(This NCD last reviewed March 2004.)

Pub. 100-3, Section 80.4
Hydrophilic Contact Lenses

Hydrophilic contact lenses are eyeglasses within the meaning of the exclusion in §1862(a)(7) of the Act and are not covered when used in the treatment of nondiseased eyes with spherical ametrophia, refractive astigmatism, and/or corneal astigmatism. Payment may be made under the prosthetic device benefit, however, for hydrophilic contact lenses when prescribed for an aphakic patient.

Contractors are authorized to accept an FDA letter of approval or other FDA published material as evidence of FDA approval. (See §80.1 of the NCD Manual for coverage of a hydrophilic lens as a corneal bandage.)

Pub. 100-3, Section 80.5
Scleral Shell

A scleral shell fits over the entire exposed surface of the eye as opposed to a corneal contact lens which covers only the central non-white area encompassing the pupil and iris. Where an eye has been rendered sightless and shrunken by inflammatory disease, a scleral shell may, among other things, obviate the need for surgical enucleation and prosthetic implant and act to support the surrounding orbital tissue.

In such a case, the device serves essentially as an artificial eye. In this situation, payment may be made for a scleral shell under §1861(s)(8) of the law.

Scleral shells are occasionally used in combination with artificial tears in the treatment of "dry eye" of diverse etiology. Tears ordinarily dry at a rapid rate, and are continually replaced by the lacrimal gland. When the lacrimal gland fails, the half-life of artificial tears may be greatly prolonged by the use of the scleral contact lens as a protective barrier against the drying action of the atmosphere. Thus, the difficult and sometimes hazardous process of frequent installation of artificial tears may be avoided. The lens acts in this instance to substitute, in part, for the functioning of the diseased lacrimal gland and would be covered as a prosthetic device in the rare case when it is used in the treatment of "dry eye."

Pub. 100-3, Section 100.6
Gastric Freezing

Since the procedure is now considered obsolete, it is not covered.

Pub. 100-3, Section 110.2
Certain Drugs Distributed by the National Cancer Institute

A physician is eligible to receive Group C drugs from the Divison of Cancer Treatment only if the following requirements are met:

- A physician must be registered with the NCI as an investigator by having completed an FD-Form 1573;
- A written request for the drug, indicating the disease to be treated, must be submitted to the NCI;
- The use of the drug must be limited to indications outlined in the NCI's guidelines; and
- All adverse reactions must be reported to the Investigational Drug Branch of the Division of Cancer Treatment.

In view of these NCI controls on distribution and use of Group C drugs, intermediaries may assume, in the absence of evidence to the contrary, that a Group C drug and the related hospital stay are covered if all other applicable coverage requirements are satisfied.

If there is reason to question coverage in a particular case, the matter should be resolved with the assistance of the Quality improvemetn organization (QIO), or if there is none, the assistance of your medical consultants.

Information regarding those drugs which are classified as Group C drugs may be obtained from:

Office of the Chief, Investigational Drug Branch
Division of Cancer Treatment, CTEP, Landow Building
Room 4C09, National Cancer Institute
Bethesda, Maryland 20205

Pub. 100-3, Section 110.3
Cytotoxic Food Tests

Prior to August 5, 1985, Medicare covered cytotoxic food tests as an adjunct to in vivo clinical allergy tests in complex food allergy problems. Effective August 5, l985, cytotoxic leukocyte tests for food allergies are excluded from Medicare coverage because available evidence does not show that these tests are safe and effective. This exclusion was published as a CMS Ruling in the "Federal Register" on July 5, 1985.

Pub. 100-3, Section 110.8
Blood Platelet Transfusions

Blood platelet transplants are safe and effective for the correction of thrombocytopenia and other blood defects. It is covered under Medicare when treatment is reasonable and necessary for the individual patient.

Pub. 100-3, Section 130.5
Treatment of Alcoholism and Drug Abuse in a Freestanding Clinic

Coverage is available for alcoholism or drug abuse treatment services (such as drug therapy, psychotherapy, and patient education) that are provided incident to a physician's professional service in a freestanding clinic to patients who, for example, have been discharged from an inpatient hospital stay for the treatment of alcoholism or drug abuse or to individuals who are not in the acute stages of alcoholism or drug abuse but require treatment. The coverage available for these services is subject to the same rules generally applicable to the coverage of clinic services. (See HCFA-Pub. 14-3, §§2020ff., and §§2050 ff.) Of course, the services also must be reasonable and necessary for the diagnosis or treatment of the individual's alcoholism or drug abuse. The Part B psychiatric limitation (see HCFA-Pub. 14-3, §2470) would apply to alcoholism or drug abuse treatment services furnished by physicians to individuals who are not hospital inpatients.

Pub. 100-3, Section 130.6
Treatment of Drug Abuse (Chemical Dependency)

Accordingly, when it is medically necessary for a patient to receive detoxification and/or rehabilitation for drug substance abuse as a hospital inpatient, coverage for care in that setting is available. Coverage is also available for treatment services that are provided in the outpatient department of a hospital to patients who, for example, have been discharged from an inpatient stay for the treatment of drug substance abuse or who require treatment but do not require the availability and intensity of services found only in the inpatient hospital setting. The coverage available for these services is subject to the same rules generally applicable to the coverage of outpatient hospital services. The services must also be reasonable and necessary for treatment of the individual's condition. Decisions regarding reasonableness and necessity of treatment, the need for an inpatient hospital level of care, and length of treatment should be made by intermediaries based on accepted medical practice with the advice of their medical consultant. (In hospitals under PSRO review, PSRO determinations of medical necessity of services and appropriateness of the level of care

at which services are provided are binding on the title XVIII fiscal intermediaries for purposes of adjudicating claims for payment.)

Pub. 100-3, Section 140.2
Breast Reconstruction Following Mastectomy

Reconstruction of the affected and the contralateral unaffected breast following a medically necessary mastectomy is considered a relatively safe and effective noncosmetic procedure. Accordingly, program payment may be made for breast reconstruction surgery following removal of a breast for any medical reason.

Program payment may not be made for breast reconstruction for cosmetic reasons. (Cosmetic surgery is excluded from coverage under §l862(a)(l0) of the Social Security Act.)

Pub. 100-3, Section 150.2
Osteogenic Stimulation

Electrical Osteogenic Stimulators

B. Nationally Covered Indications

1. Noninvasive Stimulator.

The noninvasive stimulator device is covered only for the following indications:

- Nonunion of long bone fractures;
- Failed fusion, where a minimum of nine months has elapsed since the last surgery;
- Congenital pseudarthroses; and
- Effective July 1, 1996, as an adjunct to spinal fusion surgery for patients at high risk of pseudarthrosis due to previously failed spinal fusion at the same site or for those undergoing multiple level fusion. A multiple level fusion involves 3 or more vertebrae (e.g., L3-L5, L4-S1, etc).
- Effective September 15, 1980, nonunion of long bone fractures is considered to exist only after 6 or more months have elapsed without healing of the fracture.
- Effective April 1, 2000, nonunion of long bone fractures is considered to exist only when serial radiographs have confirmed that fracture healing has ceased for 3 or more months prior to starting treatment with the electrical osteogenic stimulator. Serial radiographs must include a minimum of 2 sets of radiographs, each including multiple views of the fracture site, separated by a minimum of 90 days.

2. Invasive (Implantable) Stimulator.

The invasive stimulator device is covered only for the following indications:

- Nonunion of long bone fractures
- Effective July 1, 1996, as an adjunct to spinal fusion surgery for patients at high risk of pseudarthrosis due to previously failsed spinal fusion at the same site or for those undergoing multiple level fusion. A multiple level fusion involves 3 or more vertebrae (e.g., L3-5, L4-S1, etc.)
- Effective September 15, 1980, nonunion of long bone fractures is considered to exist only after 6 or more months have elapsed without healing of the fracture.
- Effective April 1, 2000, non union of long bone fractures is considered to exist only when serial radiographs have confirmed that fracture healing has ceased for 3 or more months prior to starting treatment with the electrical osteogenic stimulator. Serial radiographs must include a minimum of 2 sets of radiographs, each including multiple views of the fracture site, separated by a minimum of 90 days.

Effective for services performed on or after January 1, 2001, ultrasonic osteogenic stimulators are covered as medically reasonable and necessary for the treatment of non-union fractures. In demonstrating nonunion of fractures, we would expect:

- A minimum of two sets of radiographs obtained prior to starting treatment with the osteogenic stimulator, separated by a minimum of 90 days. Each radiograph must include multiple views of the fracture site accompanied with a written interpretation by a physician stating that there has been no clinically significant evidence of fracture healing between the two sets of radiographs.
- Indications that the patient failed at least one surgical intervention for the treatment of the fracture.
- Effective April 27, 2005, upon the recommendation of the ultrasound stimulation for nonunion fracture healing, CMS determins that the evidence is adequate to condlude that noninvasive ultrasound stimulation for the treatment of nonunion bone fractures prior to surfical intervention is reasonable and necessary. In demonstrating non-union fracturs, CMS expects:
- A minimum of 2 sets of radiographs, obtained prior to starting treating with the osteogenic stimulator, separated by a minimum of 90 days. Each radiograph set must include multiple views of the fracture site accompanied with a written interpretation by a physician stating that there has been no clinically significant evidence of fracture healing between the 2 sets of radiographs.

C. Nationally Non-Covered Indications

Nonunion fractures of the skull, vertebrae and those that are tumor-related are excluded from coverage.

Ultrasonic osteogenic stimulators may not be used concurrently with other non-invasive osteogenic devices.

Ultrasonic osteogenic stimulators for fresh fractures and delayed unions remain non-covered.

(This NCD last reviewed June 2005)

Pub. 100-3, Section 150.3
Bone (Mineral) Density Studies

The Following Bone (Mineral) Density Studies Are Covered Under Medicare:

A. Single Photon Absorptiometry

A non-invasive radiological technique that measures absorption of a monochromatic photon beam by bone material. The device is placed directly on the patient, uses a low dose of radionuclide, and measures the mass absorption efficiency of the energy used. It provides a quantitative measurement of the bone mineral of cortical and trabecular bone, and is used in assessing an individual's treatment response at appropriate intervals.

Single photon absorptiometry is covered under Medicare when used in assessing changes in bone density of patients with osteodystrophy or osteoporosis when performed on the same individual at intervals of 6 to 12 months.

B. Bone Biopsy

A physiologic test which is a surgical, invasive procedure. A small sample of bone (usually from the ilium) is removed, generally by a biopsy needle. The biopsy sample is then examined histologically, and provides a qualitative measurement of the bone mineral of trabecular bone. This procedure is used in ascertaining a differential diagnosis of bone disorders and is used primarily to differentiate osteomalacia from osteoporosis.

Bone biopsy is covered under Medicare when used for the qualitative evaluation of bone no more than four times per patient, unless there is special justification given. When used more than four times on a patient, bone biopsy leaves a defect in the pelvis and may produce some patient discomfort.

C. Photodensitometry(radiographic absorptiometry)

A noninvasive radiological procedure that attempts to assess bone mass by measuring the optical density of extremity radiographs with a photodensitometer, usually with a reference to a standard density wedge placed on the film at the time of exposure. This procedure provides a quantitative measurement of the bone mineral of bone, and is used for monitoring gross bone change.

The Following Bone (Mineral) Density Study Is Not Covered Under Medicare:

D. Dual Photon Absorptiometry

A noninvasive radiological technique that measures absorption of a dichromatic beam by bone material. This procedure is not covered under Medicare because it is still considered to be in the investigational stage.

Pub. 100-3, Section 150.6
Vitamin B12 Injections to Strengthen Tendons, Ligaments, ETC., of the Foot

Vitamin B12 injections to strengthen tendons, ligaments, etc., of the foot are not covered under Medicare because (1) there is no evidence that vitamin B12 injections are effective for the purpose of strengthening weakened tendons and ligaments, and (2) this is nonsurgical treatment under the subluxation exclusion. Accordingly, vitamin B12 injections are not considered reasonable and necessary within the meaning of §1862(a)(1) of the Act.

Pub. 100-3, Section 150.7
Prolotherapy, Joint Sclerotherapy, and Ligamentous Injections with Sclerosing Agents

The medical effectiveness of the above therapies has not been verified by scientifically controlled studies. Accordingly, reimbursement for these modalities should be denied on the ground that they are not reasonable and necessary as required by §1862(a)(1) of the Act.

Pub. 100-3, Section 160.2
Treatment of Motor Function Disorders with Electric Nerve Stimulation

Where electric nerve stimulation is employed to treat motor function disorders, no reimbursement may be made for the stimulator or for the services related to its implantation since this treatment cannot be considered reasonable and necessary.

NOTE: For Medicare coverage of deep brain stimulation for essential tremor and Parkinson's disease, see §65-19.

Pub. 100-3, Section 160.6
Carotid Sinus Nerve Stimulator

Implantation of the carotid sinus nerve stimulator is indicated for relief of angina pectoris in carefully selected patients who are refractory to medical therapy and who after undergoing coronary angiography study either are poor candidates for or refuse to have coronary bypass surgery. In such cases, Medicare reimbursement may be made for this device and for the related services required for its implantation.

However, the use of the carotid sinus nerve stimulator in the treatment of paroxysmal supraventricular tachycardia is considered investigational and is not in common use by the medical community. The device and related services in such cases could be considered as reasonable and necessary for the treatment of an illness or injury or to improve the functioning of a malformed body member as required by §1862(a)(1) of the law.

Pub. 100-3, Section 160.7
Electrical Nerve Stimulators

Two general classifications of electrical nerve stimulators are employed to treat chronic intractable pain: peripheral nerve stimulators and central nervous system stimulators.

A-Implanted Peripheral Nerve Stimulators

Payment may be made under the prosthetic device benefit for implanted peripheral nerve stimulators. Use of this stimulator involves implantation of electrodes around a selected peripheral nerve. The stimulating electrode is connected by an insulated lead to a receiver unit which is implanted under the skin at a depth not greater than 1/2 inch. Stimulation is induced by a generator connected to an antenna unit which is attached to the skin surface over the receiver unit. Implantation of electrodes requires surgery and usually necessitates an operating room.

NOTE: Peripheral nerve stimulators may also be employed to assess a patient's suitability for continued treatment with an electric nerve stimulator. As explained in §160.7.1, such use of the stimulator is covered as part of the total diagnostic service furnished to the beneficiary rather than as a prosthesis.

B-Central Nervous System Stimulators (Dorsal Column and Depth Brain Stimulators).The implantation of central nervous system stimulators may be covered as therapies for the relief of chronic intractable pain, subject to the following conditions:

1-Types of Implantations

There are two types of implantations covered by this instruction:

- Dorsal Column (Spinal Cord) Neurostimulation.--The surgical implantation of neurostimulator electrodes within the dura mater (endodural) or the percutaneous insertion of electrodes in the epidural space is covered.
- Depth Brain Neurostimulation.--The stereotactic implantation of electrodes in the deep brain (e.g., thalamus and periaqueductal gray matter) is covered.

2-Conditions for Coverage

No payment may be made for the implantation of dorsal column or depth brain stimulators or services and supplies related to such implantation, unless all of the conditions listed below have been met:

- The implantation of the stimulator is used only as a late resort (if not a last resort) for patients with chronic intractable pain;
- With respect to item a, other treatment modalities (pharmacological, surgical, physical, or psychological therapies) have been tried and did not prove satisfactory, or are judged to be unsuitable or contraindicated for the given patient;
- Patients have undergone careful screening, evaluation and diagnosis by a multidisciplinary team prior to implantation. (Such screening must include psychological, as well as physical evaluation);
- All the facilities, equipment, and professional and support personnel required for the proper diagnosis, treatment training, and followup of the patient (including that required to satisfy item c) must be available; and
- Demonstration of pain relief with a temporarily implanted electrode precedes permanent implantation.

Contractors may find it helpful to work with QIOs to obtain the information needed to apply these conditions to claims.

Pub. 100-3, Section 160.7.1
Assessing Patient's Suitability for Electrical Nerve Stimulation Therapy

Electrical nerve stimulation is an accepted modality for assessing a patient's suitability for ongoing treatment with a transcutaneous or an implanted nerve stimulator. Accordingly, program payment may be made for the following techniques when used to determine the potential therapeutic usefulness of an electrical nerve stimulator:

A. Transcutaneous Electrical Nerve Stimulation (TENS).

This technique involves attachment of a transcutaneous nerve stimulator to the surface of the skin over the peripheral nerve to be stimulated. It is used by the patient on a trial basis and its effectiveness in modulating pain is monitored by the physician, or physical therapist. Generally, the physician or physical therapist is able to determine whether the patient is likely to derive a significant therapeutic benefit from continuous use of a transcutaneous stimulator within a trial period of 1 month; in a few cases this determination may take longer to make. Document the medical necessity for such services which are furnished beyond the first month. (See §45-25 for an explanation of coverage of medically necessary supplies for the effective use of TENS.)

If TENS significantly alleviates pain, it may be considered as primary treatment; if it produces no relief or greater discomfort than the original pain electrical nerve stimulation therapy is ruled out. However, where TENS produces incomplete relief, further evaluation with percutaneous electrical nerve stimulation may be considered to determine whether an implanted peripheral nerve stimulator would provide significant relief from pain. (See §35-46B.)

Usually, the physician or physical therapist providing the services will furnish the equipment necessary for assessment. Where the physician or physical therapist advises the patient to rent the TENS from a supplier during the trial period rather than supplying it himself/herself, program payment may be made for rental of the TENS as well as for the services of the physician or physical therapist who is evaluating its use. However, the combined program payment which is made for the physician's or physical therapist's services and the rental of the stimulator from a supplier should not exceed the amount which would be payable for the total service, including the stimulator, furnished by the physician or physical therapist alone.

B. Percutaneous Electrical Nerve Stimulation (PEN)

This diagnostic procedure which involves stimulation of peripheral nerves by a needle electrode inserted through the skin is performed only in a physician's office, clinic, or hospital outpatient department. Therefore, it is covered only when performed by a physician or incident to physician's service. If pain is effectively controlled by percutaneous stimulation, implantation of electrodes is warranted.

As in the case of TENS (described in subsection A), generally the physician should be able to determine whether the patient is likely to derive a significant therapeutic benefit from continuing use of an implanted nerve stimulator within a trial period of 1 month. In a few cases, this determination may take longer to make. The medical necessity for such diagnostic services which are furnished beyond the first month must be documented.

NOTE: Electrical nerve stimulators do not prevent pain but only alleviate pain as it occurs. A patient can be taught how to employ the stimulator, and once this is done, can use it safely and effectively without direct physician supervision. Consequently, it is inappropriate for a patient to visit his/her physician, physical therapist, or an outpatient clinic on a continuing basis for treatment of pain with electrical nerve stimulation. Once it is determined that electrical nerve stimulation should be continued as therapy and the patient has been trained to use the stimulator, it is expected that a stimulator will be implanted or the patient will employ the TENS on a continual basis in his/her home. Electrical nerve stimulation treatments furnished by a physician in his/her office, by a physical therapist or outpatient clinic are excluded from coverage by §1862(a)(1) of the Act. (See §65-8 for an explanation of coverage of the therapeutic use of implanted peripheral nerve stimulators under the prosthetic devices benefit. See §60-20 for an explanation of coverage of the therapeutic use of TENS under the durable medical equipment benefit.)

Pub. 100-3, Section 160.12
Neuromuscular Electrical Stimulaton (NMES)

Treatment of Muscle Atrophy

Coverage of NMES to treat muscle atrophy is limited to the treatment of patients with disuse atrophy where the nerve supply to the muscle is intact, including brain, spinal cord and peripheral nerves and other non-neurological reasons for disuse atrophy. Examples include casting or splinting of a limb, contracture due to scarring of soft tissue as in burn lesions, and hip replacement surgery (until orthotic training begins). (See CIM 45-25 for an explanation of coverage of medically necessary supplies for the effective use of NMES).

Use for Walking in Patients with Spinal Cord Injury (SCI)

The type of NMES that is used to enhance the ability to walk of SCI patients is commonly referred to as functional electrical stimulation (FES). These devices are surface units that use electrical impulses to activate paralyzed or weak muscles in precise sequence. Coverage for the use of NMES/FES is limited to SCI patients, for walking, who have completed a training program, which consists of at least 32 physical therapy sessions with the device over a period of 3 months. The trial period of physical therapy will enable the physician treating the patient for his or her spinal cord injury to properly evaluate the person's ability to use these devices frequently and for the long term. Physical therapy sessions are only covered in the inpatient hospital, outpatient hospital, comprehensive outpatient rehabilitation facilities, and outpatient rehabilitation facilities. The physical therapy necessary to perform this training must be directly performed by the physical therapist as part of a one-on-one training program; this service cannot be done unattended.

The goal of physical therapy must be to train SCI patients on the use of NMES/FES devices to achieve walking, not to reverse or retard muscle atrophy.

Coverage for NMES/FES for walking will be limited to SCI patients with all of the following characteristics:

1) persons with intact lower motor units (L1 and below) (both muscle and peripheral nerve);

2) persons with muscle and joint stability for weight bearing at upper and lower extremities that can demonstrate balance and control to maintain an upright support posture independently;

3) persons that demonstrate brisk muscle contraction to NMES and have sensory perception of electrical stimulation sufficient for muscle contraction;

4) persons that possess high motivation, commitment and cognitive ability to use such devices for walking;

5) persons that can transfer independently and can demonstrate independent standing tolerance for at least 3 minutes;

6) persons that can demonstrate hand and finger function to manipulate controls;

7) persons with at least 6-month post recovery spinal cord injury and restorative surgery;

8) persons without hip and knee degenerative disease and no history of long bone fracture secondary to osteoporosis; and

9) persons who have demonstrated a willingness to use the device long-term.

NMES/FES for walking will not be covered in SCI patients with any of the following:

1) persons with cardiac pacemakers;

2) severe scoliosis or severe osteoporosis;

3) skin disease or cancer at area of stimulation;

4) irreversible contracture; or

5) autonomic dysreflexia.

The only settings where therapists with the sufficient skills to provide these services are employed, are inpatient hospitals, outpatient hospitals, comprehensive outpatient rehabilitation facilities and outpatient rehabilitation facilities. The physical therapy necessary to perform this training must be part of a one-on-one training program.

Additional therapy after the purchase of the DME would be limited by our general policies on coverage of skilled physical therapy.

All other uses of NMES remain non-covered.

Pub. 100-3, Section 160.13
Supplies Used in the Delivery of Transcutaneous Electrical Nerve Stimulation (TENS) and Neuromuscular Electrical Stimulation (NMES)

A form-fitting conductive garment (and medically necessary related supplies) may be covered under the program only when:

1. It has received permission or approval for marketing by the Food and Drug Administration;

2. It has been prescribed by a physician for use in delivering covered TENS or NMES treatment; and

3. One of the medical indications outlined below is met:

- The patient cannot manage without the conductive garment because there is such a large area or so many sites to be stimulated and the stimulation would have to be delivered so frequently that it is not feasible to use conventional electrodes, adhesive tapes and lead wires;
- The patient cannot manage without the conductive garment for the treatment of chronic intractable pain because the areas or sites to be stimulated are inaccessible with the use of conventional electrodes, adhesive tapes and lead wires;
- The patient has a documented medical condition such as skin problems that preclude the application of conventional electrodes, adhesive tapes and lead wires;
- The patient requires electrical stimulation beneath a cast either to treat disuse atrophy, where the nerve supply to the muscle is intact, or to treat chronic intractable pain; or
- The patient has a medical need for rehabilitation strengthening (pursuant to a written plan of rehabilitation) following an injury where the nerve supply to the muscle is intact.

A conductive garment is not covered for use with a TENS device during the trial period specified in §35-46 unless:

4. The patient has a documented skin problem prior to the start of the trial period; and

5. The carrier's medical consultants are satisfied that use of such an item is medically necessary for the patient.

Pub. 100-3, Section 160.23
Sensory Nerve Conduction Threshold Test (sNCT)

B. Nationally Covered Indications

Not applicable.

C. Nationally Noncovered Indications

All uses of sNCT to diagnose sensory neuropathies or radiculopathies are noncovered.

(This NCD last reviewed June 2004.)

Pub. 100-3, Section 180.2
Enteral and Parenteral Nutritional Therapy

Coverage of nutritional therapy as a Part B benefit is provided under the prosthetic device benefit provision, which requires that the patient must have a permanently inoperative internal body organ or function thereof. (See Intermediary Manual, §3110.4.) Therefore, enteral and parenteral nutritional therapy are not covered under Part B in situations involving temporary impairments. Coverage of such therapy, however, does not require a medical judgment that the impairment giving rise to the therapy will persist throughout the patient's remaining years. If the medical record, including the judgment of the attending physician, indicates that the impairment will be of long and indefinite duration, the test of permanence is considered met.

If the coverage requirements for enteral or parenteral nutritional therapy are met under the prosthetic device benefit provision, related supplies, equipment and nutrients are also covered under the conditions in the following paragraphs [see Parenteral Nutrition Therapy, Enteral Nutrition Therapy, and Nutritional Supplementation] and the Medicare Benefit Policy Manual, Chapter 15, "Covered Medical and Other Health Services, " §120.

Parenteral Nutrition Therapy

Daily parenteral nutrition is considered reasonable and necessary for a patient with severe pathology of the alimentary tract which does not allow absorption of sufficient nutrients to maintain weight and strength commensurate with the patient's general condition.

Since the alimentary tract of such a patient does not function adequately, an indwelling catheter is placed percutaneously in the subclavian vein and then advanced into the superior vena cava where intravenous infusion of nutrients is given for part of the day. The catheter is then plugged by the patient until the next infusion. Following a period of hospitalization which is required to initiate parenteral nutrition and to train the patient in catheter care, solution preparation, and infusion technique, the parenteral nutrition can be provided safely and effectively in the patient's home by nonprofessional persons who have undergone special training. However, such persons cannot be paid for their services, nor is payment available for any services furnished by nonphysician professionals except as services furnished incident to a physician's service.

For parenteral nutrition therapy to be covered under Part B, the claim must contain a physician's written order or prescription and sufficient medical documentation to permit an independent conclusion that the requirements of the prosthetic device benefit are met and that parenteral nutrition therapy is medically necessary. An example of a condition that typically qualifies for coverage is a massive small bowel resection resulting in severe nutritional deficiency in spite of adequate oral intake. However, coverage of parenteral nutrition therapy for this and any other condition must be approved on an individual, case-by-case basis initially and at periodic intervals of no more than three months by the carrier's medical consultant or specially trained staff, relying on such medical and other documentation as the carrier may require. If the claim involves an infusion pump, sufficient evidence must be provided to support a determination of medical necessity for the pump. Program payment for the pump is based on the reasonable charge for the simplest model that meets the medical needs of the patient as established by medical documentation.

Nutrient solutions for parenteral therapy are routinely covered. However, Medicare pays for no more than one month's supply of nutrients at any one time. Payment for the nutrients is based on the reasonable charge for the solution components unless the medical record, including a signed statement from the attending physician, establishes that the beneficiary, due to his/her physical or mental state, is unable to safely or effectively mix the solution and there is no family member or other person who can do so. Payment will be on the basis of the reasonable charge for more expensive premixed solutions only under the latter circumstances.

Enteral Nutrition Therapy

Enteral nutrition is considered reasonable and necessary for a patient with a functioning gastrointestinal tract who, due to pathology to, or nonfunction of, the structures that normally permit food to reach the digestive tract, cannot maintain weight and strength commensurate with his or her general condition. Enteral therapy may be given by nasogastric, jejunostomy, or gastrostomy tubes and can be provided safely and effectively in the home by nonprofessional persons who have undergone special training. However, such persons cannot be paid for their services, nor is payment available for any services furnished by nonphysician professionals except as services furnished incident to a physician's service.

Typical examples of conditions that qualify for coverage are head and neck cancer with reconstructive surgery and central nervous system disease leading to interference with the neuromuscular mechanisms of ingestion of such severity that the beneficiary cannot be maintained with oral feeding. However, claims for Part B coverage of enteral nutrition therapy for these and any other conditions must be approved on an individual, case-by-case basis. Each claim must contain a physician's written order or prescription and sufficient medical documentation (e.g., hospital records, clinical findings from the attending physician) to permit an independent conclusion that the patient's condition meets the requirements of the prosthetic device benefit and that enteral nutrition therapy is medically necessary. Allowed claims are to be reviewed at periodic intervals of no more than 3 months by the contractor's medical consultant or specially trained staff, and additional medical documentation considered necessary is to be obtained as part of this review.

Medicare pays for no more than one month's supply of enteral nutrients at any one time.

If the claim involves a pump, it must be supported by sufficient medical documentation to establish that the pump is medically necessary, i.e., gravity feeding is not satisfactory due to aspiration, diarrhea, dumping syndrome. Program payment for the pump is based on the reasonable charge for the simplest model that meets the medical needs of the patient as established by medical documentation.

Nutritional Supplementation

Some patients require supplementation of their daily protein and caloric intake. Nutritional supplements are often given as a medicine between meals to boost protein-caloric intake or the mainstay of a daily nutritional plan. Nutritional supplementation is not covered under Medicare Part B.

Pub. 100-3, Section 190.2
Diagnostic Pap Smears

A diagnostic pap smear and related medically necessary services are covered under Medicare Part B when ordered by a physician under one of the following conditions:

- Previous cancer of the cervix, uterus, or vagina that has been or is presently being treated;
- Previous abnormal pap smear;
- Any abnormal findings of the vagina, cervix, uterus, ovaries, or adnexa;
- Any significant complaint by the patient referable to the female reproductive system; or
- Any signs or symptoms that might in the physician's judgment reasonably be related to a gynecologic disorder.

Screening Pap Smears and Pelvic Examinations for Early Detection of Cervical or Vaginal Cancer

(For screening pap smears, effective for services performed on or after July 1, 1990. For pelvic examinations including clinical breast examination, effective for services furnished on or after January 1, 1998.)

A screening pap smear (use HCPCS code P3000 Screening Papanicolaou smear, cervical or vaginal, up to three smears; by technician under physician supervision or P3001 Screening Papanicolaou smear, cervical or vaginal, up to three smears requiring interpretation by physician). (Use HCPCS codes G0123 Screening Cytopathology, cervical or vaginal (any reporting system), collected in preservative fluid, automated thin layer preparation, screening by cytotechnologist under physician supervision or G0124 Screening Cytopathology, cervical or vaginal (any reporting system) collected in preservative fluid, automated thin layer preparation, requiring interpretation by physician) and related medically necessary services provided to a woman for the early detection of cervical cancer (including collection of the sample of cells and a physician's interpretation of the test results) and pelvic examination (including clinical breast examination) (use HCPCS code G0101 cervical or vaginal cancer screening; pelvic and clinical breast examination) are covered under Medicare Part B when ordered by a physician (or authorized practitioner) under one of the following conditions

She has not had such a test during the preceding three years or is a woman of childbearing age (§1861(nn) of the Act).

- There is evidence (on the basis of her medical history or other findings) that she is at high risk of developing cervical cancer and her physician (or authorized practitioner) recommends that she have the test performed more frequently than every 3 years.

High risk factors for cervical and vaginal cancer are:

- Early onset of sexual activity (under 16 years of age);
- Multiple sexual partners (five or more in a lifetime);
- History of sexually transmitted disease (including HIV infection);
- Fewer than three negative or any pap smears within the previous seven years; and
- DES (diethylstilbestrol) - exposed daughters of women who took DES during pregnancy.

NOTE: Claims for pap smears must indicate the beneficiary's low or high risk status by including the appropriate ICD-9-CM diagnosis code as required by claims processing instructions.

Definitions

A woman as described in §1861(nn) of the Act is a woman who is of childbearing age and has had a pap smear test during any of the preceding three years that indicated the presence of cervical or vaginal cancer or other abnormality, or is at high risk of developing cervical or vaginal cancer.

A woman of childbearing age is one who is premenopausal and has been determined by a physician or other qualified practitioner to be of childbearing age, based upon the medical history or other findings.

Other "qualified practitioner," as defined in 42 CFR 410.56(a) includes a certified nurse midwife (as defined in §1861(gg) of the Act), or a physician assistant, nurse practitioner, or clinical nurse specialist (as defined in §1861(aa) of the Act) who is authorized under State law to perform the examination.

Screening Pelvic Examination

Section 4102 of the Balanced Budget Act of 1997 provides for coverage of screening pelvic examinations (including a clinical breast examination) for all female beneficiaries, subject to certain frequency and other limitations. A screening pelvic examination (including a clinical breast examination) should include at least seven of the following eleven elements:

- Inspection and palpation of breasts for masses or lumps, tenderness, symmetry, or nipple discharge
- Digital rectal examination including sphincter tone, presence of hemorrhoids, and rectal masses. Pelvic examination (with or without specimen collection for smears and cultures) including:
  - External genitalia (for example, general appearance, hair distribution, or lesions).
  - Urethral meatus (for example, size, location, lesions, or prolapse).
  - Urethra (for example, masses, tenderness, or scarring).
  - Bladder (for example, fullness, masses, or tenderness).
  - Vagina (for example, general appearance, estrogen effect, discharge lesions, pelvic support, cystocele, or rectocele).
  - Cervix (for example, general appearance, lesions, or discharge).
  - Uterus (for example, size, contour, position, mobility, tenderness, consistency, descent, or support).
  - Adnexa/parametria (for example, masses, tenderness, organomegaly, or nodularity).
  - Anus and perineum.

This description is from Documentation Guidelines for Evaluation and Management Services, published in May 1997 and was developed by the Centers for Medicare & Medicaid Services and the American Medical Association.

Pub. 100-3, Section 190.6

Hair Analysis

Hair analysis to detect mineral traces as an aid in diagnosing human disease is not a covered service under Medicare.

The correlation of hair analysis to the chemical state of the whole body is not possible at this time, and therefore this diagnostic procedure cannot be considered to be reasonable and necessary under §1862(a)(1) of the Act.

Pub. 100-3, Section 210.1
Prostate Cancer Screening Tests

A. General.--Section 4103 of the Balanced Budget Act of 1997 provides for coverage of certain prostate cancer screening tests subject to certain coverage, frequency, and payment limitations. Effective for services furnished on or after January 1, 2000. Medicare will cover prostate cancer screening tests/procedures for the early detection of prostate cancer. Coverage of prostate cancer screening tests includes the following procedures furnished to an individual for the early detection of prostate cancer:

- Screening digital rectal examination; and

- Screening prostate specific antigen blood test

B. Screening Digital Rectal Examinations.--Screening digital rectal examinations (HCPCS code G0102) are covered at a frequency of once every 12 months for men who have attained age 50 (at least 11 months have passed following the month in which the last Medicare-covered screening digital rectal examination was performed). Screening digital rectal examination means a clinical examination of an individual's prostate for nodules or other abnormalities of the prostate. This screening must be performed by a doctor of medicine or osteopathy (as defined in §1861(r)(1) of the Act), or by a physician assistant, nurse practitioner, clinical nurse specialist, or certified nurse midwife (as defined in §1861(aa) and §1861(gg) of the Act) who is authorized under State law to perform the examination, fully knowledgeable about the beneficiary's medical condition, and would be responsible for using the results of any examination performed in the overall management of the beneficiary's specific medical problem.

C. Screening Prostate Specific Antigen Tests.--Screening prostate specific antigen tests (code G0103) are covered at a frequency of once every 12 months for men who have attained age 50 (at least 11 months have passed following the month in which the last Medicare-covered screening prostate specific antigen test was performed). Screening prostate specific antigen tests (PSA) means a test to detect the marker for adenocarcinoma of prostate. PSA is a reliable immunocytochemical marker for primary and metastatic adenocarcinoma of prostate. This screening must be ordered by the beneficiary's physician or by the beneficiary's physician assistant, nurse practitioner, clinical nurse specialist, or certified nurse midwife (the term "attending physician" is defined in §1861(r)(1) of the Act to mean a doctor of medicine or osteopathy and the terms "physician assistant, nurse practitioner, clinical nurse specialist, or certified nurse midwife" are defined in §1861(aa) and §1861(gg) of the Act) who is fully knowledgeable about the beneficiary's medical condition, and who would be responsible for using the results of any examination (test) performed in the overall management of the beneficiary's specific medical problem.

Pub. 100-3, Section 210.3
Colorectal Cancer Screening Tests

Section 4104 of the Balanced Budget Act of 1997 provides for coverage of screening colorectal cancer procedures under Medicare Part B. Medicare currently covers: 1) annual fecal occult blood tests (FOBTs); (2) flexible sigmoidoscopy over 4 years; (3) screening colonoscopy for persons at average risk for colorectal cancer every 10 years, or for persons at high risk for colorectal cancer every 2 years; (4) barium enema every 4 years as an alternative to flexible sigmoidoscopy, or every 2 years as an alternative to colonoscopy for persons at high risk for colorectal cancer; and, (5) other procedures the Secretary finds appropriate based on consultation with appropriate experts and organizations.

Coverage of the above screening examinations was implemented in regulations through a final rule that was published on October 31, 1997 (62 FR 59079), and was effective January 1, 1998. At that time, based on consultation with appropriate experts and organizations, the definition of the term "FOBT" was defined in 42 CFR §410.37(a)(2) of the regulation to mean a "guaiac-based test for peroxidase activity, testing two samples from each of three consecutive stools.

In the 2003 Physician Fee Schedule Final Rule (67 FR 79966) effective March 1, 2003, CMS amended the FOBT screening test regulation definition at 42 CFR §410.37(a)(2) to provide that it could include either: (1) a guaiac-based FOBT, or, (2) other tests determined by the Secretary through a national coverage determination.

A. Covered Indications

Fecal Occult Blood Tests (FOBT) (effective for services performed on or after January 1, 2004)

1. History

In 1998, Medicare began reimbursement for guaiac FOBTs, but not immunoassay type tests for colorectal cancer screening. Since the fundamental process is similar for other iFOBTs, CMS evaluated colorectal cancer screening using immunoassay FOBTs in general.

2. Expanded Coverage

Medicare covers one screening FOBT per annum for the early detection of colorectal cancer. This means that Medicare will cover one guaiac-based (gFOBT) **or** one immunoassay-based (iFOBT) at a frequency of every 12 months; i.e., at least 11 months have passed following the month in which the last covered screening FOBT was performed, for beneficiaries aged 50 years and older. The beneficiary completes the existing gFOBT by taking samples from two different sites of three consecutive stools; the beneficiary completes the iFOBT by taking the appropriate number of stool samples according to the specific manufacturer's instructions. This screening requires a written order from the beneficiary's attending physician. ("Attending physician means a doctor of medicine or osteopathy (as defined in §1861(r)(1) of the Social Security Act) who is fully knowledgeable about the beneficiary's medical condition, and who would be responsible for using the results of any examination performed in the overall management of the beneficiary's specific medical problem.)

B. Noncovered Indications

All other indications for colorectal cancer screening not otherwise specified above remain noncovered.

(This NCD last reviewed December 2003.)

Pub. 100-3, Section 220.6
PET Scans

The following indications may be covered for PET under certain circumstances. Details of Medicare PET coverage are discussed later in this section. Unless otherwise indicated, the clinical conditions below are covered when PET utilizes FDG as a tracer.

NOTE: This manual section lists all Medicare-covered uses of PET scans. A particular use of PET scans is not covered unless this manual specifically provides that such use is covered. Although this section lists some non-covered uses of PET scans, it does not constitute an exhaustive list of all non-covered uses.

Clinical Condition	Effective Date	Coverage
Solitary Pulmonary Nodules (SPNs)	January 1, 1998	Characterization
Lung Cancer (Non Small Cell)	January 1, 1998	Initial staging
Lung Cancer (Non Small Cell)	July 1, 2001	Diagnosis, staging and restaging
Esophageal Cancer	July 1, 2001	Diagnosis, staging and restaging
Colorectal Cancer	July 1, 1999	Determining location of tumors if rising CEA level suggests recurrence
Colorectal Cancer	July 1, 2001	Diagnosis, staging and restaging
Lymphoma	July 1, 1999	Staging and restaging only when used as an alternative to Gallium scan
Lymphoma	July 1, 2001	Diagnosis, staging and restaging
Melanoma	July 1, 1999	Evaluating recurrence prior to surgery as an alternative to a Gallium scan
Melanoma	July 1, 2001	Diagnosis, staging and restaging; Non-covered for evaluating regional nodes
Breast Cancer	October 1, 2002	As an adjunct to standard imaging modalities for staging patients with distant metastasis or restaging patients with locoregional recurrence or metastasis; as an adjunct to standard imaging modalities for monitoring tumor response to treatment for women with locally advanced and metastatic breast cancer when a change in therapy is anticipated.
Head and Neck Cancers (excluding CNS and thyroid)	July 1, 2001	Diagnosis, staging and restaging
Thyroid Cancer	October 1, 2003	Restaging of recurrent or residual thyroid cancers of follicular cell origin that have been previously treated by thyroidectomy and

		radioiodine ablation and have a serum thyroglobulin >10ng/ml and negative I-131 whole body scan performed
Myocardial Viability	July 1, 2001 to September 30, 2002	Covered only following inconclusive SPECT
Myocardial Viability	October 1, 2001	Primary or initial diagnosis, or following an inconclusive SPECT prior to revascularization. SPECT may not be used following an inconclusive PET scan
Refractory Seizures	July 1, 2001	Covered for pre-surgical evaluation only
Perfusion of the heart using Rubidium 82* tracer	March 14, 1995	Covered for noninvasive imaging of the perfusion of the heart
Perfusion of the heart using ammonia N-13* tracer	October 1, 2003	Covered for noninvasive imaging of the perfusion of the heart

*Not FDG-PET.

EFFECTIVE JANUARY 28, 2005: This manual section lists Medicare-covered uses of PET scans effective for services performed on or after January 28, 2005. Except as set forth below in cancer indications listed as "coverage with evidence development", a particular use of PET scans is not covered unless this manual specifically provides that such use is covered. Although this section 220.6 lists some non-covered uses of PET scans, it does not constitute an exhaustive list of all non-covered uses.

For cancer indications listed as "coverage with evidence development" CMS determines that the evidence is sufficient to conclude that an FDG PET scan is reasonable and necessary only when the provider is participating in, and patients are enrolled in, one of the following types of prospective clinical studies that is designed to collect additional information at the time of the scan to assist in patient management:

- A clilnical trial of FDG PET that meets the requirements of Food and Drug Administration (FDA) category B investigational device exemption (42 CFR 405.201);
- An FDG PET clinical study that is designed to collect additional information at the time of the scan to assist in patient management. Qualifying clinical studies must ensure that specific hypotheses are addressed; appropriate data elements are collected; hospitals and providers are qualified to provide the PET scan and interpret the results; participating hospitals and providers accurately report data on all enrolled patients not included in other qualifying trials through adequate auditing mechanisms; and, all patient confidentiality, privacy, and other Federal laws must be followed.

Effective January 28, 2005: For PET services identified as "Coverage with Evidence Development. Medicare shall notify providers and beneficiaries where theses services can be accessed, as they become available, via the following:

- Federal Register Notice
- CMS coverage Web site at: www.cms.gov/coverage

Indication	Covered[1]	Nationally Non-Covered[2]	Coverage with Evidence Development[3]
Brain			X
Breast			
-Diagnosis			
-Initial staging of axillary nodes	X	X	
-Staging of distant metastasis	X	X	
-Restaging, monitoring*			
Cervical			
-Staging as adjunct to conventional imaging	X		
-Other staging			X
-Diagnosis, restaging, monitoring*			X
Colorectal			
-Diagnosis, staging, restaging	X		X
-Monitoring*			
Esophagus			
-Diagnosis, staging, restaging	X		X
-Monitoring*			
Head and Neck (non-CNS/thyroid			
-Diagnosis, staging, restaging	X		X
-Monitoring*			
Lymphoma			
-Diagnosis, staging, restaging	X		X
-Monitoring*			
Melanoma			
-Diagnosis, staging, restaging	X		X
-Monitoring*			
Non-small Cell Lung			
-Diagnosis, staging, restaging	X		X
-Monitoring*			
Ovarian			X
Pancreatic			X
Small Cell Lung			X
Soft Tissue Sarcoma			S
Solitary Pulmonary Nodule (characterization)	X		
Thyroid			
-Staging of follicular cell tumors			X
-Restaging of medullary cell tumors	X		X
-Diagnosis, other staging & restaging			X
-Monitoring*			
Testicular			X
All other cancers not listed herein (all indications)			X

[1] Covered nationally based on evidence of benefit. Refer to National Coverage Determination Manual Section 220.6 in its entirety for specific coverage language and limitations for each indication.

[2] Non-covered nationally based on evidence of harm or no benefit.

[3] Covered only in specific settings discussed above if certain patient safeguards are provided. Otherwise, non-covered nationally based on lack of evidence sufficient to establish either benefit or harm or no prior decision addressing this cancer. Medicare shall notify providers and beneficiaries where these services can be accessed, as they become available, via the following:

- Federal Register Notice

CMS coverage Web site at: www.cms.gov/coverage

*Monitoring = monitoring response to treatment when a change in therapy is anticipated.

II. General Conditions of Coverage for FDG PET

    A. Allowable FDG PET Systems
        1. Definitions: For purposes of this section,
            a. "Any FDA approved" means all systems approved or cleared for marketing by the FDA to image radionuclides in the body.
            b. "FDA approved" means that the system indicated has been approved or cleared for marketing by the FDA to image radionuclides in the body.
            c. "Certain coincidence systems" refers to the systems that have all the following features:
                • Crystal at least 5/8-inch thick

- Techniques to minimize or correct for scatter and/or randoms, and
- Digital detectors and iterative reconstruction.

Scans performed with gamma camera PET systems with crystals thinner than 5/8-inch will not be covered by Medicare. In addition, scans performed with systems with crystals greater than or equal to 5/8-inch in thickness, but that do not meet the other listed design characteristics are not covered by Medicare.

2. Allowable PET systems by covered clinical indication:

Covered Clinical Condition	Allowable Type of FDG PET System		
	Prior to July 1, 2001	July 1, 2001 through December 31, 2001	On or after January 1, 2002
Characterization of single pulmonary nodules	Effective 1/1/1998, any FDA approved	Any FDA approved	FDA approved: Full ring Partial ring Certain coincidence systems
Initial staging of lung cancer (non small cell)	Effective 1/1/1998, any FDA approved	Any FDA approved	FDA approved: Full ring Partial ring Certain coincidence systems
Evaluating recurrence of melanoma prior to surgery as an alternative to a gallium scan	Effective 7/1/1999, any FDA approved.	Any FDA approved	FDA approved: Full ring Partial ring Certain coincidence systems
Diagnosis, staging, and restaging of colorectal cancer	Not covered by Medicare	Full ring	FDA approved: Full ring Partial ring
Diagnosis, staging, and restaging of esophageal cancer	Not covered by Medicare	Full ring	FDA approved: Full ring Partial ring
Diagnosis, staging, and restaging of head and neck cancers (excluding CNS and thyroid)	Not covered by Medicare	Full ring	FDA approved: Full ring Partial ring
Diagnosis, staging, and restaging of lung cancer (non small cell)	Not covered by Medicare	Full ring	FDA approved: Full ring Partial ring
Diagnosis, staging, and restaging of lymphoma	Not covered by Medicare	Full ring	FDA approved: Full ring Partial ring
Diagnosis, staging, and restaging of melanoma (noncovered for evaluating regional nodes)	Not covered by Medicare	Full ring	FDA approved: Full ring Partial ring
Determination of myocardial viability only following an inconclusive SPECT	Not covered by Medicare	Full ring	FDA approved: Full ring Partial ring
Presurgical evaluation of refractory seizures	Not covered by Medicare	Full ring	FDA approved: Full ring Partial ring
Breast Cancer	Not covered	Not covered	Effective October 1, 2002, full and partial ring
Thyroid Cancer	Not covered	Not covered	Effective October 1, 2003, full and partial ring
Myocardial Viability Primary or initial diagnosis prior to revascularization	Not covered	Not covered	Effective October 1, 2002, full and partial ring

B. Regardless of any other terms or conditions, all uses of FDG PET scans, in order to be covered by the Medicare program, must meet the following general conditions prior to June 30, 2001:

1. Submission of claims for payment must include any information Medicare requires to assure that the PET scans performed were: (a) medically necessary, (b) did not unnecessarily duplicate other covered diagnostic tests, and (c) did not involve investigational drugs or procedures using investigational drugs, as determined by the Food and Drug Administration (FDA).
2. The PET scan entity submitting claims for payment must keep such patient records as Medicare requires on file for each patient for whom a PET scan claim is made.

C. Regardless of any other terms or conditions, all uses of FDG PET scans, in order to be covered by the Medicare program, must meet the following general conditions as of July 1,2001:

1. The provider of the PET scan should maintain on file the doctor's referral and documentation that the procedure involved only FDA approved drugs and devices, as is normal business practice.
2. The ordering physician is responsible for documenting the medical necessity of the study and that it meets the conditions specified in the instructions. The physician should have documentation in the beneficiary's medical record to support the referral to the PET scan provider.

III. Covered Indications for PET Scans and Limitations/Requirements for Usage

For all uses of PET relating to malignancies the following conditions apply:

1. Diagnosis: PET is covered only in clinical situations in which the PET results may assist in avoiding an invasive diagnostic procedure, or in which the PET results may assist in determining the optimal anatomical location to perform an invasive diagnostic procedure. In general, for most solid tumors, a tissue diagnosis is made prior to the performance of PET scanning. PET scans following a tissue diagnosis are performed for the purpose of staging, not diagnosis. Therefore, the use of PET in the diagnosis of lymphoma, esophageal, and colorectal cancers as well as in melanoma should be rare. PET is not covered for other diagnostic uses, and is not covered for screening (testing of patients without specific signs and symptoms of disease).
2. Staging and or Restaging: PET is covered in clinical situations in which 1) (a) the stage of the cancer remains in doubt after completion of a standard diagnostic workup, including conventional imaging (computed tomography, magnetic resonance imaging, or ultrasound) or (b) the use of PET would also be considered reasonable and necessary if it could potentially replace one or more conventional imaging studies when it is expected that conventional study information is insufficient for the clinical management of the patient and 2) clinical management of the patient would differ depending on the stage of the cancer identified. PET will be covered for restaging after the completion of treatment for the purpose of detecting residual disease, for detecting suspected recurrence or to determine the extent of a known recurrence. Use of PET would also be considered reasonable and necessary if it could potentially replace one or more conventional imaging studies when it is expected that conventional study information is insufficient for the clinical management of the patient.
3. Monitoring: Use of PET to monitor tumor response during the planned course of therapy (i.e. when no change in therapy is being contemplated) is not covered except for breast cancer. Restaging only occurs after a course of treatment is completed, and this is covered, subject to the conditions above.

NOTE: In the absence of national frequency limitations, contractors, should, if necessary, develop frequency requirements on any or all of the indications covered on and after July 1, 2001.

(This NCD last reviewed December 2004.)

Pub. 100-3, Section 230.1
Treatment of Kidney Stones

In addition to the traditional surgical/endoscopic techniques for the treatment of kidney stones, the following lithotripsy techniques are also covered for services rendered on or after March 15, 1985.

A. Extracorporeal Shock Wave Lithotripsy.--Extracorporeal Shock Wave Lithotripsy (ESWL) is a non-invasive method of treating kidney stones using a device called a lithotriptor. The lithotriptor uses shock waves generated outside of the body to break up upper urinary tract stones. It focuses the shock waves specifically on stones under X-ray visualization, pulverizing them by repeated shocks. ESWL is covered under Medicare for use in the treatment of upper urinary tract kidney stones.

B. Percutaneous Lithotripsy.--Percutaneous lithotripsy (or nephrolithotomy) is an invasive method of treating kidney stones by using ultrasound, electrohydraulic or mechanical lithotripsy. A probe is inserted through an incision in the skin directly over the kidney and applied to the stone. A form of lithotripsy is then used to fragment the stone. Mechanical or electrohydraulic lithotripsy may be used as an alternative or adjunct to ultrasonic lithotripsy. Percutaneous lithotripsy of kidney stones by ultrasound or by the related techniques of electrohydraulic or mechanical lithotripsy is covered under Medicare.

The following is covered for services rendered on or after January 16, 1988.

C. Transurethral Ureteroscopic Lithotripsy.--Transurethral ureteroscopic lithotripsy is a method of fragmenting and removing ureteral and renal stones through a cystoscope. The cystoscope is inserted through the urethra into the bladder. Catheters are passed through the scope into the opening where the ureters enter the bladder. Instruments passed through this opening into the ureters are used to manipulate and ultimately disintegrate stones, using either mechanical crushing, transcystoscopic electrohydraulic shock waves, ultrasound or laser. Transurethral ureteroscopic lithotripsy for the treatment of urinary tract stones of the kidney or ureter is covered under Medicare.

Pub. 100-3, Section 230.5
Gravlee Jet Washer

The use of this device is indicated where the patient exhibits clinical symptoms or signs suggestive of endometrial disease, such as irregular or heavy vaginal bleeding.

Program payment cannot be made for the washer or the related diagnostic services when furnished in connection with the examination of an asymptomatic patient. Payment for routine physical checkups is precluded under the statute. (See §1862(a)(7) of the Act.)

Pub. 100-3, Section 230.6
Vabra Aspirator

Program payment cannot be made for the aspirator or the related diagnostic services when furnished in connection with the examination of an asymptomatic patient. Payment for routine physical checkups is precluded under the statute (§1862(a)(7) of the Act).

Pub. 100-3, Section 230.7
Water Purification and Softening Systems Used in Conjunction with Home Dialysis

A. Water Purification Systems.--Water used for home dialysis should be chemically free of heavy trace metals and/or organic contaminants which could be hazardous to the patient. It should also be as free of bacteria as possible but need not be biologically sterile. Since the characteristics of natural water supplies in most areas of the country are such that some type of water purification system is needed, such a system used in conjunction with a home dialysis (either peritoneal or hemodialysis) unit is covered under Medicare.
There are two types of water purification systems which will satisfy these requirements:
Deionization--The removal of organic substances, mineral salts of magnesium and calcium (causing hardness), compounds of fluoride and chloride from tap water using the process of filtration and ion exchange; or
Reverse Osmosis--The process used to remove impurities from tap water utilizing pressure to force water through a porous membrane.
Use of both a deionization unit and reverse osmosis unit in series, theoretically to provide the advantages of both systems, has been determined medically unnecessary since either system can provide water which is both chemically and bacteriologically pure enough for acceptable use in home dialysis. In addition, spare deionization tanks are not covered since they are essentially a precautionary supply rather than a current requirement for treatment of the patient.
Activated carbon filters used as a component of water purification systems to remove unsafe concentrations of chlorine and chloramines are covered when prescribed by a physician.

B. Water Softening System.--Except as indicated below, a water softening system used in conjunction with home dialysis is excluded from coverage under Medicare as not being reasonable and necessary within the meaning of §1862(a)(1) of the law. Such a system, in conjunction with a home dialysis unit, does not adequately remove the hazardous heavy metal contaminants (such as arsenic) which may be present in trace amounts.
A water softening system may be covered when used to pretreat water to be purified by a reverse osmosis (RO) unit for home dialysis where:
   • The manufacturer of the RO unit has set standards for the quality of water entering the RO (e.g., the water to be purified by the RO must be of a certain quality if the unit is to perform as intended);
   • The patient's water is demonstrated to be of a lesser quality than required; and
   • The softener is used only to soften water entering the RO unit, and thus, used only for dialysis. (The softener need not actually be built into the RO unit, but must be an integral part of the dialysis system.)

C. Developing Need When a Water Softening System is Replaced with a Water Purification Unit in an Existing Home Dialysis System.--The medical necessity of water purification units must be carefully developed when they replace water softening systems in existing home dialysis systems. A purification system may be ordered under these circumstances for a number of reasons. For example, changes in the medical community's opinions regarding the quality of water necessary for safe dialysis may lead the physician to decide the quality of water previously used should be improved, or the water quality itself may have deteriorated. Patients may have dialyzed using only an existing water softener previous to Medicare ESRD coverage because of inability to pay for a purification system. On the other hand, in some cases, the installation of a purification system is not medically necessary. Thus, when such a case comes to your attention, ask the physician to furnish the reason for the changes. Supporting documentation, such as the supplier's

recommendations or water analysis, may be required. All such cases should be reviewed by your medical consultants.

Pub. 100-3, Section 230.8
Non-Implantable Pelvic Floor Electrical Stimulator

Pelvic floor electrical stimulation with a non-implantable stimulator is covered for the treatment of stress and/or urge urinary incontinence in cognitively intact patients who have failed a documented trial of pelvic muscle exercise (PME) training.

A failed trial of PME training is defined as no clinically significant improvement in urinary continence after completing 4 weeks of an ordered plan of pelvic muscle exercises designed to increase periurethral muscle strength.

Pub. 100-3, Section 230.10
Incontinence Control Devices

A. Mechanical/Hydraulic Incontinence Control Devices.--Mechanical/hydraulic incontinence control devices are accepted as safe and effective in the management of urinary incontinence in patients with permanent anatomic and neurologic dysfunctions of the bladder. This class of devices achieves control of urination by compression of the urethra. The materials used and the success rate may vary somewhat from device to device. Such a device is covered when its use is reasonable and necessary for the individual patient.

B. Collagen Implant.--A collagen implant, which is injected into the submucosal tissues of the urethra and/or the bladder neck and into tissues adjacent to the urethra, is a prosthetic device used in the treatment of stress urinary incontinence resulting from intrinsic sphincter deficiency (ISD). ISD is a cause of stress urinary incontinence in which the urethral sphincter is unable to contract and generate sufficient resistance in the bladder, especially during stress maneuvers.

Prior to collagen implant therapy, a skin test for collagen sensitivity must be administered and evaluated over a 4 week period.

In male patients, the evaluation must include a complete history and physical examination and a simple cystometrogram to determine that the bladder fills and stores properly. The patient then is asked to stand upright with a full bladder and to cough or otherwise exert abdominal pressure on his bladder. If the patient leaks, the diagnosis of ISD is established.

In female patients, the evaluation must include a complete history and physical examination (including a pelvic exam) and a simple cystometrogram to rule out abnormalities of bladder compliance and abnormalities of urethral support. Following that determination, an abdominal leak point pressure (ALLP) test is performed. Leak point pressure, stated in cm H2O, is defined as the intra-abdominal pressure at which leakage occurs from the bladder (around a catheter) when the bladder has been filled with a minimum of 150 cc fluid. If the patient has an ALLP of less than 100 cm H2O, the diagnosis of ISD is established.

To use a collagen implant, physicians must have urology training in the use of a cystoscope and must complete a collagen implant training program.

Coverage of a collagen implant, and the procedure to inject it, is limited to the following types of patients with stress urinary incontinence due to ISD:

   • Male or female patients with congenital sphincter weakness secondary to conditions such as myelomeningocele or epispadias;
   • Male or female patients with acquired sphincter weakness secondary to spinal cord lesions;
   • Male patients following trauma, including prostatectomy and/or radiation; and
   • Female patients without urethral hypermobility and with abdominal leak point pressures of 100 cm H2O or less.

Patients whose incontinence does not improve with 5 injection procedures (5 separate treatment sessions) are considered treatment failures, and no further treatment of urinary incontinence by collagen implant is covered. Patients who have a reoccurrence of incontinence following successful treatment with collagen implants in the past (e.g., 6-12 months previously) may benefit from additional treatment sessions. Coverage of additional sessions may be allowed but must be supported by medical justification.

C. Non-Implantable Pelvic Floor Electrical Stimulator.--(See §60-24.)

Pub. 100-3, Section 230.12
Dimethyl Sulfoxide (DMSO)

The Food and Drug Administration has determined that the only purpose for which DMSO is safe and effective for humans is in the treatment of the bladder condition, interstitial cystitis. Therefore, the use of DMSO for all other indications is not considered to be reasonable and necessary. Payment may be made for its use only when reasonable and necessary for a patient in the treatment of interstitial cystitis.

Pub. 100-3, Section 230.16
Bladder Stimulators (Pacemakers)
The use of spinal cord electrical stimulators, rectal electrical stimulators, and bladder wall stimulators is not considered reasonable and necessary. Therefore, no program payment may be made for these devices or for their implantation.

Pub. 100-3, Section 230.17
Urinary Drainage Bags

Urinary collection and retention system are covered as prosthetic devices that replace bladder function in the case of permanent urinary incontinence. Urinary drainage bags that can be used either as bedside or leg drainage bags may be either multi-use or single use systems. Both the multi-use and the single use bags have a system that prevents urine backflow. However, the single use system is non-drainable. There is insufficient evidence to support the medical necessity of a single use system bag rather than the multi-use bag. Therefore, a single use drainage system is subject to the same coverage parameters as the multi-use drainage bags.

Pub. 100-3, Section 230.19
Levocarnitine for use in the Treatment of Carnitine Deficiency in ESRD Patients
Intravenous levocarnitine, for one of the following indications, will only be covered for those ESRD patients who have been on dialysis for a minimum of three months. Patients must have documented carnitine deficiency, defined as a plasma free carnitine level <◻40 micromol/L (determined by a professionally accepted method as recognized in current literature), along with signs and symptoms of: <ol class="red" type="1"><li class="double">Erythropoietin-resistant anemia (persistent hematocrit <◻30% with treatment) that has not responded to standard erythropoietin dosage (that which is considered clinically appropriate to treat the particular patient) with iron replacement, and for which other causes have been investigated and adequately treated, or </li><li class="double">Hypotension on hemodialysis that interferes with delivery of the intended dialysis despite application of usual measures deemed appropriate (e.g., fluid management). Such episodes of hypotension must have occurred during at least 2 dialysis treatments in a 30-day period. </li></ol> Continued use of levocarnitine will not be covered if improvement has not been demonstrated within 6 months of initiation of treatment. All other indications for levocarnitine are non-covered in the ESRD population. For a patient currently receiving intravenous levocarnitine, Medicare will cover continued treatment if: <ol class="red" type="1"><li class="double">Levocarnitine has been administered to treat erythropoietin-resistent anemia (persistent hematocrit <◻30 percent with treatment) that has not responded to standard erythropoietin dosage (that which is considered clinically appropriate to treat the particular patient) with iron replacement, and for which other causes have been investigated and adequately treated, or hypotension on hemodialysis that interferes with delivery of the intended dialysis despite application of usual measures deemed appropriate (e.g., fluid management) and such episodes of hypotension occur during at least 2 dialysis treatments in a 30-day period; and </li><li class="double">The patient's medical record documents a pre-dialysis plasma free carnitine level <◻40 micromol/L prior to the initiation of treatment; or </li><li class="double">The treating physician certifies (documents in the medical record) that in his/her judgment, if treatment with levocarnitine is discontinued, the patient's pre-dialysis carnitine level would fall below 40 micromol/L and the patient would have recurrent erythropoietin-resistant-anemia or intradialytic hypotension. </li></ol>

Pub. 100-3, Section 240.2
Home Use of Oxygen

A. <u>General</u>

<u>Medicare coverage of home oxygen and oxygen equipment under the durable medical equipment (DME) benefit (see §1861(s)(6)of the Act) is considered reasonable and necessary only for patients with significant hypoxemia who meet the medical documentation, laboratory evidence, and health conditions specified in subsections B, C, and D. This section also includes special coverage criteria for portable oxygen systems. Finally, a statement on the absence of coverage of the professional services of a respiratory therapist under the DME benefit is included in subsection F.</u>

B. <u>Medical documentation</u>.

<u>Initial</u> claims for oxygen services <u>must</u> include a completed span Form CMS-484 (Form HCFA-484 (Certificate of Medical Necessity: Oxygen)to establish whether coverage criteria are met and to ensure that the oxygen services provided are consistent with the physician's prescription or other medical documentation. The treating physician's prescription or other medical documentation must indicate that other forms of treatment (e.g., medical and physical therapy directed at secretions, bronchospasm and infection) have been tried, have not been sufficiently successful, and oxygen therapy is still required. While there is no substitute for oxygen therapy, each patient must receive optimum therapy before long-term home oxygen therapy is ordered. Use Form HCFA-484 for recertifications. (See Medicare Program Integrity Manual, Chapter 5, for completion of Form CMS-484.)

The medical and prescription information in section B of Form CMS-484 can be completed only by the treating physician, the physician's employee, or another clinician (e.g., nurse, respiratory therapist, etc.) as long as that person is not the DME supplier. Although hospital discharge coordinators and medical social workers may assist in arranging for physician-prescribed home oxygen, they do not have the authority to prescribe the services. Suppliers may not enter this information. While this section may be completed by nonphysician clinician or a physician employee, it must be reviewed and the form CMS-484 signed by the attending physician.

A physician's certification of medical necessity for oxygen equipment must include the results of specific testing before coverage can be determined.

Claims for oxygen <u>must</u> also be supported by medical documentation in the patient's record. Separate documentation is used with electronic billing. (See Medicare Carriers Manual, Part 3,§4105.5.) This documentation may be in the form of a prescription written by the patient's attending physician who has recently examined the patient (normally within a month of the start of therapy) and must specify:

- A diagnosis of the disease requiring home use of oxygen;
- The oxygen flow rate; and

- An estimate of the frequency, duration of use (e.g., 2 liters per minute, 10 minutes per hour, 12 hours per day), and duration of need (e.g., 6 months or lifetime).

NOTE: A prescription for "Oxygen PRN" or "Oxygen as needed" does not meet this last requirement. Neither provides any basis for determining if the amount of oxygen is reasonable and necessary for the patient.

A member of the carrier's medical staff should review all claims with oxygen flow rates of more than 4 liters per minute before payment can be made.

The attending physician specifies the type of oxygen delivery system to be used (i.e., gas, liquid, or concentrator) by signing the completed form CMS-484. In addition the supplier or physician may use the space in section C for written confirmation of additional details of the physician's order. The additional order information contained in section C may include the means of oxygen delivery (mask, nasal, cannula, etc.), the specifics of varying flow rates, and/or the noncontinuous use of oxygen as appropriate. The physician confirms this order information with their signature in section D.

New medical documentation written by the patient's attending physician must be submitted to the carrier in support of revised oxygen requirements when there has been a change in the patient's condition and need for oxygen therapy.

Carriers are required to conduct periodic, continuing medical necessity reviews on patients whose conditions warrant these reviews and on patients with indefinite or extended periods of necessity as described in Program Integrity Manual, Chapter 5, "Items and Services Having Special DMERC Review Considerations,". When indicated, carriers may also request documentation of the results of a repeat arterial blood gas or oximetry study.

NOTE: Section 4152 of OBRA 1990 requires earlier recertification <u>and retesting</u> of oxygen patients who begin coverage with an arterial blood gas result at or above a partial pressure of 55 or an arterial oxygen saturation percentage at or above 89. (See Medicare Claims Processing Manual, Chapter 20, "Durable Medical Equipment, Prosthetics and Orthotics, and Supplies (DMEPOS)," §100.2.3 for certification and retesting schedules.)

C. <u>Laboratory Evidence.</u>-- <u>Initial</u> claims for oxygen therapy <u>must</u> also include the results of a blood gas study that has been ordered and evaluated by the attending physician. This is <u>usually</u> in the form of a measurement of the partial pressure of oxygen (PO_2) in arterial blood. (See Medicare Carriers Manual, Part 3, §2070.1 for instructions on clinical laboratory tests.) A measurement of arterial oxygen saturation obtained by ear or pulse oximetry, however, is also acceptable when ordered and evaluated by the attending physician <u>and</u> performed under his or her supervision or when performed by a qualified provider or supplier of laboratory services. When the arterial blood gas and the oximetry studies are both used to document the need for home oxygen therapy and the results are conflicting, the arterial blood gas study is the preferred source of documenting medical need. A DME supplier is not considered a qualified provider or supplier of laboratory services for purposes of these guidelines. This prohibition does not extend to the results of blood gas test conducted by a hospital certified to do such tests. The conditions under which the laboratory tests are performed must be specified in writing and submitted with the <u>initial</u> claim, i.e., at rest, during exercise, or during sleep.

The preferred sources of laboratory evidence are existing physician and/or hospital records that reflect the patient's medical condition. Since it is expected that virtually all patients who qualify for home oxygen coverage for the first time under these guidelines have recently been discharged from a hospital where they submitted to arterial blood gas tests, the carrier needs to request that such test results be submitted in support of their initial claims for home oxygen. If more than one arterial blood gas test is performed during the patient's hospital stay, the test result obtained closest to, but no earlier than 2 days prior to the hospital discharge date is required as evidence of the need for home oxygen therapy.

For those patients whose initial oxygen prescription did not originate during a hospital stay, blood gas studies should be done while the patient is in the chronic stable state, i.e., not during a period of an acute illness or an exacerbation of their underlying disease."

Carriers may accept a attending physician's statement of recent hospital test results for a particular patient, when appropriate, in lieu of copies of actual hospital records.

A repeat arterial blood gas study is appropriate when evidence indicates that an oxygen recipient has undergone a <u>major</u> change in their condition relevant to home use of oxygen. If the carrier has reason to believe that there has been a major change in the patient's physical condition, it may ask for documentation of the results of another blood gas or oximetry study.

D. <u>Health Conditions</u>.--Coverage is available for patients with significant hypoxemia in the chronic stable state if: (1) the attending physician has determined that the patient has a health condition outlined in subsection D.1, (2) the patient meets the blood gas evidence requirements specified in subsection D.3, and (3) the patient has appropriately tried other alternative treatment measures without complete success. (See subsection B.)

1. <u>Conditions for Which Oxygen Therapy May Be Covered</u>.--

o A severe lung disease, such as chronic obstructive pulmonary disease, diffuse interstitial lung disease, whether of known or unknown etiology; cystic fibrosis bronchiectasis; widespread pulmonary neoplasm; or

o Hypoxia-related symptoms or findings that might be expected to improve with oxygen therapy. Examples of these symptoms and findings are pulmonary hypertension, recurring congestive heart failure due to chronic cor pulmonale, erythrocytosis, impairment of the cognitive process, nocturnal restlessness, and morning headache.

2. <u>Conditions for Which Oxygen Therapy Is Not Covered</u>.--

o Angina pectoris in the absence of hypoxemia. This condition is generally not the result of a low oxygen level in the blood, and there are other preferred treatments;

o Breathlessness without cor pulmonale or evidence of hypoxemia. Although intermittent oxygen use is sometimes prescribed to relieve this condition, it is potentially harmful and psychologically addicting;

o Severe peripheral vascular disease resulting in clinically evident desaturation in one or more extremities. There is no evidence that increased PO_2 improves the oxygenation of tissues with impaired circulation; or

o Terminal illnesses that do not affect the lungs.

3. <u>Covered Blood Gas Values</u>.--If the patient has a condition specified in subsection D.1, the carrier must review the medical documentation and laboratory evidence that has been submitted for a particular patient (see subsections B and C) and determine if coverage is available under one of the three group categories outlined below.

a. <u>Group I</u>.--Except as modified in subsection d, coverage is provided for patients with significant hypoxemia evidenced by <u>any</u> of the following:

(1) An arterial PO_2 at or below 55 mm Hg, or an arterial oxygen saturation at or below 88 percent, <u>taken at rest</u>, breathing room air.

(2) An arterial PO_2 at or below 55 mm Hg, or an arterial oxygen saturation at or below 88 percent, taken <u>during sleep</u> for a patient who demonstrates an arterial PO_2 at or above 56 mm Hg, or an arterial oxygen saturation at or above 89 percent, while awake; or a greater than normal fall in oxygen level <u>during sleep</u> (a decrease in arterial PO_2 more than 10 mm Hg, or decrease in arterial oxygen saturation more than 5 percent) associated with symptoms or signs reasonably attributable to hypoxemia (e.g., impairment of cognitive processes and nocturnal restlessness or insomnia). In either of these cases, coverage is provided <u>only</u> for use of oxygen during sleep, and then only one type of unit will be covered. Portable oxygen, therefore, would not be covered in this situation.

(3) An arterial PO_2 at or below 55 mm Hg or an arterial oxygen saturation at or below 88 percent, taken <u>during exercise</u> for a patient who demonstrates an arterial PO_2 at or above 56 mm Hg, or an arterial oxygen saturation at or above 89 percent, during the day while at rest. In this case, supplemental oxygen is provided for <u>during exercise</u> if there is evidence the use of oxygen improves the hypoxemia that was demonstrated during exercise when the patient was breathing room air.

b. <u>Group II</u>.--Except as modified in subsection d, coverage is available for patients whose arterial PO_2 is 56-59 mm Hg or whose arterial blood oxygen saturation is 89 percent, <u>if</u> there is evidence of:

(1) Dependent edema suggesting congestive heart failure;
(2) Pulmonary hypertension or cor pulmonale, determined by measurement of pulmonary artery pressure, gated blood pool scan, echocardiogram, or "P" pulmonale on EKG (P wave greater than 3 mm in standard leads II, III, or AVFL; or
(3) Erythrocythemia with a hematocrit greater than 56 percent.

c. <u>Group III</u>.--Except as modified in subsection d, carriers <u>must</u> apply a rebuttable presumption that a home program of oxygen use is not medically necessary for patients with arterial PO_2 levels at or above 60 mm Hg, or arterial blood oxygen saturation at or above 90 percent. In order for claims in this category to be reimbursed, the carrier's reviewing physician needs to review any documentation submitted in rebuttal of this presumption and grant specific approval of the claims. HCFA expects few claims to be approved for coverage in this category.

d. <u>Variable Factors That May Affect Blood Gas Values</u>.--In reviewing the arterial PO_2 levels and the arterial oxygen saturation percentages specified in subsections D. 3. a, b and c, the carrier's medical staff must take into account variations in oxygen measurements that may result from such factors as the patient's age, the altitude level, or the patient's decreased oxygen carrying capacity.

E. <u>Portable Oxygen Systems</u>.--A patient meeting the requirements specified below may qualify for coverage of a portable oxygen system either (1) by itself or (2) to use in addition to a stationary oxygen system. A portable oxygen system is covered for a particular patient if:

o The claim meets the requirements specified in subsections A-D, as appropriate; and

o The medical documentation indicates that the patient is mobile in the home and would benefit from the use of a portable oxygen system in the home. Portable oxygen systems are not covered for patients who qualify for oxygen solely based on blood gas studies obtained during sleep.

F. <u>Respiratory Therapists</u>.--Respiratory therapists' services are <u>not covered</u> under the provisions for coverage of oxygen services under the Part B durable medical equipment benefit as outlined above. This benefit provides for coveravge of home use of oxygen and oxygen equipment, but does not include a professional component in the delivery of such services.

Pub. 100-3, Section 240.4
Continuous Positive Airway Pressure (CPAP)

B. Nationally Covered Indications

The use of CPAP is covered under Medicare when used in adult patients with moderate or severe OSA for whom surgery is a likely alternative to CPAP. The use of CPAP devices must be ordered and prescribed by the licensed treating physician to be used in adult patients with moderate to severe OSA if either of the following criterion using the Apnea-Hypopnea Index (AHI) are met:

- AHI greater than or equal to 15 events per hour, or
- AHI greater than or equal to 5 and less than or equal to 14 events per hour with documented symptoms of excessive daytime sleepiness, impaired cognition, mood disorders or insomnia, or documented hypertension, ischemic heart disease, or history of stroke.

The AHI is equal to the average number of episodes of apnea and hypopnea per hour and must be based on a minimum of 2 hours of sleep recorded by polysomnography using actual recorded hours of sleep (i.e., the AHI may not be extrapolated or projected).

Apnea is defined as cessation of airflow for least 10 seconds. Hypopnea is defined as an abnormal respiratory event lasting at least 10 seconds with at least 30 percent reduction in thoracoabdominal movement or aiflow as compared to baseline, and with at least a 4 percent oxygen desaturation.

The polysomnography must be performed in a facility - based sleep study laboratory, and not in the home or in a mobile facility.

Initial claims must be supported by medical documentation (separate documentation where electronic billing is used), such as prescription written by the patient's attending physician that specifies:

- A diagnosis of moderate or severe obstructive sleep apnea, and
- Surgery is a likely alternative.

The claim must also certify that the documentation supporting a diagnosis of OSA (described above) is available.

C. Nationally Non-covered Indications

Effective April 4, 2005, the Centers for Medicare & Medicaid Services determined that upon reconsideration of the current policy, there is not sufficient evidence to conclude that unattended portable multi-channel sleep study testing is reasonable and necessary in the diagnosis of OSA for CPAP therapy, and these tests will remain noncovered for this purpose.

D. Other

N/A

(This NCD last reviewed April 2005)

Pub. 100-3, Section 240.5
Intrapulmonary Percussive Ventilator (IPV)
Studies do not demonstrate any advantage of IPV over that achieved with good pulmonary care in the hospital environment and there are no studies in the home setting. There are no data to support the effectiveness of the device. Therefore, IPV in the home setting is not covered.

Pub. 100-3, Section 260.3
Pancreas Transplants

B. National Covered Indications

CMS determines that whole organ pancreas transplantation will be nationally covered by Medicare only when performed siumltaneous with or after a kidney transplant. If the pancreas transplant occurs after the kidney transplant, immunosuppressive therapy will begin with the date of discharge from the inpatient stay for the pancrease transplant.

C. Nationally Noncovered Indications

CMS determines that the following procedures are not considered reasonable and necessary within the meaning of section 1862(a)(1)(A) of the Social Security Act:

1. Pancreas transplantation for diabetic patients who have not experienced end stage renal failure secondary to diabetes.

2. Transplantation of partial pancreatic tissue or islet cells (except in the context of a clinical trial (see section 260.3.1 of the NCD Manual)).

D. Other

Not applicable

(This NCD last reviewed July 2004.)

Pub. 100-3, Section 260.6
Dental Examination Prior to Kidney Transplantation

Despite the "dental services exclusion" in §1862(a)(12) of the Act (see the Medicare Benefit Policy Manual,Chapter 16, "General Exclusions from Coverage" §140), an oral or dental examination performed on an inpatient basis as part of a comprehensive workup prior to renal transplant surgery is a covered service. This is because the purpose of the examination is not for the care of the teeth or structures directly supporting the teeth. Rather, the examination is for the identification, prior to a complex surgical procedure, of existing medical problems where the increased possibility of infection would not only reduce the chances for successful surgery but would also expose the patient to additional risks in undergoing such surgery.

Such a dental or oral examination would be covered under Part A of the program if performed by a dentist on the hospital's staff, or under Part B if performed by a physician. (When performing a dental or oral examination, a dentist is not recognized as a physician under §1861(r) of the law.)(See the Mediacre Geneal Information, Eligibility and Entitlement Manual, Chapter 15, "Covered Medical and Other Health Services," §150)

Pub. 100-3, Section 260.7
Lymphocyte Immune Globulin, Anti-Thymocyte Globulin (Equine)

The FDA has approved one lymphocyte immune globulin preparation for marketing, lymphocyte immune globulin, anti-thymocyte globulin (equine). This drug is indicated for the management of allograft rejection episodes in renal transplantation. It is covered under Medicare when used for this purpose. Other forms of lymphocyte globulin preparation which the FDA approves for this indication in the future may be covered under Medicare.

Pub. 100-3, Section 270.1
Electrical Stimulation (ES) and Electromagnetic Therapy for the Treatment of Wounds
A. *Nationally Covered Indications*

The use of ES and electromagnetic therapy for the treatment of wounds are considered adjunctive therapies, and will only be covered for chronic Stage III or Stage IV pressure ulcers, arterial ulcers, diabetic ulcers, and venous stasis ulcers. Chronic ulcers are defined as ulcers that have not healed within 30 days of occurrence. ES or electromagnetic therapy will be covered only after appropriate standard wound therapy has been tried for at least 30 days and there are no measurable signs of improved healing. This 30-day period may begin while the wound is acute.

Standard wound care includes: optimization of nutritional status, debridement by any means to remove devitalized tissue, maintenance of a clean, moist bed of granulation tissue with appropriate moist dressings, and necessary treatment to resolve any infection that may be present. Standard wound care based on the specific type of wound includes: frequent repositioning of a patient with pressure ulcers (usually every 2 hours), offloading of pressure and good glucose control for diabetic ulcers, establishment of adequate circulation for arterial ulcers, and the use of a compression system for patients with venous ulcers.

Measurable signs of improved healing include: a decrease in wound size (either surface area or volume), decrease in amount of exudates, and decrease in amount of necrotic tissue. ES or electromagnetic therapy must be discontinued when the wound demonstrates 100% epitheliliazed wound bed.

ES and electromagnetic therapy services can only be covered when performed by a physician, physical therapist, or incident to a physician service. Evaluation of the wound is an integral part of wound therapy. When a physician, physical therapist, or a clinician incident to a physician, performs ES or electromagnetic therapy, the practitioner must evaluate the wound and contact the treating physician if the wound worsens. If ES or electromagnetic therapy is being used, wounds must be evaluated at least monthly by the treating physician.

B. *Nationally Noncovered Indications*

1. ES and electromagnetic therapy will not be covered as an initial treatment modality.

2. Continued treatment with ES or electromagnetic therapy is not covered if measurable signs of healing have not been demonstrated within any 30-day period of treatment.

3. Unsupervised use of ES or electromagnetic therapy for wound therapy will not be covered, as this use has not been found to be medically reasonable and necessary.
C. *Other*

All other uses of ES and electromagnetic therapy not otherwise specified for the treatment of wounds remain at local contractor discretion.

(This NCD last reviewed March 2004.)

Pub. 100-3, Section 270.2
Noncontact Normothermic Wound Therapy (NNWT)
There is insufficient scientific or clinical evidence to consider this device as reasonable and necessary for the treatment of wounds within the meaning of §1862(a)(1)(A) of the Social Security Act and will not be covered by Medicare.

Pub. 100-3, Section 280.1
Durable Medical Equipment Reference List

The durable medical equipment (DME) list which follows is designed to facilitate your processing of DME claims. This section is designed to be used as a quick reference tool for determining the coverage status of certain pieces of DME and especially for those items which are commonly referred to by both brand and generic names. The information contained herein is applicable (where appropriate) to all DME coverage determinations discussed in the DME portion of this manual. The list is organized into two columns. The first column lists alphabetically various generic categories of equipment on which national coverage decisions have been made by CMS; and the second column notes the coverage status of each equipment category.

In the case of equipment categories that have been determined by CMS to be covered under the DME benefit, the list outlines the conditions of coverage that must be met if payment is to be allowed for the rental or purchase of the DME by a particular patient, or cross-refers to another section of the manual where the applicable coverage criteria are described in more detail. With respect to equipment categories that cannot be covered as DME, the list includes a brief explanation of why the equipment is not covered. This DME list will be updated periodically to reflect any additional national coverage decisions that CMS may make with regard to other categories of equipment.

When you receive a claim for an item of equipment which does not appear to fall logically into any of the generic categories listed, you have the authority and responsibility for deciding whether those items are covered under the DME benefit. These decisions must be made by each contractor based on the advice of its medical consultants, taking into account:

The Medicare Claims Processing Manual, Chapter 20, "Durable Medical Equipment, Prosthetics and Orthotics, and Supplies (DMEPOS)".

- Whether the item has been approved for marketing by the Food and Drug Administration (FDA) and is otherwise generally considered to be safe and effective for the purpose intended; and
- Whether the item is reasonable and necessary for the individual patient.

Durable Medical Equipment Reference List:

Item	Coverage Status
Air Cleaners	- deny--environmental control equipment; not primarily medical in nature (§1861(n) of the Act)
Air Conditioners	- deny--environmental control equipment; not primarily medical in nature (§1861(n) of the Act)
Air-Fluidized Bed	- (See §60-19.)
Alternating Pressure Pads, and Matresses and Lambs Wool Pads	- covered if patient has, or is highly susceptible to, decubitus ulcers and patient's physician has specified that he will be supervising its use in connection with his course of treatment.
Audible/Visible Signal Pacemaker Monitor	- (See Self-Contained Pacemaker Monitor.)
Augmentative Communication Device	-- (See Speech Generating Devices, §60-23.)
Bathtub Lifts	- deny--convenience item; not primarily medical in nature (§1861(n) of the Act)
Bathtub Seats	- deny--comfort or convenience item; hygienic equipment; not primarily medical in nature (§1861(n) of the Act)
Bead Bed	- (See §60-19.)
Bed Baths (home type)	- deny--hygienic equipment; not primarily medical in nature (§1861(n) of the Act)
Bed Lifter (bed elevator)	- deny--not primarily medical in nature (§1861(n) of the Act.
Bedboards	- deny--not primarily medical in nature (§1861(n) of the Act)
Bed Pans (autoclavable hospital type)	- covered if patient is bed confined
Bed Side Rails	- (See Hospital Beds, §60-l8.)

Beds-Lounge (power or manual)	- deny--not a hospital bed; comfort or convenience item; not primarily medical in nature (§186l(n) of the Act)	Disposable Sheets and Bags	-- deny--nonreusable disposable supplies (§1861(n) of the Act)
Beds--Oscillating	- deny--institutional equipment; inappropriate for home use	Elastic Stockings	-- deny--nonreusable supply; not rental-type items (§1861(n) of the Act)
Bidet Toilet Seat	- (See Toilet Seats.)	Electric Air Cleaners	-- deny--(See Air Cleaners.) (§1861(n) of the Act)
Blood Glucose Analyzer Reflectance Colorimeter	- deny--unsuitable for home use (See §60-11.)	Electric Hospital Beds	-- (See Hospital Beds §60-18.)
Blood Glucose Monitor	- covered if patient meets certain conditions (See §60-11.)	Electrical Stimulation for Wounds	-- deny--inappropriate for home use
Braille Teaching Texts	- deny--educational equipment; not primarily medical in nature (§1861(n) of the Act)	Electrostatic Machines	-- deny--(See Air Cleaners and Air Conditioners.) (§1861(n) of the Act)
		Elevators	-- deny--convenience item; not primarily medical in nature (§1861(n) of the Act)
Canes	- covered if patient's condition impairs ambulation (See §60-3.)	Emesis Basins	-- deny--convenience item; not primarily medical in nature (§1861(n) of the Act)
Carafes	- deny--convenience item; not primarily medical in nature (§1861(n) of the Act)	Esophageal Dilator	-- deny--physician instrument; inappropriate for patient use
Catheters	- deny--nonreusable disposable supply (§1861(n) of the Act)	Exercise Equipment	-- deny--not primarily medical in nature (§1861(n) of the Act)
Commodes	- covered if patient is confined to bed or room	Fabric Supports	-- deny--nonreusable supplies; not rental-type it (§1861(n) of the Act)
	NOTE: The term "room confined" means that the patient's condition is such that leaving the room is medically contraindicated. The accessibility of bathroom facilities generally would not be a factor in this determination. However, confinement of a patient to his home in a case where there are no toilet facilities in the home may be equated to room confinement. Moreover, payment may also be made if a patient's medical condition confines him to a floor of his home and there is no bathroom located on that floor (See hospital beds in §60-18 for definition of "bed confinement".)	Face Masks (oxygen)	-- covered if oxygen is covered (See § 60-4.)
		Face Masks (surgical)	-- deny--nonreusable disposable items (§1861(n) of the Act)
		Flowmeter	(See Medical Oxygen Regulators)
		Fluidic Breathing Assister	(See IPPB Machines.)
		Fomentation Device	(See Heating Pads.)
		Gel Flotation Pads and Mattresses	(See Alternating Pressure Pads and Mattresses.)
Communicator	-- (See §60-23, Speech Generating Devices)	Grab Bars	deny--self-help device; not primarily medical in nature (§1861(n) of the Act)
Continuous Passive Motion	-- Continuous passive motion devices are devices covered for patients who have received a total knee replacement. To qualify for coverage, use of the device must commence within 2 days following surgery. In addition, coverage is limited to that portion of the three week period following surgery during which the device is used in the patient's home.	Heat and Massage Foam Cushion Pad	deny--not primarily medical in nature; personal comfort item (§§ 1861(n) and 1862(a)(6) of the Act)
		Heating and Cooling Plants	deny--environmental control equipment; not primarily medical in nature(§1861(n) of the Act)
	There is insufficient evidence to justify coverage of these devices for longer periods of time or for other applications.	Heating Pads	covered if the contractor's medical staff determines patient's medical condition is one for which the application of heat in the form of a heating pad is therapeutically effective.
Continuous Positive Airway Pressure (CPAP)	-- (See §60-17.)	Heat Lamps	covered if the contractor's medical staff determines patient's medical condition is one for which the application of heat in the form of a heat lamp is therapeutically effective.
Crutches	-- covered if patient's condition impairs Ambulation		
Cushion Lift Power Seat	-- (See Seat Lifts.)		
Dehumidifiers (room or central heating system type)	-- deny--environmental control equipment; not primarily medical in nature (§1861(n) of the Act	Hospital Beds	(See § 60-18.)
		Hot Packs	(See Heating Pads.)
Diathermy Machines (standard pulses wave types)	-- deny--inappropriate for home use (See and §35-41.)	Humidifiers	(oxygen) (See Oxygen Humidifiers.)
		Humidifiers (room or central heating system types)	deny--environmental control equipment; not medical in nature (§1861(n) of the Act)
Digital Electronic Pacemaker Monitor	-- (See Self-Contained Pacemaker Monitor.)	Hydraulic Lift	(See Patient Lifts.)

Incontinent Pads	deny--nonreusable supply; hygienic item (§l861(n) of the Act.)
Infusion Pumps	For external and implantable pumps, see §60-14. If the pump is used with an enteral or parenteral ralnutritional therapy system, see §§65-10 - 65.10.2 0.2 for special coverage rules.
Injectors (hypodermic jet devices for injection of insulin)	deny-- noncovered self-administered drug supply, §1861(s)(2)(A) of the Act)
IPPB Machines	covered if patient's ability to breathe is severely impaired
Iron Lungs	(See Ventilators.)
Irrigating Kit	deny--nonreusable supply; hygienic equipment (§l861(n) of the Act)
Lambs Wool Pads	covered under same conditions as alternating pressure pads and mattresses
Leotards	deny--(See Pressure Leotards.) (§l861(n)of the Act)
Lymphedema Pumps	covered (See §60-16.)(segmental and non-segmental therapy types)
Massage Devices	deny--personal comfort items; not primarily medical in nature (§§l861(n) and l862(a)(6) of the Act)
Mattress	covered only where hospital bed is medically necessary (Separate Charge for replacement mattresss should not be allowed where hospital bed with mattress is rented.) (See §60-18.)
Medical Oxygen Regulators	covered if patient's ability to breathe is severely impaired (See §60-4.)
Mobile Geriatric Chair	(See Rolling Chairs.)
Motorized Wheelchairs	(See Wheelchairs (power operated).)
Muscle Stimulators	Covered for certain conditions (See §35-77.)
Nebulizers	covered if patient's ability to breathe is severely impaired
Oscillating Beds	deny--institutional equipment--inappropriate for home use
Overbed Tables	deny--convenience item; not primarily medical in nature (§l861(n) of the Act)
Oxygen	covered if the oxygen has been prescribed for use in connection with medically necessary durable medical equipment (See §60-4.)
Oxygen Humidifiers	covered if a medical humidifier has been prescribed for use in connection with medically necessary durable medical equipment for purposes of moisturizing oxygen (See §60-4.)
Oxygen Regulators (Medical)	(See Medical Oxygen Regulators.)
Oxygen Tents	(See § 60-4.)
Paraffin Bath Units (Portable)	(See Portable Paraffin Bath Units.)
Paraffin Bath Units (Standard)	deny--institutional equipment; inappropriate for home use
Parallel Bars	deny--support exercise equipment; primarily for institutional use; in the home setting other devices (e.g., a walker) satisfy the patient's need
Patient Lifts	covered if contractor's medical staff determines patient's condition is such that periodic movement is necessary to effect improvement or to arrest or retard deterioration in his condition.
Percussors	covered for mobilizing respiratory tract secretions in patients with chronic obstructive lung disease, chronic bronchitis, or emphysema, when patient or operator of powered percussor has received appropriate training by a physician or therapist, and no one competent to administer manual therapy is available.
Portable Oxygen Systems: 1. Regulated (adjustable flow rate) 2. Preset (flow rate not adjustable)	--covered under conditions specified in §60-4. Refer all claims to medical staff for this determination. --deny--emergency, first-aid, or precautionary equipment; essentially not therapeutic in nature
Portable Paraffin Bath Units	covered when the patient has undergone a successful trial period of paraffin therapy ordered by a physician and the patient's condition is expected to be relieved by long term use of this modality.
Portable Room Heaters	deny--environmental control equipment; not primarily medical in nature (§l861(n) of the Act)
Portable Whirlpool Pumps	deny--not primarily medical in nature; personal comfort items (§§l861(n) and l862(a)(6) of the Act)
Postural Drainage Boards	covered if patient has a chronic pulmonary condition
Preset Portable Oxygen Units	deny--emergency, first-aid, or precautionary equipment; essentially not therapeutic in nature
Pressure Leotards	deny--nonreusable supply, not rental-type item (§l861(n) of the Act)
Pulse Tachometer	deny--not reasonable or necessary for monitoring pulse of homebound patient with or without a cardiac pacemaker
Quad-Canes	(See Walkers.)
Raised Toilet Seats	deny--convenience item; hygienic equipment; not primarily medical in nature (§l861(n) of the Act)
Reflectance Colorimeters	(See Blood Glucose Analyzers.)
Respirators	(See Ventilators.)
Rolling Chairs	covered if the contractor's medical staff determines that the patient's condition is such that there is a medical need for this item and it has been prescribed by the patient's physician in lieu of a wheelchair. Coverage is limited to those rollabout chairs having casters of at least 5 inches in diameter and specifically designed to meet the needs of ill, injured, or otherwise impaired individuals. Coverage is denied for the wide range of chairs with smaller casters as are found in general use in homes, offices, and institutions for many purposes not related to the care or treatment of ill or injured persons. This type is not primarily medical in nature. (§l861(n) of the Act)
Safety Roller	(See §60-15.)

Sauna Baths	deny--not primarily medical in nature; personal comfort items (§§1861(n) and (1862(a)(6) of the Act)
Seat Lift	covered under the conditions specified in §60-8. Refer all to medical staff for this determination.
Self-Contained Pacemaker Monitor	covered when prescribed by a physician for a patient with a cardiac pacemaker (See §§50-1C and 60-7.)
Sitz Bath	covered if the contractor's medical staff determines patient has an infection or injury of the perineal area and the item has been prescribed by the patient's physician as a part of his planned regimen of treatment in the patient's home.
Spare Tanks of Oxygen	deny--convenience or precautionary supply
Speech Teaching Machine	deny--education equipment; not primarily medical in nature (§1861(n) of the Act)
Stairway Elevators	deny--(See Elevators.) (§1861(n) of the Act)
Standing Table	deny--convenience item; not primarily medical in nature (§1861(n) of the Act)
Steam Packs	these packs are covered under the same condition as a heating pad (See Heating Pads.)
Suction Machine	covered if the contractor's medical staff determines that the machine specified in the claim is medically required and appropriate for home use without technical or professional supervision.
Support Hose	deny (See Fabric Supports.) (§1861(n) of the Act)
Surgical Leggings	deny--nonreusable supply; not rental-type item (§1861(n) of the Act)
Telephone Alert Systems	deny--these are emergency communications systems and do not serve a diagnostic or therapeutic purpose
Telephone Arms	deny--convenience item; not medical in nature (§1861(n) of the Act)
Toilet Seats	deny--not medical equipment (§1861(n) of the Act)
Traction Equipment	covered if patient has orthopedic impairment requiring traction equipment which prevents ambulation during the period of use (Consider covering devices usable during ambulation; e.g., cervical traction collar, under the brace provision)
Trapeze Bars	covered if patient is bed confined and the patient needs a trapeze bar to sit up because of respiratory condition, to change body position for other medical reasons, or to get in and out of bed.
Treadmill Exerciser	deny--exercise equipment;not primarily medical in nature(§1861(n) of the Act)
Ultraviolet Cabinet	covered for selected patients with generalized intractable psoriasis. Using appropriate consultation, the contractor should determine whether medical and other factors justify treatment at home rather than at alternative sites, e.g., outpatient department of a hospital.

Urinals (autoclavable hospital type)	covered if patient is bed confined
Vaporizers	covered if patient has a respiratory illness
Ventilators	covered for treatment of neuromuscular diseases, thoracic restrictive diseases, and chronic respiratory failure consequent to chronic obstructive pulmonary disease. Includes both positive and negative pressure types.
Walkers	covered if patient's condition impairs ambulation (See also §60-15.)
Water and Pressure Pads and Mattresses	(See Alternating Pressure Pads and Mattresses.)
Wheelchairs	covered if patient's condition is such that without the use of a wheelchair he would otherwise be bed or chair confined. An individual may qualify for a wheelchair and still be considered bed confined.
Wheelchairs (power operated) and wheelchairs with other special features	covered if patient's condition is such and that a wheelchair is medically necessary and the patient is unable to operate the wheelchair manually. Any claim involving a power wheelchair or a wheelchair with other special features should be referred for medical consultation since payment for the special features is limited to those which are medically required because of the patient's condition. (See §60-5 for power operated and §60-6 for specially sized wheelchairs.) NOTE: A power-operated vehicle that may appropriately be used as a wheelchair can be covered. (See §60-5 for coverage details.)
Whirlpool Bath Equipment (standard)	covered if patient is homebound and has a condition for which the whirlpool bath can be expected to provide substantial therapeutic benefit justifying its cost. Where patient is not homebound but has such a condition, payment is restricted to the cost of providing the services elsewhere; e.g., an outpatient department of a participating hospital, if that alternative is less costly. In all cases, refer claim to medical staff for a determination.
Whirlpool Pumps	deny--(See Portable Whirlpool Pumps.) (§1861(n) of the Act)
White Cane	deny--(See §60-3.)

Pub. 100-3, Section 280.2
White Cane For Use By A Blind Person

A white cane for use by a blind person is more an identifying and self-help device rather than an item which makes a meaningful contribution in the treatment of an illness or injury.

Pub. 100-3, Section 280.3
Mobility Assistive Equipment

B. Nationally Covered IndicationsEffective May 5, 2005, CMS findes that the evidence is adequate to determine that MAE is reasonable and necessary for beneficiaries who have a personal mobility deficit sufficient to impair their participation in mobility-related activities of daily living (MRADLs) such as toileting, feeding, dressing, grooming, and bathing in customary locations within the home. Determination of the presence of a mobility deficit will be made by an algorithmic process, Clinical Criteria for MAE Coverage, to provide the appropriate MAE to correct the mobility deficit.Clinical Criteria for MAE CoverageThe beneficiary, the beneficiary's family or other caregiver, or a clinician, will usually initiate the discussion and consideration of MAE use. Sequential consideration of the questions below provides clinical guidance fo the coverage of equipment of appropriate type and complexity to restore the beneficiary's ability to participate in MRADLs such toileting, feeding, dressing, grooming, and bathing in customary locations in the home. These questions correspond to the numbered decision points on the accompanying flow chart. In the individual cases where the beneficiary's condition clearly and unambiguously precludes the reasonable use of a device, it is not necessary to undertake a trial of that device for that beneficiary.1. Does the beneficiary have a mobility limitation that significantly impairs his/her ability to participate in one or more MRADLs in the home A mobility limitation is one that:a. Prevents the beneficiary from accomplishing the MRADLs entirely, or, b. Places the beneficiary at reasonably determined heightened risk of morbidity or mortality secondary to the attempts to participate in MRADLs, or,c. Prevents the beneficiary from completeing the MRADLs within a reasonable time fram.2. Are there other conditions that limit the beneficiary's ability to participate in MRADLs at the home a. Some examples are significant impairement of cognition of judment and/or visionb. For these beneficiaries, the provision of MAE might not enable them to participate in MRADLs if the comorbidity prevents effective us of the wheelchair or reasonable completion of the tasks even with MAE.3. If these other limitations exist, can they be ameliorated or compensated sufficiently such that the additional provision of MAE will be reasonably expected to significanly improve the beneficiary's ability to perform or obtain assistance to participate in MRADLs in the home a. A caregiver, for example a family member, may be compensatory, if consistently available in the beneficiary's home and willing and able to safely operate and transfer the beneficiary to and from the wheelchair and to transport the beneficiary using the wheelchair. The caregiver's need to use a wheelchair toassis the beneficiary in the MRADLs is to be considered in this determination.b. If the amelioration or compensation requires the beneficiary's compliance with treatment, for example medications or therapy, substantive non-compliance, whether willing or involuntary, can be grounds for denial of MAE coverage if it results in the beneficiary continuing to have a significant limitation. It may be determined that partial compliance results in adequate amelioration or compensation for the appropriate use of MAE.4. Does the beneficiary or caregiver demonstrate the capability and the willingness to consistently operate the MAE safely a. Safety considerations include personal risk to the beneficiary as well as risk to others. The determination of safety may need to occur several times during the process as the consideration focuses on a specific device.b. A history of unsafe behavior in other venues may be considered.5. Can the functional mobility deficit be sufficiently resolved by the prescription of a cane or walker a. The cane or walker should be appropriately fitted to the beneficiary for this evaluation.b. Assess the beneificiary's ability to safely use a cane or walker.6. Does the beneficiary's typical environment support the use of wheelchairs including scooters/power-operated vehicles (POVs) a. Determine whether the beneficiary's envirnment will support the use of these types of MAE.b. Keep in mind such factors as physical layout, surfaces, and obstacles, which may render MAE unusable in the beneficiary's home.7. Does the beneficiary have sufficient upper extremity function to propel a manual wheelchair in the home to participate in MRADLs during a typical day The manual wheelchair should be optimally configured (seating options, wheelbase, device weight, and other appropriate accessories) for this determination.a. Limitations of strength, endurance, range of motion, coordination, and absence or deformity in one or both upper extremities are relevent.b. A beneficiary with sufficient upper extremity function may qualify for a manual wheelchair. The appropriate type of manual wheelchair, i.e. light weight, etc., should be determined based on the beneficiary's physical characteristics and anticipated intensity of use.c. The beneficiary's home should provide adequate access, maneuvering space and surfaces for the operation of a manual wheelchair.d. Assess the beneficiary's ability to safely use a manual wheelchair.NOTE: If the beneficiary is unable to self-propel a manual wheelchair, and if there is a caregiver who is available, willing and able to provide assistance, a manual wheelchair may be appropriate.8. Does the beneficiary have sufficient strength and postural stability to operate a POV/scooter a. A POV is a 3-or 4-wheeled device with tiller steering and limited seat modification capabilities. The beneficiary must be able to maintain stability and position for adequate operation.b. The beneficiary's home should provide adequate access, maneuvering space and surfaces for the operation of a POV.c. Assess the beneficiary's ability to safely use a POV/scooter.9. Are the additional features provided by a power wheelchair needed to allow the beneficiary to participate in one or more MRADLs a. The pertinent features of a power wheelchair compared to a POV are typically control by a joystick or alternative input device, lower seat height for slide transfers, and the ability to accommodate a variety of seating needs.b. The type of wheelchair and options provided should be appropriate for the degree of the beneficiary's functional impairments.c. The beneficiary's home should provide adequate access, maneuvering space and surfaces for the operation of a power wheelchair.d. Assess the beneficiary's ability to safely use the wheelchair.NOTE: If the beneficiary is unable to use a power wheelchair, and if there is a caregiver who is available, willing, and able to provide assistance, a manual wheelchair is appropriate. A caregiver's inability to operate a manual wheechair can be considered in covering a power wheelchair so that the caregiver can assis the beneficiary.C. Nationally Non-Covered IndicationsMedicare beneficiaries not meeting the clinical criteria for prescribing MAE as outlined above, and as documented by the beneficiary's physiciain, would not be eligible for Medicare coverage of the MAE.D. OtherAll other durable medical equipment (DME) not meeting the definition of MAE as described in this instruction will continue to be covered, or noncovered, as is currently described in the NCD Manual, in Section 280, Medical and Surgical Supplies. Also, all other sections not altered here and the corresponding policies regarding MAEs which have not been discussed here remain unchanged.(This NCD last reviewed May 2005).Cross ReferenceSee Section 280.1 Durable Medical Equipment (DME) Reference List.

Pub. 100-3, Section 280.4
Seat Lift

Reimbursement may be made for the rental or purchase of a medically necessary seat lift when prescribed by a physician for a patient with severe arthritis of the hip or knee and patients with muscular dystrophy or other neuromuscular diseases when it has been determined the patient can benefit therapeutically from use of the device. In establishing medical necessity for the seat lift, the evidence must show that the item is included in the physician's course of treatment, that it is likely to effect improvement, or arrest or retard deterioration in the patient's condition, and that the severity of the condition is such that the alternative would be chair or bed confinement.

Coverage of seat lifts is limited to those types which operate smoothly, can be controlled by the patient, and effectively assist a patient in standing up and sitting down without other assistance. Excluded from coverage is the type of lift which operates by a spring release mechanism with a sudden, catapult-like motion and jolts the patient from a seated to a standing position. Limit the payment for units which incorporate a recliner feature along with the seat lift to the amount payable for a seat lift without this feature.

Pub. 100-3, Section 280.5
Safety Roller

They may be appropriate, and therefore covered, for some patients who are obese, have severe neurological disorders, or restricted use of one hand, which makes it impossible to use a wheeled walker that does not have the sophisticated braking system found on safety rollers.

In order to assure that payment is not made for a safety roller when a less expensive standard wheeled walker would satisfy the patient's medical needs, carriers refer safety roller claims to their medical consultants. The medical consultant determines whether some or all of the features provided in a safety roller are necessary, and therefore covered and reimbursable. If it is determined that the patient could use a standard wheeled walker, the charge for the safety roller is reduced to the charge of a standard wheeled walker.

Some obese patients who could use a standard wheeled walker if their weight did not exceed the walker's strength and stability limits can have it reinforced and its wheel base expanded. Such modifications are routine mechanical adjustments and justify a moderate surcharge. In these cases the carrier reduces the charge for the safety roller to the charge for the standard wheeled walker plus the surcharge for modifications. In the case of patients with medical documentation showing severe neurological disorders or restricted use of one hand which makes it impossible for them to use a wheeled walker that does not have a sophisticated braking system, a reasonable charge for the safety roller may be determined without relating it to the reasonable charge for a standard wheeled walker. (Such reasonable charge should be developed in accordance with the instructions in The Medicare Claims Processing Manual, Chapter 23)

Pub. 100-3, Section 280.6
Pneumatic Compression Devices

Pneumatic devices are covered for the treatment of lymphedema or for the treatment of chronic venous insufficiency with venous stasis ulcers.

Lymphedema

Lymphedema is the swelling of subcutaneous tissues due to the accumulation of excessive lymph fluid. The accumulation of lymph fluid results from impairment to the normal clearing function of the lymphatic system and/or from an excessive production of lymph. Lymphedema is divided into two broad classes according to etiology. Primary lymphedema is a relatively uncommon, chronic condition which may be due to such causes as Milroy's Disease or congenital anomalies. Secondary lymphedema, which is much more common, results from the destruction of or damage to formerly functioning lymphatic channels, such as surgical removal of lymph nodes or post radiation fibrosis, among other causes.

Pneumatic compression devices are covered in the home setting for the treatment of lymphedema if the patient has undergone a four-week trial of conservative therapy and the treating physician determines that there has been no significant improvement or if significant symptoms remain after the trial. The trial of conservative therapy must include use of an appropriate compression bandage system or compression garment, exercise, and elevation of the limb. The garment may be prefabricated or custom-fabricated but must provide adequate graduated compression.

Chronic Venous Insufficiency With Venous Stasis Ulcers

Chronic venous insufficiency (CVI) of the lower extremities is a condition caused by abnormalities of the venous wall and valves, leading to obstruction or reflux of blood flow in the veins. Signs of CVI include hyperpigmentation, stasis dermatitis, chronic edema, and venous ulcers.

Pneumatic compression devices are covered in the home setting for the treatment of CVI of the lower extremities only if the patient has one or more venous stasis ulcer(s) which have failed to heal after a 6 month trial of conservative therapy directed by the treating physician. The trial of conservative therapy must include a compression bandage system or compression garment, appropriate dressings for the wound, exercise, and elevation of the limb.

General Coverage Criteria

Pneumatic compression devices are covered only when prescribed by a physician and when they are used with appropriate physician oversight, i.e., physician evaluation of the patient's condition to determine medical necessity of the device, assuring suitable instruction in the operation of the machine, a treatment plan defining the pressure to be used and the frequency and duration of use, and ongoing monitoring of use and response to treatment.

The determination by the physician of the medical necessity of a pneumatic compression device must include (1) the patient's diagnosis and prognosis; (2) symptoms and objective findings, including measurements which establish the severity of the condition; (3) the reason the device is required, including the treatments which have been tried and failed; and (4) the clinical response to an initial treatment with the device. The clinical response includes the change in pre-treatment measurements, ability to tolerate the treatment session and parameters, and ability of the patient (or caregiver) to apply the device for continued use in the home.

The only time that a segmented, calibrated gradient pneumatic compression device (HCPCs code E0652) would be covered is when the individual has unique characteristics that prevent them from receiving satisfactory pneumatic compression treatment using a nonsegmented device in conjunction with a segmented appliance or a segmented compression device without manual control of pressure in each chamber.

Pub. 100-3, Section 280.7
Hospital Beds

A. <u>General Requirements for Coverage of Hospital Beds.</u>--A physician's prescription, and such additional documentation as the contractors' medical staffs may consider necessary, including medical records and physicians' reports, must establish the medical necessity for a hospital bed due to one of the following reasons:
- The patient's condition requires positioning of the body; e.g., to alleviate pain, promote good body alignment, prevent contractures, avoid respiratory infections, in ways not feasible in an ordinary bed; or
- The patient's condition requires special attachments that cannot be fixed and used on an ordinary bed.

B. <u>Physician's Prescription.</u>--The physician's prescription, which must accompany the initial claim, and supplementing documentation when required, must establish that a hospital bed is medically necessary. If the stated reason for the need for a hospital bed is the patient's condition requires positioning, the prescription or other documentation must describe the medical condition, e.g., cardiac disease, chronic obstructive pulmonary disease, quadriplegia or paraplegia, and also the severity and frequency of the symptoms of the condition, that necessitates a hospital bed for positioning.

If the stated reason for requiring a hospital bed is the patient's condition requires special attachments, the prescription must describe the patient's condition and specify the attachments that require a hospital bed.

C. <u>Variable Height Feature.</u>--In well documented cases, the contractors' medical staffs may determine that a variable height feature of a hospital bed, approved for coverage under subsection A above, is medically necessary and, therefore, covered, for one of the following conditions:
- Severe arthritis and other injuries to lower extremities; e.g., fractured hip. The condition requires the variable height feature to assist the patient to ambulate by enabling the patient to place his or her feet on the floor while sitting on the edge of the bed;
- Severe cardiac conditions. For those cardiac patients who are able to leave bed, but who must avoid the strain of "jumping" up or down;
- Spinal cord injuries, including quadriplegic and paraplegic patients, multiple limb amputee and stroke patients. For those patients who are able to transfer from bed to a wheelchair, with or without help; or
- Other severely debilitating diseases and conditions, if the variable height feature is required to assist the patient to ambulate.

D. <u>Electric Powered Hospital Bed Adjustments.</u>--Electric powered adjustments to lower and raise head and foot may be covered when the contractor's medical staff determines that the patient's condition requires frequent change in body position and/or there may be an immediate need for a change in body position (i.e., no delay can be tolerated) and the patient can operate the controls and cause the adjustments. Exceptions may be made to this last requirement in cases of spinal cord injury and brain damaged patients.

E. <u>Side Rails.</u>--If the patient's condition requires bed side rails, they can be covered when an integral part of, or an accessory to, a hospital bed.

Pub. 100-3, Section 280.8
Air-Fluidized Bed

Medicare payment for home use of the air-fluidized bed for treatment of pressure sores can be made if such use is reasonable and necessary for the individual patient.

A decision that use of an air-fluidized bed is reasonable and necessary requires that:

- The patient has a stage 3 (full thickness tissue loss) or stage 4 (deep tissue destruction) pressure sore;
- The patient is bedridden or chair bound as a result of severely limited mobility;
- In the absence of an air-fluidized bed, the patient would require institutionalization;
- The air-fluidized bed is ordered in writing by the patient's attending physician based upon a comprehensive assessment and evaluation of the patient after completion of a course of conservative treatment designed to optimize conditions that promote wound healing. This course of treatment must have been at least one month in duration without progression toward wound healing. This month of prerequisite conservative treatment may include some period in an institution as long as there is documentation available to verify that the necessary conservative treatment has been rendered.
- Use of wet-to-dry dressings for wound debridement, begun during the period of conservative treatment and which continue beyond 30 days, will not preclude coverage of air-fluidized bed. Should additional debridement again become necessary, while a patient is using an air-fluidized bed (after the first 30-day course of conservative treatment) that will not cause the air-fluidized bed to become non-covered. In all instances documentation verifying the continued need for the bed must be available.

- Conservative treatment must include:
  - Frequent repositioning of the patient with particular attention to relief of pressure over bony prominences (usually every 2 hours);
  - Use of a specialized support surface (Group II) designed to reduce pressure and shear forces on healing ulcers and to prevent new ulcer formation;
  - Necessary treatment to resolve any wound infection;
  - Optimization of nutrition status to promote wound healing;
  - Debridement by any means (including wet to dry dressings-which does not require an occlusive covering) to remove devitalized tissue from the wound bed;
  - Maintenance of a clean, moist bed of granulation tissue with appropriate moist dressings protected by an occlusive covering, while the wound heals.
- A trained adult caregiver is available to assist the patient with activities of daily living, fluid balance, dry skin care, repositioning, recognition and management of altered mental status, dietary needs, prescribed treatments, and management and support of the air-fluidized bed system and its problems such as leakage;
- A physician directs the home treatment regimen, and reevaluates and recertifies the need for the air-fluidized bed on a monthly basis; and
- All other alternative equipment has been considered and ruled out.

Home use of the air-fluidized bed is <u>not covered</u> under any of the following circumstances:

- The patient has coexisting pulmonary disease (the lack of firm back support makes coughing ineffective and dry air inhalation thickens pulmonary secretions);
- The patient requires treatment with wet soaks or moist wound dressings that are not protected with an impervious covering such as plastic wrap or other occlusive material; an air-fluidized bed;
- The caregiver is unwilling or unable to provide the type of care required by the patient on an air-fluidized bed;
- Structural support is inadequate to support the weight of the air-fluidized bed system (it generally weighs 1600 pounds or more);
- Electrical system is insufficient for the anticipated increase in energy consumption; or
- Other known contraindications exist.

Coverage of an air-fluidized bed is limited to the equipment itself. Payment for this covered item may only be made if the written order from the attending physician is furnished to the supplier prior to the delivery of the equipment. Payment is not included for the caregiver or for architectural adjustments such as electrical or structural improvement.

Pub. 100-3, Section 280.9
Power-Operated Vehicles That May Be Used as Wheelchairs

Power-operated vehicles that may be appropriately used as wheelchairs are covered under the durable medical equipment provision.

These vehicles have been appropriately used in the home setting for vocational rehabilitation and to improve the ability of chronically disabled persons to cope with normal domestic, vocational and social activities. They may be covered if a wheelchair is medically necessary and the patient is unable to operate a wheelchair manually.

A specialist in physical medicine, orthopedic surgery, neurology, or rheumatology must provide an evaluation of the patient's medical and physical condition and a prescription for the vehicle to assure that the patient requires the vehicle and is capable of using it safely. When an intermediary determines that such a specialist is not reasonably accessible, e.g., more than 1 day's round trip from the beneficiary's home, or the patient's condition precludes such travel, a prescription from the beneficiary's physician is acceptable.

The intermediary's medical staff reviews all claims for a power-operated vehicle, including the specialists' or other physicians' prescriptions and evaluations of the patient's medical and physical conditions, to insure that all coverage requirements are met.

Pub. 100-3, Section 280.11
Corset Used as Hernia Support

A hernia support (whether in the form of a corset or truss) which meets the definition of a brace is covered under Part B under §1861(s)(9) of the Act.

Pub. 100-3, Section 280.12
Sykes Hernia Control

Based on professional advice, it has been determined that the sykes hernia control (a spring-type, U-shaped, strapless truss) is not functionally more beneficial than a conventional truss. Make program reimbursement for this device only when an ordinary truss would be covered. (Like all trusses, it is only of benefit when dealing with a reducible hernia.) Thus, when a charge for this item is substantially in excess of that which would be reasonable for a conventional truss used for the same condition, base reimbursement on the reasonable charges for the conventional truss.

See also the Medicare Benefit Policy Manual, Chapter 15, §130.

Pub. 100-3, Section 280.13
Transcutaneous Electrical Nerve Stimulators (TENS)

Payment for TENS may be made under the durable medical equipment benefit. (See §45-25 for an explanation of coverage of medically necessary supplies for the effective use of TENS and §45-19 for an explanation of coverage of TENS for acute post-operative pain.)

Pub. 100-3, Section 280.14
Infusion Pumps

B. Nationally Covered Indications

THE FOLLOWING INDICATIONS FOR TREATMENT USING INFUSION PUMPS ARE COVERED UNDER MEDICARE:

1. External Infusion Pumps.--

a. Iron Poisoning (Effective for Services Performed On or After September 26, 1984).--When used in the administration of deferoxamine for the treatment of acute iron poisoning and iron overload, only external infusion pumps are covered.

b. Thromboembolic Disease (Effective for Services Performed On or After September 26, 1984).--When used in the administration of heparin for the treatment of thromboembolic disease and/or pulmonary embolism, only external infusion pumps used in an institutional setting are covered.

c. Chemotherapy for Liver Cancer (Effective for Services Performed On or After January 29, 1985).--The external chemotherapy infusion pump is covered when used in the treatment of primary hepatocellular carcinoma or colorectal cancer where this disease is unresectable or where the patient refuses surgical excision of the tumor.

d. Morphine for Intractable Cancer Pain (Effective for Services Performed On or After April 22, 1985).--Morphine infusion via an external infusion pump is covered when used in the treatment of intractable pain caused by cancer (in either an inpatient or outpatient setting, including a hospice).

e. Continuous subcutaneous Insulin Infusion (CSII) Pumps (Effective for Services Performed On or After December 17, 2004)

Continuous subcutaneous insuline infusion (CSII) and related drugs/supplies are covered as medically reasonable and necessary in the home setting for the treatment of diabetic patients who: (1) either meet the updated fasting C-Peptide testing requirement, or, are beta cell autoantibody podsitive; and, (2) satisfy the remaining criteria for insulin pump therapy as described below. Patients must meet either Criterion A or B as follows:

Criterion A: The patient has completed a comprehensive diabetes education program, and has been on a program of multiple daily injections of insulin (i.e. at least 3 injections per day), with frequent self-adjustments of insulin dose for at least 6 months prior to initiation of the insulin pump, and has documented frequency of glucose self-testing an average of at least 4 times per day during the 2 months prior to initiation of the insulin pump, and meets one or more of the following criteria while on the multiple daily injection regimen:

- Glycosylated hemoglobin level (HbAlc) > 7.0 percent
- History of recurring hypoglycemia
- Wide fluctuations in blood glucose before mealtime
- Dawn phenomenon with fasting blood sugars frequently exceeding 200 mg/dl
- History of severe glycemic excursions

Criterion B The patient with diabetes has been on a pump prior to enrollment in Medicare and has documented frequency of glucose self-testing average of at least 4 times per day during the month prior to Medicare enrollment.

General CSII Criteria

In addition to meeting Criterion A or B above, the following general requirements must be met:

The patient with diabetes must be insulinopenic per the updated fasting C-peptide testing requirement, or, as an alternative, must be beta cell autoantibody positive.

Update fasting C-peptide testing requirment:

- Insuliopenia is defined as a fasting C-peptide level that is less than or equal to 110% of the lower limit of normal of the laboratory's measurement method.
- For patients with renal insufficiency and creatinine clearance (actual or calculated from age, gender, weight, and serum creatinine) <50 ml/minue, insulinopenia is defined as a fasting C-peptide level that is less than or equal to 200% of the lower limit of normal of the laboratory's measurement method.
- Fasting C-peptide levels will only be considered valid with a concurrently obtained fasting glucose <225 mg/dl.
- Levels only need to be documented once in the medical records.

Continued coverage of the insulin pump would require that the patient has been seen and evaluated the treating physician at least every 3 months.

The pump must be ordered by and follow-up care of the patient must be managed by a physician who manages multiple patients with CSII and who works closely with a team including nurses, diabetes educators, and dietitians who are knowledgeable in the use of CSII.

Other Uses of CSII

The CMS will continue to allow coverage of all other uses of CSII in accordance with the Category B investigational device exemption (IDE) clinical trials regulation (42 CFR 405.201) or as a routine cost umder the clinical trials policy (Medicare National Coverage Determination (NCD) Manual 310.1).

f. Other uses of external infusion pumps are covered if the contractor's medical staff verifies the appropriateness of the therapy and of the prescribed pump for the individual patient.

NOTE: Payment may also be made for drugs necessary for the effective use of an external infusion pump as long as the drug being used with the pump is itself reasonable and necessary for the patient's treatment.

2. Implantable Infusion Pumps.--

a. Chemotherapy for Liver Cancer (Effective for Services Performed On or After September 26, 1984)

The implantable infusion pump is covered for intra-arterial infusion of 5-FUdR for the treatment of liver cancer for patients with primary hepatocellular carcinoma or Duke's Class D colorectal cancer, in whom the metastases are limited to the liver, and where (1) the disease is unresectable or (2) where the patient refuses surgical excision of the tumor.

b. Anti-Spasmodic Drugs for Severe Spasticity.

An implantable infusion pump is covered when used to administer anti-spasmodic drugs intrathecally (e.g., baclofen) to treat chronic intractable spasticity in patients who have proven unresponsive to less invasive medical therapy as determined by the following criteria:

As indicated by at least a 6-week trial, the patient cannot be maintained on noninvasive methods of spasm control, such as oral anti-spasmodic drugs, either because these methods fail to control adequately the spasticity or produce intolerable side effects, and prior to pump implantation, the patient must have responded favorably to a trial intrathecal dose of the anti-spasmodic drug.

c. Opioid Drugs for Treatment of Chronic Intractable Pain.

An implantable infusion pump is covered when used to administer opioid drugs (e.g., morphine) intrathecally or epidurally for treatment of severe chronic intractable pain of malignant or nonmalignant origin in patients who have a life expectancy of at least 3 months and who have proven unresponsive to less invasive medical therapy as determined by the following criteria:

The patient's history must indicate that he/she would not respond adequately to non-invasive methods of pain control, such as systemic opioids (including attempts to eliminate physical and behavioral abnormalities which may cause an exaggerated reaction to pain); and a preliminary trial of intraspinal opioid drug administration must be undertaken with a temporary intrathecal/epidural catheter to substantiate adequately acceptable pain relief and degree of side effects (including effects on the activities of daily living) and patient acceptance.

d. Coverage of Other Uses of Implanted Infusion Pumps

Determinations may be made on coverage of other uses of implanted infusion pumps if the contractor's medical staff verifies that:

- The drug is reasonable and necessary for the treatment of the individual patient;
- It is medically necessary that the drug be administered by an implanted infusion pump; and
- The Food and Drug Administration (FDA)- approved labelling for the pump must specify that the drug being administered and the purpose for which it is administered is an indicated use for the pump.

e. Implantation of Infusion Pump Is Contraindicated.

The implantation of an infusion pump is contraindicated in the following patients:

- with a known allergy or hypersensitivity to the drug being used (e.g., oral baclofen, morphine, etc.);
- who have an infection;
- whose body size is insufficient to support the weight and bulk of the device; andwith other implanted programmable devices since crosstalk between devices may inadvertently change the prescription.

NOTE: Payment may also be made for drugs necessary for the effective use of an implantable infusion pump as long as the drug being used with the pump is itself reasonable and necessary for the patient's treatment.

C. Nationall Noncovered Indications

THE FOLLOWING INDICATIONS FOR TREATMENT USING INFUSION PUMPS ARE NOT COVERED UNDER MEDICARE:

1. External Infusion Pumps.--

a. Vancomycin (Effective for Services Beginning On or After September 1, 1996).

Medicare coverage of vancomycin as a durable medical equipment infusion pump benefit is not covered. There is insufficient evidence to support the necessity of using an external infusion pump, instead of a disposable elastomeric pump or the gravity drip method, to administer vancomycin in a safe and appropriate manner.

2. Implantable Infusion Pump.--

a. Thromboembolic Disease (Effective for Services Performed On or After September 26, 1984).

According to the Public Health Service, there is insufficient published clinical data to support the safety and effectiveness of the heparin implantable pump. Therefore, the use of an implantable infusion pump for infusion of heparin in the treatment of recurrent thromboembolic disease is not covered.

b. Diabetes

Implanted infusion pumps for the infusion of insulin to treat diabetes is not covered. The data do not demonstrate that the pump provides effective administration of insulin.

D. Other

Not applicable

(This NCD last reviewed January 2005.)

Pub. 100-3, Section 300.1
Obsolete or Unreliable Diagnostic Tests

A. Diagnostic Tests (Effective for services performed on or after May 15, 1980).--Do not routinely pay for the following diagnostic tests because they are obsolete and have been replaced by more advanced procedures. The listed tests may be paid for only if the medical need for the procedure is satisfactorily justified by the physician who performs it. When the services are subject to PRO review, the PRO is responsible for determining that satisfactory medical justification exists. When the services are not subject to PRO review, the intermediary or carrier is responsible for determining that satisfactory medical justification exists. This includes:

- Amylase, blood isoenzymes, electrophoretic,
- Chromium, blood,
- Guanase, blood,
- Zinc sulphate turbidity, blood,
- Skin test, cat scratch fever,
- Skin test, lymphopathia venereum,
- Circulation time, one test,
- Cephalin flocculation,
- Congo red, blood,
- Hormones, adrenocorticotropin quantitative animal tests,
- Hormones, adrenocorticotropin quantitative bioassay,
- Thymol turbidity, blood,
- Skin test, actinomycosis,
- Skin test, brucellosis,
- Skin test, psittacosis,
- Skin test, trichinosis,
- Calcium, feces, 24-hour quantitative,
- Starch, feces, screening,
- Chymotrypsin, duodenal contents,
- Gastric analysis, pepsin,
- Gastric analysis, tubeless,
- Calcium saturation clotting time,
- Capillary fragility test (Rumpel-Leede),
- Colloidal gold,
- Bendien's test for cancer and tuberculosis,
- Bolen's test for cancer,
- Rehfuss test for gastric acidity, and
- Serum seromucoid assay for cancer and other diseases.

B. Cardiovascular Tests (Effective for services performed on or after January 1, 1997).--Do not pay for the following phonocardiography and vectorcardiography diagnostic tests because they have been determined to be outmoded and of little clinical value. They include:

- CPT code 93201, Phonocardiogram with or without ECG lead; with supervision during recording with interpretation and report (when equipment is supplied by the physician),
- CPT code 93202, Phonocardiogram; tracing only, without interpretation and report (e.g., when equipment is supplied by the hospital, clinic),
- CPT code 93204, Phonocardiogram; interpretation and report,
- CPT code 93205, Phonocardiogram with ECG lead, with indirect carotid artery and/or jugular vein tracing, and/or apex cardiogram; with interpretation and report,
- CPT code 93208, Phonocardiogram; without interpretation and report,
- CPT code 93209, Phonocardiogram; interpretation and report only,
- CPT code 93210, Intracardiac,
- CPT code 93220, Vectorcardiogram (VCG), with or without ECG; with interpretation and report,
- CPT code 93221, Vectorcardiogram; tracing only, without interpretation and report, and
- CPT code 93222, Vectorcardiogram; interpretation and report only.

Pub. 100-4, Chapter 1, Section 30.3.5

Effect of Assignment Upon Purchase of Cataract Glasses From Participating Physician or Supplieron Claims Submitted to Carriers

B3-3045.4

A pair of cataract glasses is comprised of two distinct products: a professional product (the prescribed lenses) and a retail commercial product (the frames). The frames serve not only as a holder of lenses but also as an article of personal apparel. As such, they are usually selected on the basis of personal taste and style. Although Medicare will pay only for standard frames, most patients want deluxe frames. Participating physicians and suppliers cannot profitably furnish such deluxe frames unless they can make an extra (noncovered) charge for the frames even though they accept assignment.

Therefore, a participating physician or supplier (whether an ophthalmologist, optometrist, or optician) who accepts assignment on cataract glasses with deluxe frames may charge the Medicare patient the difference between his/her usual charge to private pay patients for glasses with standard frames and his/her usual charge to such patients for glasses with deluxe frames, in addition to the applicable deductible and coinsurance on glasses with standard frames, if all of the following requirements are met:

A. The participating physician or supplier has standard frames available, offers them for sale to the patient, and issues and ABN to the patient that explains the price and other differences between standard and deluxe frames. Refer to Chapter 30.

B. The participating physician or supplier obtains from the patient (or his/her representative) and keeps on file the following signed and dated statement:

_____

Name of Patient Medicare Claim Number

Having been informed that an extra charge is being made by the physician or supplier for deluxe frames, that this extra charge is not covered by Medicare, and that standard frames are available for purchase from the physician or supplier at no extra charge, I have chosen to purchase deluxe frames.

_____

Signature Date

C. The participating physician or supplier itemizes on his/her claim his/her actual charge for the lenses, his/her actual charge for the standard frames, and his/her actual extra charge for the deluxe frames (charge differential).

Once the assigned claim for deluxe frames has been processed, the carrier will follow the ABN instructions as described in §60.

Pub. 100-4, Chapter 8, Section 60.4.2
Epoetin Alfa (EPO) Supplier Billing Requirements (Method II) on the Form CMS-1500

(Rev 118, 03-05-04)

A. Claims with dates of service prior to January 1, 2004:

For claims with dates of service prior to January 1, 2004, the correct EPO code to use is the one that indicates the patient's most recent hematocrit (HCT) (rounded to the nearest whole percent) or hemoglobin (Hgb) (rounded to the nearest g/dl) prior to the date of service of the EPO. For example, if the patient's most recent hematocrit was 20.5 percent, bill Q9921; if it was 28.4 percent, bill Q9928.

To convert actual hemoglobin to corresponding hematocrit for Q code reporting, multiply the Hgb value by 3 and round to the nearest whole number. For example, if Hgb = 8.4, report as Q9925 (8.4 X 3 = 25.2, rounded down to 25).

One unit of service of EPO is reported for each 1000 units dispensed. For example if 20,000 units are dispensed, bill 20 units. If the dose dispensed is not an even multiple of 1,000, rounded down for 1 - 499 units (e.g. 20,400 units dispensed = 20 units billed), round up for 500 - 999 units (e.g. 20,500 units dispensed = 21 units billed).

Q9920 Injection of EPO, per 1,000 units, at patient HCT of 20 or less

Q9921 Injection of EPO, per 1,000 units, at patient HCT of 21

Q9922 Injection of EPO, per 1,000 units, at patient HCT of 22

Q9923 Injection of EPO, per 1,000 units, at patient HCT of 23

Q9924 Injection of EPO, per 1,000 units, at patient HCT of 24

Q9925 Injection of EPO, per 1,000 units, at patient HCT of 25

Q9926 Injection of EPO, per 1,000 units, at patient HCT of 26

Q9927 Injection of EPO, per 1,000 units, at patient HCT of 27

Q9928 Injection of EPO, per 1,000 units, at patient HCT of 28

Q9929 Injection of EPO, per 1,000 units, at patient HCT of 29

Q9930 Injection of EPO, per 1,000 units, at patient HCT of 30

Q9931 Injection of EPO, per 1,000 units, at patient HCT of 31

Q9932 Injection of EPO, per 1,000 units, at patient HCT of 32

Q9933 Injection of EPO, per 1,000 units, at patient HCT of 33

Q9934 Injection of EPO, per 1,000 units, at patient HCT of 34

Q9935 Injection of EPO, per 1,000 units, at patient HCT of 35

Q9936 Injection of EPO, per 1,000 units, at patient HCT of 36

Q9937 Injection of EPO, per 1,000 units, at patient HCT of 37

Q9938 Injection of EPO, per 1,000 units, at patient HCT of 38

Q9939 Injection of EPO, per 1,000 units, at patient HCT of 39

Q9940 Injection of EPO, per 1,000 units, at patient HCT of 40 or above.

B. Claims with Dates of Service January 1, 2004 and after

The above codes were replaced effective January 1, 2004 by Q4055. This Q code is for the injection of EPO furnished to ESRD Beneficiaries on Dialysis. The new code does not include the hematocrit. See §60.7.

Q4055 – Injection, Epoetin alfa, 1,000 units (for ESRD on Dialysis).

The DMERC shall return to provider (RTP) assigned claims for EPO, Q4055, that do not contain a HCT value. For unassigned claims, the DMERC shall deny claims for EPO, Q4055 that do not contain a HCT value.

DMERCs must use the following messages when payment for the injection (Q4055) does not meet the coverage criteria and is denied:

MSN Message 6.5—English: Medicare cannot pay for this injection because one or more requirements for coverage were not met

MSN Message 6.5—Spanish: Medicare no puede pagar por esta inyeccion porque uno o mas requisitos para la cubierta no fueron cumplidos. (MSN Message 6.5 in Spanish).

Adjustment Reason Code B:5 Payment adjusted because coverage/program guidelines were not met or were exceeded.

The DMERCs shall use the following messages when returning as unprocessable assigned claims without a HCT value:

ANSI Reason Code 16 – Claim/service lacks information, which is needed for adjudication.

Additional information is supplied using remittance advice remarks codes whenever appropriate.

Remark Code M58 – Missing/incomplete/invalid claim information. Resubmit claim after corrections.

Deductibles and coinsurance apply.

Pub. 100-4, Chapter 8, Section 70
Payment for Home Dialysis

A3-3644, PRM-1-2706.1.E, PRM-1-2706.2, A3-3169, RO-2 3440.2, B3-4270.1

Home dialysis is dialysis performed by an appropriately trained dialysis patient at home. Hemodialysis, CCPD, IPD and CAPD may be performed at home. For all dialysis services furnished by an ESRD facility, the facility must accept assignment, and only the facility may be paid by the Medicare program. Method II suppliers can receive payment for patients selecting Method II. The Method II supplier must accept assignment. Method II suppliers receive payment for supplies and equipment only.

For purposes of home dialysis, a skilled nursing facility (SNF) may qualify as a beneficiary's home. The services are excluded from SNF consolidated billing for its inpatients. The home dialysis services are billed either by the ESRD facility or the supplier depending on the Method selection made by the beneficiary.

Pub. 100-4, Chapter 8, Section 80
Home Dialysis Method I Billing to the Intermediary

A3-3644.A, PRM-1-2710, PRM-1-2710.4, A3-3169, RDF-318, RO2-3440, B3-4270, B3-4271

If the Medicare home dialysis patient chooses Method I, the dialysis facility with which the Medicare home patient is associated assumes responsibility for providing all home dialysis equipment and supplies, and home support services. For these services, the facility receives the same Medicare dialysis payment rate as it would receive for an in-facility patient under the composite rate system. The beneficiary is responsible for paying any unmet Part B deductible and the 20-percent coinsurance. After the beneficiary's Part B deductible is met, the FI pays 80 percent of the specific facility's composite rate for each in-facility outpatient maintenance dialysis treatment.

Under Method I items and services included in the composite rate must be furnished by the facility, either directly or under arrangement. The cost of an item or service is included under the composite rate unless specifically excluded. Therefore, the determination as to whether an item or service is covered under the composite rate payment does not depend on the frequency that dialysis patients require the item or service, or the number of patients who require it. If the facility fails to provide (either directly or under arrangement) any part of the items and services covered under the rate, the facility cannot be paid any amount for the items and services that it does furnish.

New items or services developed after the rate applicable for that particular year was computed are included in the composite rate payments. As such, ESRD facilities assume the responsibility for providing a dialysis service and must decide whether a particular item or service is medically appropriate and cost effective. Since the composite rate is adjusted, as necessary, based on the most recent cost data available to CMS, the costs of new items and services are taken into account in setting future rates. Similarly, any savings attributable to advancements in the treatment of ESRD accrue to the facility because no adjustment to any individual facility's rate is made.

Pub. 100-4, Chapter 8, Section 90
Method II Billing

A3-3644.A, RO-2-3440.C, B3-4270, B3-4271, B3-4270.1, B3-4270.2, B3-34271, PRM-1-2740, A3-3644.3

Physicians and independent laboratories, must submit claims (Form CMS-1500 or electronic equivalent) to their local carrier for services furnished to end stage renal disease (ESRD) beneficiaries. Suppliers of Method II dialysis equipment and supplies will submit their claims (Form CMS-1500 or electronic equivalent) to the appropriate Durable Medical Equipment Regional Carriers (DMERCs). All ESRD facilities must submit their claims to their appropriate FI.

The amount of Medicare payment under Method II for home dialysis equipment and supplies may NOT exceed $1974.45 for continuous cycling peritoneal dialysis (CCPD) and $1490.85 for all other methods of dialysis.

All laboratory tests furnished to home dialysis patients who have selected payment Method II (see §70.1 above), are billed to and paid by the carrier at the fee schedule, if the tests are performed by an independent laboratory for an independent dialysis facility patient.

If the beneficiary elects to deal directly with a supplier and make arrangements for securing the necessary supplies and equipment to dialyze at home, and chooses Method II, he/she deals directly with a supplier of home dialysis equipment and supplies (this supplier is not a dialysis facility). A supplier other than a facility bills the DMERC. There can be only one supplier per beneficiary, and the supplier must accept assignment. The beneficiary is responsible for any unmet Part B deductible and the 20 percent coinsurance.

Only a supplier that is not a dialysis facility may submit a claim to a DMERC for home dialysis supplies and equipment. Suppliers will submit these claims on Form CMS-1500, or electronic equivalent. Under Method II, beneficiaries may not submit any claims and cannot receive payment for any benefits for home dialysis equipment and supplies.

The supplier must have a written agreement with a Medicare approved dialysis facility that will provide all necessary support, backup, and emergency dialysis services. The dialysis facility will not receive a regular per treatment payment for a patient who chooses Method II.

However, if the facility provides any support services, backup, and emergency dialysis services to a beneficiary who selects this option, the facility is reimbursed for the items or services it furnishes. Hospital-based facilities are paid the reasonable cost of support services, subject to the lesser of cost or charges provisions of §1833(a)(2)(A) of the Act. Independent facilities are paid on a reasonable charge basis for any home dialysis support services they furnish.

A - Description of Support Services

Support services specifically applicable to home patients include but are not limited to:

- Surveillance of the patient's home adaptation, including provisions for visits to the home in accordance with a written plan prepared and periodically reviewed by a team that includes the patient's physician and other professionals familiar with the patient's condition;
- Furnishing dialysis-related emergency services;
- Consultation for the patient with a qualified social worker and a qualified dietician;
- Maintaining a record-keeping system which assures continuity of care;
- Maintaining and submitting all required documentation to the ESRD network;
- Assuring that the water supply is of the appropriate quality;
- Assuring that the appropriate supplies are ordered on an ongoing basis;
- Arranging for the provision of all ESRD laboratory tests;
- Testing and appropriate treatment of water used in dialysis;
- Monitoring the functioning of dialysis equipment;
- All other necessary dialysis services as required under the ESRD conditions for coverage;
- Watching the patient perform CAPD and assuring that it is done correctly, and reviewing with the patient any aspects of the technique he/she may have forgotten, or informing the patient of modification in apparatus or technique;
- Documenting whether the patient has or has not had peritonitis that requires physician intervention or hospitalization, (unless there is evidence of peritonitis, a culture for peritonitis is not necessary);
- Inspection of the catheter site; and
- Since home dialysis support services include maintaining a medical record for each home dialysis patient, the Method II supplier must report to the support service dialysis facility within 30 days all items and services that it furnished to the patient so that the facility can record this information in the patient's medical record.

The services must be furnished in accordance with the written plan required for home dialysis patients. See the Medicare Benefit Policy Manual, Chapter 15, for coverage of telehealth services, and this manual, Chapter 12 for billing telehealth.

Each of the support services may be paid routinely at a frequency of once per month. Any support services furnished in excess of this frequency must be documented for being reasonable and necessary. For example, the patient may contract peritonitis and require an unscheduled connecting tube change.

B - Reasonableness Determinations

Support services (which include the laboratory services included under the composite rate for in-facility patients) are paid on a reasonable charge basis to independent facilities and a reasonable cost basis to hospital-based facilities, subject to the Method II payment cap (refer to §140). A reasonable cost/charge determination must be made for each individual support service furnished to home patients. With respect to the connecting tube change, facilities may bill Medicare for the personnel services required to change the connecting tube, but must look to the Method II supplier for payment for the connecting tube itself.

The payment cap is not a payment rate that is paid automatically each month. Accordingly, in no case may the FI routinely pay any monthly amount for support services without a claim that shows the services actually furnished.

Pub. 100-4, Chapter 8, Section 90.1
DMERC Denials for Beneficiary Submitted Claims Under Method II

A3-3170.6, A3-3644.3, A3-3644.3.A - E, HO-238.2.C, HO-238.3, HO-238.3.A, B32231.3.A and B, B3-2231, B3-4270.1, PRM-1-2709.2.A

Under Method II, beneficiaries may not submit any claims and cannot receive payment for any benefits for home dialysis equipment and supplies. DMERCs must deny unassigned and beneficiary submitted claims with the following MSN messages.

MSN # 16.6: "This item or service cannot be paid unless the provider accepts assignment."

Spanish: "Este articulo o servicio no se pagar a menos de que el proveedor acepte asignaci n."

MSN # 16.7: "Your provider must complete and submit your claim."

Spanish: "Su proveedor debe completar y someter su reclamaci n."

MSN # 16.36: "If you have already paid it, you are entitled to a refund from this provider."

Spanish: "Si usted ya lo ha pagado, tiene derecho a un reebolso de su proveedor."

Pub. 100-4, Chapter 8, Section 90.3.2
Home Dialysis Supplies and Equipment HCPCS Codes Used to Bill the DMERC

PM B-01-56, B3-4270 updated 11-16-01(CR 1799)

A - HCPCS Codes

Prior to January 1, 2002, suppliers billed for dialysis supplies using codes describing "kits" of supplies. The use of kit codes such as A4820, A4900, A4901, A4905, and A4914 allows suppliers to bill for supply items without separately identifying the supplies that are being furnished to the patient. Effective January 1, 2002, these kit codes were deleted and suppliers are now required to bill for dialysis supplies using existing and newly developed HCPCS codes for individual dialysis items. Refer to the LMRP for the HCPCS codes for dialysis supplies and equipment that are effective for claims received on or after January 1, 2002.

A4651	A4652	A4656	A4657	A4660	A4663	A4680	A4690	A4706
A4707	A4708	A4709	A4712	A4714	A4719	A4720	A4721	A4722
A4723	A4724	A4725	A4726	A4730	A4736	A4737	A4740	A4750
A4755	A4760	A4765	A4766	A4770	A4771	A4772	A4773	A4774
A4801	A4802	A4860	A4870	A4911	A4913	A4918	A4927	A4928
A4929	E1500	E1510	E1520	E1530	E1540	E1550	E1560	E1570
E1575	E1580	E1590	E1592	E1594	E1600	E1610	E1615	E1620
E1625	E1630	E1632	E1635	E1636	E1637	E1638	E1639	E1699

DMERCs gap-fill reasonable charge amounts for 2002 for all of the applicable codes other than codes A4913 and E1699, the codes used for miscellaneous supplies and equipment that do not fall under any of the other HCPCS codes. The gap-filled amounts should be established using price lists in effect as of December 31, 2000 if available. These gap-filled payment amounts will apply to all claims with dates of service from January 1, 2002, through December 31, 2002.

Codes A4650 - A4927 and E1510 - E1702 may be used only for supplies and equipment relating to home dialysis. In particular, items not related to dialysis should not be included in the supply kit codes (A4820, A4900, A4901, A4905) or listed in the miscellaneous codes (A4910, A4913, E1699). Conversely, supplies and equipment relating to home dialysis should not be billed using other HCPCS codes.

Dialysis supply kits (A4820, A4900, A4901, A4905) billed by an individual supplier must contain the same type and quantity of supplies each time that it is billed. One unit of service would represent the typical amount of supplies needed for one month of dialysis. The content of the kit may not vary from patient to patient or in a single patient from month to month unless the 52 modifier is used (see below). If more than this typical amount of supplies is needed in one month, the excess supplies should be billed using other dialysis supply codes. If significantly less than the usual amount is needed for 1 month, the 52 modifier should be added to the code and the submitted charge reduced accordingly. A listing of the components of each kit billed by a supplier must be available for review by the DMERC.

For items before January 1, 2002, dialysis solutions (A4700, A4705) should not be included in the supply kit but should be separately billed. One unit of service for these codes is for one liter of dialysis solution.

For items before January 1, 2002, items not included in kits must be billed separately, using either a specific code (A4650 - A4927) or miscellaneous code (A4910, A4913, E1699).

Code A4901 and/or E1594 should be billed for each month that the patient receives CCPD.

An EM modifier should be added to a dialysis supply code when it represents emergency reserve supplies over and above the typical monthly amount.

B - Modifiers

Method II suppliers must maintain documentation to support the existence of a written agreement with a Medicare certified support service facility within a reasonable distance from the beneficiary's home.

Effective July 1, 2002, suppliers must use "KX" modifier on the line item level for all Method II home dialysis claims to indicate that they have this documentation on file, and must provide it to the DMERC upon request. As of July 1, 2002, DMERCs must front end reject any Method II claims that do not have the "KX" modifier at the line level. The supplier may correct and resubmit the claim with the appropriate modifier. DMERCs and the shared systems must make all systems changes necessary to reject Method II claims that do not have the "KX" modifier.

The following listed modifiers are frequently used to identify the service/charges billed for Dialysis Supplies.

CC-Procedure code change - Used by the carrier when the procedure code submitted was changed either for administrative reasons or because an incorrect procedure code was filed. Do not use this modifier when filing claims to Palmetto GBA.

EJ-Subsequent Claim (for Erythropoietin Alpha-EPO injection only)

EM-Emergency reserve supply [for End Stage Renal Disease (ESRD) benefit only]

KY-Specific requirements found in the Documentation section of the Medical Policy have been met and evidence of this is available in the supplier's record. Effective July 1, 2002, suppliers must use the " KY" modifier on the line item level for all Method II home dialysis claims.

NU-New Equipment - Used when purchasing new equipment.

RR-Initial Rental - Rental (use the -RR modifier when DME is to be rented).

UE-Used durable medical equipment

ZU-Advance notice of possible medical necessity denial on file (this modifier will be discontinued with the implementation of HIPAA)

ZY-Potentially noncovered item or service billed for denial or at the beneficiary's request (not to be used for medical necessity denials) (this modifier will be discontinued with the implementation of HIPAA)

Pub. 100-4, Chapter 8, Section 120.1
Payment for Immunosuppressive Drugs Furnished to Transplant Patients

PRM-1-2711.5, B3-4471, AB-01-10

A. General

Effective January 1, 1987, Medicare pays for FDA approved self-administered immunosuppressive drugs. Generally, under this benefit, payment is made for self-administered immunosuppressive drugs that are specifically labeled and approved for marketing as such by the FDA, as well as those prescription drugs, such as prednisone, that are used in conjunction with immunosuppressive drugs as part of a therapeutic regimen reflected in FDA approved labeling for immunosuppressive drugs. This benefit is subject to the Part B deductible and coinsurance provision. There is no time limitation on the coverage of these drugs; however, if a beneficiary loses Medicare coverage as a result of the transplant, the drugs are no longer covered. When the beneficiary reaches the age of 65 and becomes entitled, that person can have the drugs covered again. The hospital pharmacy must ask the physician to furnish the patient with a non-refillable 30-day prescription for the immunosuppressive drugs. This is because the dosage of these drugs frequently diminishes over a period of time, and it is not uncommon for the physician to change the prescription from one drug to another because of the patient's needs. Also, these drugs are expensive, and the coinsurance liability on unused drugs could be a financial burden to the beneficiary. Unless there are special circumstances, the FI and carrier do not consider a supply of drugs in excess of 30 days to be reasonable and necessary and limits payment accordingly.

B. Payment

Payment is made on a reasonable cost basis if the beneficiary is the outpatient of a participating hospital. In all other cases, payment is made on an allowable charge basis.

C. FDA Approved Drugs

Some of the most commonly prescribed immunosuppressive drugs are:

- Sandimmune (cyclosporine), Sandoz Pharmaceutical (oral or parenteral),
- Imuran (azathioprine), Burroughs Wellcome Vial (oral),
- Atgam (antithymocyte/globulin), Upjohn (parenteral); and
- Orthoclone OKT3 (muromonab - CD3) Ortho Pharmaceutical (parenteral).

Also covered are prescription drugs used in conjunction with immunosuppressive drugs as part of a therapeutic regimen reflected in FDA approved labeling for immunosuppressive drugs.

The payment for the drug is limited to the cost of the most frequently administered dosage of the drug (adjusted for medical factors as determined by the physician).

Consult such sources as the Drug Topics Red Book, American Druggists Blue Book, and Medispan, realizing that substantial discounts are available.

Pub. 100-4, Chapter 8, Section 130
Physicians and Supplier (Nonfacility) Billing for ESRD Services - General

B3-4270 updated with Transmittal 1729

Payment for renal-related physicians' services to ESRD patients is made in either of the following ways:

- Under the Monthly Capitation Payment (MCP) (see §140 below for an explanation of the MCP); or
- Using the daily codes for ESRD services (CPT codes 90922-90925) with units that represent the number of days services were furnished.
- Under the Initial method (IM)

The carrier receives bills (Form CMS-1500 or electronic equivalent) from physicians for services furnished ESRD beneficiaries. DMERCs receive bills for equipment and supplies for Method II beneficiaries. Intermediaries receive bills from ESRD facilities. Lab bills from CLIA certified independent dialysis facilities were billed to the carrier before September 1, 1997, and to the FI beginning on that date. Other certified labs continue to bill the carrier.

Pub. 100-4, Chapter 12, Section 30.4
Echocardiography Services (Codes 93303 - 93350)

B3-15360

Effective October 1, 2000, physicians may separately bill for contrast agents used in echocardiography. Physicians should use HCPCS Code A9700 (Supply of injectable contrast material for use in echocardiography, per study). The type of service code is 9. This code will be carrier-priced.

Pub. 100-4, Chapter 12, Section 30.6.1.1
Initial Preventive Physical Examination (HCPCS Codes G0344, G0366, G0367 and G0368)

A – Definition

The initial preventive physical examination (IPPE), or "Welcome to Medicare Visit", is a preventive evaluation and management service (E/M) that includes: (1) review of the individual's medical and social history with attention to modifiable risk factors for disease detection, (2) review of the individual's potential (risk factors) for depression or other mood disorders, (3) review of the individual's functional ability and level of safety; (4) a physical examination to include measurement of the individual's height, weight, blood pressure, a visual acuity screen, and other factors as deemed appropriate by the examining physician or qualified nonphysician practitioner (NPP), (5) performance and interpretation of an electrocardiogram (EKG); (6) education, counseling, and referral, as deemed appropriate, based on the results of the review and evaluation services described in the previous 5 elements, and (7) education, counseling, and referral including a brief written plan (e.g., a checklist or alternative) provided to the individual for obtaining the appropriate screening and other preventive services, which are separately covered under Medicare Part B benefits. (For billing requirements, refer to Pub. 100-04, Chapter 18, Section 80.)

B – Who May Perform

The IPPE may be performed by a doctor of medicine or osteopathy as defined in section 1861 (r)(1) of the Social Security Act or by a qualified NPP (nurse practitioner, physician assistant and clinical nurse specialist). The carrier will pay the appropriate physician fee schedule amount based on the rendering UPIN/PIN.

C – Eligibility

Medicare will pay for one IPPE per beneficiary per lifetime. A beneficiary is eligible when he first enrolls in Medicare Part B on or after January 1, 2005, and receives the IPPE benefit within the first 6 months of the effective date of the initial Part B coverage period.

D – The EKG Component

If the physician or qualified NPP is not able to perform both the examination and the screening EKG, an arrangement may be made to ensure that another physician or entity performs the screening EKG and reports the EKG separately using the appropriate HCPCS G code. The primary physician or qualified NPP shall document the results of the screening EKG into the beneficiary's medical record to complete and bill for the IPPE benefit. **NOTE:** Both components of the IPPE (the examination and the screening EKG) must be performed before the claims can be submitted by the physician, qualified NPP and/or entity.

E – Codes Used to Bill the IPPE

The physician or qualified NPP shall bill HCPCS code G0344 for the physical examination performed face-to-face and HCPCS code G0366 for performing a screening EKG that includes both the interpretation and report. If the primary physician or qualified NPP performs only the examination, he/she shall bill HCPCS code G0344 only. The physician or entity that performs the screening EKG that includes both the interpretation and report shall bill HCPCS code G0366. The physician or entity that performs the screening EKG tracing only (without interpretation and report) shall bill HCPCS code G0367. The physician or entity that performs the interpretation and report only (without the EKG tracing) shall bill HCPCS code G0368. Medicare will pay for a screening EKG only as part of the IPPE. **NOTE:** For an IPPE performed during the global period of surgery refer to section 30.6.6, chapter 12, Pub 100-04 for reporting instructions.

F – Documentation

The physician and qualified NPP shall use the appropriate screening tools typically used in routine physician practice. As for all E/M services, the 1995 and 1997 E/M documentation guidelines (http://www.cms.hhs.gov/medlearn/emdoc.asp) should be followed for recording the appropriate clinical information in the beneficiary's medical record. All referrals and a written medical plan must be included in this documentation.

G – Reporting A Medically Necessary E/M at Same IPPE Visit

When the physician or qualified NPP provide a medically necessary E/M service in addition to the IPPE, CPT codes 99201 – 99215 may be used depending on the clinical appropriateness of the circumstances. CPT Modifier –25 shall be appended to the medically necessary E/M service identifying this service as a separately identifiable service from the IPPE code G0344 reported. **NOTE:** Some of the components of a medically necessary E/M service (e.g., a portion of history or physical exam portion) may have been part of the IPPE and should not be included when determining the most appropriate level of E/M service to be billed for the medically necessary E/M service.

Pub. 100-4, Chapter 12, Section 70
Payment Conditions for Radiology Services

B3-15022

See Chapter 13 for claims processing instructions for radiology.

Pub. 100-4, Chapter 12, Section 210.1
Application of Limitation

B3-2472 - 2472.5

A - Status of Patient

The limitation is applicable to expenses incurred in connection with the treatment of an individual who is not an inpatient of a hospital. Thus, the limitation applies to mental health services furnished to a person in a physician's office, in the patient's home, in a skilled nursing facility, as an outpatient, and so forth. The term "hospital" in this context means an institution, which is primarily engaged in providing inpatients, by or under the supervision of physician(s):

- Diagnostic and therapeutic services for medical diagnosis, treatment and care of injured, disabled, or sick persons;
- Rehabilitation services for injured, disabled, or sick persons; or
- Psychiatric services for the diagnosis and treatment of mentally ill patients.

B - Disorders Subject to Limitation

The term "mental, psychoneurotic, and personality disorders" is defined as the specific psychiatric conditions described in the American Psychiatric Association's (APA) "Diagnostic and Statistical Manual of Mental Disorders, Third Edition - Revised (DSM-III-R)."

When the treatment services rendered are both for a psychiatric condition as defined in the DSM-III-R and one or more nonpsychiatric conditions, separate the expenses for the psychiatric aspects of treatment from the expenses for the nonpsychiatric aspects of treatment. However, in any case in which the psychiatric treatment component is not readily distinguishable from the nonpsychiatric treatment component, all of the expenses are allocated to whichever component constitutes the primary diagnosis.

1. Diagnosis Clearly Meets Definition - If the primary diagnosis reported for a particular service is the same as or equivalent to a condition described in the APA's DSM-III-R, the expense for the service is subject to the limitation except as described in subsection D.

2. Diagnosis Does Not Clearly Meet Definition - When it is not clear whether the primary diagnosis reported meets the definition of mental, psychoneurotic, and personality disorders, it may be necessary to contact the practitioner to clarify the diagnosis. In deciding whether contact is necessary in a given case, give consideration to such factors as the type of services rendered, the diagnosis, and the individual's previous utilization history.

C - Services Subject to Limitation

Carriers apply the limitation to claims for professional services that represent mental health treatment furnished to individuals who are not hospital inpatients by physicians, clinical psychologists, clinical social workers, and other allied health professionals. Items and supplies furnished by physicians or other mental health practitioners in connection with treatment are also subject to the limitation. (The limitation also applies to CORF claims processed by intermediaries.)

Carriers apply the limitation only to treatment services. It does not apply to diagnostic services as described in subsection D. Testing services performed to evaluate a patient's progress during treatment are considered part of treatment and are subject to the limitation.

D - Services Not Subject to Limitation

1. Diagnosis of Alzheimer's Disease or Related Disorder - When the primary diagnosis reported for a particular service is Alzheimer's Disease (coded 331.0 in the "International Classification of Diseases, 9th Revision") or Alzheimer's or other disorders coded 290.XX in the APA's DSM-III-R, carriers look to the nature of the service that has been rendered in determining whether it is subject to the limitation. Typically, treatment provided to a patient with a diagnosis of Alzheimer's Disease or a related disorder represents medical management of the patient's condition (rather than psychiatric treatment) and is not subject

to the limitation. However, when the primary treatment rendered to a patient with such a diagnosis is psychotherapy, it is subject to the limitation.

2. Brief Office Visits for Monitoring or Changing Drug Prescriptions - Brief office visits for the sole purpose of monitoring or changing drug prescriptions used in the treatment of mental, psychoneurotic and personality disorders are not subject to the limitation. These visits are reported using HCPCS code M0064 (brief office visit for the sole purpose of monitoring or changing drug prescriptions used in the treatment of mental, psychoneurotic, and personality disorders). Claims where the diagnosis reported is a mental, psychoneurotic, or personality disorder (other than a diagnosis specified in subsection A) are subject to the limitation except for the procedure identified by HCPCS code M0064.

3. Diagnostic Services - Carriers do not apply the limitation to tests and evaluations performed to establish or confirm the patient's diagnosis. Diagnostic services include psychiatric or psychological tests and interpretations, diagnostic consultations, and initial evaluations.

An initial visit to a practitioner for professional services often combines diagnostic evaluation and the start of therapy. Such a visit is neither solely diagnostic nor solely therapeutic. Therefore, carriers deem the initial visit to be diagnostic so that the limitation does not apply. Separating diagnostic and therapeutic components of a visit is not administratively feasible, unless the practitioner already has separately identified them on the bill. Determining the entire visit to be therapeutic is not justifiable since some diagnostic work must be done before even a tentative diagnosis can be made and certainly before therapy can be instituted. Moreover, the patient should not be disadvantaged because therapeutic as well as diagnostic services were provided in the initial visit. In the rare cases where a practitioner's diagnostic services take more than one visit, carriers do not apply the limitation to the additional visits. However, it is expected such cases are few. Therefore, when a practitioner bills for more than one visit for professional diagnostic services, carriers request documentation to justify the reason for more than one diagnostic visit.

4. Partial Hospitalization Services Not Directly Provided by Physician - The limitation does not apply to partial hospitalization services that are not directly provided by a physician. These services are billed by hospitals and community mental health centers (CMHCs) to intermediaries.

E - Computation of Limitation

Carriers determine the Medicare allowed payment amount for services subject to the limitation. They:

- Multiply this amount by 0.625;
- Subtract any unsatisfied deductible; and,
- Multiply the remainder by 0.8 to obtain the amount of Medicare payment.

The beneficiary is responsible for the difference between the amount paid by Medicare and the full allowed amount.

EXAMPLE A

A beneficiary is referred to a Medicare participating psychiatrist who performs a diagnostic evaluation that costs $350. Those services are not subject to the limitation, and they satisfy the deductible. The psychiatrist then conducts 10 weekly therapy sessions for which he/she charges $125 each. The Medicare allowed amount is $90 each, for a total of $900.

Apply the limitation by multiplying 0.625 times $900, which equals $562.50.

Apply regular 20 percent coinsurance by multiplying 0.8 times $562.50, which equals $450 (the amount of Medicare payment).

The beneficiary is responsible for $450 (the difference between Medicare payment and the allowed amount).

EXAMPLE B

A beneficiary was an inpatient of a psychiatric hospital and was discharged on January 1, 1992. During his/her inpatient stay he/she was diagnosed and therapy was begun under a treatment team that included a clinical psychologist. He/she received post-discharge therapy from the psychologist for 12 sessions, at which point the psychologist administered testing that showed the patient had recovered sufficiently to warrant termination of therapy. The allowed amount for the therapy sessions was $80 each, and the amount for the testing was $125, for a total of $1085. All services in 1992 were subject to the limitation, since the diagnosis had been completed in the hospital and the subsequent testing was a part of therapy.

Apply the limitation by multiplying 0.625 times $1085, which gives $678.13.

Since the deductible must be met for 1992, subtract $100 from $678.13, for a remainder of $578.13.

Determine Medicare payment by multiplying the remainder by 0.8, which equals $462.50.

The beneficiary is responsible for $622.50.

Pub. 100-4, Chapter 13, Section 20
Payment Conditions for Radiology Services

B3-15022

Pub. 100-4, Chapter 13, Section 60
Positron Emission Tomography (PET) Scans– GeneralInformation

Positron emission tomography (PET) is a noninvasive imaging procedure that assesses perfusion and the level of metabolic activity in various organ systems of the human body. A positron camera (tomograph) is used to produce cross-sectional tomographic images which are obtained by detecting radioactivity from a radioactive tracer substance (radiopharmaceutical) that emits a radioactive tracer substance (radiopharmaceutical FDG) such as 2 –[F-18] flouro-D-glucose FDG, that is administered intravenously to the patient.

The Medicare National Coverage Determinations *(NCD)* Manual, Chapter 1, §220.6, contains additional coverage instructions to indicate the conditions under which a PET scan is performed.

A – Definitions

For all uses of PET, excluding Rubidium 82 for perfusion of the heart, myocardial viability and refractory seizures, the following definitions apply:

Diagnosis: PET is covered only in clinical situations in which the PET results may assist in avoiding an invasive diagnostic procedure, or in which the PET results may assist in determining the optimal anatomical location to perform an invasive diagnostic procedure. In general, for most solid tumors, a tissue diagnosis is made prior to the performance of PET scanning. PET scans following a tissue diagnosis are *generally* performed for the purpose of staging, *rather than* diagnosis. Therefore, the use of PET in the diagnosis of lymphoma, esophageal and colorectal cancers, as well as in melanoma, should be rare. PET is not covered for other diagnostic uses, and is not covered for screening (testing of patients without specific signs and symptoms of disease).

Staging: PET is covered in clinical situations in which (1) (a) the stage of the cancer remains in doubt after completion of a standard diagnostic workup, including conventional imaging (computed tomography, magnetic resonance imaging, or ultrasound) or, (b) the use of PET would also be considered reasonable and necessary if it could potentially replace one or more conventional imaging studies when it is expected that conventional study information is insufficient for the clinical management of the patient and, (2) clinical management of the patient would differ depending on the stage of the cancer identified.

Restaging: PET will be covered for restaging: *(1)* after the completion of treatment for the purpose of detecting residual disease, *(2)*for detecting suspected recurrence, or *metastasis,* *(3)*to determine the extent of a known recurrence, or *(4) if it could potentially replace one or more conventional imaging studies when it is expected that conventional study information isto determine the extent of a known recurrence, or if study information is insufficient for the clinical management of the patient.* Restaging applies to testing after a course of treatment is completed and is covered subject to the conditions above.

Monitoring: Use of PET to monitor tumor response to treatment during the planned course of therapy (i.e., when *a* change in therapy is *anticipated*).

B - Limitations

For staging and restaging: PET is covered in either/or both of the following circumstances:

The stage of the cancer remains in doubt after completion of a standard diagnostic workup, including conventional imaging (computed tomography, magnetic resonance imaging, or ultrasound); and/or

The clinical management of the patient would differ depending on the stage of the cancer identified. PET will be covered for restaging after the completion of treatment for the purpose of detecting residual disease, for detecting suspected recurrence, or to determine the extent of a known recurrence. Use of PET would also be considered reasonable and necessary if it could potentially replace one or more conventional imaging studies when it is expected that conventional study information is insufficient for the clinical management of the patient.

The PET is not covered for other diagnostic uses, and is not covered for screening (testing of patients without specific symptoms). Use of PET to monitor tumor response during the planned course of therapy (i.e. when no change in therapy is being contemplated) is not covered.

Pub. 100-4, Chapter 13, Section 60.14
Billing Requirements for PET Scans for Non-Covered Indications

For services performed on or after January 28, 2005, contractors shall accept claims with the following HCPCS code for non-covered PET indications:

- G0235: PET imaging, any site not otherwise specified

Short Descriptor: PET not otherwise specified

Type of Service: 4

NOTE: This code is for a non-covered service.

Pub. 100-4, Chapter 13, Section 90
Services of Portable X-Ray Suppliers

B3-2070.4, B3-15022.G, B3-4131, B3-4831

Services furnished by portable x-ray suppliers may have as many as four components. Carriers must follow the following rules.

Pub. 100-4, Chapter 13, Section 90.3
Transportation Component (HCPCS Codes R0070 - R0076)

This component represents the transportation of the equipment to the patient. Establish local RVUs for the transportation R codes based on carrier knowledge of the nature of the service furnished. Carriers *shall* allow only a single transportation payment for each trip the portable x-ray supplier makes to a particular location. When more than one Medicare patient is x-rayed at the same location, e.g., a nursing home, prorate the single fee schedule transportation payment among all patients receiving the services. For example, if two patients at the same location receive x-rays, make one-half of the transportation payment for each.

R0075 must be billed in conjunction with the CPT radiology codes (7000 series) and only when the x-ray equipment used was actually transported to the location where the x-ray was taken. R0075 would not apply to the x-ray equipment stored in the location where the x-ray was done (e.g., a nursing home) for use as needed.

Below are the definitions for each modifier that must be reported with R0075. Only one of these five modifiers shall be reported with R0075. **NOTE**: If only one patient is served, R0070 should be reported with no modifier since the descriptor for this code reflects only one patient seen.

UN - Two patients served

UP - Three patients served

UQ - Four patients served

UR - Five Patients served

US - Six or more patients served

Payment for the above modifiers must be consistent with the definition of the modifiers. Therefore, for R0075 reported with modifiers, -UN, -UP, -UQ, and –UR, the total payment for the service shall be divided by 2, 3, 4, and 5 respectively. For modifier –US, the total payment for the service shall be divided by 6 regardless of the number of patients served. For example, if 8 patients are served, R0075 would be reported with modifier –US and the total payment for this service would be divided by 6.

The units field for R0075 shall always be reported as "1" except in extremely unusual cases. The number in the units field should be completed in accordance with the provisions of 100-04, chapter 23, section 10.2 item 24 G which defines the units field as the number of times the patient has received the itemized service during the dates listed in the from/to field. The units field must never be used to report the number of patients served during a single trip. Specifically, the units field must reflect the number of services that the specific beneficiary received, not the number of services received by other beneficiaries.

As a carrier priced service, carriers must initially determine a payment rate for portable x-ray transportation services that is associated with the cost of providing the service. In order to determine an appropriate cost, the carrier should, at a minimum, cost out the vehicle, vehicle modifications, gasoline and the staff time involved in only the transportation for a portable x-ray service. A review of the pricing of this service should be done every five years.

Direct costs related to the vehicle carrying the x-ray machine are fully allocable to determining the payment rate. This includes the cost of the vehicle using a recognized depreciation method, the salary and fringe benefits associated with the staff who drive the vehicle, the communication equipment used between the vehicle and the home office, the salary and fringe benefits of the staff who determine the vehicles route (this could be proportional of office staff), repairs and maintenance of the vehicle(s), insurance for the vehicle(s), operating expenses for the vehicles and any other reasonable costs associated with this service as determined by the carrier. The carrier will have discretion for allocating indirect costs (those costs that cannot be directly attributed to portable x-ray transportation) between the transportation service and the technical component of the x-ray tests.

Suppliers may send carriers unsolicited cost information. The carrier may use this cost data as a comparison to its carrier priced determination. The data supplied should reflect a year's worth (either calendar or corporate fiscal) of information. Each provider who submits such data is to be informed that the data is subject to verification and will be used to supplement other information that is used to determine Medicare's payment rate.

Carriers are required to update the rate on an annual basis using independently determined measures of the cost of providing the service. A number of readily available measures (e.g., ambulance inflation factor, the Medicare economic index) that are used by the Medicare program to adjust payment rates for other types of services may be appropriate to use to update the rate for years that the carrier does not recalibrate the rate. Each carrier has the flexibility to identify the index it will use to update the rate. In addition, the carrier can consider locally identified factors that are measured independently of CMS as an adjunct to the annual adjustment.

NOTE: No transportation charge is payable unless the portable x-ray equipment used was actually transported to the location where the x-ray was taken. For example, carriers do not allow a transportation charge when the x-ray equipment is stored in a nursing home for use as needed. However, a set-up payment (see §90.4, below) is payable in such situations. Further, for services furnished on or after January 1, 1997, carriers may not make separate payment under HCPCS code R0076 for the transportation of EKG equipment by portable x-ray suppliers or any other entity.

Pub. 100-4, Chapter 13, Section 90.4
Set-Up Component (HCPCS Code Q0092)

Carriers must pay a set-up component for each radiologic procedure (other than retakes of the same procedure) during both single patient and multiple patient trips under Level II

HCPCS code Q0092. Carriers do not make the set-up payment for EKG services furnished by the portable x-ray supplier.

Pub. 100-4, Chapter 13, Section 140
Bone Mass Measurements

SNF-533.5 B3-4181, A3-3631.n

Sections 1861(s)(15) and (rr)(1) of the Act (as added by §4106 of the Balanced Budget Act (BBA) of 1997) standardize Medicare coverage of medically necessary bone mass measurements by providing for uniform coverage under Medicare Part B. This coverage is effective for claims with dates of service furnished on or after July 1, 1998.

Pub. 100-4, Chapter 16, Section 10
Background

B3-2070, B3-2070.1, B3-4110.3, B3-5114

Diagnostic X-ray, laboratory, and other diagnostic tests, including materials and the services of technicians, are covered under the Medicare program. Some clinical laboratory procedures or tests require Food and Drug Administration (FDA) approval before coverage is provided.

A diagnostic laboratory test is considered a laboratory service for billing purposes, regardless of whether it is performed in:

A physician's office, by an independent laboratory;

By a hospital laboratory for its outpatients or nonpatients;

In a rural health clinic; or

In an HMO or Health Care Prepayment Plan (HCPP) for a patient who is not a member.

When a hospital laboratory performs laboratory tests for nonhospital patients, the laboratory is functioning as an independent laboratory, and still bills the fiscal intermediary (FI). Also, when physicians and laboratories perform the same test, whether manually or with automated equipment, the services are deemed similar.

Laboratory services furnished by an independent laboratory are covered under SMI if the laboratory is an approved Independent Clinical Laboratory. However, as is the case of all diagnostic services, in order to be covered these services must be related to a patient's illness or injury (or symptom or complaint) and ordered by a physician. A small number of laboratory tests can be covered as a preventive screening service.

See the Medicare Benefit Policy Manual, Chapter 15, for detailed coverage requirements.

See the Medicare Program Integrity Manual, Chapter 10, for laboratory/supplier enrollment guidelines.

See the Medicare State Operations Manual for laboratory/supplier certification requirements.

Pub. 100-4, Chapter 16, Section 10.1
Definitions

B3-2070.1, B3-2070.1.B, RHC-406.4

"Independent Laboratory" - An independent laboratory is one that is independent both of an attending or consulting physician's office and of a hospital that meets at least the requirements to qualify as an emergency hospital as defined in §1861(e) of the Social Security Act (the Act.) (See the Medicare Benefits Policy Manual, Chapter 15, for detailed discussion.)

"Physician Office Laboratory" – A physician office laboratory is a laboratory maintained by a physician or group of physicians for performing diagnostic tests in connection with the physician practice.

"Clinical Laboratory"- See the Medicare Benefits Policy Manual, Chapter 15.

"Qualified Hospital Laboratory" - A qualified hospital laboratory is one that provides some clinical laboratory tests 24 hours a day, 7 days a week, to serve a hospital's emergency room that is also available to provide services 24 hours a day, 7 days a week. For the qualified hospital laboratory to meet this requirement, the hospital must have physicians physically present or available within 30 minutes through a medical staff call roster to handle emergencies 24 hours a day, 7 days a week; and hospital laboratory technologists must be on duty or on call at all times to provide testing for the emergency room.

"Hospital Outpatient" - See the Medicare Benefit Policy Manual, Chapter 2.

"Referring laboratory" - A Medicare-approved laboratory that receives a specimen to be tested and that refers the specimen to another laboratory for performance of the laboratory test.

"Reference laboratory" - A Medicare-enrolled laboratory that receives a specimen from another, referring laboratory for testing and that actually performs the test.

"Billing laboratory" - The laboratory that submits a bill or claim to Medicare.

"Service" - A clinical diagnostic laboratory test. Service and test are synonymous.

"Test" - A clinical diagnostic laboratory service. Service and test are synonymous.

"CLIA" - The Clinical Laboratory Improvement Act and CMS implementing regulations and processes.

"Certification" - A laboratory that has met the standards specified in the CLIA.

"Draw Station' - A place where a specimen is collected but no Medicare-covered clinical laboratory testing is performed on the drawn specimen.

"Medicare-approved laboratory - A laboratory that meets all of the enrollment standards as a Medicare provider including the certification by a CLIA certifying authority.

Pub. 100-4, Chapter 16, Section 60
Specimen Collection Fee and Travel Allowance

B3-5114.1

Pub. 100-4, Chapter 16, Section 110.4
Carrier Contacts With Independent Clinical Laboratories

B3-2070.1.F

An important role of the carrier is as a communicant of necessary information to independent clinical laboratories. Failure to inform independent laboratories of Medicare regulations and claims processing procedures may have an adverse effect on prosecution of laboratories suspected of fraudulent activities with respect to tests performed by, or billed on behalf of, independent laboratories. United States Attorneys often must prosecute under a handicap or may refuse to prosecute cases where there is no evidence that a laboratory has been specifically informed of Medicare regulations and claims processing procedures.

To assure that laboratories are aware of Medicare regulations and carrier's policy, notification must be sent to independent laboratories when any changes are made in coverage policy or claims processing procedures. Additionally, to completely document efforts to fully inform independent laboratories of Medicare policy and the laboratory's responsibilities, previously issued newsletters should be periodically re-issued to remind laboratories of existing requirements.

Some items which should be discussed are the requirements to have the same charges for Medicare and private patients, to document fully the medical necessity for collection of specimens from a skilled nursing facility or a beneficiary's home, and, in cases when a laboratory service is referred from one independent laboratory to another independent laboratory, to identify the laboratory actually performing the test.

Additionally, when carrier professional relations representatives make personal contacts with particular laboratories, they should prepare and retain reports of contact indicating dates, persons present, and issues discussed.

Pub. 100-4, Chapter 17, Section 80.2
Oral Anti-Emetic Drugs Used as Full Replacement for Intravenous Anti-Emetic Drugs as Part of a Cancer Chemotherapeutic Regimen

B3-4460, A3-3660.15, PM A-98-5

See the Medicare Benefits Policy Manual ,Chapter 15, for detailed coverage requirements.

Effective for dates of service on or after January 1, 1998, FIs and carriers pay for oral anti-emetic drugs when used as full therapeutic replacement for intravenous dosage forms as part of a cancer chemotherapeutic regimen when the drug(s) is administered or prescribed by a physician for use immediately before, at, or within 48 hours after the time of administration of the chemotherapeutic agent.

The allowable period of covered therapy includes day one, the date of service of the chemotherapy drug (beginning of the time of treatment), plus a period not to exceed two additional calendar days, or a maximum period up to 48 hours. Some drugs are limited to 24 hours; some to 48 hours. The hour limit is included in the narrative description of the HCPCS code.

The oral anti-emetic drug(s) should be prescribed only on a per chemotherapy treatment basis. For example, only enough of the oral anti-emetic(s) for one 24 or 48 hour dosage regimen (depending upon the drug) should be prescribed/supplied for each incidence of chemotherapy treatment. These drugs may be supplied by the physician in the office, by an inpatient or outpatient provider (e.g., hospital, CAH, SNF, etc.), or through a supplier (e.g., a pharmacy).

The physician must indicate on the prescription that the beneficiary is receiving the oral anti-emetic drug(s) as full therapeutic replacement for an intravenous anti-emetic drug as part of a cancer chemotherapeutic regimen. Where the drug is provided by a facility, the beneficiary's medical record maintained by the facility must be documented to reflect that the beneficiary is receiving the oral anti-emetic drug(s) as full therapeutic replacement for an intravenous anti-emetic drug as part of a cancer chemotherapeutic regimen.

Payment for these drugs is made under Part B. Payment is based on the lower of the actual charge on the Medicare claim or 95 percent of the lesser of the median average wholesale price, as reflected in the SDP, for all sources of the generic forms of the drug or lowest priced brand name product. Deductible and coinsurance apply

HCPCS codes shown in §80.2.1 are used.

CWF edits claims with these codes to assure that the beneficiary is receiving the oral anti-emetic(s) as part of a cancer chemotherapeutic regimen by requiring a diagnosis of cancer.

Most drugs furnished as an outpatient hospital service are packaged under OPPS. However, chemotherapeutic agents and the supportive and adjunctive drugs used with them are paid separately.

Pub. 100-4, Chapter 18, Section 50

Prostate Cancer Screening Tests and Procedures

B3-4182, A3-3616

Sections 1861(s)(2)(P) and 1861(oo) of the Act (as added by §4103 of the Balanced Budget Act of 1997), provide for Medicare Part B coverage of certain prostate cancer screening tests subject to certain coverage, frequency, and payment limitations. Effective for services furnished on or after January 1, 2000, Medicare Part B covers prostate cancer screening tests/procedures for the early detection of prostate cancer. Coverage of prostate cancer screening tests includes the following procedures furnished to an individual for the early detection of prostate cancer:

Screening digital rectal examination, and

Screening prostate specific antigen (PSA) blood test.

Each test may be paid at a frequency of once every 12 months for men who have attained age 50 (i.e., starting at least one day after they have attained age 50), if at least 11 months have passed following the month in which the last Medicare-covered screening digital rectal examination was performed (for digital rectal exams) or PSA test was performed (for PSA tests).

Pub. 100-4, Chapter 20, Section 20
Calculation and Update of Payment Rates

B3-5017, PM B-01-54, 2002 PEN Fee Schedule

Section1834 of the Act requires the use of fee schedules under Medicare Part B for reimbursement of durable medical equipment (DME) and for prosthetic and orthotic devices, beginning January 1 1989. Payment is limited to the lower of the actual charge for the equipment or the fee established.

Beginning with fee schedule year 1991, CMS calculates the updates for the fee schedules and national limitation amounts and provides the contractors with the revised payment amounts. The CMS calculates most fee schedule amounts and provides them to the carriers, DMERCs, FIs and RHHIs. However, for some services CMS asks carriers to calculate local fee amounts and to provide them to CMS to include in calculation of national amounts. These vary from update to update, and CMS issues special related instructions to carriers when appropriate.

Parenteral and enteral nutrition services paid on and after January 1, 2002 are paid on a fee schedule. This fee schedule also is furnished by CMS. Prior to 2002, payment amounts for PEN were determined under reasonable charge rules, including the application of the lowest charge level (LCL) restrictions.

The CMS furnishes fee schedule updates (DMEPOS, PEN, etc.) at least 30 days prior to the scheduled implementation. FIs use the fee schedules to pay for covered items, within their claims processing jurisdictions, supplied by hospitals, home health agencies, and other providers. FIs consult with DMERCs and where appropriate with carriers on filling gaps in fee schedules.

The CMS furnishes the fee amounts annually, or as updated if special updates should occur during the year, to carriers and FIs, including DMERCs and RHHIs, and to other interested parties (including the Statistical Analysis DMERC (SADMERC), Railroad Retirement Board (RRB), Indian Health Service, and United Mine Workers).

Pub. 100-4, Chapter 20, Section 20.4
Contents of Fee Schedule File

PM A-02-090

The fee schedule file provided by CMS contains HCPCS codes and related prices subject to the DMEPOS fee schedules, including application of any update factors and any changes to the national limited payment amounts. The file does not contain fees for drugs that are necessary for the effective use of DME. It also does not include fees for items for which fee schedule amounts are not established. See Chapter 23 for a description of pricing for these. The CMS releases via program issuance, the gap-filled amounts and the annual update factors for the various DMEPOS payment classes:

IN = Inexpensive/routinely purchased...DME;

FS = Frequency Service...DME;

CR = Capped Rental... DME;

OX = Oxygen and Oxygen Equipment... OXY;

OS = Ostomy, Tracheostomy and Urologicals...P/O;

S/D = Surgical Dressings...S/D;

P/O = Prosthetics and Orthotics...P/O;

SU = Supplies...DME; and

TE = TENS...DME,

RHHIs need to retrieve data from all of the above categories. Regular FIs need to retrieve data only from categories P/O, S/D and SU. FIs need to retrieve the SU category in order to be able to price supplies on Part B SNF claims.

Pub. 100-4, Chapter 20, Section 40.1
General

B3-5102.2.G, B3-5102.3

Contractors pay for maintenance and servicing of purchased equipment in the following classes:

inexpensive or frequently purchased,

customized items, other prosthetic and orthotic devices, and

capped rental items purchased in accordance with §30.5.2 or §30.5.3.

They do not pay for maintenance and servicing of purchased items that require frequent and substantial servicing, or oxygen equipment. (Maintenance and servicing may be paid for purchased items in these two classes if they were purchased prior to June 1, 1989). Reasonable and necessary charges include only those made for parts and labor that are not otherwise covered under a manufacturer's or supplier's warranty. Contractors pay on a lump-sum, as needed basis based on their individual consideration for each item. Payment may not be made for maintenance and servicing of rented equipment other than maintenance and servicing for PEN pumps (under the conditions of §40.3) or the maintenance and servicing fee established for capped rental items in §40.2.

Servicing of equipment that a beneficiary is purchasing or already owns is covered when necessary to make the equipment serviceable. The service charge may include the use of "loaner" equipment where this is required. If the expense for servicing exceeds the estimated expense of purchasing or renting another item of equipment for the remaining period of medical need, no payment can be made for the amount of the excess. Contractors investigate and deny cases suggesting malicious damage, culpable neglect or wrongful disposition of equipment as discussed in BPM Chapter 15 where they determine that it is unreasonable to make program payment under the circumstances. Such cases are referred to the program integrity specialist in the RO.

Pub. 100-4, Chapter 20, Section 100
General Documentation Requirements

B3-4107.1, B3-4107.8, HHA-463, Medicare Handbook for New Suppliers: Getting Started, B-02-31

Benefit policies are set forth in the Medicare Benefit Policy Manual, Chapter 15, §§110-130.

Program integrity policies for DMEPOS are set forth in the Medicare Program Integrity Manual, Chapter 5.

See Chapter 21 for applicable MSN messages.

See Chapter 22 for Remittance Advice coding.

Pub. 100-4, Chapter 20, Section 100.2
Certificates of Medical Necessity (CMN)

B3-3312

For certain items or services billed to the DME Regional Carrier (DMERC), the supplier must receive a signed Certificate of Medical Necessity (CMN) from the treating physician. CMNs are not required for the same items when billed by HHAs to RHHIs. Instead, the items must be included in the physician's signed orders on the home health plan of care. See the Medicare Program Integrity Manual, Chapter 6.

The FI will inform other providers (see §01 for definition pf provider) of documentation requirements.

Contractors may ask for supporting documentation beyond a CMN.

Refer to the local DMERC Web site described in §10 for downloadable copies of CMN forms.

See the Medicare Program Integrity Manual, Chapter 5, for specific Medicare policies and instructions on the following topics:

Requirements for supplier retention of original CMNs

CMN formats, paper and electronic

List of currently approved CMNs and items requiring CMNs

Supplier requirements for submitting CMNs

Requirements for CMNs to also serve as a physician's order

Civil monetary penalties for violation of CMN requirements

Supplier requirements for completing portions of CMNs

Physician requirements for completing portions of CMNs

Pub. 100-4, Chapter 20, Section 100.2.2
Evidence of Medical Necessity for Parenteral and Enteral Nutrition (PEN) Therapy

B3-3324, B3-4450

PEN coverage is determined by information provided by the treating physician and the PEN supplier. A completed certification of medical necessity (CMN) must accompany and support initial claims for PEN to establish whether coverage criteria are met and to ensure that the PEN therapy provided is consistent with the attending or ordering physician's prescription. Contractors ensure that the CMN contains pertinent information from the treating physician. Uniform specific medical data facilitate the review and promote consistency in coverage determinations and timelier claims processing.

The medical and prescription information on a PEN CMN can be most appropriately completed by the treating physician or from information in the patient's records by an employee of the physician for the physician's review and signature. Although PEN suppliers

sometimes may assist in providing the PEN services, they cannot complete the CMN since they do not have the same access to patient information needed to properly enter medical or prescription information. Contractors use appropriate professional relations issuances, training sessions, and meetings to ensure that all persons and PEN suppliers are aware of this limitation of their role.

When properly completed, the PEN CMN includes the elements of a prescription as well as other data needed to determine whether Medicare coverage is possible. This practice will facilitate prompt delivery of PEN services and timely submittal of the related claim.

Pub. 100-4, Chapter 20, Section 130.2
Billing for Inexpensive or Other Routinely Purchased DME

A3-3629, B3-4107.8

This is equipment with a purchase price not exceeding $150, or equipment that the Secretary determines is acquired by purchase at least 75 percent of the time, or equipment that is an accessory used in conjunction with a nebulizer, aspirator, or ventilators that are either continuous airway pressure devices or intermittent assist devices with continuous airway pressure devices. Suppliers and providers other than HHAs bill the DMERC or, in the case of implanted DME only, the local carrier. HHAs bill the RHHI.

Effective for items and services furnished after January 1, 1991, Medicare DME does not include seat lift chairs. Only the seat lift mechanism is defined under Medicare as DME. Therefore, seat lift coverage is limited to the seat lift mechanism. If a seat lift chair is provided to a beneficiary, contractors pay only for the lift mechanism portion of the chair. Some lift mechanisms are equipped with a seat that is considered an integral part of the lift mechanism. Contractors do not pay for chairs (HCPCS code E0620) furnished on or after January 1, 1991. The appropriate HCPCS codes for seat lift mechanisms are E0627, E0628, and E0629.

For TENS, suppliers and providers other than HHAs bill the DMERC. HHAs bill the RHHI using revenue code 0291 for the 2-month rental period (see §30.1.2), billing each month as a separate line item and revenue code 0292 for the actual purchase along with the appropriate HCPCS code.

Pub. 100-4, Chapter 20, Section 130.3
Billing for Items Requiring Frequent and Substantial Servicing

A3-3629, B3-4107.8

These are items such as intermittent positive pressure breathing (IPPB) machines and ventilators, excluding ventilators that are either continuous airway pressure devices or intermittent assist devices with continuous airway pressure devices.

Suppliers and providers other than HHAs bill the DMERC. HHAs bill the RHHI.

Pub. 100-4, Chapter 20, Section 130.4
Billing for Certain Customized Items

A3-3629, B3-4107.8

Due to their unique nature (custom fabrication, etc.), certain customized DME cannot be grouped together for profiling purposes. Claims for customized items that do not have specific HCPCS codes are coded as E1399 (miscellaneous DME). This includes circumstances where an item that has a HCPCS code is modified to the extent that neither the original terminology nor the terminology of another HCPCS code accurately describes the modified item.

Suppliers and providers other than HHAs bill the DMERC or local carrier. HHAs bill their RHHI, using revenue code 0292 along with the HCPCS.

Pub. 100-4, Chapter 20, Section 130.5
Billing for Capped Rental Items (Other Items of DME)

A3-3629, B3-4107.8

These are DME items, other than oxygen and oxygen equipment, not covered by the above categories. Suppliers and providers other than HHAs bill the DMERC. HHAs bill the RHHIs.

Pub. 100-4, Chapter 32, Section 11.1
Electrical Stimulation

A - Coding Applicable to Carriers & Fiscal Intermediaries (FIs)

Effective April 1, 2003, a National Coverage Decision was made to allow for Medicare coverage of Electrical Stimulation for the treatment of certain types of wounds. The type of wounds covered are chronic Stage III or Stage IV pressure ulcers, arterial ulcers, diabetic ulcers and venous stasis ulcers. All other uses of electrical stimulation for the treatment of wounds are not covered by Medicare. Electrical stimulation will not be covered as an initial treatment modality.

The use of electrical stimulation will only be covered after appropriate standard wound care has been tried for at least 30 days and there are no measurable signs of healing. If electrical stimulation is being used, wounds must be evaluated periodically by the treating physician but no less than every 30 days by a physician. Continued treatment with electrical stimulation is not covered if measurable signs of healing have not been demonstrated within any 30-day period of treatment. Additionally, electrical stimulation must be discontinued when the wound demonstrates a 100% epithelialzed wound bed.

Coverage policy can be found in Pub. 100-03, Medicare National Coverage Determinations Manual, Chapter 1, Section 270.1 (http://www.cms.hhs.gov/manuals/103_cov_determ/ncd103index.asp)

The applicable Healthcare Common Procedure Coding System (HCPCS) code for Electrical Stimulation and the covered effective date is as follows:

HCPCS	Definition	Effective Date
G0281	Electrical Stimulation, (unattended), to one or more areas for chronic Stage III and Stage IV pressure ulcers, arterial ulcers, diabetic ulcers and venous stasis ulcers not demonstrating measurable signs of healing after 30 days of conventional care as part of a therapy plan of care.	04/01/2003

Medicare will not cover the device used for the electrical stimulation for the treatment of wounds. However, Medicare will cover the service. Unsupervised home use of electrical stimulation will not be covered.

B - FI Billing Instructions

The applicable types of bills acceptable when billing for electrical stimulation services are 12X, 13X, 22X, 23X, 71X, 73X, 74X, 75X, and 85X. Chapter 25 of this manual provides general billing instructions that must be followed for bills submitted to FIs. FIs pay for electrical stimulation services under the Medicare Physician Fee Schedule for a hospital, Comprehensive Outpatient Rehabilitation Facility (CORF), Outpatient Rehabilitation Facility (ORF), Outpatient Physical Therapy (OPT) and Skilled Nursing Facility (SNF).

Payment methodology for independent Rural Health Clinic (RHC), provider-based RHCs, free-standing Federally Qualified Health Center (FQHC) and provider based FQHCs is made under the all-inclusive rate for the visit furnished to the RHC/FQHC patient to obtain the therapy service. Only one payment will be made for the visit furnished to the RHC/FQHC patient to obtain the therapy service. As of April 1, 2005, RHCs/FQHCs are no longer required to report HCPCS codes when billing for these therapy services.

Payment Methodology for a Critical Access Hospital (CAH) is on a reasonable cost basis unless the CAH has elected the Optional Method and then the FI pays115% of the MPFS amount for the professional component of the HCPCS code in addition to the technical component.

In addition, the following revenues code must be used in conjunction with the HCPCS code identified:

Revenue Code	Description
420	Physical Therapy
430	Occupational Therapy
520	Federal Qualified Health Center *
521	Rural Health Center *
977, 978	Critical Access Hospital- method II CAH professional services only

* NOTE: As of April 1, 2005, RHCs/FQHCs are no longer required to report HCPCS codes when billing for these therapy services.

C - Carrier Claims

Carriers pay for Electrical Stimulation services billed with HCPCS codes G0281 based on the MPFS. Claims for Electrical Stimulation services must be billed on Form CMS-1500 or the electronic equivalent following instructions in chapter 12 of this manual (http://www.cms.hhs.gov/manuals/104_claims/clm104c12.pdf).

D - Coinsurance and Deductible

The Medicare contractor shall apply coinsurance and deductible to payments for these therapy services except for services billed to the FI by FQHCs. For FQHCs, only co-insurance applies.

Pub. 100-8, Chapter 5, Section 5.1.1.2
Written Orders

Written orders are acceptable for all transactions involving DMEPOS. Written orders may take the form of a photocopy, facsimile image, electronically maintained, or original "pen-and-ink" document. (See Chapter 3, Section 3.4.1.1.B.)

All orders must clearly specify the start date of the order.

For items that are dispensed based on a verbal order, the supplier must obtain a written order that meets the requirements of this section.

If the written order is for supplies that will be provided on a periodic basis, the written order should include appropriate information on the quantity used, frequency of change, and duration of need. (For example, an order for surgical dressings might specify one 4 x 4 hydrocolloid dressing that is changed 1-2 times per week for 1 month or until the ulcer heals.)

The written order must be sufficiently detailed, including all options or additional features that will be separately billed or that will require an upgraded code. The description can be either a narrative description (e.g., lightweight wheelchair base) or a brand name/model number.

If the order is for a rented item or if the coverage criteria in a policy specify length of need, the order must include the length of need.

If the supply is a drug, the order must specify the name of the drug, concentration (if applicable), dosage, frequency of administration, and duration of infusion (if applicable).

Someone other than the physician may complete the detailed description of the item. However, the treating physician must review the detailed description and personally sign and date the order to indicate agreement.

If a supplier does not have a faxed, photocopied, electronic or pen & ink signed order in their records before they can submit a claim to Medicare (i.e., if there is no order or only a verbal order), the claim will be denied. If the item is one that requires a written order prior to delivery (see Section 5.1.1.2.1), the claim will be denied as not meeting the benefit category. If the claim is for an item for which an order is required by statute (e.g., therapeutic shoes for diabetics, oral anticancer drugs, oral antiemetic drugs which are a replacement for intravenous antiemetic drugs), the claim will be denied as not meeting the benefit category and is therefore not appealable by the supplier (see MCM Section 12000 for more information on appeals). For all other items, if the supplier does not have an order that has been both signed and dated by the treating physician before billing the Medicare program, the item will be denied as not reasonable and necessary

If an item requires a *Certificate of Medical Necessity (CMN)* and the supplier does not have a faxed, photocopied, electronic, or pen & ink signed CMN in their records before they submit a claim to Medicare, the claim will be denied. If the CMN is used to verify that statutory benefit requirements have been met, then the claim will be denied as not meeting the benefit category. If the CMN is used to verify that medical necessity criteria have been met, the claim will be denied as not reasonable and necessary.

Medical necessity information (e.g., an ICD-9-CM diagnosis code, narrative description of the patient's condition, abilities, limitations, etc.) is NOT in itself considered to be part of the order although it may be put on the same document as the order.

APPENDIX 5 — HCPCS CODES FOR WHICH CPT CODES SHOULD BE REPORTED

CPT (HCPCS Level I)	PM/Transmittal	Source	HCPCS Level II
21077			L8042
21087			L8040
21088			L8041, L8042, L8044, L8046
38210-38213	AB-02-163		G0267
45300-45387 (mutually exclusive)		CCI	Comprehensive code G0105
45300-45387, 46604, 46608, 46614 (mutually exclusive)		CCI	Comprehensive code G0104
69210 for non-Medicare only	A-02-129		G0268
71555		Medicare Claims Processing Manual, Ch. 13, Sec. 40.1.2 (Rev. 10/1/03)	C8909-C8911
72198	A-03-051	Medicare Claims Processing Manual, Ch. 13, Sec. 40.1.2 (Rev. 10/1/03)	C8918-C8920
74270, 74280 (mutually exclusive)		CCI	Comprehensive code G0106
76090	Hospital Manual, Ch. 10, Sec. 458	—	G0206
76091	Hospital Manual, Ch. 10, Sec. 458	—	G0202-G0206
82270	R80CP	Pub 100-04	G0328
82270 (mutually exclusive)		CCI	Comprehensive code G0107
84153, 84154 (mutually exclusive)		CCI	Comprehensive code G0103
88160-88161		Transmittal 800, CCI	Comprehensive code P3000
88174	AB-02-163		G0144
88175	AB-02-163		G0145
88240	AB-02-163		G0265
88241	AB-02-163		G0266
90471-90472	B-03-001		G0008, G0009, G0010
90919, 90920, 90921		68FR63216	G0308-G0327
99183 (carrier requires) hyperbaric oxygen therapy)	AB-702-183		C1300 (report for hospital outpatient)
Included in E & M code 99201-99456 & 99499		CCI	G0102

APPENDIX 6 — NEW, CHANGED, DELETED, AND REINSTATED HCPCS CODES FOR 2006

NEW CODES

A0998	A4218	A4233	A4234	A4235	A4236	A4411
A4412	A4604	A5120	A5512	A5513	A6457	A6513
A6530	A6531	A6532	A6533	A6534	A6535	A6536
A6537	A6538	A6539	A6540	A6541	A6542	A6543
A6544	A6549	A9275	A9281	A9282	A9535	A9536
A9537	A9538	A9539	A9540	A9541	A9542	A9543
A9544	A9545	A9546	A9547	A9548	A9549	A9550
A9551	A9552	A9553	A9554	A9555	A9556	A9557
A9558	A9559	A9560	A9561	A9562	A9563	A9564
A9565	A9566	A9567	A9698	B4185	C2637	C8950
C8951	C8952	C8953	C8954	C8955	C8956	C8957
C9224	C9225	C9723	C9724	C9725	E0170	E0171
E0172	E0485	E0486	E0641	E0642	E0705	E0762
E0764	E0911	E0912	E1812	E2207	E2208	E2209
E2210	E2211	E2212	E2213	E2214	E2215	E2216
E2217	E2218	E2219	E2220	E2221	E2222	E2223
E2224	E2225	E2226	E2371	E2372	G0235	G0235
G0332	G0333	G0372	G0375	G0376	G0378	G0379
G8006	G8007	G8008	G8009	G8010	G8011	G8012
G8013	G8014	G8015	G8016	G8017	G8018	G8019
G8020	G8021	G8022	G8023	G8024	G8025	G8026
G8027	G8028	G8029	G8030	G8031	G8032	G8033
G8034	G8035	G8036	G8037	G8038	G8039	G8040
G8041	G8051	G8052	G8053	G8054	G8055	G8056
G8057	G8058	G8059	G8060	G8061	G8062	G8075
G8076	G8077	G8078	G8079	G8080	G8081	G8082
G8093	G8094	G8099	G8100	G8103	G8104	G8106
G8107	G8108	G8109	G8110	G8111	G8112	G8113
G8114	G8115	G8116	G8117	G8126	G8127	G8128
G8129	G8130	G8131	G8135	G8152	G8153	G8154
G8155	G8156	G8157	G8158	G8159	G8160	G8161
G8162	G8163	G8164	G8165	G8166	G8167	G8170
G8171	G8172	G8182	G8183	G8184	G8185	G8186
G9050	G9051	G9052	G9053	G9054	G9055	G9056
G9057	G9058	G9059	G9060	G9061	G9062	G9063
G9064	G9065	G9066	G9067	G9068	G9069	G9070
G9071	G9072	G9073	G9074	G9075	G9076	G9077
G9078	G9079	G9080	G9081	G9082	G9083	G9084
G9085	G9086	G9087	G9088	G9089	G9090	G9091
G9092	G9093	G9094	G9095	G9096	G9097	G9098
G9099	G9100	G9101	G9102	G9103	G9104	G9105
G9106	G9107	G9108	G9109	G9110	G9111	G9112
G9113	G9114	G9115	G9116	G9117	G9118	G9119
G9120	G9121	G9122	G9123	G9124	G9125	G9126
G9127	G9128	G9129	G9130	J0132	J0133	J0278
J0365	J0795	J0881	J0882	J0885	J0886	J1162
J1265	J1451	J1566	J1567	J1675	J1751	J1752
J1945	J2278	J2325	J2425	J2503	J2504	J2513
J2805	J3285	J3471	J3472	J7188	J7189	J7306
J7341	J8498	J8515	J8540	J8597	J9025	J9027
J9175	J9225	J9264	K0730	L0491	L0492	L0621
L0622	L0623	L0624	L0625	L0626	L0627	L0628
L0629	L0630	L0631	L0632	L0633	L0634	L0635
L0636	L0637	L0638	L0639	L0640	L0859	L2034
L2387	L3671	L3672	L3673	L3702	L3763	L3764
L3765	L3766	L3905	L3913	L3919	L3921	L3933
L3935	L3961	L3967	L3971	L3973	L3975	L3976
L3977	L3978	L5858	L5971	L6621	L6677	L6883
L6884	L6885	L7400	L7401	L7402	L7403	L7404
L7405	L7600	L8609	L8681	L8682	L8683	L8684
L8685	L8686	L8687	L8688	L8689	Q0480	Q0481
Q0482	Q0483	Q0484	Q0485	Q0486	Q0487	Q0488
Q0489	Q0490	Q0491	Q0492	Q0493	Q0494	Q0495
Q0496	Q0497	Q0498	Q0499	Q0500	Q0501	Q0502
Q0503	Q0504	Q0505	Q0510	Q0511	Q0512	Q0513
Q0514	Q0515	Q4079	Q4080	Q9945	Q9945	Q9946
Q9946	Q9947	Q9947	Q9948	Q9948	Q9949	Q9949
Q9950	Q9950	Q9951	Q9951	Q9952	Q9952	Q9953
Q9953	Q9954	Q9954	Q9955	Q9955	Q9956	Q9956
Q9957	Q9957	Q9958	Q9959	Q9960	Q9961	Q9962
Q9963	Q9964	S0133	S0142	S0142	S0143	S0143
S0145	S0146	S0197	S0197	S0198	S0265	S0595
S0595	S0613	S0625	S0625	S2068	S2075	S2076
S2077	S2078	S2079	S2114	S2117	S2900	S3005
S3005	S3626	S3854	S8270	S8434	S8434	S8940
S8940	V2788					

CHANGED CODES

A4215	A4216	A4372	A4630	A4641	A4642	A6550
A7032	A7033	A9500	A9502	A9503	A9504	A9505
A9507	A9508	A9510	A9512	A9516	A9517	A9521
A9524	A9526	A9528	A9529	A9530	A9531	A9532
A9600	A9605	A9699	B4149	C2634	C2635	E0116
E0637	E0638	E0935	E0971	E1038	E1039	G0333
G9041	G9042	G9043	G9044	J7340	J7342	J7343
J7344	J7350	J7626	K0669	L1832	L1843	L1844
L1845	L1846	L2036	L2037	L2038	L2405	L3170
L3215	L3216	L3217	L3219	L3221	L3222	L3230
L3906	L3923	L7600				

DELETED CODES

A4254	A4260	A4643	A4644	A4645	A4646	A4647
A4656	A5119	A5509	A5511	A6551	A9511	A9513
A9514	A9515	A9519	A9520	A9522	A9523	A9525
A9533	A9534	B4184	B4186	C1079	C1080	C1081
C1082	C1083	C1091	C1092	C1093	C1122	C1200
C1201	C1305	C1775	C9000	C9007	C9008	C9009
C9013	C9102	C9103	C9105	C9112	C9123	C9126
C9200	C9201	C9202	C9203	C9205	C9206	C9211
C9212	C9218	C9400	C9401	C9402	C9403	C9404
C9405	C9410	C9411	C9413	C9414	C9415	C9417
C9418	C9419	C9420	C9421	C9422	C9423	C9424
C9425	C9426	C9427	C9428	C9429	C9430	C9431
C9432	C9433	C9435	C9436	C9437	C9438	C9439
C9704	C9713	C9718	C9719	C9720	C9721	C9722
E0169	E0590	E0752	E0754	E0756	E0757	E0758
E0759	E0953	E0954	E0972	E0996	E1000	E1001
E1019	E1021	E1025	E1026	E1027	E1210	E1211
E1212	E1213	G0030	G0031	G0032	G0033	G0034
G0035	G0036	G0037	G0038	G0039	G0040	G0041
G0042	G0043	G0044	G0045	G0046	G0047	G0110
G0111	G0112	G0113	G0114	G0115	G0116	G0125
G0210	G0211	G0212	G0213	G0214	G0215	G0216
G0217	G0218	G0220	G0221	G0222	G0223	G0224
G0225	G0226	G0227	G0228	G0229	G0230	G0231
G0232	G0233	G0234	G0242	G0244	G0253	G0254
G0258	G0263	G0264	G0279	G0280	G0296	G0336
G0338	G0345	G0346	G0347	G0348	G0349	G0350
G0351	G0353	G0354	G0355	G0356	G0357	G0358
G0359	G0360	G0361	G0362	G0363	G0369	G0370
G0371	G9021	G9022	G9023	G9024	G9025	G9026
G9027	G9028	G9029	G9030	G9031	G9032	J0880
J1563	J1564	J1750	J2324	J7051	J7616	J7617
K0064	K0066	K0067	K0068	K0074	K0075	K0076
K0078	K0102	K0104	K0106	K0415	K0416	K0452
K0600	K0618	K0619	K0620	K0628	K0629	K0630
K0631	K0632	K0633	K0634	K0635	K0636	K0637
K0638	K0639	K0640	K0641	K0642	K0643	K0644
K0645	K0646	K0647	K0648	K0649	K0670	K0671
L0860	L1750	L2039	L3963	L8100	L8110	L8120
L8130	L8140	L8150	L8160	L8170	L8180	L8190
L8195	L8200	L8210	L8220	L8230	L8239	L8620
Q0136	Q0137	Q0187	Q1001	Q1002	Q2001	Q2002
Q2003	Q2005	Q2006	Q2007	Q2008	Q2011	Q2012
Q2013	Q2014	Q2018	Q2019	Q2020	Q2021	Q2022
Q3000	Q3002	Q3003	Q3004	Q3005	Q3006	Q3007
Q3008	Q3009	Q3010	Q3011	Q3012	Q4054	Q4055
Q4075	Q4076	Q4077	Q9941	Q9942	Q9943	Q9944
S0071	S0072	S0114	S0168	S0173	S2082	S2090
S2091	S2215	S8095	T2006			

REINSTATED CODES

A4363	E1392	J0480	J1430	J1640	J2850	J3355
J7620	J7627	J7640	L5703	L8623	L8624	L8680

APPENDIX 7 — PLACE OF SERVICE AND TYPE OF SERVICE

PLACE OF SERVICE CODES FOR PROFESSIONAL CLAIMS

Database (last updated March 29, 2004)

Listed below are place of service codes and descriptions. These codes should be used on professional claims to specify the entity where service(s) were rendered. Check with individual payers (e.g., Medicare, Medicaid, other private insurance) for reimbursement policies regarding these codes. If you would like to comment on a code(s) or description(s), please send your request to posinfo@cms.hhs.gov.

01-02   UNASSIGNED
N/A

03   SCHOOL
A facility whose primary purpose is education.

04   HOMELESS SHELTER
A facility or location whose primary purpose is to provide temporary housing to homeless individuals (e.g., emergency shelters, individual or family shelters).

05   INDIAN HEALTH SERVICE FREE-STANDING FACILITY
A facility or location, owned and operated by the Indian Health Service, which provides diagnostic, therapeutic (surgical and non-surgical), and rehabilitation services to American Indians and Alaska Natives who do not require hospitalization.

06   INDIAN HEALTH SERVICE PROVIDER-BASED FACILITY
A facility or location, owned and operated by the Indian Health Service, which provides diagnostic, therapeutic (surgical and non-surgical), and rehabilitation services rendered by, or under the supervision of, physicians to American Indians and Alaska Natives admitted as inpatients or outpatients.

07   TRIBAL 638   FREE-STANDING FACILITY
A facility or location owned and operated by a federally recognized American Indian or Alaska Native tribe or tribal organization under a 638 agreement, which provides diagnostic, therapeutic (surgical and non-surgical), and rehabilitation services to tribal members who do not require hospitalization.

08   TRIBAL 638   PROVIDER-BASED FACILITY
A facility or location owned and operated by a federally recognized American Indian or Alaska Native tribe or tribal organization under a 638 agreement, which provides diagnostic, therapeutic (surgical and non-surgical), and rehabilitation services to tribal members admitted as inpatients or outpatients.

09-10   UNASSIGNED
N/A

11   OFFICE
Location, other than a hospital, skilled nursing facility (SNF), military treatment facility, community health center, State or local public health clinic, or intermediate care facility (ICF), where the health professional routinely provides health examinations, diagnosis, and treatment of illness or injury on an ambulatory basis.

12   HOME
Location, other than a hospital or other facility, where the patient receives care in a private residence.

13   ASSISTED LIVING FACILITY
Congregate residential facility with self-contained living units providing assessment of each resident's needs and on-site support 24 hours a day, 7 days a week, with the capacity to deliver or arrange for services including some health care and other services. (effective 10/1/03)

14   GROUP HOME *
A residence, with shared living areas, where clients receive supervision and other services such as social and/or behavioral services, custodial service, and minimal services (e.g., medication administration).

15   MOBILE UNIT
A facility/unit that moves from place-to-place equipped to provide preventive, screening, diagnostic, and/or treatment services.

16-19   UNASSIGNED
N/A

20   URGENT CARE FACILITY
Location, distinct from a hospital emergency room, an office, or a clinic, whose purpose is to diagnose and treat illness or injury for unscheduled, ambulatory patients seeking immediate medical attention.

21   INPATIENT HOSPITAL
A facility, other than psychiatric, which primarily provides diagnostic, therapeutic (both surgical and nonsurgical), and rehabilitation services by, or under, the supervision of physicians to patients admitted for a variety of medical conditions.

22   OUTPATIENT HOSPITAL
A portion of a hospital which provides diagnostic, therapeutic (both surgical and nonsurgical), and rehabilitation services to sick or injured persons who do not require hospitalization or institutionalization.

23   EMERGENCY ROOM - HOSPITAL
A portion of a hospital where emergency diagnosis and treatment of illness or injury is provided.

24   AMBULATORY SURGICAL CENTER
A freestanding facility, other than a physician's office, where surgical and diagnostic services are provided on an ambulatory basis.

25   BIRTHING CENTER
A facility, other than a hospital's maternity facilities or a physician's office, which provides a setting for labor, delivery, and immediate post-partum care as well as immediate care of new born infants.

26   MILITARY TREATMENT FACILITY
A medical facility operated by one or more of the Uniformed Services. Military Treatment Facility (MTF) also refers to certain former U.S. Public Health Service (USPHS) facilities now designated as Uniformed Service Treatment Facilities (USTF).

27-30   UNASSIGNED
N/A

31   SKILLED NURSING FACILITY
A facility which primarily provides inpatient skilled nursing care and related services to patients who require medical, nursing, or rehabilitative services but does not provide the level of care or treatment available in a hospital.

32   NURSING FACILITY
A facility which primarily provides to residents skilled nursing care and related services for the rehabilitation of injured, disabled, or sick persons, or, on a regular basis, health-related care services above the level of custodial care to other than mentally retarded individuals.

33   CUSTODIAL CARE FACILITY
A facility which provides room, board and other personal assistance services, generally on a long-term basis, and which does not include a medical component.

34   HOSPICE
A facility, other than a patient's home, in which palliative and supportive care for terminally ill patients and their families are provided.

35-40   UNASSIGNED
N/A

41   AMBULANCE - LAND
A land vehicle specifically designed, equipped and staffed for lifesaving and transporting the sick or injured.

42   AMBULANCE - AIR OR WATER
An air or water vehicle specifically designed, equipped and staffed for lifesaving and transporting the sick or injured.

43-48   UNASSIGNED
N/A

49   INDEPENDENT CLINIC
A location, not part of a hospital and not described by any other Place of Service code, that is organized and operated to provide preventive, diagnostic, therapeutic, rehabilitative, or palliative services to outpatients only. (effective 10/1/03)

50   FEDERALLY QUALIFIED HEALTH CENTER
A facility located in a medically underserved area that provides Medicare beneficiaries preventive primary medical care under the general direction of a physician.

51   INPATIENT PSYCHIATRIC FACILITY
A facility that provides inpatient psychiatric services for the diagnosis and treatment of mental illness on a 24-hour basis, by or under the supervision of a physician.

52   PSYCHIATRIC FACILITY-PARTIAL HOSPITALIZATION
A facility for the diagnosis and treatment of mental illness that provides a planned therapeutic program for patients who do not require full time hospitalization, but who need broader programs than are possible from outpatient visits to a hospital-based or hospital-affiliated facility.

53   COMMUNITY MENTAL HEALTH CENTER
A facility that provides the following services: outpatient services, including specialized outpatient services for children, the elderly, individuals who are chronically ill, and residents of the CMHC's mental health services area who have been discharged from inpatient treatment at a mental health facility; 24 hour a day emergency care services; day treatment, other partial hospitalization services, or psychosocial rehabilitation services; screening for patients being considered for admission to State mental health facilities to determine the appropriateness of such admission; and consultation and education services.

54   INTERMEDIATE CARE FACILITY/MENTALLY RETARDED
A facility which primarily provides health-related care and services above the level of custodial care to mentally retarded individuals but does not provide the level of care or treatment available in a hospital or SNF.

55   RESIDENTIAL SUBSTANCE ABUSE TREATMENT FACILITY
A facility which provides treatment for substance (alcohol and drug) abuse to live-in residents who do not require acute medical care. Services include individual and group therapy and counseling, family counseling, laboratory tests, drugs and supplies, psychological testing, and room and board.

56   PSYCHIATRIC RESIDENTIAL TREATMENT CENTER
A facility or distinct part of a facility for psychiatric care which provides a total 24-hour therapeutically planned and professionally staffed group living and learning environment.

57   NON-RESIDENTIAL SUBSTANCE ABUSE TREATMENT FACILITY
A location which provides treatment for substance (alcohol and drug) abuse on an ambulatory basis. Services include individual and group therapy and counseling, family counseling, laboratory tests, drugs and supplies, and psychological testing. (effective 10/1/03)

58-59   UNASSIGNED
N/A

60   MASS IMMUNIZATION CENTER
A location where providers administer pneumococcal pneumonia and influenza virus vaccinations and submit these services as electronic media claims, paper claims, or using the roster billing method. This generally takes place in a mass immunization setting, such as, a public health center, pharmacy, or mall but may include a physician office setting.

61   COMPREHENSIVE INPATIENT REHABILITATION FACILITY
A facility that provides comprehensive rehabilitation services under the supervision of a physician to inpatients with physical disabilities. Services include physical therapy, occupational therapy, speech pathology, social or psychological services, and orthotics and prosthetics services.

62   COMPREHENSIVE OUTPATIENT REHABILITATION FACILITY
A facility that provides comprehensive rehabilitation services under the supervision of a physician to outpatients with physical disabilities. Services include physical therapy, occupational therapy, and speech pathology services.

63-64   UNASSIGNED
N/A

65   END-STAGE RENAL DISEASE TREATMENT FACILITY
A facility other than a hospital, which provides dialysis treatment, maintenance, and/or training to patients or caregivers on an ambulatory or home-care basis.

66-70   UNASSIGNED
N/A

71   PUBLIC HEALTH CLINIC
A facility maintained by either State or local health departments that provides ambulatory primary medical care under the general direction of a physician. (effective 10/1/03)

72   RURAL HEALTH CLINIC
A certified facility which is located in a rural medically underserved area that provides ambulatory primary medical care under the general direction of a physician.

73-80   UNASSIGNED
N/A

81   INDEPENDENT LABORATORY
A laboratory certified to perform diagnostic and/or clinical tests independent of an institution or a physician's office.

82-98   UNASSIGNED
N/A

99   OTHER PLACE OF SERVICE
Other place of service not identified above.

* Revised, effective April 1, 2004.

TYPE OF SERVICE

COMMON WORKING FILE TYPE OF SERVICE (TOS) INDICATORS

For submitting a claim to the Common Working File (CWF), use the following table to assign the proper TOS. Some procedures may have more than one applicable TOS. For claims received on or after April 3, 1995, CWF will produce alerts on codes with incorrect TOS designations. Effective July 3, 1995, CWF is rejecting codes with incorrect TOS designations.

The only exceptions to this table are:

- Surgical services billed with the ASC facility service modifier SG must be reported as TOS F. The indicator F does not appear on the TOS table because its use is dependent upon the use of the SG modifier.

- Surgical services billed with an assistant-at-surgery modifier (80-82, AS,) must be reported with TOS 8. The 8 indicator does not appear on the TOS table because its use is dependent upon the use of the appropriate modifier. (See Medicare Claims Processing Manual, Chapter 12, "Physician/Practitioner Billing," for instructions on when assistant-at-surgery is allowable.)

- Psychiatric treatment services that are subject to the outpatient mental health treatment limitation should be reported with TOS T.

- TOS H appears in the list of descriptors. However, it does not appear in the table. In CWF, "H" is used only as an indicator for hospice. The carrier should not submit TOS H to CWF at this time.

- When these specific transfusion medicine codes appear on the claim (86880, 86885, 86886, 86900, 86903, 86904, 86905, and 86906) that also contains a blood product (P9010-P9022)), the transfusion medicine codes are paid under reasonable charge. When these services are to be paid under reasonable charge, use TOS 1. When paid under reasonable charge, tests are paid at 80 percent. Coinsurance and deductible also apply.

NOTE: For injection codes with more than one possible TOS designation, use the following guidelines when assigning the TOS:

When the choice is L or 1,

- Use TOS L when the drug is used related to ESRD; or

- Use TOS 1 when the drug is not related to ESRD and is administered in the office.

When the choice is G or 1:

- Use TOS G when the drug is an immunosuppressive drug; or

- Use TOS 1 when the drug is used for other than immunosuppression.

When the choice is P or 1,

- Use TOS P if the drug is administered through durable medical equipment (DME); or

- Use TOS 1 if the drug is administered in the office.

The place of service or diagnosis may be considered when determining the appropriate TOS. The descriptors for each of the TOS codes listed in the following table are:

0	Whole Blood
1	Medical Care
2	Surgery
3	Consultation
4	Diagnostic Radiology
5	Diagnostic Laboratory
6	Therapeutic Radiology
7	Anesthesia
8	Assistant at Surgery
9	Other Medical Items or Services
A	Used DME
B	High Risk Screening Mammography
C	Low Risk Screening Mammography
D	Ambulance
E	Enteral/Parenteral Nutrients/Supplies
F	Ambulatory Surgical Center (Facility Usage for Surgical Services)
G	Immunosuppressive Drugs
H	Hospice
J	Diabetic Shoes
K	Hearing Items and Services
L	ESRD Supplies
M	Monthly Capitation Payment for Dialysis
N	Kidney Donor
P	Lump Sum Purchase of DME, Prosthetics, Orthotics
Q	Vision Items or Services
R	Rental of DME
S	Surgical Dressings or Other Medical Supplies
T	Outpatient Mental Health Treatment Limitation
U	Occupational Therapy
V	Pneumococcal/Flu Vaccine
W	Physical Therapy

BERENSON-EGGERS TYPE OF SERVICE (BETOS) CODES

The BETOS coding system was developed primarily for analyzing the growth in Medicare expenditures. The coding system covers all HCPCS codes; assigns a HCPCS code to only one BETOS code; consists of readily understood clinical categories (as opposed to statistical or financial categories); consists of categories that permit objective assignment; is stable over time; and is relatively immune to minor changes in technology or practice patterns.

BETOS CODES AND DESCRIPTIONS:

1. Evaluation And Management
   1. M1A Office Visits—New
   2. M1B Office Visits—Established
   3. M2A Hospital Visit—Initial
   4. M2B Hospital Visit—Subsequent
   5. M2C Hospital Visit—Critical Care
   6. M3 Emergency Room Visit
   7. M4A Home Visit
   8. M4B Nursing Home Visit
   9. M5A Specialist—Pathology
   10. M5B Specialist—Psychiatry
   11. M5C Specialist—Ophthalmology
   12. M5D Specialist—Other
   13. M6 Consultations

2. Procedures
   1. P0 Anesthesia
   2. P1A Major Procedure—Breast
   3. P1B Major Procedure—Colectomy
   4. P1C Major Procedure—Cholecystectomy
   5. P1D Major Procedure—Turp
   6. P1E Major Procedure—Hysterectomy
   7. P1F Major Procedure—Explor/Decompr/Excisdisc
   8. P1G Major Procedure—Other
   9. P2A Major Procedure, Cardiovascular—CABG
   10. P2B Major Procedure, Cardiovascular—Aneurysm Repair
   11. P2C Major Procedure, Cardiovascular—Thromboendarterectomy
   12. P2D Major Procedure, Cardiovascular—Coronary Angioplasty (PTCA)

13. P2E Major Procedure, Cardiovascular—Pacemaker Insertion
14. P2F Major Procedure, Cardiovascular—Other
15. P3Aa Major Procedure, Orthopedic—Hip Fracture Repair
16. P3B Major Procedure, Orthopedic—Hip Replacement
17. P3C Major Procedure, Orthopedic—Knee Replacement
18. P3D Major Procedure, Orthopedic—Other
19. P4A Eye Procedure—Corneal Transplant
20. P4B Eye Procedure—Cataract Removal/Lens Insertion
21. P4C Eye Procedure—Retinal Detachment
22. P4D Eye Procedure—Treatment Of Retinal Lesions
23. P4E Eye Procedure—Other
24. P5A Ambulatory Procedures—Skin
25. P5B Ambulatory Procedures—Musculoskeletal
26. P5C Ambulatory Procedures—Inguinal Hernia Repair
27. P5D Ambulatory Procedures—Lithotripsy
28. P5E Ambulatory Procedures—Other
29. P6A Minor Procedures—Skin
30. P6B Minor Procedures—Musculoskeletal
31. P6C Minor Procedures—Other (Medicare Fee Schedule)
32. P6D Minor Procedures—Other (Non-Medicare Fee Schedule)
33. P7A Oncology—Radiation Therapy
34. P7B Oncology—Other
35. P8A Endoscopy—Arthroscopy
36. P8B Endoscopy—Upper Gastrointestinal
37. P8C Endoscopy—Sigmoidoscopy
38. P8D Endoscopy—Colonoscopy
39. P8E Endoscopy—Cystoscopy
40. P8F Endoscopy—Bronchoscopy
41. P8G Endoscopy—Laparoscopic Cholecystectomy
42. P8H Endoscopy—Laryngoscopy
43. P8I Endoscopy—Other
44. P9A Dialysis Services (Medicare Fee Schedule)
45. P9B Dialysis Services (Non-Medicare Fee Schedule)

3. Imaging
1. I1A Standard Imaging—Chest
2. I1B Standard Imaging—Musculoskeletal
3. I1C Standard Imaging—Breast
4. I1D Standard Imaging—Contrast Gastrointestinal
5. I1E Standard Imaging—Nuclear Medicine
6. I1F Standard Imaging—Other
7. I2A Advanced Imaging—CAT: Head
8. I2B Advanced Imaging—CAT: Other
9. I2C Advanced Imaging—MRI: Brain
10. I2D Advanced Imaging—MRI: Other
11. I3A Echography—Eye
12. I3B Echography—Abdomen/Pelvis
13. I3C Echography—Heart
14. I3D Echography—Carotid Arteries
15. I3E Echography—Prostate, Transrectal
16. I3F Echography—Other
17. I4A Imaging/Procedure—Heart,Including Cardiac Catheterization
18. I4B Imaging/Procedure—Other

4. Tests
1. T1A Lab Tests—Routine Venipuncture (Non-Medicare Fee Schedule)
2. T1B Lab Tests—Automated General Profiles
3. T1C Lab Tests—Urinalysis
4. T1D Lab Tests—Blood Counts
5. T1E Lab Tests—Glucose
6. T1F Lab Tests—Bacterial Cultures
7. T1G Lab Tests—Other (Medicare Fee Schedule)
8. T1H Lab Tests—Other (Non-Medicare Fee Schedule)
9. T2A Other Tests—Electrocardiograms
10. T2B Other Tests—Cardiovascular Stress Tests
11. T2C Other Tests—Ekg Monitoring
12. T2D Other Tests—Other

5. Durable Medical Equipment
1. D1A Medical/Surgical Supplies
2. D1B Hospital Beds
3. D1C Oxygen And Supplies
4. D1D Wheelchairs
5. D1E Other DME
6. D1F Orthotic Devices

6. Other
1. O1A Ambulance
2. O1B Chiropractic
3. O1C Enteral And Parenteral
4. O1D Chemotherapy
5. O1E Other Drugs
6. O1F Vision, Hearing And Speech Services
7. O1G Influenza Immunization

7. Exceptions/Unclassified
1. Y1 Other—Medicare Fee Schedule
2. Y2 Other—Non-Medicare Fee Schedule
3. Z1 Local Codes
4. Z2 Undefined Codes